Talley & O'Connor's
examination
MEDICINE

Talley & O'Connor's
examination
MEDICINE

9th edition

A guide to physician training

- -

Nicholas J Talley

MD, PhD, FRACP, FAFPHM, FRCP (Lond.), FRCP (Edin.), FACP, FAHMS
Laureate Professor, University of Newcastle and Senior Staff Specialist,
John Hunter Hospital, NSW, Australia; Adjunct Professor, Mayo Clinic, Rochester,
MN, USA; Adjunct Professor, University of North Carolina, Chapel Hill, NC, USA;
Foreign Guest Professor, Karolinska Institutet, Stockholm, Sweden

Simon O'Connor

FRACP, DDU, FCSANZ
Cardiologist, The Canberra Hospital; Clinical Senior Lecturer, Australian National
University Medical School, Canberra, ACT, Australia

ELSEVIER

ELSEVIER

Elsevier Australia. ACN 001 002 357
(a division of Reed International Books Australia Pty Ltd)
Tower 1, 475 Victoria Avenue, Chatswood, NSW 2067

ISBN: 978-0-7295-4386-6

Notice

Practitioners and researchers must always rely on their own experience and knowledge in evaluating and using any information, methods, compounds or experiments described herein. Because of rapid advances in the medical sciences, in particular, independent verification of diagnoses and drug dosages should be made. To the fullest extent of the law, no responsibility is assumed by Elsevier, authors, editors or contributors for any injury and/or damage to persons or property as a matter of products liability, negligence or otherwise, or from any use or operation of any methods, products, instructions, or ideas contained in the material herein.

National Library of Australia Cataloguing-in-Publication Data

A catalogue record for this book is available from the National Library of Australia

Head of Content: Larissa Norrie
Content Project Manager: Shubham Dixit
Edited by Chris Wyard
Proofread by Tim Learner
Cover design by Alice Weston
Internal Design by Stan Lamond
Index by Innodata Indexing
Typeset by New Best-set Typesetters Ltd
Printed in Singapore by KHL Printing Co Pte Ltd

Contents

Foreword by Catherine Yelland

The first edition of *Examination medicine* was published in 1986, the year after I passed the RACP examination. We wondered how we had managed without it, and now, 34 years and many physicians later, it is up to its ninth edition. Students rely on *Clinical examination* – the undergraduate counterpart. Those who undertake physician training depend on *Examination medicine* for guidance about just how much they need to master, from a seemingly infinite amount of medical information. The books are now part of the medical classics, and the various editions are known by the colour of their covers.

Each new edition contains updated medical knowledge and is presented with contemporary educational methods. The clinical examination may have changed in its format slightly over the thirty-five years since I sat it, but the basics are the same – the ability to take a complete medical history, including the relevant social and behavioural factors, to conduct a physical examination reliably and efficiently, and then to synthesise a diagnosis and an appropriate management plan – all in an hour for the long case. For the short case, a thorough and focused clinical examination and interpretation of investigations is assessed to ensure that our next generation of physicians is able to elicit and interpret physical signs reliably.

These skills are the foundation of most physician practice, and what is mastered in the lead-up to the examination is used for the rest of the young doctor's career. An examination should assess what the candidate needs to be able to do, and this is the enduring rationale for what is a stressful time for our basic trainees. Both Professor Talley and Dr O'Connor are practising physicians, and this is evident in their book. The examiners are also clinicians who are there to ensure that all who go on to advanced training in a specialty have mastered the essential skills of a physician.

Examination medicine, or 'Talley and O'Connor', as it is fondly known, is a great comfort as well as a guide. This is how it is done in Australia and New Zealand; this is written for you, the examination candidates. Although no book can cover everything, *Examination medicine* is a solid guide and if diligently used, with lots of time spent with real patients, it will stand our trainees in good stead for the rest of their medical careers.

Dr Catherine Yelland
PSM, MBBS, FRACP
Past President of the Royal Australasian College of Physicians
Medical Director of the Medicine Service Line, Redcliffe Hospital

Foreword by Jennifer Martin

We are remembered best by the lives we touch, those of our patients and our students.

It is now over 30 years since I left an inner-city state high school and entered into the hallowed lecture halls of Otago Medical School, with energy and enthusiasm to 'cure' patients and 'fix' our health system. One by one, as idealism of the vision to 'do' and to 'fix' became trounced by the reality that 'doing' could result in more harm, and trying to make more efficient an underfunded public health system ended in burnout and annoying senior administrators who were responsible for the likelihood of my ever getting a physician job, I became increasingly and interestingly aware of how different patients with the same disease responded variably to the continuum of observation, investigation and intervention in the wards around me. This seemed to be even more obvious at night, when it was often clear that the day plan was not working. The quote *'a good physician treats the disease, the great physician treats the patient who has the disease'* became imprinted into my actions as it seemed to explain observed variability and also the effect socioeconomic and demographic factors had on disease incidence, trajectory and response to interventions.

Against that variability and the overwhelming lack of the wisdom and experience that comes later, in those junior doctor and physician training years, Talley and O'Connor (or affectionately known as 'T and O') provided a methodical and calm process for junior doctors to manage complicated and co-morbid patients, distilled from years of their and others' experience of elicitation and interpretation of signs, symptoms and likely diagnostic lists in an Australian setting. It provided a platform for prognostication, management and treatment and enabled space for the 'unknowns' to be considered. As well as carrying my colleagues and I through the practicalities of undergraduate medicine examinations, and house surgeon, residency and basic physician training, T and O has remained a staple to many physicians who cannot always recall the prioritised list of the common causes of, for example, a peripheral neuropathy on a ward round, but do remember there is one.

Thirty-four years post the first edition, the fact that this edition is still edited by T and O – Australian practising physicians – ensures that the differentials, laboratory and radiology testing and management including specific geographical and demographical characteristics remain very relevant to an Australasian setting. Even the process of the chapter updating and writing is a truly 'down under' experience, a truly collaborative approach to including or excluding information that might be useful or relevant as important negatives, to a practising junior doctor or physician, as opposed to information of academic interest only. From that perspective, we have referred to it as a 'functional' tome, with the line 'What does T and O have to say?'

Although the knowledge has changed over the years, and requirements for physician practice now encompass listening and reflective skills, patient-centred care, ethical considerations, teamwork and collaborative skills, the patient–physician skills are the same – history, examination, diagnosis and management plan, in the context of the current health system. The format of examinations and clinical training has also changed; however, an appropriate history, examination and interpretation, as laid out in 'T and O', is and always will be key.

Examination medicine, the new edition of the much loved and treasured 'T and O', continues to be the most relevant and up-to-date examination textbook for physicians, physician trainees and junior doctors, particularly in the Australasian setting.

Professor Jennifer Martin
MBChB, MA (Oxon.), FRACP, PhD, GAICD
Director of the Centre for Drug Repurposing and Medicines Research,
    The University of Newcastle
Chair of Clinical Pharmacology, School of Medicine and Public Health,
    The University of Newcastle

Preface to the 9th edition

Welcome to a new edition of *Examination Medicine*. The skills physicians must acquire have never been more important in caring for patients with complex life-threatening diseases. We write this Preface at a time of great uncertainty in medicine and society, at a time when an infectious disease pandemic (SARS-CoV-2) has severely strained, even broken, healthcare systems and, in an unprecedented fashion, shut down countries around the world. We applaud all the healthcare heroes in the front line including the physicians and trainees who have risked their lives to care for COVID-19 patients, and honour all those who have died in this terrible outbreak.

We work on the front line in medicine and recognise how important the skills we acquired as basic physician trainees – the same skills needed to pass the Royal Australasian College of Physicians (RACP) examinations – remain to practising excellent medicine. This has only been reinforced during the pandemic. This book was written to help guide physician trainees learn and practise these core clinical skills. A mature clinical approach requires you to understand each patient's unique personal and social environment, and complex medical problem-solving must be considered in this context; we have written our book with this key principle in mind.

Since its initial publication in 1986, we have been proud that examination candidates not only in internal medicine but also across many other specialties have turned to our book for guidance on approaching long and short cases. We even know of RACP examiners who use the book to refresh their knowledge before examining. Senior medical students have also told us the book is very useful for approaching long cases and objective structured clinical examinations (OSCEs), although it is aimed at medical registrars sitting their barrier examinations.

In this edition, we have updated all of the long cases and added new material into the short cases. The book has again undergone peer review to help us avoid errors and maximise clarity and usefulness. We always welcome any feedback.

We wrote in 2014 '*Practising medicine of the highest standard is both art and science; physicians are meant to think and think deeply. Use this book as a help for your preparation, not something to be learned by heart.*' We stand by these words.

Careful preparation and constant practice are the keys to succeeding in clinical examinations. We wish you every success.

Nicholas J Talley, AC
Simon O'Connor
Newcastle and Canberra, 2020

Authors' statement

Distinguished Laureate Professor Nick Talley AC is a Past President of the Royal Australasian College of Physicians, a local RACP examiner and Editor-in-Chief of the *Medical Journal of Australia*. Dr Simon O'Connor is a member of the RACP Senior Examination Panel (SEP).

Examination medicine, first published in 1986, is not an RACP publication, nor is it endorsed by the RACP. Trainees should directly consult the College website to obtain up-to-date information about all policies and procedures as these are subject to regular change.

Acknowledgements

The authors and publishers thank all of the reviewers and colleagues who have provided feedback on this new edition and all past editions.

We in particular wish to thank the following for their assistance with the preparation of *Examination medicine* 9th edition:

Clinical Associate Professor Adrian Gillin, Senior Staff Specialist, Royal Prince Alfred Hospital, Sydney;

Dr Mudar Zand Irani MD, Advanced Trainee in General Medicine, John Hunter Hospital, Newcastle; Conjoint Fellow, School of Medicine and Public Health, University of Newcastle;

Dr Dima Hamed MBBS, Advanced Trainee in Respiratory and Sleep Medicine, John Hunter Hospital, Newcastle; Conjoint Fellow, School of Medicine and Public Health, University of Newcastle;

Dr Alexander Gordon MBBS, Advanced Trainee in Respiratory and Sleep Medicine, John Hunter Hospital, Newcastle; Conjoint Fellow, School of Medicine and Public Health, University of Newcastle;

Dr Simon O'Hare BMBS, Advanced Trainee in Acute and General Medicine, John Hunter Hospital, Newcastle; Conjoint Fellow, School of Medicine and Public Health, University of Newcastle.

Abbreviations

AALF	acalculia, agraphia, left–right disorientation, finger agnosia
ABP	ambulatory blood pressure
ABVD	adriamycin, bleomycin, vinblastine and dacarbazine
ACE	angiotensin-converting enzyme
ACEI	angiostensin-converting enzyme inhibitor
AChR	acetylcholine receptor
ACPA	anti-citrullinated protein antibody
ACTH	adrenocorticotrophic hormone
ADL	activities of daily living
ADP	adenosine diphosphate
ADPKD	autosomal dominant polycystic kidney disease
AF	atrial fibrillation
AFB	acid-fast bacilli
AHI	apnoea hypopnoea index
AICD	automatic implantable cardioverter-defibrillator
AIDS	acquired immunodeficiency syndrome
AIHA	autoimmune haemolytic anaemia
ALK1	activin receptor-like kinase type I
ALL	acute lymphocytic leukaemia
ALT	alanine aminotransferase
AMA	antimitochondrial antibody
AMC	Australian Medical Council
AML	acute myeloid leukaemia
AMSAP	Adult Medicine Self-Assessment Programme
ANA	antinuclear antibody
ANCA	antineutrophil cytoplasmic antibody
anti-LKM1	anti-liver and kidney microsomes type 1
anti-Xa	anti-factor Xa
AP	anteroposterior
APC	activated protein C
APD	automated peritoneal dialysis
apo E2	apolipoprotein E2
APRI	AST to platelet ratio index
aPTT	activated partial thromboplastin time
AR	aortic regurgitation / angiotensin receptor
ARB	angiotensin II receptor blocker
AS	aortic stenosis
ASAP	Australian Self-Assessment Programme
ASCA	anti-*Saccharomyces cerevisiae* antibodies
ASD	atrial septal defect
ASH	asymmetrical hypertrophy
ASMA	anti-smooth muscle antibody
AST	aspartate aminotransferase
AT	antithrombin
ATP	antitachycardia pacing
AV	atrioventricular
β_2-GP-1	beta$_2$-glycoprotein-1

BCG	bacille Calmette–Guérin
BD	twice a day
BGL	blood glucose level
BiPAP	bilevel positive airways pressure
BMD	bone mineral density
BMI	body mass index
BMPR	bone morphogenetic protein receptor type 2
BMS	bare metal stent
BNP	B-type natriuretic peptide
BPPV	benign paroxysmal positional vertigo
BSL	blood sugar level
CABG	coronary artery bypass graft
CAD	coronary artery disease
CAIHA	cold autoimmune haemolytic anaemia
CAPD	continuous ambulatory peritoneal dialysis
CCF	congestive cardiac failure
CCP	citrullinated cyclic peptide
CEA	carcinoembryonic antigen
CFE	Committee for Examinations
CIDP	chronic inflammatory demyelinating polyradiculoneuropathy
CKD	chronic kidney disease
CLD	chronic liver disease
CMC	carpometacarpal
CML	chronic myeloid leukaemia
CMT	Charcot–Marie–Tooth
CMV	cytomegalovirus
CNI	calcineurin inhibitor
CNS	central nervous system
COP	cryptogenic organising pneumonia
COPD	chronic obstructive pulmonary disease
COX-2	cyclo-oxygenase 2
CPAP	continuous positive airways pressure
CPT	Committee for Physician Training
Cr	creatinine
CRAB	hypercalcaemia, renal disease, anaemia and bone lytic lesions
CREST	calcinosis cutis; Raynaud's phenomenon; (o)esophageal involvement; sclerodactyly; telangiectasia
CRH	corticotrophin-releasing hormone
CRP	C-reactive protein
CRT	cardiac resynchronisation therapy
CS	coronary sinus
CSF	cerebrospinal fluid
CSII	continuous subcutaneous infusion
CT	computed tomography
CTEPH	chronic thromboembolic pulmonary hypertension
CTPA	computed tomography pulmonary angiogram
CVA	cerebrovascular accident
CVP	cyclophosphamide, vincristine and prednisone
CXR	chest X-ray
DAF	decay-accelerating factors

DAP	3,4-diaminopyridine
DAPT	dual anti-platelet treatment
DC	direct current
DCD	donation after cardiac death
dcSSc	diffuse cutaneous systemic sclerosis
DES	drug-eluting stent
DEXA	dual-energy X-ray absorptiometry
DIC	disseminated intravascular coagulation
DIP	distal interphalangeal
DLCO	diffusion capacity for carbon monoxide
DLE	discoid lupus erythematosus
DMARD	disease-modifying, antirheumatic drug
DMOAD	diabetes insipidus, diabetes mellitus, optic atrophy and deafness
DOAC	direct oral anticoagulant
DOT	direct observed treatment
DPE	Director of Physician Education
DPP-IV	dipeptidyl peptidase IV
DPT	Director of Physician Training
dsDNA	double-stranded DNA
DVT	deep venous thrombosis
DWI	diffusion-weighted image
EBV	Epstein–Barr virus
ECG	electrocardiogram
ECOG	Eastern Cooperative Oncology Group
EF	ejection fraction
EGPA	eosinophilic granulomatosis with polyangiitis
EIA	enzyme immunoassay
ELISA	enzyme-linked immunosorbent assay
EMG	electromyogram
EMQ	extended matching question
ENA	extractable nuclear antigen
EPG	electrophoretogram
EPS	electrophysiological studies
ERCP	endoscopic retrograde cholangiopancreatography
ES	educational supervisor
ESA	erythropoietin-stimulating agent
ESR	erythrocyte sedimentation rate
FAP	familial adenomatous polyposis
FBC	full blood count
FET	forced expiratory time
FEV_1	forced expiratory volume in 1 second
FFP	fresh frozen plasma
FHH	familial hypocalciuric hypercalcaemia
FODMAP	fermentable oligosaccharides, disaccharides, monosaccharides and polyols
FRACP	Fellow of the Royal Australasian College of Physicians
FS	fractional shortening
FSGS	focal segmental glomerulosclerosis
FSH	follicle-stimulating hormone / facioscapulohumeral
5FU	5-fluorouracil

FVC	forced vital capacity
G6PD	glucose-6-phosphate dehydrogenase
GADA	glutamic acid decarboxylase antibody
GALS	gait, arms, legs and spine
GBM	glomerular basement membrane
GFR	glomerular filtration rate
GGT	gamma-glutamyl transferase
GH	growth hormone
GI	glycaemic index / gastrointestinal
GIT	gastrointestinal tract
GLP-1	glycogen-like peptide
GM-CSF	granulocyte-macrophage colony stimulating factor
GN	glomerulonephritis
GOLD	Global Initiative for Chronic Obstructive Lung Disease
GORD	gastro-oesophageal reflux disease
GPI	glycosylphosphatidylinositol
GTH	general teaching hospital
GUG	get up and go
GVHD	graft versus host disease
HAART	highly active antiretroviral therapy
Hb	haemoglobin
HB_C	hepatitis B core
HB_S	hepatitis B surface
HBV	hepatitis B virus
HCC	hepatocellular carcinoma
HCM	hypertrophic cardiomyopathy
HCV	hepatitis C virus
HD	haemodialysis
HDL	high-density lipoprotein
HELLP	haemolysis, elevated liver enzymes, low platelets
Hib	*Haemophilus influenzae* type b
HIV	human immunodeficiency virus
HLA	human leukocyte antigen
HMG-CoA	hydroxymethylglutaryl coenzyme A
HMSN	hereditary motor and sensory neuropathy
HNPCC	hereditary non-polyposis colon cancer
HPL	human placental lactogen
HPO	hypertrophic pulmonary osteoarthropathy
HRCT	high-resolution computed tomography
HRS	hepatorenal syndrome
HSV	herpes simplex virus
HT	hypertension
HUS	haemolytic uraemic syndrome
HZV	herpes zoster virus
IA-2	insulinoma-associated protein 2 antibody
IAA	insulin autoantibody
IBD	inflammatory bowel disease
IBS	irritable bowel syndrome
ICD	implantable cardioverter-defibrillator
ICU	intensive care unit

IDEAL	Initiating Dialysis Early and Late
IDL	intermediate-density lipoprotein
IEPG	immunoelectrophoretogram
IFN-λ	interferon gamma
Ig	immunoglobulin
IGF-I	insulin-like growth factor I
IHD	ischaemic heart disease
IIP	idiopathic interstitial pneumonia
IL-1	interleukin 1
ILD	interstitial lung disease
INR	international normalised ratio
IPF	idiopathic pulmonary fibrosis
IPH	idiopathic pulmonary hypertension
IPI	International Prognostic Index
IPH	idiopathic pulmonary hypertension
IRTC	Independent Review of Training Committee
ITP	idiopathic thrombocytopenic purpura
IUD	intrauterine device
IVP	intravenous pyelogram
JCV	John Cunningham (JC) virus
JME	juvenile myoclonic epilepsy
JVP	jugular venous pressure
KUB	kidneys, ureters, bladder
LA	left atrium
LAD	left anterior descending
LAHB	left anterior hemi-block
LAM	lymphangioleiomyomatosis
LBBB	left bundle branch block
LCAT	lecithin cholesterol acyltransferase
lcSSc	limited cutaneous systemic sclerosis
LDH	lactate dehydrogenase
LDL	low-density lipoprotein
LEO	local exam organiser
LFT	liver function test
LH	luteinising hormone
LIMA	left internal mammary artery
LKM1	liver and kidney microsomes type 1
LNA	learning needs analysis
LOAF	lateral two lumbricals, opponens pollicis, abductor pollicis brevis, flexor pollicis brevis
Lp(a)	lipoprotein A
LV	left ventricle / left ventricular
LVEDD	left ventricular end-diastolic dimension
LVH	left ventricular hypertrophy
LVOT	left ventricular outflow tract
LVPW	left ventricular posterior wall
MAC	*Mycobacterium avium* complex
MALT	mucosa-associated lymphoid tissue
MAP	MuTYH-associated polyposis
MCP	metacarpophalangeal

MCQ	multiple-choice question
MCTD	mixed connective tissue disease
MCV	mean corpuscular volume
MELD	model for end-stage liver disease
MEN	multiple endocrine neoplasia
MEO	Medical Education Officer
MET	metabolic equivalent of task
MGUS	monoclonal gammopathies of uncertain significance
mini-CEX	mini-clinical evaluation exercise
MKSAP	Medical Knowledge Self-Assessment Program
MODY	maturity onset diabetes of the young
6MP	6-mercaptopurine
MPO	myeloperoxidase
MR	mitral regurgitation / magnetic resonance
MRC	Medical Research Council
MRCP	magnetic resonance cholangiopancreatography
MRI	magnetic resonance imaging
MS	multiple sclerosis
MSF	multi-source feedback
MSI	microsatellite instability
MTP	melphalan, thalidomide and prednisone / metatarsophalangeal
MTX	methotrexate
MuSK	muscle-specific kinase antibodies
MV	mitral valve
MVP	mitral valve prolapse
NAFLD	non-alcoholic fatty liver disease
NAP	neutrophil alkaline phosphatase
NASH	non-alcoholic steatohepatitis
NEP	National Examination Panel
NHMRC	National Health and Medical Research Council
NOAC	novel oral anticoagulant
non-STEMI	non-ST elevation myocardial infarction
nRNP	nuclear ribonucleoprotein
NSAID	non-steroidal anti-inflammatory drug
NSIP	non-specific interstitial pneumonia
NSTEACS	non-ST elevation acute coronary syndrome
NYHA	New York Heart Association
OA	osteoarthritis
OAT	Open Artery Trial
OSA	obstructive sleep apnoea
OSCE	objective structured clinical examination
OTP	overseas-trained physician
PA	plasma aldosterone / posteroanterior
PACE PODS	polymyositis, alcohol, carcinoma, endocrine, periodic paralysis, osteomalacia, drugs, sarcoidosis
PAD	peripheral artery disease
PAH	pulmonary arterial hypertension
PAN	polyarteritis nodosa
p-ANCA	perinuclear antineutrophil cytoplasmic antibodies
PAP	pulmonary artery pressure

PAS	para-aminosalicylic acid / periodic acid–Schiff
PBS	Pharmaceutical Benefits Scheme
PCH	pulmonary capillary haemangiomatosis
PCR	polymerase chain reaction
PCWP	pulmonary capillary wedge pressure
PD	peritoneal dialysis
PDA	patent ductus arteriosus / professional development advisor
PE	pulmonary embolism
PET	positron emission tomography
PFO	patent foramen ovale
Ph	Philadelphia
PIE	pulmonary infiltrate and eosinophilia
PIP	proximal interphalangeal
PJP	*Pneumocystis jirovecii* pneumonia
PKE	paired kidney exchange
PLCH	pulmonary Langerhans cell histiocytosis
PML	progressive multifocal leukoencephalopathy
PNES	psychogenic non-epileptic seizure
PNH	paroxysmal nocturnal haemoglobinuria
POEMS	polyneuropathy, organomegaly, endocrinopathy, monoclonal gammopathy, skin changes
PPD	purified protein derivative
PPI	proton pump inhibitor
PPMS	primary progressive multiple sclerosis
PRA	plasma renin activity
PREP	Physician Readiness for Expert Practice
PSA	prostate-specific antigen
PSCK9	proprotein convertase subtilisin kexin
PTH	parathyroid hormone
PTLD	post-transplant lymphoproliferative disease
PTTK	prolonged partial thromboplastin time with kaolin
PUO	pyrexia of unknown origin
PV	per vaginam
PVC	polyvinyl chloride
PVD	peripheral vascular disease
PVOD	pulmonary veno-occlusive disease
PY1	Postgraduate Year 1
RA	rheumatoid arthritis
RAA	right atrial abnormality
RACP	Royal Australasian College of Physicians
RAD	right-axis deviation
RANKL	receptor activator of nuclear factor kappa-B ligand
RAPD	relative afferent pupillary defect
RBBB	right bundle branch block
RBILD	respiratory bronchiolitis interstitial lung disease
RCHOP	rituximab, doxorubicin, cyclophosphamide, vincristine and prednisone
RCVP	rituximab, cyclophosphamide, vincristine and prednisone
RDW	red cell distribution width
REM	rapid eye movement

RF	rheumatoid factor
RFA	radiofrequency ablation
RIMA	right internal mammary artery
RLS	restless legs syndrome
RNP	ribonucleoprotein
RRMS	relapsing–remitting multiple sclerosis
RSV	respiratory syncytial virus
rtPA	recombinant tissue plasminogen activator
RV	right ventricle / right ventricular
SAAG	serum-to-ascites albumin gradient
SAC	Specialist Advisory Committee
SAM	systolic anterior motion
SBP	spontaneous bacterial peritonitis
SC	subcutaneous
SCA	spinocerebellar ataxia
SE	supplementary examination
SEP	Senior Examination Panel
SGLT-2	sodium–glucose cotransporter 2
SIAT	Significant Incident Analysis Tool
SLE	systemic lupus erythematosus
SLL	small lymphocytic lymphoma
Sm	Smith
SPMS	secondary progressive multiple sclerosis
SRP	signal recognition protein
SSA / SSB	Sjögren's syndrome A / B
ssDNA	single-strand DNA
SSRI	selective serotonin reuptake inhibitor
STEMI	ST elevation myocardial infarction
STIR	short tau (T1) inversion recovery (an MRI fat suppression technique)
SVC	superior vena cava
SVG	saphenous vein graft
SVR	sustained virological response
SVT	supraventricular tachycardia
T_4	thyroxine
TACE	transarterial chemo-embolisation
TB	tuberculosis
TFT	thyroid function test
TIA	transient ischaemic attack
TIPS	transjugular intrahepatic portosystemic shunt
TKI	tyrosine kinase inhibitor
TNF	tumour necrosis factor
TNM	tumour node metastases
TOE	transoesophageal echocardiography
TOR	target of rapamycin
TPHA	*Treponema pallidum* haemagglutination assay
TPMT	thiopurine methyltransferase
TR	tricuspid regurgitation
TSH	thyroid-stimulating hormone
tTG	tissue transglutaminase
TTP	thrombotic thrombocytopenic purpura

TZD	thiazolidinedione
UC	ulcerative colitis
UIP	usual interstitial pneumonia
UKPDS	United Kingdom Prognosis in Diabetes Study
UTH	university teaching hospital
UTI	urinary tract infection
VC	vital capacity
VDRL	venereal disease research laboratory
VF	ventricular fibrillation
VGEF	vascular endothelial growth factor
VLDL	very-low-density lipoprotein
VMP	bortezomib, melphalan and prednisone
VOR	vestibulo-ocular reflex
VSD	ventricular septal defect
VT	ventricular tachycardia
VTE	venous thromboembolism
VVI	ventricular-ventricular inhibited
VWF	von Willebrand factor
WAIHA	warm antibody immunohaemolytic anaemia
WC	ward consultant
WCC	white cell count
WPW	Wolff–Parkinson–White
ZnT8	zinc transporter 8

Note to candidate: Abbreviations can be confusing, even misleading (e.g. 'AR' can be used for 'aortic regurgitation' or 'angiotensin receptor': which do you mean?). Minimise their use in your presentations (and letters to referring doctors), and you will practise better medicine (and not upset your examiners). Join the 'I hate abbreviations' club today!

Chapter 1

Basic physician training

I would live to study, and not study to live.
Francis Bacon (1561–1626)

There is nothing more rewarding and exciting than working as a consultant physician. Physicians are specialists who expertly diagnose and look after patients with complicated medical problems. They typically see patients referred to them for specialised advice and treatment by other doctors, and manage complex patients admitted to hospital. Accurate diagnosis is the key to optimal management outcomes in medicine, and when there is uncertainty or multisystem disease, colleagues turn to physicians for answers and guidance. As a consultant physician you will have the opportunity to change the lives of your patients for the better.

Physicians have the option to specialise in general medicine and look after patients who may have single organ problems or complex co-morbidities and diagnostic dilemmas; this may be in a rural, regional or urban hospital. Physicians may choose to train in another specialty specific to an organ or system, such as cardiology or endocrinology. Interventional work is frequently carried out by physicians from all specialties, even those who shudder at the thought of being a surgeon, and is often seen as an extension of their thoughtful diagnosis and skilled management of complex patients.

Training to become a physician may be perceived as long, complicated and difficult, yet it is a highly rewarding experience. Training requirements differ across the world, but particularly in Australasia, the United Kingdom and South East Asia, physicians are required to have a solid grounding in the basics of general medicine before they can begin sub-specialty training. In Australasia this means at least 3 years of work as a junior medical officer and registrar in hospitals, including a written theory examination and a clinical examination. Both the rotations and the hospital need to be accredited by the Royal Australasian College of Physicians (RACP) to be accepted for training purposes by the RACP. All trainees are required to complete formative (ongoing) assessments under the PREP (Physician Ready for Expert Practice) guidelines, before completing their training.

Historical note

The RACP was established in 1938 with a core responsibility to train future medical specialists, including adult physicians and paediatricians. The RACP was originally a branch of the Royal College of Physicians established in London in 1518 by means of a royal charter from Henry VIII.

The RACP appoints supervisors who provide the training required before candidates may sit their exams. This period is called *basic training*. All registered basic trainees who have paid their fees are now members of the College and can vote in College elections (and you should, to shape the future of your College).

Success in the written and clinical exams (which are both barrier examinations) enables a trainee to enter *advanced training* in an area of specialty medicine. This usually takes another 3 years. Successful completion of advanced training enables the trainee to be admitted to the College as a physician and use the prestigious letters FRACP (Fellow of the Royal Australasian College of Physicians) after their name, often colloquially described as 'getting your ticket'. There is currently no summative examination at the end of advanced training. In other countries (e.g. UK, USA), end-of-training examinations are required for sub-specialties.

Basic training

To be eligible for basic training in the RACP, candidates must have a medical degree, accredited by the Australian Medical Council (AMC) or the Medical Council of New Zealand, have completed an intern year (the first year after graduation) and have secured an appointment in a training position in a College-accredited basic physician training hospital, which is approved by the local Director of Physician Education (DPE). You must formally apply (as directed on the College Website: www.racp.edu.au). With the surge in medical student training in recent years, these positions have become even more competitive. International medical graduates must meet the same requirements. A list of accredited training sites in Australia and New Zealand is available on the College website. The College has no current role in obtaining training positions for people wanting to enter basic training.

During the core 36 months (full-time equivalent) of basic training, trainees work in different areas within accredited hospitals. There are certain requirements that candidates work in a variety of different medical teams before they are allowed to sit the written examination. A total of 24 months must be spent in what are referred to as core training rotations, including general and acute medicine, and at least a year in the other medical specialties (e.g. 6 months in neurology and cardiology – both highly recommended rotations if available). Up to 12 months can be spent in non-core training rotations (e.g. 6 months in emergency medicine and 6 months in psychiatry). At least 12 months must be spent at a level 3 teaching hospital and at least 3 months outside a level 3 teaching hospital. No more than 6 months can be spent in any one specialty. Specialty training time must include at least two of these three areas:
- inpatient care
- outpatient clinics
- ward consults.

An Advanced Life Support course needs to be completed (and certified), usually in the first year.

Training supervision under the RACP is provided by the DPE, a professional develop-ment advisor, educational supervisors, and term supervisors on the wards (Box 1.1).

Box 1.1 A basic trainee's helpers

- Director of Physician Education
- Educational supervisor
- Professional development advisor
- Ward / service consultant (term supervisor – 1 per rotation)

Box 1.2 A basic trainee's year

- 2 learning needs analyses
- 2 professional qualities reflections
- 2–4 ward / service consultant reports (1 per rotation)
- 4 mini-CEXs
- 2 progress supervisor's reports

Table 1.1 Summary of required teaching and learning activities and assessments under physician readiness for expert practice (PREP)

AUSTRALIA AND NEW ZEALAND
Learning needs analysis (2 per year)
Professional qualities reflection (2 per year)
'FORMATIVE ASSESSMENTS'
Mini-CEX (4 per year) – ideally 1 per term
Ward / service consultant report (1 per rotation)
'SUMMATIVE ASSESSMENTS'
2 progress reports (DPE or education supervisor) (1 mid-year and 1 annual)
Written exam (after 24 months)
Clinical exam
Mini-CEX = mini clinical evaluation exercise; DPE = Director of Physician Education.

For those with postgraduate overseas experience in internal medicine, this may be counted towards training and a formal application process is available.

The period of basic training in Australasia is closely supervised by the RACP (Box 1.2) and candidates must report their progress to the College regularly. Each year, trainees must submit at least two 'learning needs analyses' and at least two 'professional qualities reflections'. These are submitted online to the college via the basic training portal and the candidate's supervisor will help. For each rotation a 'ward / service consultant report' is also required. A detailed curriculum is available and provides an excellent guide to the examination. The details of basic training are set out in detail on the College website (www.racp.edu.au). The specifics of training requirements differ minimally from Australia to New Zealand. Please refer to the website for all current information as the particulars do change over time.

For the trainee's idle moments, another important innovation is the PREP assessments (Table 1.1). The mini clinical evaluation exercise (mini-CEX) requires trainees to assess a patient in their own hospital while being watched by an assessor. The trainee will be guided to a specific aspect of history-taking, examination or assessment. Before the trainee evaluates the patient, the trainee and assessor spend some time discussing what should occur. The trainee then spends 15–20 minutes with the patient and another

10–15 minutes afterwards with the assessor, again to discuss the performance. The idea is to simulate a normal clinical encounter in which a targeted history or examination or both are performed. A number of competencies are possible to assess in addition to those in interviewing and detecting physical signs in different exercises, including professionalism, clinical judgement and counselling.

Fees

On entering basic training, candidates pay an annual fee, which is currently (in 2020) $3646 (AUD) in Australia and $4192.90 (NZD) in New Zealand (excluding GST). The fee for the written examination is $1986 AUD and $NZD 2283.90, respectively. The fee for the clinical examination is $2972 AUD and $NZD 3417.80, respectively. The annual fee during advanced training is $3646 AUD or $4192.90 NZD. The fees change (increase) annually.

The written examination

The *written examination* is described in more detail in Chapter 2. It is an examination of theoretical medical knowledge at a high standard. People who are serious about physician training need to begin preparation for this examination at least 18 months before they sit. You will be eligible to sit the written and clinical examination after 24 months of certified basic training (i.e. in your third year).

The clinical examination

Physicians are particularly concerned that patients' treatment is of the highest standard and that physicians must have not only theoretical knowledge, but also the ability to assess patients clinically and come to a sensible diagnosis. This means being able to take a thorough history and expertly interpret the information, as well as perform an accurate physical examination. As a physician you should be able to manage patients as individuals who are all different from each other. There is continuing concern among senior physicians that too many doctors in practice do not take adequate histories, often perform rather cursory physical examinations (or none at all of the relevant system), and fail to consider a list of sensible differential diagnoses, to patients' detriment. Fundamentally, it is our job to ensure our patients always come first. There has also been a disturbing trend to manage patients by *protocol* rather than by the use of skilled clinical assessment and judgement. An example would be the performance of a series of routine tests on every patient who complains of chest or abdominal pain, without making an attempt to assess the individual patient's risks and circumstances so as to identify the relevant (and reversible) problems. Physician training is designed to educate physicians so that they do not practise in this way. This is why the *clinical examination* is as important as the written theoretical part (many in the College would argue that it is even more important than the written part – it is certainly the most memorable part).

The clinical examination for physician trainees is an extension of types of examination experienced by most undergraduate students.

The short case

Currently the clinical examination is not based on a system of objective structured clinical examinations (OSCEs) (as arguably these are too rigid and fail to reflect complex clinical practice). Rather, it includes a more intense *short-case* type of exam where the candidate's ability to perform a rapid and accurate physical examination of a certain system or part of the body is observed by the examiners (15 minutes are allowed in the RACP clinical exam – this includes presenting the findings). The emphasis is on the detection of important clinical signs and the candidate's approach to the patient. Candidates currently see four short-case patients during a whole day of examination. This means that a number of different systems can and will be tested (e.g. a cranial nerve examination, assessment of gait, a heart murmur, palpation of abdominal masses, etc.). It is usually very clear to the examiners when a candidate has sufficiently practised the particular examination asked for; these candidates look self-assured and smooth (even if they feel less than confident). This indeed is the point of the short case: to ensure candidates are practised in and able to perform an examination of any part of the body with excellent technique that will identify, as reliably as possible, key clinical signs, even when they are under stress. Successful candidates will have spent at least several months diligently practising their examination technique and seeing patients with a very large variety of clinical signs. A good trainee will have seen almost all the important physical signs and will identify them on the test day.

The long case

The other component of the clinical exam that is also applied in most undergraduate medical programs is the *long case*. Each candidate will see two long cases during the RACP exam day. Here the candidate is left alone with the patient for an hour. Patients are chosen who have a number of different medical problems. These tend to be chronic problems such as ischaemic heart disease, diabetes mellitus, inflammatory bowel disease, etc. The exam organisers are asked to find patients with two or three (or more) chronic medical problems and to include acute problems if possible. Most patients who come to the exams, however, are outpatients and generally have chronic rather than acute medical problems.

Candidates are expected to take a very detailed history from the patient and to perform an accurate examination. A summary of the patient's history and examination findings is then presented to the examiners (who have also seen the patient). This presentation is expected to take about 12 minutes. The examiners ask questions about management of the patient's problems over the remaining time. Again, the emphasis is on treating the patient as an individual and not by protocol. Candidates are expected to show that they know how to manage complex patients.

This type of exam tests the broad range of general skills required by a physician. It is our view that the clinical examination is among the most rigorous in the world and the standard expected is appropriately high. Many argue that this barrier exam explains the very high standard of physician practice in Australasia.

Success at the clinical examination is not recognised as a specialist qualification. To be admitted to Fellowship of the College, the candidate must be successful in both examinations and complete both basic and advanced training.

Passing the exam

Determination to pass both the written and clinical examinations on the first attempt is an important part of preparation. Currently, candidates are permitted only a maximum of three attempts at the written examination and three attempts at the clinical examination, and basic training must be completed within 8 years of commencement. Hence a candidate who was successful in the written examination in 2020 on the first attempt has until 2025 to pass the clinical examination. Please refer to the College website for a full review of the rules and any updates. If you are an overseas-trained physician it is essential to refer to the College website for more information about applying for the Fellowship.

There used to be no limit to the number of times candidates could sit the entire examination. Some persistent individuals sat many times (the record, we believe, is 11, and the candidate passed). More than 90 per cent of those who continue to sit do eventually get through, if they have the stamina. The pass rates for the last several years for the written and the clinical examination are each around 70 per cent, and the results are published by the College on their website.

HINT

Read the basic training curriculum and work on a study plan as soon as you start basic training.

Rationale for the FRACP exam

There are a number of competencies that will be expected to have been achieved by the end of basic training (see the College website). Medical knowledge across a broad range of medical conditions and some depth in the specialties are key components, but not the only ones. Diagnosing and managing common medical problems (and knowing when to refer) is a skill you must acquire. Other core competencies include excellent communication skills with colleagues, patients and families (both oral and written), an understanding of the social determinants of health, including cultural awareness and the special needs of vulnerable groups (e.g. indigenous populations) and the ability to work in (and eventually lead) a team that manages very complex medical problems. The highest level of professionalism will be expected of you as a physician.

We would argue there are additional competencies that should be acquired by consultant physicians over and above a very high level of clinical expertise, excellent communication skills and teamwork. Physicians should understand research methodology enough to be able to interpret expertly the ever-growing medical literature and include advances as appropriate in their clinical practice (doing and publishing research is the best way to acquire these skills). A lifelong love of learning remains an essential skill and maintaining competence will be an area of increasing attention for medical regulators. We would like to think that physicians are experts on the medical system and will become medical leaders who will advocate for appropriate system change in the interests of the community and all patients ('medical systems engineering'). Who else is going to do it and do it well if we don't?

This book was first published over 30 years ago as a guide to the FRACP exams. The basic skills needed for a candidate to perform well in short- and long-case examinations are also used by senior medical students and trainees in other specialties, including anaesthetics, emergency medicine, general practice and even psychiatry. The acquisition of the ability to take a history from patients accurately (and quickly) and examine them competently remains as important today as it did when we started, despite the availability of better and better testing. We believe the approach set out in the rest of the book should be helpful for all practising clinicians who aspire to clinical excellence.

For further information, contact the following (from the College website):

Basic training units

The Basic Training Units in Australia and New Zealand are the first point of contact for any training-related enquiries.

Australia
Basic Training Unit
Education Services
The Royal Australasian College of Physicians
145 Macquarie Street
SYDNEY NSW 2000
Phone: +61 2 9256 5454
Email: prep_bt@racp.edu.au

New Zealand
Basic Training Unit
PO Box 10601
WELLINGTON 6143
or
4th Floor
99 The Terrace
WELLINGTON 6143
Phone: +64 4 472 6713
Email: basic.training@racp.org.nz

Trainees' committee

Australia
Email: traineescommittee@racp.edu.au

New Zealand
Email: traineescommittee@racp.org.nz

Medical education officers

Medical Education Officers (MEOs) are also available in each Australian state and New Zealand to answer queries and conduct on-site workshops.

Australia
Email: supervisor@racp.edu.au

New Zealand
Email: meo@racp.org.nz

Examinations unit

Enquiries regarding applying for and sitting the written and clinical examinations should be directed to the Examinations Unit in Australia or the Basic Training Unit in New Zealand.

Australia
Email: examinations@racp.edu.au

New Zealand
Email: basic.training@racp.org.nz

Chapter 2

The written examination

No man's opinions are better than his information.
Paul Getty (1960)

The examination format

The written examination is a screening examination to select candidates for further testing. Only three attempts are now permitted. It is usually held in February in Australia and New Zealand with results released in March. There are two papers, which are both taken on the same day. The written examination is an objective multiple-choice examination. It is proposed that the written exam will be held twice a year in the near future.

The basic training curriculum

An outline of what candidates are expected to know is set out in the curriculum. It is due for further revision in 2020. Candidates can judge which specialties are currently most influential in the college by noting the length of the various specialty sections. Cardiology comes first in the list of specialties, but this may be an alphabetical phenomenon rather than a reflection of the influence of humble cardiologists. Throughout the curriculum there is emphasis on the implications of the disease on patients themselves, their relatives and communities.

Paper 1

The first paper, Medical (basic) Sciences (Paper 1), is set with an emphasis on medical sciences and relevant basic science. It contains 70 questions to be answered in 2 hours. The majority of the questions are 'A-type' questions where five alternatives are given, but only one is correct.

Paper 2

The second paper, Clinical Applications (Paper 2), contains 100 questions to be answered in 3 hours. Marks are not deducted for wrong answers in either paper and therefore it is no longer possible to score a negative mark for the total paper. An incorrect or omitted answer will score zero. This is meant to encourage candidates to attempt to answer all questions.

Extended matching questions

Extended matching questions (EMQs) are now included in both papers, and are aimed at testing problem-solving and clinical reasoning. Currently there are four in Medical Sciences and eight in the Clinical Applications paper. Each EMQ comprises a theme that may be a symptom or sign, investigation, diagnosis or treatment. There are usually two or more clinical vignettes (the stems, typically a case history with symptoms, signs and/or test results). The problem includes an option list (i.e. eight possible answers from A to H, of which one is correct), and a lead-in question (such as: 'for each patient, choose the most useful test' or 'for each of these patients, select the most likely diagnosis'). One answer is chosen for each stem. Examples are available on the College website.

Although their reliability and validity are similar to that of traditional multiple-choice questions (MCQs), EMQs are thought to be superior to traditional MCQs in assessing candidates' problem-solving and clinical-reasoning abilities.[1]

ORGANISATION

EMQs are organised into four parts:

- **A theme** – this can include a symptom, investigation, diagnosis or treatment (e.g. back pain, chest pain, lung function tests, MRI scan, ulcerative colitis, diabetes, immunosuppression).
- **A list of possible answers (options)** – this is a list of eight possible answers, marked A–H. The answer for the question will come from this list and should be written on the answer sheet.
- **The question (lead-in statement)** – this outlines the clinical picture and patient history, and asks for the question to be matched with the option.
- **A clinical problem, or vignette (the stem)** – this will usually consist of a clinical problem. There may be more than one clinical vignette for each theme.

EXAMPLES OF EXTENDED MATCHING QUESTIONS

The following (rather easy) examples of EMQs consist of:

- an option list
- a lead-in statement
- two stems.

For each stem, the candidate should choose the most appropriate option from A to H on the answer sheet. An option can be correct for more than one question.

Example 1:

Theme: Chest pain

Option list:

A. Costochondritis.

B. Aortic dissection.

C. Pericarditis.

D. Oesophageal reflux.

E. Herpes zoster.

---

[1]S M Case, D B Swanson. Extended-matching items: a practical alternative to free-response questions. *Teaching and Learning in Medicine* 1993; 5:107–15.

F. Acute coronary syndrome.

G. Angina.

H. Pulmonary embolus.

Lead-in statement:

For each patient with chest pain, select the most likely diagnosis.

Stems:

QUESTION 1

A 33-year-old man has a 12-hour history of central chest pain. His pain is predominantly in the front of the chest and does not radiate. The pain is worse when he lies down or breathes deeply, and more comfortable when he sits up and leans forward. There has been little relief from narcotic analgesics. Examination of the heart and lungs is normal. (Answer: **C**)

QUESTION 2

A 70-year-old man has had 3 months of episodes of chest pain, which he describes as tightness across his chest. Episodes occur predictably when he walks up a hill. If he keeps going the sensation is relieved quickly when he reaches the top. Episodes come on with less exertion after he has eaten and in the cold weather. The cardiac examination and ECG are normal. (Answer: **G**)

Example 2:

Theme: Dyspnoea

Option list:

A. Cardiac failure.

B. Anaemia.

C. Angina.

D. Aortic stenosis.

E. Chronic obstructive pulmonary disease.

F. Asthma.

G. Interstitial lung disease.

H. Pulmonary embolism.

Lead-in statement:

For each patient with dyspnoea, select the most likely diagnosis.

Stems:

QUESTION 1

A 75-year-old woman with a history of 15 packet years of smoking until 3 years ago has become gradually more breathless on exertion. She has a dry cough that is not severe. She has not noticed any wheezing. She has no occupational dust exposure. On examination, she is breathless undressing but is able to lie flat. She is cyanosed. There is finger clubbing. On auscultation of the lungs, fine middle and late inspiratory crackles are audible at the bases of the lungs up to the middle zones. Hoover's sign is negative. (Answer: **G**)

QUESTION 2

A 50-year-old man has had increasing dyspnoea for 3 months, which was diagnosed as asthma. There has been no improvement with bronchodilators. He is sometimes wheezy. He stopped drinking alcohol 3 weeks ago because he felt unwell, but had drunk two bottles of a wine a day for several years. He is a current smoker with a history of 20 packet years of smoking. For four nights he has only been able to sleep sitting up in a chair because of severe breathlessness when he lies flat. He appears breathless on minimal exertion and cannot lie flat. His breath sounds are slightly reduced, but the lungs are clear. The apex beat is not palpable. On auscultation of the heart there are no murmurs, but a third heart sound is audible.

(Answer: **A**)

Example 3:

Theme: Abdominal distension

Option list:

A. Ascites.

B. Obesity.

C. Renal transplant.

D. Splenomegaly alone.

E. Hepatosplenomegaly.

F. Polycystic kidney disease.

G. Constipation.

H. Irritable bowel syndrome.

Lead-in statement:

For each patient with abdominal distension, select the most likely diagnosis.

Stems:

QUESTION 1

A 30-year-old woman with a history of hypertension presents with slowly worsening abdominal fullness and discomfort. Her blood pressure is 175/100 mmHg despite antihypertensive treatment. On abdominal examination her abdomen is distended and two masses with irregular surfaces are palpable in the flanks. They can both be balloted. Her eGFR is 43 mL/min.

(Answer: **F**)

QUESTION 2

A 70-year-old man presents with increasing abdominal girth over the past several months. He has also been tired and somewhat breathless on exertion. There are no signs of portal hypertension. Masses are palpable in the right and left upper quadrants. On the right a firm edge is palpable 3 cm below the costal margin and on the left a mass moves below the costal margin on inspiration.

(Answer: **E**)

Exam timing and make-up

Although most candidates report that the time limit is sufficient for the completion of Paper 1, this is not the case for Paper 2, which is considerably more rushed. Some candidates have reported difficulty in completing Paper 2 within the time allowed. The questions in Paper 2 are clinical scenarios and often contain long preambles, which may include a clinical history and the results of numerous investigations. They can be spread over several paragraphs. The clinical application questions are designed to include tests that a practising clinician must be able to interpret. Various X-ray films (including chest radiographs, computed tomography (CT) and magnetic resonance imaging (MRI) scans), blood films (actual photographs or reports, or both), photographs of urinary sediments and histopathology slides (e.g. renal biopsies) may be included. The preamble to the question will usually give a good idea of what the scan or specimen is likely to demonstrate. Be familiar with interpreting common CT and MRI findings, ECGs, lung function tests, sleep studies and nuclear medicine scans. Photographs (both black-and-white and colour) are usually of high quality. Interpretation of biochemistry results (e.g. liver function tests, blood gases) is also examined. Normal values are always supplied. Recently the examination has had rather shorter preambles than in previous years, providing more time to complete the paper.

A pencil is provided for a paper test, as well as a well-used eraser. It is advisable, however, to bring a pencil sharpener, a spare soft (B) pencil and a good eraser, particularly if you are indecisive.

Marking

All questions are approved by a test committee. About one-third of the questions on each paper come from previous papers. These are questions that have been found to be particularly discriminating. In the past there was no predetermined pass mark and statistical methods were employed to separate candidates into high-performing and less-well-performing groups. Now the pass mark is set using a criterion-based reference standard – see the College website for details. The pass mark is not set according to the number of places that are available in the clinical examinations. It is expected that about two-thirds of candidates will continue to pass the written examination each year.

Approaching multiple-choice questions

By the time most candidates sit this examination, they will have had considerable experience with MCQs. However, it is worth stating a few relevant points:
- Ensure that you estimate in advance the amount of time you have for each question.
- The questions are complicated and each one tests several items of knowledge. The correct answer may be a number of steps removed from the initial statement. This means that it is important to read each question with great care, noting or underlining the salient points that may be helpful, and looking out especially for negatives and double negatives.
- It is worth remembering that the words 'always' and 'never' do not often apply in medicine. The word 'recognised' means that an association has been described, whereas 'characteristic' implies that the given factor is important to the condition and essential to the diagnosis.
- It is always better to guess at an answer when the question is obscure rather than leave it out entirely.
- To avoid coming to the end of the paper and finding an unexpected unfilled space on the answer sheet, keep a constant check that question and answer numbers match.

Preparation for the written examination

Reading

Review the college curriculum and use this as an outline of what is expected of you. It is worth carefully reading one of the major textbooks and key journals. We recommend concentrating on the latest edition of a standard textbook (e.g. the most recent edition of *Harrison's principles of internal medicine* or the *Oxford textbook of medicine*); it is a most satisfactory method of preparation. Another useful textbook is *Essentials of internal medicine* 4rd edition (edited by Talley, Frankum and O'Connor), which has been specifically written for FRACP candidates.

There are a number of general medical journals that candidates should read regularly. These currently include (roughly in order of usefulness):

- *New England Journal of Medicine*
- *JAMA*
- *Annals of Internal Medicine*
- *Lancet*
- *Internal Medicine Journal*
- *British Medical Journal*
- *Medical Journal of Australia*

We recommend concentrating on review articles. Study of specialist journals is not required.

Practising exam questions

There is great value in practising answering multiple-choice questions. Sample questions from past papers are available from the College. These are taken from papers that have been used in recent years. The College has a large bank of questions that are adjusted annually. The Written Examination Committee adds new questions and updates and improves old questions. Many candidates find it helpful to practise multiple-choice questions in a study group of three or four to discuss the various options.

Many candidates avail themselves of past papers and recall papers. Recall papers are written by sitters of the written exam shortly after the exam. They are often shared amongst trainees. The book *Passing the FRACP* by Jonathan Gleadle and colleagues is still a popular choice for practice questions, even if it is beginning to age a little. It is important to bear in mind that while there are certainly common persistent themes to be found in the FRACP written exam each year, the matching correct answer for each question in past papers may no longer be valid as the literature and evidence continues to grow.

The *Medical Knowledge Self-Assessment Program* (*MKSAP*) of the American College of Physicians is in our view very useful. It contains brief, up-to-date accounts of most areas of internal medicine. It clearly indicates the currently fashionable topics on which questions are likely to be set and has a comprehensive series of multiple-choice questions (and excellent critiques) based on the text. We also recommend that you read the *Board basics 3* book or app in the series – it is an excellent source of tricks and tips! However, only some of these questions are of a similar standard to the written examination questions. Another learning tool is the *Internal medicine review core curriculum* (18th edition) from MedStudy.

Trial examinations

Many hospitals conduct their own trial examinations, with questions written by staff. Also available on the market are books of multiple-choice questions based on other postgraduate examinations such as the MRCP, but these are of less value.

Exam courses

Each year, postgraduate institutions hold courses on various topics, which some candidates find helpful. A course of lectures lasting 34 weeks (one night per week for 17 weeks per year over 2 years) is available for candidates in Sydney. Short but comprehensive courses are also available in Australia (e.g. at the Royal Prince Alfred Hospital, Sydney) and New Zealand (e.g. in Dunedin), and can be particularly useful for revision.

The Physician Education Program, a thorough lecture series given by the Victorian State Committee of the RACP, running over 40 weeks of the year and held once a week in the evening for 3 hours, is now video-conferenced widely across Australia. The series covers the entirety of the syllabus in 1 year. This is particularly useful for trainees in regional centres. Details can be obtained from the RACP Department of Education.

For the clinical examination, courses are also available to assist candidates. For example, the *Canberra Course* is held most years in May at the Canberra Hospital. It includes lectures from experienced examiners. Recorded long cases are shown to the audience and the candidate is marked by the audience. There is the discussion with the audience from experienced examiners about the mark that was awarded. This method is used in the local and national calibration sessions undertaken each year by examiners. Short and long cases are also conducted in front of the audience (live) by brave volunteers from the attendees and marked and discussed in a similar way. The idea is to give candidates insight into the way examiners think. A number of these cases are available with this book. Other courses include a weekend and one-week program in Dunedin by the Department of Medicine in April, and a one-day program in Melbourne in May.

Listening

A number of audio programs are available on medical topics. The Audio Digest Internal Medicine programs are available in many libraries and provide updates of topics, but are mostly from a North American perspective and of somewhat patchy quality. The American College of Physicians sells recordings of Board Review Courses in Internal Medicine that contain excellent summaries of recent topics. The Mayo Clinic Board review video lecture series and multiple-choice questions is another excellent resource.

General advice

In summary, here are a number of conventional but important suggestions for the written examination:

- Be well rested and avoid travelling long distances on the day of the examination. Make sure you know exactly where the examination centre is situated.
- Be familiar with the format of the paper and know how much time to allow for each question.
- Work through the paper at a leisurely, deliberate pace and return to troublesome questions at the end. Inspiration may well come from other questions.
- First, careful impressions are important, but change your answer if on review you see a flaw – the data suggest that well-prepared candidates are more likely to change a wrong answer to a right answer (50% increase their test score), rather than a right answer to a wrong one (25% decrease their test scores, although rather more memorable).[2]
- Check every tenth question or so to be sure that answer numbers match the question numbers.

Have a short rest after the written examination before beginning work for the 'viva' examination, as time between the two parts of the examination is limited.

---

[2]L Di Milia. Benefiting from multiple-choice exams: the positive impact of answer switching. *Educational Psychology* 2007; 27(5):607–15.

Chapter 3

The clinical examination

This is a very testing part. It is more difficult than the written test.

Nick Talley and Simon O'Connor (1986)

The examination format

The clinical examination is divided into two sessions (morning and afternoon), each comprising two parts (one long case and two short cases), and now takes up a whole, rather exhausting, day. There is evidence to suggest that lengthening a clinical examination improves its reliability.

Candidates are notified of the starting time of the ordeal after their success in the written examination. Be on time for the clinical examination: it runs to a strict timetable and no allowances can be made for late arrivals.

The organisation of the clinical examination is an enormous enterprise. More than 800 candidates sit the exam in adult medicine each year. There are over 150 examiners from the national examiners panel (NEP) and senior examiners panel (SEP) – these are examiners who have been examining for more than 7 years, but apparently retain their enthusiasm, who travel round the country for the exam cycle. Over 90 hospitals run the exam, with between 8 and 16 candidates. Up to 20 examiners (local and national) turn up at each examining centre expecting everything to run smoothly. Up to 8 short- and 8 long-case patients have to be organised for both the morning and the afternoon sessions. The organising registrar (now called a LEO – local exam organiser) is always warned that several back-up patients are required. Examiners may see a short- or long-case patient and decide that he or she is not suitable; a replacement has to be found quickly. Organisers sometimes look ready to panic when several patients back out on the day before the exam (which is usual).

Short- and long-case rooms and an examiners' room (for the long-case interview) have to be provided. There is little time between cases for the examiners and these rooms all need to be close to each other. Assistants have to be found to make sure the examiners don't get lost. Tearooms have to be provided for the examiners and candidates. Both examiners and candidates prefer that these be separate.

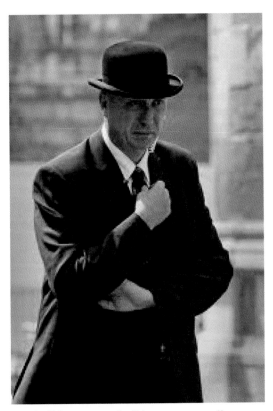

Figure 3.1 **An Oxbridge bulldog. RACP bulldogs are usually younger and not so well dressed.**

Other logistical problems include trying to ensure candidates and examiners are not standing outside the hospital in the same taxi queue, which is embarrassing for both. In some smaller centres there may be only one restaurant and candidates and examiners find themselves at adjacent tables the night before the exam.

In some towns there is only one flight out on the morning after the exam. Candidates think examiners will know, as they stand together in the taxi queue or sit beside each other on the aeroplane, whether they have passed or failed. However, examiners do not know who has passed or failed, and it would be the exceptional examiner who could remember the mark they themselves gave a particular candidate on a case. The new CLEAR marking system ensures examiners really do not know who has passed or failed.

On the exam day

For half of the candidates the first session begins with a long case. At the appropriate moment, each candidate is escorted to the patient by a proctor attendant or 'bulldog' (a term derived from the name of proctor attendants at the universities of Oxford and Cambridge) (Fig. 3.1).

The bulldog is usually a resident medical officer working at the examining hospital who has an interest in sitting the clinical examination. The bulldog introduces the candidate to the patient and then leaves. If ever you have the opportunity to work as a bulldog you should take it. There is no better way to come to understand what is expected of candidates in the exam.

The bulldogs are given clear instructions from the examinations committee when they register to help. They are also addressed by one of the national examiners for the day at the beginning of the exam day. They are reminded to be helpful to their candidate but not intrusive. It is their job to make sure their candidate gets to the various examination rooms on time. They are told not to discuss the candidate's performance – good or bad – with the candidate. They are not allowed to help candidates with timing during their short- and long-case presentations.

There are never any examiners in the room during a long case. The time is limited to 60 minutes with the patient. A 5-minute warning is given after 55 minutes. At the end, the candidate is escorted by his or her bulldog from the patient's room to a chair outside the examiners' room. Ten minutes are allowed for candidates to pull themselves together and get to the examination room. A glass of water or weak orange juice is usually offered at this stage. If not, do ask for a drink if you need one.

A bell then rings and the candidate is taken in, seated and introduced to the examiners. Try to appear self-assured (even if you are weak at the knees), but don't give an air of nonchalance (e.g. by slouching in your chair). By the time the last long-case candidate of the day has arrived, it may be the examiners who are slouching in their chairs.

As a rule there are two examiners in the room, but there may be three (one a provisional examiner only) and there may be a bulldog sitting in as well. At least one examiner will be a National Examination Panel member or Senior Examination Panel member and the other will be an experienced examiner who is a local physician (a co-opted examiner), perhaps even the DPE. In the afternoon the provisional examiner will usually examine and always with an NEP.

Immediately before the examination, the examiners interview the long-case patient. Usually one examiner does this 'blind' – that is, without reference to the patient's problem list. Patient notes are no longer provided to the examiners, who have only a summary of the patient's problems to look at. This ensures that the history is up to date, helps gauge any difficulty in terms of the patient's ability to give a history and enables the examiners to assess the physical signs. If the examiners cannot agree with each other, or don't agree with the summary about signs, they do not expect a candidate to find those signs.

The long case

The examiners assess the candidate's ability to take a detailed history and complete the examination. They also assess the candidate's ability to identify the patient's active problems and to recognise priorities for investigation and management. The examiners are very interested in finding out whether the candidate recognises the effect of the patient's disease on the patient and his or her family.

LONG-CASE MARKING

The examiners mark the candidate's performance in each of five 'domains' according to set key criteria from 1 (very poor) to 6 (outstanding) (Box 3.1). Remember that the various 'domains' do not have the same weighting and the relative importance of each will differ from one case to another. Do check the RACP website for any updates on the criteria as the examiners take these seriously. Try to ensure you meet the criteria in each domain as you undertake long cases in mock exams.

Concise, standard and generally 'open' questions will usually be asked. Only two examiners will ask questions; one 'leads' the discussion and the other follows near the end for 5–7 minutes. The lead examiner will usually introduce him- or herself and the other examiner and then ask you whether there were any problems during your time

Box 3.1 Long case 'domains'

First domain: accuracy of history

1 (Very poor performance) = No clear structure; focused on single problem; minimal detail[a]
2 (Well below expected standard) = Omission of many key points; inaccuracies or lack of detail; repetitive, poorly structured; historical details not clarified
3 (Below expected standard) = Poorly organised; omission of some key problems; need to clarify important details
4 (Expected standard) = Complete and accurate history; minimal need to clarify details; timely and well structured; some interpretation
5 (Better than expected standard) = Emphasis on appropriate details; appreciates subtleties; interprets significant aspects of the history
6 (Superior) = Sophisticated interpretation of the history; focuses on key problems; shows perceptiveness in extracting difficult information

Second domain: accuracy of the clinical examination

1 = Minimal attention to detail with the examination
2 = Many significant signs not recognised
3 = Omission or incorrect reporting of some important signs
4 = Correctly identifies all important physical signs
5 = Includes important relevant negative signs; appreciates significance of more subtle signs
6 = Actively seeks subtle signs that might enhance the diagnosis; superior organisation of difficult examination

Third domain: synthesis and prioritisation of clinical problems

1 = Most key management problems unverified; no attempt to establish priority
2 = Poor understanding of significant problems; requires substantial prompting
3 = Problems poorly prioritised; significant problems undervalued
4 = Identifies all problems; identifies problems in order of priority
5 = Confidently identifies essential problems; shows maturity in recognising lesser ones
6 = Identifies all major and minor problems; very careful prioritisation which includes a long-term view; recognises the social effect of disease

Fourth domain: understanding the effect of the illness on the patient and family

1 = Effect of disease not explored at all, or unable to be discussed
2 = Poor understanding of the effect of the disease on the patient and family; shows little concern about psychological aspects
3 = Fails to recognise some important aspects of the disease on the patient or family; misses some aspects affecting function or reaction to illness
4 = Understands the patient's physical and psychological functioning in relation to disease; appreciates the effect of treatment and prognosis on the patient <u>and</u> family
5 = Shows persistence in exploring subtle psychological issues, or issues that affect the patient or family
6 = Shows mature understanding of subtle, difficult, or intimate aspects of patient's functioning; demonstrates balance when discussing issues and sophisticated use of external social support

Continued

Box 3.1 **Continued**

Fifth domain: development and discussion of an appropriate management plan

1 = Poorly directed management plan without consideration of major problems; very poor ordering of investigations without consideration of expense or potential complications; no attempt to interpret investigations; no understanding of side-effects of treatment

2 = Inappropriate or poorly directed management plan; poor understanding of useful investigations; inability to interpret investigations; major inability to appreciate side effects of treatment

3 = Some errors in arranging a management plan; erratic and non-discriminatory use of investigations; errors in the interpretation of tests; lacking some appreciation of complications of treatment

4 = Proposes an appropriate management plan for the major issues; provides a sensible balanced approach to investigations; interprets investigations appropriately; recognises important side-effects of proposed treatment

5 = Proposes an appropriate management plan with good understanding of social effects, lifestyle and psychological aspects of disease; good use of discriminating investigations; and accurate interpretation of results

6 = Superior construction of management plan, including long-term effect; highly developed and discriminating use of investigations; mature recognition and interpretation of inconsistent results

ªAs there is no mark lower than 1, candidates must get this just for turning up.
Source: https://www.racp.edu.au/docs/default-source/default-document-library/clear-adult-medicine-long-and-short-cases-rubric.pdf?sfvrsn=d8e60b1a_0.

with the patient. For reasons of fairness, it is unusual for specialists to 'lead' the examination of a candidate on a patient with problems in their own field. Examiners will not lead if they know the patient or the candidate. Twenty-five minutes are spent with the examiners, presenting the case and discussing diagnosis and management.

It is generally expected that the history and examination findings will be presented in about 12 minutes. Presenting for longer than this will usually result in the examiners' telling you to finish up and get on to your list of problems, because the next and most important stage is analysing how you think.

You *cannot* pass the exam if you do not allow enough time for the examiners to ask you questions and discuss the case. It is important when practising long-case presentations to get the timing right. When a patient's history is long and complicated, a good candidate can still distil this into 12 minutes. The discussion period is critical to passing (or failing).

Candidates are generally expected to finish their initial presentation with a list of the patient's problems that they wish to discuss. One of the examiners' marking domains is this list of priorities and whether it agrees with theirs. Some candidates are tempted to embellish the problems list by adding some discussion about each problem as it is listed – for example 'Number 3: bone health. I would really like to know the results of the recent DEXA scan and think her risk of falls and steroid treatment pose a considerable risk …'. We don't recommend doing this – save it for answering the questions that will follow.

At the end of the time a bell will ring and the candidate is taken to begin the short-case examination. There are a few minutes available, however, for drinking weak orange juice or water.

Some candidates ask the bulldog about their performance. Apart from the fact that they are forbidden to discuss this, we believe this to be an unwise policy, as the resident medical officer is usually junior to the examinee and so is liable to give an incorrect assessment or an inappropriate cryptic remark, such as 'You were very unlucky this time'.

The short case (Fig. 3.2)

The candidate is then introduced to the short-case examiners. The examiners for the first short case are never the same as those who examined for the long case, but you may see the long-case examining team for your second short case. Again, one examiner in each team will be a member of the NEP. Fifteen minutes are allowed for the first short case; a second short case is then examined after a 5- or 10-minute break.

The examination system does not allow for more than two short cases per session. This, and the extension of time to 15 minutes for each case, means that examination of each patient is a little less rushed. However, the result of this extra time means that there is a greater opportunity for the examiners to ask questions related to the physical findings. The examiners assess five domains during the short-case examination (Box 3.2).

The key criteria and the skills that are required to achieve a satisfactory standard are available from the College or the DPE. Examining centres have also been told to have X-rays, CT scans, MRI scans and electrocardiograms (ECGs) available for discussion.

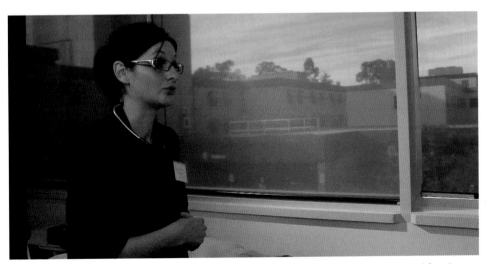

Figure 3.2 **A candidate presents her short-case findings – this short-case video is available at Student Consult (studentconsult.inkling.com).**

Box 3.2 Short-case domains

First domain: the way the candidate approaches the patient (interaction with the patient)[a]

1 = Examiner needs to intervene [to protect the patient]

2 = Rough or clumsy, causes pain without adjustment or apology

3 = Inappropriate and insensitive approach to the patient

4 = Introduces him- or herself to patient; shows respect for patient as indicated by preservation of patient's modesty, seeking permission for sensitive parts of the examination; recognises and modifies examination when it appears to be painful

5 = Meets expected standard

6 = Exceeds expected standard

Second domain: examination technique

1 = Slow examination not completed in appropriate time; cannot perform appropriate examination of the system

2 = Very slow and requires substantial prompting and guidance

3 = Examination incomplete or lacking fluency or systematic approach

4 = Undertakes systematic examination of required area without unnecessary duplication; demonstrates confidence in the examination; completes assigned tasks in appropriate time

5 = Fluent and accurate and within time; makes adjustment to routine where appropriate

6 = Fluent and accurate and within time; makes adjustment to routine where appropriate

Third domain: examination accuracy

1 = Misses all essential signs; finds abnormalities that are not present; fails to look for important negative findings

2 = Misses essential signs; finds abnormalities that are not present; fails to look for or mention important negative findings

3 = Misses essential signs; fails to look for or mention important negative findings

4 = Detects all essential signs; reports significant negative findings; does not find major signs that are not present

5 = Correctly identifies all essential and most desirable signs

6 = Correctly identifies all essential and desirable signs

Fourth domain: interpretation and synthesis of physical findings

1 = Unable to suggest a reasonable diagnosis; unable to interpret the physical signs elicited

2 = Unable to suggest a reasonable diagnosis; may advance diagnoses inconsistent with signs; requires substantial prompting; unable to reconsider additional information which may alter the diagnosis

3 = Not confident with the diagnosis; list of differential diagnoses poorly developed; unable to consider alternative explanations for the findings; requires more than minor prompting to reconsider options

4 = Provides appropriate interpretation of signs; recognises inconsistencies in interpretation and findings; provides sensible priorities in diagnosis; discusses appropriate alternative diagnoses

5 = Identifies most likely diagnosis and provides reasonable differential diagnoses based on physical findings

6 = Establishes most likely diagnosis on basis of examination; considers all likely alternatives

> **Box 3.2 Continued**
>
> ### Fifth domain: investigations and management
> 1 = Unable to suggest reasonable investigations; misinterprets information provided
> 2 = Unable to use investigations to assist in diagnosis; inappropriate dependence on investigations
> 3 = Does not suggest appropriate investigations; misinterprets or is unable to integrate investigations with examination findings
> 4 = Accurately interprets investigations in context; suggests appropriate line of investigation and integrates them with examination findings
> 5 = Correctly interprets all major investigations
> 6 = Correctly interprets investigations and integrates them with examination findings without prompting; recognises and discusses areas of doubt; uses results to support differential diagnosis and discussions

[a]Many candidates ask 'if I am really nice and considerate to the patient, is that enough for me to pass despite other failings?' Answer 'No'.
Source: https://www.racp.edu.au/docs/default-source/default-document-library/clear-adult-medicine-long-and-short-cases-rubric.pdf?sfvrsn=d8e60b1a_0.

If technology has achieved anything, it has made it more difficult to find X-rays and scans for candidates. Most hospitals have electronic storage of scans. There is often a problem logging on to the system and preventing the screen from turning itself off every few minutes. This tends to cause episodes of panic for the bulldog and organisers (and sometimes the examiners).

The other half of the candidates does this routine in the reverse order. After lunch the second session begins, and this time the order of the short and long cases is reversed for each candidate.

The marking system yesterday and today

The way the exam is marked is under constant revision. Until 2019 the mark awarded for each short case was out of 7, as follows:

1. very poor performance
2. well short of expected standard
3. short of expected standard
4. expected standard
5. better than expected standard
6. much better than expected standard
7. exceptional performance.

In 2006 part-marks were introduced for the short case, so that for both long and short cases the scoring system incorporated positives and negatives (part marks) between 1 and 7, giving a 19-point scale. The use of part-marks helped some candidates who were very close to a pass overall. For example, if the examiners agree that a candidate's performance was better than a 4 but not deserving of a 5, a 4+ was awarded, while if the candidate's performance was much better than a 4 but not deserving of a 5, the mark would have been a 5−. When the marks were added up at the end of the day, for example, 4+ would be 4.33 and 5− would be 4.67. Once a 'raw score' out of 7 was awarded, it was weighted; the long-case scores were multiplied by 3. This means that it had been possible to pass the exam with two good long-case scores, but without passing any short case.

Each long case was worth 21 marks and each short case was worth 7 marks. Because there were plus and minus marks for all cases the marks were again multiplied by 3 – so the total mark possible was 210. The mark required to pass the examination was 120. The introduction of part marks made the marking more complicated but increased the pass rate somewhat. It also left room for compromise between examiners who found it difficult to agree about the mark.

The examiners subsequently began to suspect that some candidates had decided preparation for the short case was not very important and had been concentrating on their long cases. From a candidate's point of view this may seem a reasonable strategy, but it may mean suffering embarrassing humiliation in front of the short-case examiners and it defeated the underlying purpose of the examination: to determine whether candidates were fully ready for advanced training. In 2014 the rules were changed so that candidates had to pass at least one short case and one long case to obtain an overall pass. We wonder whether this is still too lax (historically, to pass overall, candidates had to pass every case, both the long and two shorts, largely explaining the relatively low pass rates in the past).

In 2018 a new marking system was tried out and in 2019 was formally introduced. The CLEAR marking system has only 6 marks (for both long and short cases).
- 6 = excellent performance
- 5 = better than expected
- 4 = expected standard (a pass)
- 3 = below expected standard (a fail)
- 2 = well below expected standard
- 1 = very poor performance.

The candidates' short- and long-case marks are put into a grid, with the long-case scores on the X-axis and the short-case scores on the Y-axis (Fig. 3.3).

Rather than there being an absolute mark required for a pass, the long- and short-case scores have become interdependent. The idea is to make sure there is still a higher weighting for long cases but at least one short and one long case must be passed. This wasn't quite true for the 2019 exam but the diagonal line that determines a candidate's fate can be adjusted from year to year – but not, the College assures us, after the examination has been held.

This CLEAR system makes marking quicker – there are fewer options – but also makes compromise more difficult between examiners. The difference between marks 4 and 3 is large and important – unlike that between 4 and 4–. There is also the potential risk that the pass mark might be manipulated. To date, analyses of results from previous years and from the trial of the CLEAR system in 2018 suggest that the overall pass rate is the same but that the candidates who pass and fail are not quite the same. There is also the difficulty that some candidates may pass when others with a higher raw mark fail. We therefore wonder whether in a few years the examinations committee will say 'Why don't we make the marking system a bit more subtle and introduce part marks?'

The new system will be thoroughly evaluated and this is part of continuing efforts to make the exam as fair as possible. For this reason, please refer to the College website for any updates in the year you sit.

The examiners try very hard to be fair. Each candidate's performance is discussed at the end of each long- and short-case session. Each examiner scores independently; if there is disagreement about a mark, this is discussed and a consensus mark is chosen. If the examiners cannot agree, the NEP member has the final say. Examiners record any special considerations that may have caused difficulties for the candidate (and flag the assessment sheet). This used to be done with the infamous 'red dot' but now a section at the top of each marking sheet is filled in with details of any minor problem (e.g. the

Long Case #2 Score	Long Case #1 Score: 1	2	3	4	5	6
1	0	0	0	0	1	2
2	0	0	0	1	2	3
3	0	0	0	2	3	4
4	0	1	2	3	4	4
5	1	2	3	4	4	5
6	2	3	4	4	5	5

0	Band 0: Does not meet Standard
1	Band 1: SC Passed ≥3 AND SC Aggregate Score ≥19
2	Band 2: SC Passed ≥2 AND SC Aggregate Score ≥15
3	Band 3: SC Passed ≥2 AND SC Aggregate Score ≥13
4	Band 4: SC Passed ≥1 AND SC Aggregate Score ≥13
5	Band 5: SC Passed ≥1 AND SC Aggregate Score ≥12

Figure 3.3 **RACP divisional clinical examination score combination grid. (SC = short case.)**

long-case patient went briefly to the bathroom during the candidate's time with him or her). A more serious problem (e.g. the prolonged absence of the patient) is recorded in detail on a separate sheet. The examiners are asked to record whether they felt the problem led to a significant difficulty for the candidate and whether this was taken in to account when the score was decided. The chief examiner of the day (always a member of the NEP) is responsible for collecting the marked score sheets and dealing with any procedural matters. These matters can be considered later by the executive, if necessary.

The chief examiner can, in rare cases, halt the examination for a period. For example, if a patient becomes very ill and a substitute has to be found, the whole examination can be stopped for a period and restarted.

The examiners do not know the candidate's marks in other sections of the exam (including the written examination), and therefore they do not know the effect of their own mark on the candidate's overall success or failure. The examiners see the same short case four times with four candidates. They give a mark at the end of each session and cannot change this after assessing the other candidates' attempts at the same case. The examination is not meant to be competitive. This means that every candidate can pass if the required standard is achieved.

Rather than trying to pass candidates (as at undergraduate level), the examiners are trying to evaluate the true standard of each candidate. Examinees must prove to the College that they are 'good enough'; that is, they must demonstrate that they have mastered the material and have reached the required standard. The standards are very high, but the College emphasises to the examiners that the standard is that required for a person to enter advanced training and not the standard expected of a consultant physician. The rationale for this approach is that trainees who are likely to begin training in a sub-specialty should know how to examine all the systems of the body properly and have a sensible approach to the management of medical problems outside their specialty. A senior chest physician, for example, will always be able to boast that he or she once knew how to examine the cranial nerves expertly.

To achieve uniform standards, the CFE has been constantly working on improvements. Senior members of the CFE examine more often with less-experienced examiners. The CFE also holds regular formal calibration exercises, in which all examiners view video recordings and mark a candidate's performance. A general discussion is then held to try to develop a uniform approach. The calibration is far from perfect; however, the CFE is working towards eliminating obvious mistakes.

NEP examiners are given a chart showing where each of them sits as to the average mark he or she awards. There is surprisingly little variation between examiners considered to be hawkish and those with a reputation as doves. Experienced examiners submit reports on their junior colleagues at the end of the exam period. This helps the examinations committee choose new members for the NEP. If there is a disagreement between examiners about the suitable consensus mark (a rare event), the NEP member can override the co-opted local examiner.

Local examiners and NEP and CFE members all undergo 'calibration' exercises before they examine. Even experienced examiners are not allowed to examine unless they have been 'calibrated' that year.

The overall pass rate (for the written *and* viva examinations) in any one year in the past was between 30% and 40%. The eventual pass rate after success at the written examination and over four vivas (the old system) approached 85%. Under the new system, the pass rate has increased to 70% or more for the clinical examination each year.

The mini-CEX

In 2008 the mini-CEX was introduced for basic trainees in their final year and is now used in all years of basic training. This is quite separate from the clinical examination and, although it has to be performed, it does *not* count towards marks in the formal clinical examination. The trainee undertakes four mini-CEX exams a year, usually in the trainee's own hospital and marked by the Director of Physician Training (DPT) or a suitably trained delegate. Each exam lasts about 30 minutes and is a cross between a long and short case. The trainee is introduced to a patient and given a clinical problem – for example, 'Mr Smith has had problems with dyspnoea for a year and has noticed a recent deterioration in his symptoms. Please take a relevant history and examine him.' The trainee is expected to ask directed questions about the symptoms and then examine the relevant system or systems of the body. This is all observed by the examiner. The trainee then presents the findings and a differential diagnosis, and suggests investigations and possible treatment.

Preparation for the clinical examination

For one mistake made for not knowing, ten mistakes are made for not looking.

J A Lindsay

The clinical examination aims to test not only clinical ability but also attitudes and interpersonal skills. For most candidates a successful approach to the viva depends on seeing a large number of long and short practice cases (Fig. 3.4a and b). It is usually too late to start practising these cases after passing the written examination; preparation should start at least several months beforehand.

Read the stem

The stem for the short case in Fig. 3.4(a) is 'This man has noticed some enlargement of his hands. Please examine him.'

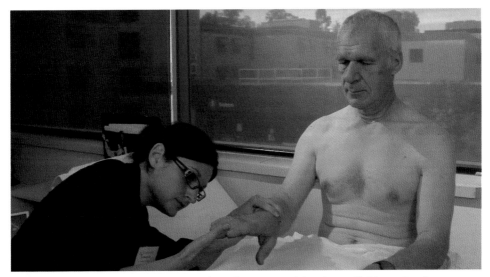

Figure 3.4(a) **Short-case practice – this short-case video is available at Student Consult (studentconsult.inkling.com).**[1]

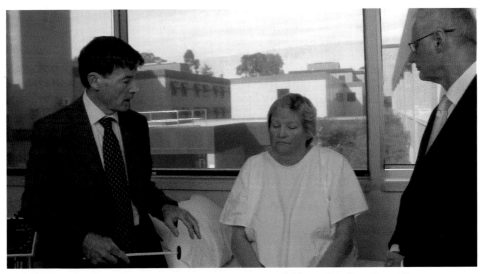

Figure 3.4(b) **Long case – this long-case video is available at Student Consult (studentconsult.inkling.com) and see p. 401 for details (guess who the examiners are).**[2]

---

[1]Diagnosis? See p. 293 (Fig. 10.6) for an answer.
[2]The examiners are Simon O'Connor, holding the patella hammer, and Nick Talley observing intently.

This usually means acromegaly.

The examiners expect the candidate to make the correct diagnosis and subsequently proceed to demonstrating or looking for systemic signs of the disease itself or relating to treatment complications.

Examine the hands and look for the important signs of acromegaly (p. 292). Signs of activity must also be noticed. In this case there were numerous skin tags.

Practise, practise!

To practise for the long cases, try to set aside a regular time each week. Most physicians, if approached, are only too willing to test-run candidates. Being exposed to many different examiners (of variable severity) is desirable. It will help to iron out mistakes and provide practice in answering different types of questions. Although most teaching hospitals have a training scheme in which long cases are examined by consultants or senior registrars, this is not enough. It is difficult to quote numbers, but we believe 75 formal long cases (across all disciplines) in which different specialists and senior registrars act as examiners represents the bare minimum requirement for preparation.

Practice examiners have not usually interviewed the patient and are therefore not quite like the real examiners. This does make a difference to the way they will mark your case.

Remember also that, each time a patient is admitted to hospital, practice can be gained in the long-case technique – this turns over time into useful preparation time. Practising cases is also critical in order to be able to cope with management problems in Paper 2 of the written examination.

Many candidates now video-record their long-case presentation practice cases. This can be a useful way of assessing your technique. A number of recorded cases are available from the College. The cases in this book are available via Inkling with our enhanced eBook edition and via Student Consult with the print book.

Practice for the short cases is also important. More examinees used to fail these than the long cases, although this has changed now that the short cases are receiving more emphasis. It is valuable to have senior colleagues, as well as peers, take you on short cases. Travelling to other hospitals to practise is also worthwhile, because you have to examine patients in strange surroundings while mastering short-case drilling. It also relieves the boredom somewhat.

The best practice examiner is the one who frightens candidates a little but does not demolish them when they make an error. Seek out constructive criticism while being watched by unfamiliar examiners. Many candidates practise in pairs, with each person taking turns to be the examiner. Practising being an examiner helps you to appreciate the bad habits that annoy the real examiners.

Clinical exam courses

For the clinical examination, courses are also available to assist candidates. For example, the *Canberra Course* is held most years in May at the Canberra Hospital. It includes lectures from experienced examiners. Recorded long cases are shown to the audience and the candidate is marked by the audience. Then there is a discussion with the audience from experienced examiners about the mark that was awarded. This method is used in the local and national calibration sessions undertaken each year by examiners.

Equipment

Equipment is always provided at the hospital where the examination is held. However, it is important to take the following:

- a familiar stethoscope that you have used for a long time. Do not buy a new, fancier stethoscope the day before the test; it takes time to get used to a new instrument. Electronic stethoscopes are not generally allowed unless a candidate has a hearing problem and has obtained permission from the College
- a hand-held eye card – obtainable from Optical Prescription Spectacle Makers (OPSM) for a moderate charge and essential for cranial nerve or eye examinations (see Ch 16)
- a red-tipped hatpin – you can buy a plain one and paint the top with nail polish; this is invaluable for visual field testing (see Ch 16)
- paper and pens.

It is debatable whether candidates should take in their own bags of instruments. Many favour bringing their own ophthalmoscope and pocket torch (with fresh or recharged batteries in both). Others also like to have cotton wool, neurology pins (an unused one for each case) and spatulas, as well as tuning forks (256 Hz and 128 Hz) and a patella hammer, which is too much to carry in the pockets. This has led to a trend for leather briefcases to house all the equipment (Fig. 3.5). However, the occasional difficult examiner

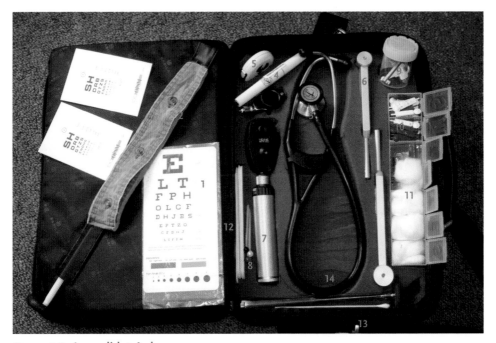

Figure 3.5 **A candidate's bag.**

1. Eye charts
2. Buttons and long patella hammer (underneath)
3. Stethoscope
4. Torch
5. Tape measure
6. Tuning forks
7. Ophthalmoscope and auriscope
8. Hatpins (red and white)
9. Jar with lid (containing key for key grip assessment)
10. Disposable neurology pins
11. Cotton wool
12. Spatula
13. Cotton buds and spare patella hammer
14. Carefully shaped foam inserts

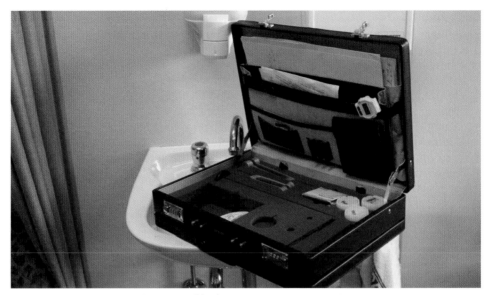

Figure 3.6 **Incorrect positioning of bag #1.**

has been known to complain about this! There is a legend about one candidate's briefcase, which was filled with such elaborate equipment, including an inverted cardigan for testing dressing apraxia, that his examiners spent their time inspecting the contents rather than watching him examine the patient (not a recommended approach). A few more cautionary tales:

- Candidates who have recently bought their bags have been known to forget the combination number needed to release the lock at the critical moment in the exam when the bag has to be opened.
- One candidate placed her open bag on the sink in the examination room for her first case, only to have the bag flooded with water when one of the examiners leaned closer to watch the examination and accidentally turned on the tap above the sink (Fig. 3.6).
- Leaving your bag on the floor might also be problematic. Many an examiner has been anxious that a candidate might walk backwards, trip over his or her bag and be impaled by a patella hammer (Fig. 3.7).
- During the assessment of the patient by the examiners, one examiner mocked the old-fashioned stethoscope of his colleague: 'You have a 19th-century stethoscope and I have a 21st-century one,' he said. On going to examine the patient with his electronic stethoscope (not usually allowed to candidates), he stopped and said, 'Ah, the battery is flat.' 'Don't worry, you can borrow mine,' said his helpful colleague. If you have permission to use one, make sure it is charged. It would be embarrassing to have to ask to borrow the examiner's.
- During practice sessions, it is always a good idea to place equipment in the same pockets each time. In the exam, you do not want to be fumbling at this crucial time – it will only create a poor impression. Consultants, other than cardiologists, carry their stethoscopes or put them in their coat pocket; rarely do they place them around their neck. This seems a sensible policy for aspiring consultants also. Candidates who do carry a briefcase into the test (and many neurologists carry one everywhere) can usually place it on the patient's bedside table and leave it open so that its contents are easily accessible.

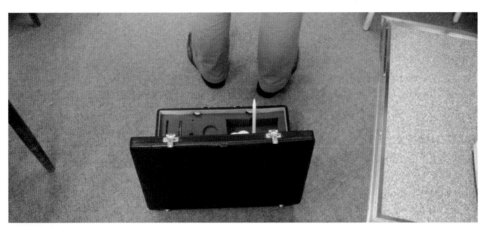

Figure 3.7 Incorrect positioning of bag #2.

Travel

Most candidates fly in to the examination city on the day before their exam. At least one candidate arriving in jeans and a T-shirt found that his luggage, containing his suit and tie, had been sent by the airline to Hawaii (or somewhere). It was too late to buy more clothes. He sat the exam in these casual clothes, having explained to the exam organisers what had happened. The story had a happy ending, but the anxiety caused by such an occurrence is probably best avoided. Carry your exam clothes onto the aeroplane with you. Check, however, that there is nothing in your exam bag that will disturb the airport security people. They are easily alarmed.

Appearance

Dress is important. The medical establishment is well known for its conservatism, and the non-verbal messages that your appearance gives should not be forgotten when dressing. Traditionally, men and women wear a conservative suit and men a non-committal tie. Almost all examiners wear suits and ties (or perhaps a bow tie). In fact, a suit (for both men and women) is a sort of uniform and by far the easiest clothing to wear. The most important thing is not to wear something that will make you feel self-conscious and distract you from performing well in the exam itself.

Other important considerations for men are having short tidy hair, a neatly trimmed beard if you cannot bear to shave it off, and a neutral smell. Dress formally, with care to project an air of quiet efficiency. White coats are never worn. However, being well dressed is no guarantee of success. There is a story of two male candidates, wearing grey suits and with recently cut hair, who were viewing with satisfaction a third examinee whose long hair was tied neatly in a bun and who was dressed in a flowing Kaftan-like garment – they felt their own success assured with such competition. However, it turned out that they were unsuccessful and their colleague passed.

It is important that clothing used in the exam fits properly. The examiners were once alarmed to see a candidate whose suit was either borrowed from a smaller person or which had not kept up with his weight gain. When he bent over to examine the patient, his shirt and trousers separated and the examiners thought he must have had a previous career as a plumber.

> **HINT**
> 1. Remember your bag lock combination number.
> 2. Do not place your bag on a sink (or behind you on the floor).
> 3. Make sure all your batteries are charged.

Nerves

Some candidates take beta-blockers on the day of the test to remain calm. An interesting story from the *Lancet* highlights this very situation. A Scottish physician refers to a British censor who had the habit of counting the temporal pulse of candidates: if he found that the pulse rate was less than 60 beats/minute, he would take this fact into account when giving his mark.[3] We are unaware of a similar practice in Australasia. However, candidates intending to use these drugs should give themselves a dose during a practice session. One doctor who did not do this learnt to his horror during the actual examination that beta-blockers caused him severe bronchospasm (he failed). Another was so bradycardic after doubling the dose to calm his exam nerves that he felt less than tip-top. Everyone is anxious before the exam starts but you need some anxiety to drive an excellent performance.

Nervous individuals with a tendency to sweat can have problems. One candidate (now a professor), who was balding and wore glasses, found that, during times of intense anxiety, rivers of sweat would roll down from his forehead and fog up his glasses, washing them from his nose. His solution was antiperspirant (unscented, of course) applied generously to the forehead (he passed).

The day before

Preparation is the key to success. Like an Olympic athlete, obtain plenty of sleep in the week before the ordeal, take no alcohol or tranquillisers in the 48 hours before it, and do not study during the final 24 hours. Make sure that you eat something before the examination and avoid taking a long trip to the examination city on the morning of or the night before the test.

The impact of COVID-19

In 2020, because of the corona virus pandemic, the clinical examination was postponed and the split. The long cases are to be conducted separately and via video conference in November with plans for short cases to be held in early 2021.

---

[3]M G Bamber. Dope test for doctors. *Lancet* 1980; ii:1308.

Chapter 4

The long case

In what manner are the examiners elected? Are they elected by the profession or any part of the profession whose interests are equal to those of the whole and are they responsible to the profession at large for their conduct?
Neither the one nor the other.
Lancet 1824; i:20

When the examiners discuss a long case with a candidate, they are expecting to find out how the candidate would manage the patient and his or her problems, and if the candidate has taken ownership of the case. They want to know whether the candidate has a practical grasp of what is required in consultant practice. Candidates are expected to have a mature and sensible approach to the patient's problems. It may help to picture yourself as the physician taking over the care of a new patient. Practising long cases trains candidates to be better clinicians.

Careful allocation of time with the patient in the long case is vital. The exact proportions will depend on the case itself but, as a rough guide, spend 25 minutes on the history-taking, 15 minutes on the examination and the rest of the time preparing discussion and reviewing vital facts with the patient. Remember, though, that you can continue to ask the patient questions as these occur to you while you are examining. Nothing is more important than ensuring you leave enough time to put your thoughts in order.

Candidates favour many different systems for recording long-case details (as an aid to memory or *aide memoire*). There are two we recommend: one is to use a pad that can be held comfortably in the hand and the pages turned unobtrusively. Most candidates now use a large card folder, one side of which is used for the history and the other for the examination findings; a second card (if necessary) is used for relevant investigations, management and short lists of facts you may wish to mention. Obviously, numbering each side is important, so as not to mix up the order of presentation. These cards are usually provided to candidates who want them at the examination site. Mixing up the cards can be a disaster. One candidate was sitting, preparing to enter the examination room, when the side door opened and a puff of wind blew the cards out of her hands.

She was then ushered straight into the examination room with the cards in random order. She began the long case badly and failed.

Candidates who do not want to rewrite the whole long-case presentation before facing the examiners (time is often a problem) may find it helpful to number the paragraphs with a red pen in the order in which they wish to present the story.

Many examination centres provide manila folders. These are large enough for candidates to be able to write out one whole long case on one folder. They do, however, seem to lead to a lot of turning backwards and forwards and folding and unfolding as candidates search to find where something was written. Practise with whatever method you choose so that it works smoothly.

The history-taking and physical examination

Once you have said, 'How do you do?' to the patient at the beginning of the long case, we suggest initially following the steps outlined below. Remember though that there is no *single right* way to conduct any part of the exam. This book is meant only to provide a framework upon which candidates can work out what suits them best. These steps may help you ascertain rapidly the patient's major problems so that you can direct further questioning more easily.

1. Explain to the patient that this is a very important examination. Gain the patient's interest and support. This is a test of bedside manner.

2. Ask the patient 'What do you see as the main problem with your health at the moment?' If he or she asks, 'Am I allowed to tell you?', look confident and firm and say, 'Yes, of course.' Candidates are entitled to all the information the patient can offer. The examiners will usually similarly instruct the patient to tell the candidates all they can. Patients are told by the examiners not to give any written information such as referral or specialist letters to the candidate. Expect more than one problem.

3. Ask the patient for a list (single word answers) of the other health problems they have. In the setting of multiple problems, confirm the main issue by asking 'What is troubling you most now?' Do record and note in your presentation the problem the patient considers most important. The problems the patient finds troubling should appear somewhere in the problems list you give to the examiners, even if some are less interesting issue in terms of the patient's health.

4. Ask why the patient is in hospital this time (i.e. is he or she an inpatient or outpatient?) and, if relevant, the presenting symptoms when he or she was admitted. The majority of patients are brought in specifically for the examination. Exam organisers have been asked to find long-case patients who have active problems suitable for discussion. This can be difficult and, certainly, patients often have no acute medical problems.

5. Review early on what medications the patient is taking. A full list should be provided for you by the examination centre. Use this list to identify any medical conditions you may have missed, and sometimes to gauge the severity or prognosis. This information is, however, not always helpful (see Table 4.1).

6. Ask the patient about any recent tests, again to obtain clues about the current problem.

7. If, as you probe, the patient stops talking, ask, 'Anything else?' and repeat as needed.

In the majority of long cases, the patient has a chronic illness about which he or she may be very well informed. It is sensible to make use of this knowledge, but remember the trap that patients may be biased in their opinions and give (inadvertently) false information. Be sceptical about patients' opinions regarding their diagnoses and ask questions that will help verify what the patient has said. For example, a patient who

Table 4.1 A medication list provided by a young adult patient with extreme interest in her medical condition

1. Azathioprine 50 mg daily	16. Oxycodone SR 10 mg mane 20 mg nocte
2. Methotrexate 25 mg weekly	17. Oxycodone 5 mg QID prn
3. Prednisone 25 mg daily	18. Vitamin B_{12} IM monthly
4. Folinic acid 50 mg IM weekly	19. Vitamin C 500 mg daily
5. Metformin 1 g daily	20. Paracetamol 1 g QID prn
6. Aciclovir 500 mg daily	21. Ibuprofen 400 mg TDS prn
7. Baclofen 12.5 mg QID	22. Citirizine 10 mg daily prn
8. Calcium carbonate 600 mg daily	Then added to this typed list by hand:
9. Mirtazepine 60 mg daily	23. Moxifloxacin
10. Esomeprazole 40 mg daily	24. Frusemide
11. Nifedipine 30 mg daily	25. Ivabradine
12. Hydroxychloroquine 200 mg daily	26. Magnesium
13. Pramipexole 250 mcg daily	27. Salbutamol
14. Oestradiol valerate 2 mg BD	28. Potassium
15. Oralube artificial saliva prn	

Although a list of medications is usually a big help, this one might cause anxiety for the examiners and candidates, and might suggest an underlying somatic symptom disorder.

says he has had five heart attacks, but has not been admitted to hospital for any of them, is probably mistaken. A candidate who merely repeats to the examiners what the patient has said without any attempt at interpretation will not pass and is not a sophisticated physician. Many experienced patients bring in a typed summary of their medical problems. The examiners have decided to tell patients to use these as an *aide memoire* for answering the candidates' questions, but not to hand them over. Candidates should exercise scepticism when patients bring in large amounts of medical information about themselves. Some patients have an exaggerated interest in their health and there have been a few suspected Munchhausen patients slip into the exams (Table 4.1). It is the sign of a mature candidate that he or she can manage 'difficult' patients.

Having established the main diagnosis early on, confirm this with specific questioning. On finding symptoms that do not fit the diagnosis, decide the likely possibilities and follow up with further questions. Never blindly believe the patient but don't upset patients by doubting them openly. One of the skills of a physician is to obtain information and explore all aspects of a patient's illness without causing upset. A history of exotic previous illnesses without a history of appropriate investigations or treatment for such conditions should prompt a careful and tactful retaking of the history.

Next, enquire about other problems. Most long-case patients are chosen because they have multiple medical problems. An example might be an elderly woman with interstitial lung disease as her major presenting illness who also has significant ischaemic heart disease, chronic kidney disease and peptic ulceration secondary to aspirin use. It is a terrible experience to discover another major illness only minutes before the end of the time. List all the important diseases chronologically and obtain full details about each one. Organise the material to present the most important (i.e. often the current) problem first, followed by the others in order of importance

It is important to appreciate the great amount of detail the examiners will expect about the patient's past history. A lot of time needs to be spent on this. Failing to uncover a medical problem from long ago that the examiners found when they saw the patient counts against the candidate. Remember that the patient's history is often well rehearsed after the examiners and perhaps another candidate have taken it.

If the patient has an illness that can become suddenly severe or life-threatening – for example, asthma or insulin-requiring diabetes – ask whether there is an *action plan*. That is, does the patient know what to do or whom to contact if he or she becomes suddenly worse? All patients should be asked about their immunisation status, including influenza, hepatitis A and B, herpes zoster and pneumococcus (depending on their age).

Do not ever forget the social history. This is especially important because the examiners (and society) are keen to have caring specialists who are fully aware of the complete social environment of their patients. The examiners will expect great detail here as well. Ask about:

- *occupation* – now and in the past
- *adequacy of income* – particularly if the patient is on a pension, whether the patient can afford medications and transport to appointments
- *current housing arrangements* – e.g. renting, mortgage
- *ability to cope and resilience at home and the quality of life* if this is a chronic disease problem – the activities of daily living (ADLs) should be assessed
- *stress points* – whether there are problems in the patient's life that make coping with the illness much more difficult, e.g. threatened loss of a driver's licence
- *depression* – it is reasonable to ask patients whether the illness or other problems have been associated with depression, loss of interest in life and even suicidal thoughts, but be tactful; also consider anxiety. Don't miss post-traumatic stress disorder in a returned war veteran
- *mobility* – particularly the number of steps that need to be climbed at home and at work, and on which floor of the building the patient lives
- *hobbies* – e.g. contact with animals, chemicals or dust
- *marital status* and number of children (from which partners)
- *sexual problems* – particularly ask about erectile dysfunction in men if indicated (e.g. patients with diabetes)
- *end-of-life decisions* – discussion of this may be appropriate if the patient has an incurable disease
- *place of birth* and *overseas travel* in relationship to the illness
- *immunisation status* and whether the patient has a general practitioner.

A family history must also be taken. This sort of information is easy to obtain and fills in discussion time neatly, but disaster can threaten if the candidate does not know it. The most important aspects of the social and family history should be outlined in the initial presentation and the rest kept in reserve to be unleashed if the examiners show an interest.

There has been recent debate about the need for candidates to take a detailed sexual history. In reality this is necessary only if it is related directly to the patient's medical problems (e.g. someone with HIV infection). It would not be usual for a doctor to take this type of history during a first consultation, except in these circumstances. If asked why you had not taken a more detailed sexual history, a reasonable answer would be that it was not directly relevant and that your usual practice is to wait until you know the patient better before asking questions of this sort.

As you examine the patient, always ask when the examiners came, what parts they examined and whether any comments were made about the signs. One candidate was told by his patient that during a fundoscopic examination the examiner had said to the other: 'Look, a Roth's spot!' However, this is no substitute for a thorough examination.

Even though you should spend most time on the relevant systems, remember that unexpected signs will sometimes crop up, such as a large breast mass, gross papilloedema or an abdominal mass. The examiners always have in front of them a list of the signs and have always gone to the trouble of checking that, in fact, these signs are present. You will be expected to have found all the important signs, so be thorough. Any equivocal findings should probably be ignored. Ask the bulldog for the results of the urinalysis and rectal examination; you are not expected to perform these personally. Also, don't forget to take the patient's blood pressure at some stage and check for a postural change, if at all relevant (e.g. diabetes mellitus).

Practise performing quick screening tests, such as GALS (gait, arms, legs and spine (Ch 9)) as a test of mobility, and have an approach to assessing diabetic patients for their possible vascular and neurological complications quickly.

At the end of the history-taking and physical examination, always ask the patient: 'Is there anything else you think I should know?' Amazingly, important information is often volunteered at this point. Then ask yourself: 'Could this be anything else?' and 'Can I tie all the multisystem problems into one disease?' (usually you can't in an older person, but this may be possible in a younger patient).

During the 20 minutes or so remaining, decide what type of case it is – that is, is it a *treatment* problem or a *diagnostic* problem, or both? Sort out the active from the inactive problems. Draft your introductory statement – for example, 'I saw Mrs J Smith, a 30-year-old woman, who presents for the treatment problem of active rheumatoid arthritis and also with the diagnostic problem of jaundice'.

Next, mentally rehearse presenting the history and examination concisely and clearly. There is a tension between detail and brevity in the presentation of the patient. Experience and practice will help you get this right. Your concluding statement should reiterate the problems (in order of importance). It is usual to end the presentation by requests for relevant investigations. Always formulate a differential diagnosis, even if the history and examination lead to a definite diagnosis. Create a list of the findings on history and examination that support (or refute) the diagnoses considered. If a positive diagnosis cannot confidently be made, try to decide on the most likely diagnosis.

The discovery of a major problem with a particular long case (e.g. a patient with obvious dementia) shouldn't lead to panic. By recognising the problem, fully examining the patient and having a plan of management (finding reversible causes, eliciting from relatives the social set-up, etc.), you will pass. One candidate who was faced with a demented patient in the long-case examination became angry and complained bitterly to his examiners. He failed.

Occasionally there are other difficulties, such as language problems (usually the candidate is supplied with an interpreter) or the patient becomes ill during the time (cardiac arrests have occurred). Be sure to inform the bulldog of any difficulties; people will go out of their way to be fair in such circumstances. The examiners will make a note of any such problems on their scoresheet, so that this can be taken into account by the executive later on. As the first question, the lead examiner will ask the candidate if there were any problems with the patient during the case. This is not the time to complain about the patient. The examiner will know if the patient was a difficult historian. However, if there were problems, such as late arrival of the patient or the patient's need to leave the room a number of times to go to the toilet, this should be mentioned, but not dwelt upon.

The presentation

Your whole presentation to the examiners should take 10–12 minutes. Never go longer. Leave out any irrelevant detail; padding the presentation never impresses. Avoid repetition – for example, mentioning various medications as a part of the history of a particular system and then later as part of a long general list. Try not to use the brand names of drugs.

The physical examination findings usually take only a few minutes to present. Avoid giving long lists of normal findings, but make sure the examination findings in the systems affected are thorough.

The examiners are only human too: sometimes they are hungry, tired or just bored after previous presentations (particularly if yours is the last long case of the afternoon). Show interest and enthusiasm while speaking. Think of yourself as a newsreader and speak at a speed that allows the examiners to keep up and take notes. Do not read your notes in a monotone. Look up from your notes to make eye contact with the examiners. The notes are meant to help your memory. Break up the pace and include a pregnant pause after you make an important point (for emphasis).

Ideally, the long case should be a discussion between consultants, with the candidate being a respectful junior colleague. The examiners only rarely interrupt during the presentation. If your presentation is taking too long and there will not be time for discussion you will usually be interrupted and asked to summarise. Remember, aim to have finished presenting the case in less than 12 minutes.

Most examiners expect the candidate to finish the presentation with a list of the main problems the candidate thinks should be discussed in order of importance. This list of priorities is one of the domains used by the examiners when marking a candidate. The examiners will expect you to have asked the patient what he or she thinks is the most important problem with his or her health at the moment (they will certainly have done so) and to put that close to or at the top of the list of problems.

It is likely that the examiners will want to discuss the patient's active problems. They will almost always want to talk about the problem the patient sees as most important. These should be the areas of management that you are best prepared for. It is very unsatisfactory for examiners to feel that they have not been told all the major problems, and what the management plan for each problem is, by the end of the discussion. At the end of your presentation, and before discussion of management, the lead examiner may ask some questions to clarify aspects of the history or examination findings. This should be no cause for alarm. After this, you are usually given the opportunity to outline a plan of management, or the examiners may ask specific questions. Examining styles differ, but you should strive to direct the discussion tactfully. Being allowed to do this is usually a good sign, but not being allowed to control the discussion is not necessarily a bad sign. Some candidates appear to think that if they speak quickly and loudly enough they may prevent the examiners from asking any questions. This strategy does not work. The exam is meant to be a discussion and if the examiners cannot ask questions the candidate cannot score marks.

When appropriate, ask for one or two important investigations relevant to the problems, rather than rattling off a rote list of routine tests. Examiners find a long list irritating and consider it a sign of an immature approach. *A reason should be given for ordering every test.* For a diagnostic problem it may be useful to ask for the results of previous investigations. Any mentioned test may have to be discussed in detail with the examiners. Sometimes the examiners will not give you the results of a test (they may not have it available), but merely ask how it would help you. We suggest that you write down the results you are told (it is embarrassing to have to ask for the figures to be repeated). Don't ignore any information that is given; for example, if the haemoglobin value is normal, comment on this and explain how it helps. Many examiners will have underlined or marked the relevant results from a printed pathology or biochemistry report. This is to avoid wasting time as a candidate wades through a series of irrelevant results. Concentrate on the marked results. Remember not to touch X-ray films or criticise the quality of the material shown. Pathological specimens are not shown in the clinical examinations.

Always prepare answers to obvious lines of questioning and try to think like a consultant physician who is in charge of the patient's care (and hypothesise that the patient is a close relative of the examiner). If there is a diagnostic dilemma, consider the tests you want and how positive and negative results will support or refute your proposed diagnoses. In a management case, prepare an outline of the suggested treatment and be able to justify it. A good approach to management if the patient is an inpatient is to ask yourself, 'What steps will be required to get this patient home?' Always set management goals for all key therapeutic interventions. The examiners may ask about theoretical aspects of the condition. Most often, they will concentrate on the testing of factual knowledge in areas that are necessary for the formulation of adequate management decisions or interpretation of test results. You should think about these areas beforehand. Always consider whether the patient's current treatment is justified and whether the diagnosis previously made is consistent with the history and examination; it may not be. Do not be afraid to contradict the current management in a restrained way, if there is clear justification. Sometimes the patient's current management seems entirely appropriate; it is quite reasonable to tell the examiners that is the case.

A common series of questions for many long cases involving chronic diseases includes aspects of how you would discuss the illness and the prognosis with the patient. The examiners might ask: 'What would you tell Mrs Smith about her prognosis and likely future treatment?' and 'What would you advise her about the safety of future pregnancies?'

The examiners will not usually ask hypothetical questions unrelated to the patient being discussed. If you are answering well, the line of questioning may change or the depth may become overwhelming. Do *not* be frightened to say, in the latter situation, 'I don't know', when asked a very difficult question. Obvious wild guesses will be detrimental. If the examiner persists in asking a question, it usually means he or she is trying to establish a basic fact. Talk sensibly around the topic – often a supplementary question will result in recall of the appropriate information. With an especially difficult issue it is reasonable to say you would consult the literature or an appropriate sub-specialist for advice. Remember that examiners are instructed to avoid making snap judgements or failing candidates because of one small mistake. The best examiners will not labour a point. If it is clear you do not know the answer they will move on to another series of questions. This does not mean you have failed, but rather gives you the opportunity to gain marks elsewhere.

You must be able to discuss sensibly anything that you mention in a viva, so don't casually allude to rare diseases that you know nothing about (e.g. kala-azar as a cause of massive splenomegaly).

When the case includes a diagnostic problem the discussion should revolve around the differential diagnosis. A good approach is to talk about the possible diagnoses, with what seems the most likely first, and to give reasons from the history, examination and test results that are in favour of or against each possibility.

The long-case rationale

The long case is a test of the candidate's ability at history-taking, physical examination, interpretation of findings and construction of a diagnosis (and differential diagnosis), and approach to management (investigation and treatment). Important and common long cases are presented in some detail in the next chapters. The list in Table 4.2 is not exhaustive, but gives an idea of the range of possible cases. Many patients do not have a single long-case problem. For example it would be unusual to see a patient with only ischaemic heart disease, but a patient with previous infarction, heart failure and ventricular arrhythmias who has diabetes would be a good long case. Most (but not all) are discussed

Table 4.2 Common long cases
CARDIOVASCULAR LONG CASES (CH 5)
1. Ischaemic heart disease
2. Revascularisation
3. Infective endocarditis
4. Congestive cardiac failure
5. Hyperlipidaemia
6. Hypertension
7. Heart transplantation
8. Cardiac arrhythmias and atrial fibrillation (AF)
9. Valvular heart disease
10. Pacemaker or implantable cardioverter-defibrillators (ICD)
RESPIRATORY LONG CASES (CH 6)
1. Bronchiectasis
2. Lung carcinoma
3. Chronic obstructive pulmonary disease (chronic airflow limitation)
4. Sleep apnoea
5. Interstitial lung disease including idiopathic pulmonary fibrosis
6. Pulmonary hypertension
7. Sarcoidosis
8. Cystic fibrosis
9. Tuberculosis
10. Lung transplantation
GASTROINTESTINAL LONG CASES (CH 7)
1. Irritable bowel syndrome
2. Peptic ulceration
3. Malabsorption and chronic diarrhoea
4. Inflammatory bowel disease
5. Colon cancer
6. Chronic liver disease
7. Hepatitis B
8. Hepatitis C
9. Liver transplantation
HAEMATOLOGICAL LONG CASES (CH 8)
1. Haemolytic anaemia
2. Thrombophilia
3. Myeloproliferative disorders, e.g. polycythaemia (rubra) vera, idiopathic myelofibrosis and essential thrombocythaemia
4. Chronic myeloid leukaemia
5. Lymphomas
6. Multiple myeloma
7. Bone marrow transplantation
8. Breast cancer (see also Ch 13)

Table 4.2 **Continued**

RHEUMATOLOGICAL LONG CASES (CH 9)

1. Rheumatoid arthritis
2. Systemic sclerosis (scleroderma)
3. Systemic lupus erythematosus
4. Ankylosing spondylitis
5. Systemic vasculitis
6. Antiphospholipid antibody syndrome

ENDOCRINE LONG CASES (CH 10)

1. Osteoporosis (and osteomalacia)
2. Hypercalcaemia
3. Paget's disease of the bone (osteitis deformans)
4. Acromegaly
5. Diabetes mellitus
6. Thyrotoxicosis
7. Hypothyroidism
8. Panhypopituitarism
9. Cushing's syndrome
10. Addison's disease
11. Phaeochromocytoma

RENAL LONG CASES (CH 11)

1. Chronic kidney disease (chronic renal failure)
2. Renal transplantation
3. Nephrotic syndrome

NEUROLOGICAL LONG CASES (CH 12)

1. Multiple sclerosis
2. Myasthenia gravis
3. Guillain–Barré syndrome
4. Syncope, seizures and 'funny turns'
5. TIA and stroke

INFECTIOUS DISEASE LONG CASES (CH 13)

1. Pyrexia of unknown origin (PUO)
2. Human immunodeficiency virus (HIV) infection / acquired immunodeficiency syndrome (AIDS)

OTHER IMPORTANT LONG CASES (CH 13)

1. Falls and risk of falls
2. The obese patient
3. The preoperative assessment
4. Carcinoma of the breast

EXAMPLES OF COMMON COMBINATION CASES

1. Diabetes mellitus / ischaemic heart disease
2. Diabetes mellitus / arthritis
3. Diabetes mellitus / chronic kidney disease
4. HIV infection or rheumatoid arthitis / ischaemic heart disease
5. Connective tissue disease / osteoporosis (malacia) / diabetes mellitus
6. Hypertension / obesity / sleep apnoea / atrial fibrillation
7. Transplant / diabetes mellitus

in Chapters 5–13. Some other relevant aspects are dealt with in Chapter 16. These cases are presented as single problems, but most patients will have a combination of problems. Some problems tend to occur together.

It would be unusual not to see at least one patient with type 2 diabetes on the examination day. These patients are often obese and have diabetic complications and problems related to their obesity, such as vascular disease or arthritis. A common question to be asked about such patients would be fitness for surgery such as for a joint replacement. Another likely case is a transplant patient. Transplant patients have many similar problems as well as the specific problems related to their particular organ failure and original illness. For example, a kidney and pancreas transplant patient may have complications of previous diabetes mellitus. Scleroderma may be a rare disease but it is common in the examination. It is worthwhile making an effort to find and assess the patients with the types of chronic diseases that repeatedly crop up, and have a systematic approach worked out for their management.

Candidates are often very well prepared for common types of long cases and are able to produce a formulaic response to a trigger word such as *diabetes* or *transplant*. The examiners are then given a rote list instead of management directed at the particular patient. It is important always to relate these management lists to the actual patient and adapt them as required. Such an approach reflects the maturity expected at this level.

Another common problem faced by the examiners is the excessively detailed social history that takes up much of the presentation. Relevant social problems should be noted and, if asked, you should be able to provide more detail and discuss the problems sensibly; however, attempting to replace the more difficult medical aspects of the patient's care with this detail will not lead to a successful long case – the examiners are on to it.

HINT

Remember the point of the long case. The examiners want to know if you can:
- take a comprehensive and accurate history in an orderly fashion
- perform a thorough and efficient physical examination without missing important signs
- work out what this particular patient's problems are in a sensible order of importance, taking into account the patient's own priorities and the effect of these problems on the patient and his or her family
- order properly thought-out investigations and interpret the results
- work out a differential diagnosis that takes into account all this information
- create a plan for the management of this patient's problems that seems sensible and makes the examiners confident you are ready to go on to advanced training and can look after new patients in hospital, clinics or rooms.

Long-case marking

The examiners are advised to look at various aspects of the case presentation called *domains*. The detailed scoring is summarised in Chapter 3. The key points include:
1. History
   - Complete and accurate.
   - Few details need to be clarified by the examiners.
   - A well-structured and timely presentation.
   - Sensible interpretation of what the patient has said.

2. Examination
   - All the important physical signs are found and important negatives noted.
3. Synthesis
   - All important problems are identified.
   - Problems are listed in a sensible order of priority.
4. Effect of the disease
   - The candidate understands how the patient functions physically and psychologically in response to the disease.
   - The candidate understands the effect that the treatment and prognosis has on the patient and their family.
5. Management
   - The candidate suggests an appropriate management plan for the major problems.
   - There is a sensible approach to investigations.
   - Investigations are thoughtfully interpreted.
   - Important side-effects of the proposed treatment are recognised.

The various domains are not necessarily of equal weight and will vary in importance from one case to another.

Types of long case

The cases in Chapters 5–13 are written as a guide to dealing with the long-case examination and are not meant to replace textbook descriptions. To pass, you must really know and understand your general medicine, be able to take an outstanding history, examine accurately and maturely synthesise all the data. Remember that usually several problems occur in the one case. A patient with an unusual diagnosis will often have one or more common problems as well.

The examiners will often ask whether you would like the results of appropriate investigations. Be prepared to interpret any results you have asked for. Electrocardiograms (ECGs), chest X-rays, and computed tomography (CT) and magnetic resonance imaging (MRI) scans may be shown to candidates. Echocardiograms are not usually shown to candidates, but you are expected to be able to interpret echocardiography reports. Some common examples are included in Chapters 5–13 and also in Chapter 16. At the end of each report is a comment that gives an idea of the sort of interpretation expected from candidates.

The key to passing any exam is obviously providing the examiners with what they want. Candidates have plenty of opportunity to find out what examiners want. Practise cases with examiners and senior registrars. The stories (sometimes exaggerated) of previous candidates and information from the College are all readily available these days.

If you can think like an examiner then you can give them exactly what they want (see Ch 14). In essence, what they want is that you should think like a physician. The College exam is successful at producing people who do think like physicians. Physicians from all internal medicine specialties have had a common training experience and this makes communication between them easier.

There is a list of basic skills and qualities that an examiner wants you to establish from your long-case presentation.
- Are you safe?
- Do you know what you are doing and what your limitations are?
- If you go on to become a cardiac electrophysiologist, starting next week, do you know enough about, say, thyrotoxicosis to cope with it, with help if necessary?

- Have you developed a competent approach to the patient who has problems involving many sub-specialties?
- Have you an approach to the patient that is sympathetic and practical? This means knowing at least enough about a patient's non-medical circumstances to understand what might affect his or her ability to have treatment and how different treatments might affect the patient – for example, financially because of a particular occupation.
- Have you recognised the problem that the patient thinks is most important?

These simple principles are worth keeping in mind as you interview and examine your long-case patient. They should help you work out what the examiners will consider important and what sorts of questions they are likely to ask.

Chapter 5

The cardiovascular long case

A rule of thumb in the matter of medical advice is to take everything any doctor says with a grain of aspirin.

Goodman Ace (1899–1982)

Ischaemic heart disease

Patients with recent acute coronary syndromes (ASCs) including myocardial infarction are always available for long cases if required. Many with more exotic medical problems will also have ischaemic heart disease. The whims of the long-case examiners may lead to concentrated questioning about the ischaemic heart disease of a patient in hospital for the management of, say, renal transplant rejection. These patients are more likely to present management rather than diagnostic problems once they reach the status of long-case patients.

The classification of patients with episodes of acute coronary ischaemia is based on electrocardiogram (ECG) changes and on the detection of markers of myocardial damage (troponins), which have prognostic as well as diagnostic usefulness for patients with chest pain. Those who present with chest pain and ECG changes of ST elevation have an ST elevation myocardial infarction (STEMI). Those without ST elevation are said to have a non-ST elevation acute coronary syndrome (NSTEACS), but once abnormal cardiac markers have been detected the diagnosis can be revised to a non-ST elevation myocardial infarction (non-STEMI). The diagnosis *unstable angina* is no longer part of this classification, but is still often used to describe patients with increasing exertional angina.

Patients with ST elevation benefit from urgent action to re-open the blocked coronary artery (angioplasty or thrombolytic treatment). Those with non-STEMI are usually treated medically in the first instance. The presence of abnormal cardiac markers indicates an adverse prognosis (increased risk of further infarction or death) and these patients benefit from early but not immediate intervention (angioplasty or coronary surgery) and from immediate aggressive antiplatelet treatment and anticoagulation with fractionated or unfractionated heparin. Non-STEMI patients who have ST depression on the ECG have a worse prognosis than do those with T wave inversion or flattening. The concept of risk stratification is based on these factors and determines the urgency and type of treatment.

The history

1. Find out whether the patient has been or is in hospital because of a recent myocardial infarction or an acute coronary syndrome, or for some other cardiac or non-cardiac reason.
2. The patients with the worst prognosis are those with chest pain and ECG changes at rest (Table 5.1). Clearly, these may represent different pathophysiological states, varying from occlusion of a coronary artery and inadequate collateral flow to rupture of a lipid-rich plaque with thrombus formation. Ask about obvious precipitating factors, such as a gastrointestinal bleed or the onset of an arrhythmia. Also ask about the character of the chest pain and what precipitated the admission.

    Remember that the diagnosis of angina can be suspected from the history, but needs to be established by investigations – an abnormal ECG or exercise test at least. You should be suspicious of the diagnosis unless it has been confirmed by investigations. The most common differential diagnosis is gastro-oesophageal reflux disease (GORD). This can be difficult to prove without endoscopy (and, if normal, oesophageal pH testing), but an excellent response to a trial of a proton pump inhibitor (PPI) is very suggestive. Oesophageal spasm is another cause of central chest pain and may respond to nitrates.
3. Detail the patient's current treatment and management history. Oral medications will probably include:
    - aspirin with or without an ADP inhibitor (clopidogrel, prasugrel, ticagrelor)
    - a beta-blocker or occasionally a calcium antagonist
    - nitrates (intravenous, oral or topical)
    - statin
    - an angiotensin-converting enzyme (ACE) inhibitor (ACEI) or angiotensin II receptor (AR) blocker (ARB).
    a. Acute coronary syndromes are managed with heparin and aspirin, and clopidogrel or ticagrelor. Remember that prasugrel should not be used in patients older than 75 or in patients who have had a haemorrhagic stroke.
    b. Thrombolytic treatment is not effective for NSTEACS. This is possibly because acute coronary syndromes are not a single pathological entity and also because a state of increased thrombogenesis may follow initial thrombolysis with these drugs.
    c. Most patients have early angiography (within 48 hours) with the intention of angioplasty to the culprit lesion if this is practical. Ask whether the patient knows details of what investigations or treatment were performed.

Table 5.1 Risk stratification in patients with ischaemic chest pain at rest

HIGHEST TO LOWEST RISK

1. ST elevation myocardial infarction
2. ST depression
3. T wave inversion
4. Non-specific ST–T wave changes
5. Normal ECG

- The risk is higher in each group if cardiac biomarkers (troponins) are elevated.
- The risk is higher in each group for patients with previous ischaemic heart disease or diabetes.
- The higher the risk, the more the benefit of aggressive treatment.

d. If the patient has had an infarct during this or previous admissions, find out about the management, which may have included primary angioplasty or thrombolysis, and treatment of complications such as arrhythmias, cardiac failure, further angina and embolic events.

e. In many hospitals a comprehensive cardiac rehabilitation program will have been offered to the patient. Ask whether this has been helpful and ask about the hospital staff's explanations to the patient about his or her condition and prognosis. Also ask questions about the effect of this illness on the patient's life and work.

4. Next, ask standard questions about risk factors in addition to age and male sex. Remember that risk factors are of vital importance to long-term prognosis, but add little to the likelihood that undiagnosed chest pain is ischaemic. Risk factors include:
- previous ischaemic heart disease or previous abnormal CT coronary angiogram or calcium score (which may over-diagnose atheroma)
- hyperlipidaemia
- diabetes mellitus (the increased risk in these patients is as high as that in non-diabetics who have already had an ischaemic event)
- hypertension
- family history (in particular, first-degree relatives with ischaemic heart disease before the age of 60; 92-year-old great-uncles with heart trouble do not count)
- smoking (how many; if stopped, how long ago – risk of infarction is no longer increased after 1 year and that of angina after 10 years)
- use of oral contraceptives or premature onset of menopause
- obesity and physical inactivity
- chronic inflammatory diseases, e.g. rheumatoid arthritis, other arthritis, HIV infection
- high serum homocysteine levels, which may have been measured if the patient has premature coronary disease and few other risk factors – levels in the top population quintile increase coronary risk twofold; trials of treatment (mostly with folate), however, have been negative and routine treatment is not recommended
- long-term use, in high doses, of cyclo-oxygenase 2 (COX-2) inhibitors or other non-steroidal anti-inflammatory drugs (NSAIDs) (which should be stopped)
- erectile dysfunction (which often precedes symptomatic ischaemic heart disease and is a marker of endothelial dysfunction). Remember that the presence of multiple risk factors is more than additive.

5. Then find out whether risk factor control has been successful. Remember the important results of recent secondary prevention trials.
a. Aggressive cholesterol lowering to below a level of 4 mmol/L of total cholesterol (low-density lipoprotein (LDL) < 1.8) is now considered appropriate for patients with established coronary disease.
b. There is some evidence that statins have beneficial effects beyond their effect on lowering cholesterol levels (via anti-inflammatory effects).

6. Find out what investigations the patient can remember.
a. An echocardiogram may have been performed to assess ventricular function and possible complications of infarction, such as a pericardial collection, a left ventricular thrombus, mitral regurgitation or a ventricular septal defect (VSD).
b. An exercise test, a sestamibi or a stress echocardiogram may have been performed to assess ischaemia or myocardial viability (MRI scan).
c. Cardiac catheterisation is perhaps the most memorable of the investigations for ischaemic heart disease and if negative suggests a cause other than coronary artery disease (e.g. pericarditis).

The patient may know how many coronaries are abnormal and whether angioplasty was performed. Ask whether a drug-eluting stent (DES) was used and for how long dual antiplatelet treatment was recommended. Bare metal stent use is now uncommon; the superiority of modern DESs is well established.

7. Complications such as acute mitral regurgitation or an infarct-related VSD are usually treated surgically but have a relatively poor prognosis. All complications are uncommon if early coronary patency and normal flow have been achieved.

The examination

Examine the cardiovascular system (see Ch 16).

1. Record the blood pressure.
2. Look for signs of valvular heart disease, cardiac failure, rhythm disturbances (e.g. atrial fibrillation (AF), frequent ectopic beats) and murmurs suggesting mitral regurgitation or a VSD caused by an infarct.
3. There may be spectacular bruises at venepuncture or femoral or radial puncture sites if the patient has had thrombolytic treatment. Abdominal wall bruising suggests subcutaneous low-molecular-weight heparin therapy. Occasionally the radial pulse may be absent after radial angioplasty. More general complications include a stroke due to embolism from the heart.

Management

Discuss the management of the presenting problem. If the patient has only recently been admitted with an infarct, this means a discussion of thrombolysis and primary angioplasty.

1. Candidates should have some knowledge of the major thrombolysis and angioplasty trials.
   a. These have shown that early treatment has improved mortality. Treatment up to 12 hours after the onset of an infarct is worthwhile.
   b. Alteplase and reteplase have been shown to produce a small survival advantage compared with streptokinase, probably because they are more effective in opening occluded vessels, but have a slightly increased risk of causing cerebral haemorrhage.
   c. Alteplase is given as a bolus followed by an infusion, and reteplase is given as a double bolus injection with a 30-minute interval. Tenecteplase is given as a single injection. In many states ambulance officers can give thrombolysis according to a rigorous protocol and usually after transmitting the patient's ECG to a central location for confirmation of ST elevation. Even when thrombolysis seems successful (resolution of symptoms and ST depression) patients are now routinely transferred so that angiography can be performed as soon as practical.
2. Urgent coronary (primary) angioplasty, if available, is of proven benefit and has been shown to reduce mortality compared with treatment with thrombolytic drugs.
   a. The advantages, theoretical and real, include definite re-opening of the infarct-related artery in more than 90% of patients (compared with < 60% of patients given thrombolytics), normal flow in the infarct-related artery in most cases, dilatation and stenting of the offending (culprit) lesion and often removal of clot, very low risk of stroke and shortening of hospital stay, often to just 3 days.
   b. Patients are treated with potent antiplatelet drugs: aspirin, clopidogrel (or ticagrelor) and sometimes with one of the platelet aggregation inhibitors, abciximab or tirofiban. Ticagrelor is more rapidly effective than clopidogrel and in most protocols is now preferred for primary angioplasty patients. It improves prognosis compared with

the other drugs. Its most common side-effect is dyspnoea, which may develop after 5–10 days.

   c. There is now trial evidence that transport of patients to a hospital where this procedure can be performed is preferable to treatment with thrombolytic drugs, if transport time is less than 2–3 hours.

   d. Rapid transport to the catheter laboratory is important and the 'door to balloon' time should be less than 90 minutes when angioplasty is available in the hospital to which the patient presented.

   e. Recent trials have not shown a benefit for routine thrombus aspiration for primary angioplasty procedures.

3. If the history has suggested complications resulting from the infarct, these will have to be discussed. Common complications include:

- ventricular arrhythmias
- bradyarrhythmias (especially following an inferior infarct)
- cardiac failure
- further ischaemia or re-infarction.

It is important to have planned an approach to the management of these problems.

Investigations

These are aimed at assessment of the infarct size, complications and presence of further ischaemia:

1. **left ventricular function** – echocardiogram (ejection fraction, wall motion abnormality), left ventriculogram
2. **complications** – echocardiogram for valvular regurgitation, left ventricular thrombus, infarct-related VSD
3. **further ischaemia** – exercise test, sestamibi stress test, cardiac catheterisation
4. **viability** – MRI scan, sestamibi scan.

Long-term treatment

1. Early revascularisation is of proven benefit for high-risk patients with acute coronary syndromes (ST elevation, troponin elevation).
2. Prognosis is improved with aspirin, beta-blockers and, for large infarcts (ejection fraction < 40%), ACE inhibitors and beta-blockers (e.g. carvedilol, bisoprolol, nebivolol and extended-release metoprolol).
3. Be prepared to discuss balloon versus stent versus surgery versus do nothing invasive. Patients with three-vessel disease and significant left ventricular damage or with left main coronary artery stenosis benefit prognostically from coronary artery bypass surgery even if their symptoms have settled on medical treatment. Those with tight proximal (before the first diagonal branch) left anterior descending lesions probably also benefit from surgery or angioplasty. Consider suggesting discussion at a heart multidisciplinary team meeting if the lesions are complex.
4. Eplerenone, an aldosterone antagonist, is indicated for patients with cardiac failure following an infarct.

Secondary prevention

1. Control of cardiac risk factors is even more important once the presence of coronary artery disease has been established. It should be a routine part of the management.
2. Dietary advice for weight and lipid reduction may be indicated. Lipid-lowering drug treatment with a statin should be introduced for all patients who can tolerate it.

3. Patients should be encouraged to take part in a cardiac rehabilitation program, if this is available, where advice about safe exercise, weight reduction and changes to dietary and smoking habits can be encouraged.

Revascularisation

For some long-case patients with ischaemic heart disease the emphasis will be on revascularisation (coronary surgery or angioplasty). These procedures are so common that many patients with other presenting problems will have had them.

The history
Similar information to that outlined in the ischaemic heart disease long case is required.
1. Careful questioning about risk factor control, both before and after surgery or angioplasty, is very important. The patient should know whether he or she has ever had an infarct and may know whether there was significant left ventricular damage.
2. Find out what procedure (or procedures) the patient has had and whether there has been complete relief of symptoms.
3. If coronary artery surgery was performed, ask how many grafts were inserted and whether internal mammary or other arterial (e.g. radial artery) conduits were used. It may be possible to work out from the history whether surgery was performed to improve symptoms or prognosis (e.g. three-vessel or left main disease), or both.
4. The patient may know how many vessels were dilated if angioplasty was performed and whether stents were inserted. The patient should know whether bare metal stents (BMSs) or drug-eluting stents were used. Ask whether the angioplasty was performed in the setting of a myocardial infarction or acute coronary syndrome. Find out for how long dual antiplatelet treatment was prescribed.

The examination
Examine the patient as for the ischaemic heart disease long case.
1. Note the presence of a median sternotomy scar. Patients who have had a left internal mammary artery (LIMA) graft often have a numb patch to the left of the sternum. This may be permanent.
2. Look at the sternal wound for signs of infection; osteomyelitis of the sternum is a rare but disastrous complication of surgery. Look and feel for sternal instability. Sternal wires are often palpable.
3. Examine the arms for the very large scar that results from radial artery harvesting.
4. Examine the legs for saphenous-vein-harvesting wounds. Infection and breakdown of these wounds are more common than for the sternal wound.

Management

SURGERY

Use of the left internal mammary artery (LIMA) to graft the left anterior descending (LAD) coronary artery has been routine for more than 20 years. Other arterial conduits are used less often, but 'all arterial revascularisation' is performed routinely in some centres or where saphenous vein grafts (SVGs) are not possible (e.g. previous coronary artery bypass graft (CABG) or varicose veins in both legs and thighs). In these cases the right internal mammary artery (RIMA) may be used, usually to graft the right coronary, or the radial artery is used as a free arterial graft. The RIMA may also be used as a free graft attached to the aorta, if that is necessary to make it reach. There is excellent evidence that LIMA grafts have a higher long-term patency rate (> 90% at 10 years) than SVGs (50% at 10 years). There is less information about other arterial conduits.

In general, CABG is better than angioplasty for patients with three-vessel disease and diabetes (improved mortality, fewer re-interventions, fewer infarcts).

In response to the increasing numbers of angioplasty procedures, surgeons have begun to perform fewer invasive bypass procedures. The most widely used alternative is the 'off-pump' LIMA graft to the LAD coronary artery. A median sternotomy incision is still used, but the LIMA is attached to the LAD coronary artery on the beating heart. A 'Y' graft from the LIMA to the circumflex and right coronaries can be performed using the RIMA attached to the LIMA. These operations avoid the need for cardiopulmonary bypass, speed recovery and possibly reduce the risk of intraoperative cerebral events. Minimally invasive bypasses are carried out in some centres. A series of lateral chest incisions are used as ports for surgery using thoracoscopic equipment. The technique is not easy and the chest wound, although small, is not necessarily less painful than a median sternotomy.

Angina may recur at any time after CABG. Very early angina suggests a technical problem, such as mammary artery spasm, thrombosis of an SVG, grafting of the wrong vessel, or grafting of the correct vessel but proximal to the area of stenosis. Sometimes revascularisation may be 'incomplete' because one or more vessels were unsuitable for grafting – usually because of distal disease in the target vessel.

Recurrence of angina is more common if risk factors have not been aggressively controlled. Low-dose aspirin has also been shown to prolong graft survival and patients with severe diffuse disease are often given dual antiplatelet treatment by their surgeons. When angina recurs, the patient usually describes symptoms similar in character to the old ones. Recurrent chest pain that is different from the old angina is less likely to be ischaemic.

ANGIOPLASTY

Angioplasty is now performed more often than surgery in many centres. It has not been shown to improve the prognosis for patients with stable angina receiving optimal medical treatment (Table 5.2).

Many angioplasties are performed to provide symptom relief for patients with one- or two-vessel disease. Patients with acute coronary syndromes, and especially those with raised troponin levels, are treated with early angioplasty. There is now good evidence that this group of patients has an improved prognosis (fewer deaths and fewer large infarcts) and a shortened hospital stay when treated aggressively in this way.

Dual antiplatelet treatment (DAPT) has made subacute stent thrombosis a rare event (< 1%). DAPT is ideally given for 48 hours before angioplasty and for at least 4 weeks afterwards; 6 months to a year is often recommended for patients who have had an acute coronary syndrome or a drug-eluting stent.

Table 5.2 Optimal medical treatment for stable angina
1. Aspirin +/− clopidogrel (for 1 year post ACS)
2. Statin – target LDL 1.8 mmol/L
3. ACEI or ARB at maximum tolerated dose
4. Beta-blocker – heart rate down to < 70
5. Hypertension treated to < 130/80
6. Exercise 3 times a week at least for > 150 minutes/week
ACS = acute coronary syndrome; ACEI = angiotensin-converting enzyme inhibitor; ARB = angiotensin II receptor blocker.

For patients treated for an infarct or acute coronary syndrome, a loading dose of 180 mg of ticagrelor or 300–600 mg of clopidogrel or 60 mg of prasugrel is given. Patients should continue with aspirin forever.

- Optimal medical treatment is as good as angioplasty in terms of prognosis when there is one- or two-vessel disease (excluding left main and proximal LAD).
- However, angina is better controlled by an angioplasty.
- If angioplasty is performed only when ischaemia has been demonstrated by measurement of the fractional flow reserve by a flow wire in the catheter laboratory, angioplasty improves outcome compared with optimal medical treatment.

FREQUENT TRIAL

Drug-eluting stents have dramatically reduced the incidence of restenosis. The currently available stents have either everolimus or sirolimus bound via a polymer to the metal surface of the stent. These antineoplastic drugs are eluted for about a month and prevent the migration of smooth muscle cells into the lumen of the vessel that is the cause of restenosis. Very low restenosis rates of a few per cent have been obtained in trials, even when diabetics are included. These stents also seem to be effective in preventing further restenosis when used in a restenosed bare metal stent. Drug-eluting stents (DESs) are more expensive but more effective than bare metal stents and are now routinely recommended for almost all patients. The current generation of DES has a lower thrombotic risk than BMS and DAPT can usually be suspended if necessary at 3 months. Their use for patients taking warfarin or a novel (non-vitamin-K antagonist) oral anticoagulant (NOAC) is complicated, but most protocols take into account bleeding risk and thrombotic risk. Generally, 1 month of triple therapy with aspirin, clopidogrel and the NOAC or of warfarin is followed by 11 months of clopidogrel and lower dose NOAC or warfarin. For patients at high bleeding risk, aspirin may be omitted. The more potent ADP agent, ticagrelor, should be avoided.

Patients presenting with a STEMI or non-STEMI who are being treated with warfarin or a NOAC present a difficult problem. Current recommendations are to continue warfarin, use a radial approach for the angioplasty if possible and then use DAPT and oral anticoagulation (increased bleeding risk) or clopidogrel and warfarin, or NOAC only.

Stents do not set off metal detectors and patients can safely have an MRI scan within a month.

It is reasonably safe to suspend a second antiplatelet drug (as long as aspirin is continued) at about 3 months for a patient to have urgent surgery when a modern DES has been used. Heparin is not a substitute for antiplatelet treatment for these patients.

Possible lines of questioning

1. How would you manage *this* patient's anticoagulation during a future presentation with an acute coronary syndrome?
2. How would you manage this patient's anticoagulation for atrial fibrillation following his recent angioplasty?

HINT

The examiners will not expect you to know how to perform an angioplasty, but they will want you to know how to manage risk factors and antiplatelet treatment.

Infective endocarditis

Patients with infective endocarditis (IE) stay in hospital for weeks, so are often available for long cases. The disease presents diagnostic, plus short-term and long-term management problems. Cases combine cardiological, microbiological and immunological problems. The diagnosis is usually known to the patient. An intravenous infusion containing antibiotics is a valuable clue.

Three-quarters of cases are caused by streptococci or staphylococci.

The history
Ask about:
1. details of presenting symptoms (e.g. malaise, fever, symptoms of anaemia)
2. symptoms suggesting embolic phenomena in large vessels (e.g. brain, viscera) or small vessels (e.g. kidney, with haematuria or loin pain)
3. recent dental, endoscopic or operative procedures – a precipitating event is identified in only about 5% of cases (the time between procedure and diagnosis may be up to 3 months); remember that *Streptococcus gallolyticus* (*S. bovis*) or *Clostridium septicus* endocarditis is associated with colonic cancer and these patients all deserve a colonoscopy
4. use of antibiotics for prophylaxis, either before an invasive procedure or for rheumatic fever, or both
5. a past history of rheumatic fever
6. a history of other heart disease or heart operations, especially valve replacement
7. a history of intravenous drug abuse, particularly for its association with tricuspid and pulmonary valve infection
8. antibiotic allergies
9. how the diagnosis was made – including the number of blood cultures and the use of transthoracic or transoesophageal echocardiography (TOE)
10. management since admission to hospital, including the names of the antibiotics used, the duration of treatment and whether the possibility of valve replacement has been discussed
11. a history of other major diseases, particularly those associated with immune suppression, such as renal transplantation or steroid use.

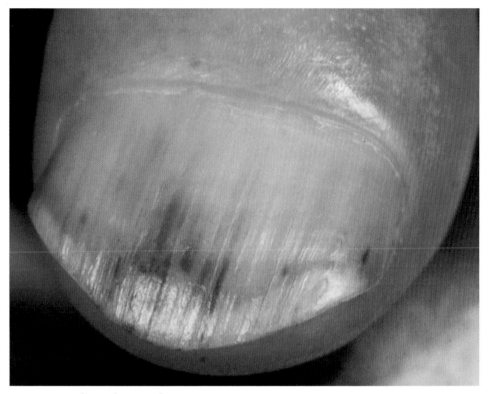

Figure 5.1 **Splinter haemorrhages.**

M H Swartz. The skin. *Textbook of physical diagnosis: history and examination.* Fig 8. Saunders, Elsevier, 2009, with permission.

The examination

1. Start by examining for the peripheral stigmata of endocarditis.
   a. **Hands:**
      - clubbing
      - splinter haemorrhages (Fig. 5.1)
      - Osler's nodes on the finger pulp (these are always painful and palpable, are probably an embolic phenomenon and are rare)
      - Janeway lesions (*non-tender* erythematous maculopapular lesions containing bacteria on the palms or pulps, which are rare).
   b. **Eyes:** Roth's spots in the fundus (Fig. 5.2), conjunctival petechiae
   c. **Abdomen:** splenomegaly (a late sign)
   d. **Urine analysis** for haematuria and proteinuria
   e. **Neurological signs** of embolic disease
   f. **Joints** (occasionally resembles rheumatic fever pattern).
2. Next examine the **heart**. Assess for predisposing cardiac lesions. These are, in order:
   a. acquired:
      - prosthetic valve (mechanical)
      - mitral regurgitation, mitral stenosis
      - aortic stenosis
      - aortic regurgitation

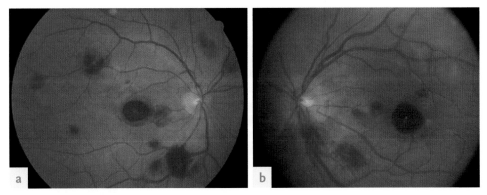

Figure 5.2 (a) Right fundus and (b) left fundus, showing multiple flame-shaped and blot haemorrhages in both eyes. Several haemorrhages are white centred, consistent with Roth spots. A retinal haemorrhage is centred on the fovea of each eye, accounting for the decreased visual acuity.

S Nazir. *Journal of AAPOS* 2008; 12(4):415–17. American Association for Pediatric Ophthalmology and Strabismus, with permission.

- prosthetic valve (tissue)
- repaired mitral valve
- mitral valve prolapse with mitral regurgitation
b. congenital:
  - bicuspid aortic valve
  - patent ductus arteriosus
  - ventricular septal defect
  - coarctation of the aorta.
Remember:
  - an atrial septal defect of the secundum type is almost never affected
  - 20% of endocarditis patients have no recognised underlying cardiac abnormality
  - coronary stents and pacemaker leads do not appear to involve any risk of endocarditis.
3. Examine for the signs of cardiac failure. Look for signs of a prosthetic valve and for scars that may be present from previous valvotomy or repair operations.
4. Look for a source of infection and take the patient's temperature.

Investigations

1. Three sets of blood cultures each from a different site over 24 hours (98% of culture-positive cases will give positive results in the first three bottles).
2. **Full blood count (FBC) and erythrocyte sedimentation rate (ESR):** look for anaemia (normochromic, normocytic), neutrophilia, an elevated ESR, which may be > 100 mm/h, and a raised C-reactive protein (CRP) level. The ESR tends to remain elevated for months, even when treatment has been successful, but the CRP level falls quite quickly and may be useful for assessing the effectiveness of treatment.
3. **Renal function:** a freshly spun urine sample will often show red cell casts but is rarely assessed these days.
4. **Chest X-ray film:** look for left ventricular (LV) or right ventricular (RV) hypertrophy, increased pulmonary artery markings, Kerley B lines, frank cardiac failure and valve calcification (lateral film). The onset of heart failure is a poor prognostic sign.

5. **ECG:** atrial fibrillation in the elderly (particularly common) and conduction defects may occur, but are not specific.
6. **Echocardiography** (Fig. 5.3) (**2-D and Doppler**): vegetations must be larger than 2 mm to be detected. This procedure cannot distinguish active from inactive lesions. Vegetations are seen in approximately 40% of cases. They tend to occur downstream of the abnormal jet (e.g. on the aortic surface of the aortic valve in cases of aortic stenosis and endocarditis). Colour Doppler examination is a very sensitive means of detecting new valvular regurgitation, which may be an important sign of endocarditis. *Transoesophageal echocardiography* allows better definition of valvular involvement and is more likely to detect vegetations. Perhaps more importantly, it is much more likely to detect such complications as valve abscesses. It is in routine use for the assessment of cases of known or suspected endocarditis.

Notes

ORGANISMS

Streptococci account for approximately half of these infections.

1. Viridans streptococci (often referred to by the pseudotaxonomic term 'Streptococcus viridans') – usually presents subacutely. Current important types for endocarditis include *S. sanguinis*, *S. gordonii* and *S. mitis*.
2. *Streptococcus faecalis* – traditionally more common in older men with prostatism and younger women with urinary tract infections, but now in intravenous drug users.
3. *Streptococcus gallolyticus (S. bovis)* – associated with colon polyps and carcinoma.
4. *Staphylococcus aureus* – particularly in intravenous drug users; usually presents acutely. Note, though, that only a small minority of *S. aureus* bacteraemias are associated with endocarditis.
5. *Staphylococcus epidermidis* – more common in patients with recent valve replacement but can be a contaminant in blood cultures.
6. Gram-negative coccobacilli – rarely a cause; more common with prosthetic valves. The responsible organisms are called the HACEK group:
   Haemophilus
   Actinobacillus
   Cardiobacterium hominis
   Eikonella spp.
   Kingella kingae
7. Fungi (e.g. *Candida*, *Aspergillus*) – particularly in intravenous drug users and immunosuppressed patients.

CAUSES OF CULTURE-NEGATIVE ENDOCARDITIS

Note: This diagnosis should be made with caution. It condemns a patient to prolonged treatment with intravenous antibiotics.

1. Previous use of antibiotics.
2. Exotic organisms (e.g. *Haemophilus parainfluenzae*, histoplasmosis, *Brucella*, *Candida*, Q fever).
3. Right-sided endocarditis (rarely).

POST-VALVE SURGERY ENDOCARDITIS

Early infection is acquired at operation; late infection occurs from another source. This condition has a worse prognosis than native valve endocarditis.

Echocardiography Report

Reason for study: AR ?; endocarditis
Study quality: Good <u>Satisfactory</u> Poor

RV	18	(mm)	(N 10–26)
Sept.	10	(mm)	(N 7–11)
LVEDD	68	(mm)	(N 36–56)
LVESD	42	(mm)	(N 20–40)
LVPW	10	(mm)	(N 7–11)
Aorta	34	(mm)	(N 20–35)
LA	36	(mm)	(N 24–40)
FS	38	%	(N 27–40)
EF	67	%	(N 55–70)

Valves

Mitral	Mild MR
Tricus.	Mild TR
Aortic	Thickened, bicuspid
Pulm.	Appears normal

Doppler – 2D

The left ventricle is dilated. The fractional shortening is in the normal range. The aortic valve is thickened and probably bicuspid. A mobile mass 2 mm in diameter is visible on the LV side of the valve and represents a probable vegetation.

Doppler – colour flow mapping

There is no aortic gradient. A large jet of aortic regurgitation is present, extending three-quarters of the way into the LV cavity. Mild-to-moderate MR is present. Mild TR. RV pressure = 28 mmHg.

Conclusions

Severe AR, probable vegetation, bicuspid valve.

Comment

The diagnosis of endocarditis cannot really be made on the basis of echocardiography alone. Even what appears to be a vegetation may be sterile. Nevertheless, a mobile mass attached to a valve in a patient with positive blood cultures makes the diagnosis of endocarditis almost certain.

An abnormal echocardiogram adds weight to the diagnosis. It also enables detection of left ventricular enlargement, which suggests haemodynamic compromise. Serial echocardiograms allow assessment of the treatment of endocarditis and help with the decision about the timing of possible surgery.

The underlying valve abnormality may be obvious. Here the aortic valve is congenitally bicuspid.

More detailed analysis of the heart is possible with transoesophageal echocardiography, which is now routine in cases of endocarditis. It enables smaller vegetations to be identified, as well as complications, such as valve ring abscesses.

Key

AR = aortic regurgitation; EF = ejection fraction; FS = fractional shortening; LA = left atrium; LVEDD = left ventricular end-diastolic dimension; LVESD = left ventricular end-systolic dimension; LVPW = left ventricular posterior wall; MR = mitral regurgitation; Pulm. = pulmonary; RV = right ventricle; Sept. = septal thickness; TR = tricuspid regurgitation; Tricus. = tricuspid.

Figure 5.3 Echocardiography report in a patient with possible infective endocarditis.

Diagnosis

The diagnosis is usually a clinical one. The modified Duke criteria are often used to assist. Two major criteria, one major and three minor, or five minor criteria secure the diagnosis.

MAJOR CRITERIA

1. Typical organisms in two separate blood cultures.
2. Evidence of endocardial involvement: echocardiogram showing a mobile intracardiac mass on a valve or in the path of a regurgitant jet, or an abscess or new valvular regurgitation.
3. Transoesophageal echocardiogram: recommended for patients with a prosthetic valve and at least possible IE by clinical criteria; recommended for other patients initially.
4. Single positive blood culture for *Coxiella burnettii* or anti-phase IgG antibody > 1 : 800.

MINOR CRITERIA

1. Predisposing cardiac condition or intravenous drug use.
2. Fever.
3. Embolic vascular phenomena or stigmata.
4. Serological or acute phase abnormalities.

Treatment

Early involvement in the management by a cardiac surgeon in a cardiac surgical unit is usually indicated, particularly for staphylococcal infection.

1. Intravenous administration of a bactericidal antibiotic. If the organism is a sensitive viridans streptococcus, give benzylpenicillin, 6–12 g daily for 4–6 weeks. If it is an enterococcus, at least 4 weeks of intravenous treatment are necessary and the choice of antibiotic depends on the organism's sensitivity (e.g. a cell wall active drug such as a beta lactam plus a synergistic aminoglycoside such as gentamicin). For prosthetic valves, 6–8 weeks of intravenous treatment are necessary.
2. Follow the progress by looking at the temperature chart, serological results and haemoglobin values.
3. The decision to go on to valve replacement is a difficult one; it is best made with the assistance of a cardiac surgeon who has been involved from the start. Indications for surgery include:
   a. resistant organisms (e.g. fungi)
   b. valvular dysfunction causing moderate-to-severe cardiac failure (e.g. acute severe aortic regurgitation)
   c. ongoing fever and persistently positive blood cultures in spite of treatment
   d. invasive paravalvular infection causing conduction disturbances, or a paravalvular abscess or fistula (detected by TOE)
   e. recurrent major embolic phenomena, although this is controversial (an isolated vegetation is not in itself an indication for surgery).

Factors suggesting a poorer prognosis

1. Shock.
2. Congestive cardiac failure.
3. Extreme age.
4. Aortic valve or multiple valve involvement.

5. Multiple organisms.
6. Culture-negative endocarditis.
7. Delay in starting treatment.
8. Prosthetic valve involvement.
9. Staphylococcal, Gram-negative and fungal infections.

Differential diagnosis
1. Atrial myxoma.
2. Occult malignant neoplasm.
3. Systemic lupus erythematosus.
4. Polyarteritis nodosa.
5. Post-streptococcal glomerulonephritis.
6. Pyrexia of unknown origin.
7. Cardiac thrombus.

Prognosis
Prior to antibiotic use this was an invariably fatal disease. Currently, more than 70% of patients with endogenous infection survive, as do 50% of those with a prosthetic valve infection. Intravenous drug users have a good prognosis.

Prophylaxis
Confusion between rheumatic fever and endocarditis prophylaxis is common. Rheumatic fever prophylaxis consists of long-term, low-dose antibiotic administration. Prophylaxis against endocarditis requires high-dose, short-term treatment only in patients with a very high risk, namely:
- a previous episode of endocarditis
- a prosthetic heart valve or prosthetic material used for valve repair
- a congenital heart malformation (unrepaired cyanotic heart disease, repaired cyanotic heart disease with residual defects or recent surgery using artificial material (within 6 months)) or
- a cardiac transplant with valve disease.

According to the latest (2007) American Heart Association guidelines, all other lesions no longer require prophylaxis.

Prophylaxis is also recommended according to the Australian (Heart Foundation) guidelines for:
- complex congenital heart disease, including patients who have had repair operations using shunts or artificial material and have persisting shunts (e.g. VSD repaired with Gortex, but with residual shunt)
- Aboriginal patients with any intermediate- or high-risk lesion.

Prophylaxis regimens are as follows (recommendations from *Therapeutic guidelines – antibiotic*):
1. **Dental procedures (e.g. periodontal procedures) or oral surgery:** amoxycillin 2 g, 1 hour before the procedure. For patients unable to take oral antibiotics, use ampicillin IV 15–30 minutes before the procedure. For those allergic to penicillin, cephalexin 2 g orally 1 hour before the procedure is adequate.
2. **Gastrointestinal or genitourinary procedures, or bronchosocopy:** no prophylaxis is recommended unless infection is already present.

Remember that the effectiveness of antibiotic prophylaxis has not been proven. Patients need to be reminded of the need for good dental hygiene and regular dental review.

Possible lines of questioning

1. What would persuade you that *this* patient now needs surgery for his or her infective endocarditis?

2. What would make you decide to treat this culture-negative patient for endocarditis?

Congestive cardiac failure

This is a common therapeutic problem, but may be a diagnostic problem; It is uncommonly the only major problem in a long case.

The history

1. It is important first to find out what may have precipitated episodes of cardiac failure. Precipitating problems include:
   a. arrhythmias (especially atrial fibrillation – these can be the cause or the result of heart failure; incessantly frequent VEBs (more than 5–10,000 in 24 hours))
   b. discontinuation of medications – usually the diuretic, e.g. on a long bus trip (particularly important)
   c. myocardial infarction
   d. anaemia
   e. infection and fever
   f. thyrotoxicosis
   g. anaesthesia and surgery
   h. pulmonary embolism
   i. high salt intake, drugs that cause salt and water retention (e.g. traditional NSAIDs, COX-2 inhibitors) or excessive physical exertion
   j. pregnancy.
   Note: Chronic lung disease can be a cause of, or a precipitating factor for, right and left ventricular failure.
2. Then ask about the symptoms of left ventricular failure, e.g.:
   a. dyspnoea
   b. orthopnoea
   c. paroxysmal nocturnal dyspnoea
   and right ventricular failure, e.g.:
   d. oedema
   e. ascites
   f. anorexia
   g. nausea.
   Ask about symptoms of ischaemic heart disease (e.g. angina). These may help distinguish dyspnoea caused by lung disease from that caused by cardiac failure.
3. Enquire about the history of previous heart disease:
   a. hypertension
   b. ischaemic heart disease – infarcts, angina
   c. rheumatic or other valve disease
   d. congenital heart disease
   e. cardiomyopathy

     f. previous cardiac surgery (e.g. coronary artery bypass grafting, valve replacement or resection of an aneurysm)

     g. cardiac transplantation.

4. Find out about coronary risk factors, in addition to previous ischaemic heart disease, age and male sex, including:

     a. hyperlipidaemia

     b. hypertension

     c. smoking

     d. diabetes mellitus

     e. family history of early coronary heart disease

     f. use of oral contraceptives or premature onset of menopause

     g. obesity

     h. physical inactivity

     i. erectile dysfunction.

5. Ascertain the risk factors for dilated cardiomyopathy:

     a. excessive alcohol intake

     b. family history of cardiomyopathy

     c. haemochromatosis.

6. Ask what medications are currently being taken.

7. Ask what investigations have been undertaken – particularly:

     a. echocardiography

     b. stress ECG testing

     c. nuclear studies

     d. cardiac catheterisation.

8. Find out how the disease affects the patient's life and ability to cope at home (e.g. climbing stairs, sexual difficulties, etc.). Remember to classify the patient according to the New York Heart Association (NYHA) guidelines.

NYHA classification

I	No limitation of physical activity. Ordinary physical activity does not cause angina / dyspnoea.
II	Angina / dyspnoea on moderate activity.
III	Angina / dyspnoea on mild activity.
IV	Angina / dyspnoea at rest.

The examination

1. Perform a detailed cardiovascular system examination.

2. Look particularly for signs of cardiac failure, the underlying causes of the problem and any precipitating factors.

3. Look for a pacemaker or defibrillator box.

4. Note wasting as a result of cardiac cachexia.

5. Take the blood pressure lying and standing. Treatment with ACE inhibitors and beta-blockers often results in mild hypotension.

Investigations

1. **Chest X-ray film** (Fig. 5.4): look for cardiomegaly and chamber size (e.g. left atrium), cardiac aneurysm, valve calcification, sternal wires suggesting previous cardiac surgery, signs of lung disease and pulmonary congestion.

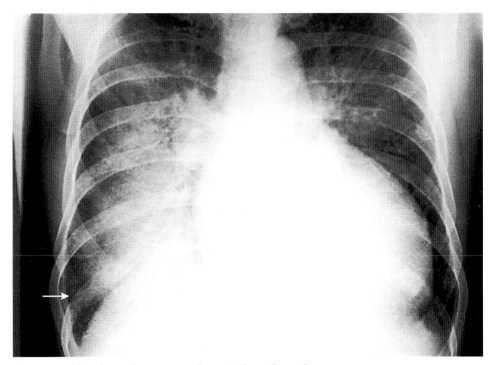

Figure 5.4 **Alveolar pulmonary oedema.** When the pulmonary venous pressure reaches 30 mmHg, oedema fluid will pass into the alveoli. This causes shadowing (patchy to confluent depending on the extent) in the lung fields. This usually occurs first around the hila and gives a bat's wing appearance. These changes are usually superimposed on interstitial oedema. A lamellar pleural effusion (arrow) is seen at the right costophrenic angle where Kerley 'B' lines are also evident.

The Canberra Hospital X-Ray Library, reproduced with permission.

2. **ECG:** look for arrhythmias, signs of ischaemia or recent or old infarction (Fig. 5.5), left ventricular hypertrophy and persisting ST elevation (aneurysm). Left bundle branch block (LBBB) is a common ECG finding in these patients (Fig. 5.6). The ECG is rarely entirely normal in a patient with heart failure.
3. **Electrolytes and creatinine levels:** to exclude hypokalaemia (as a cause of arrhythmia), hyponatraemia (which may indicate severe longstanding cardiac failure, a poor prognostic sign) and renal failure.
4. **B-type natriuretic peptide level (BNP; previously called brain natriuretic peptide):** although there is doubt about the reference range, a definitely elevated level may help distinguish cardiac from non-cardiac dyspnoea. Although BNP is raised in both diastolic and systolic heart failure, the levels are lower in diastolic heart failure. As BNP falls when heart failure is treated, trials of monitoring BNP are under way as a means of assessing the adequacy of cardiac treatment.
5. **Haemoglobin value:** to exclude anaemia as a precipitating cause.
   If the diagnosis is not already obvious, consider *dilated cardiomyopathy*. Investigations for this include those outlined below.
6. **Echocardiography** (Fig. 5.7): this will show generalised or segmental wall motion abnormalities and reduced fractional shortening. An estimate of the left ventricular

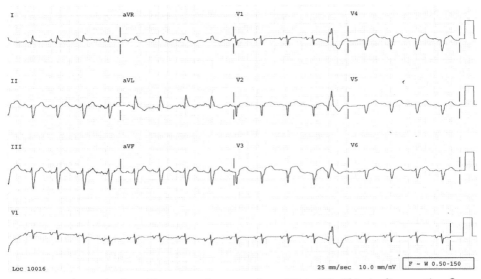

Figure 5.5 Sinus rhythm. There are Q waves from V1 to V5. This is diagnostic of an extensive old anterior infarct, which is likely to be the cause of this patient's heart failure.

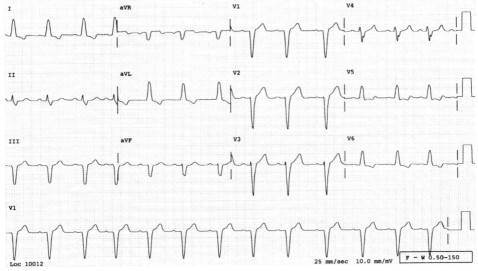

Figure 5.6 Sinus rhythm. Left bundle branch block. The QRS complexes may widen further as heart failure progresses. LBBB is a common finding in heart failure but is not diagnostic.

ejection fraction can be made. Segmental hypokinesia suggests that ischaemia is the cause of the cardiac failure. Doppler echocardiography will usually show at least some mitral and tricuspid regurgitation in these patients. The presence of more severe valvular disease suggests a different aetiology for the cardiac failure. Serial echocardiograph measurements of left and right ventricular dimensions can be useful for following the patient's progress.

7. **Cardiac MRI or CT** can help assess LV and RV function and MRI, myocardial viability.
8. **Coronary angiography:** this is often necessary to exclude coronary artery disease.
9. **Right ventricular biopsy:** this may help determine the aetiology in selected patients.

Treatment

1. Remove precipitating causes. Atrial fibrillation and other incessant tachycardias can be a cause of cardiac failure – tachycardia-induced cardiomyopathy. The prognosis is good if normal heart rate can be restored. Very frequent ventricular ectopic beats (VEBs; more than 5000 in 24 hours) can be a cause of heart failure.

Echocardiography Report

Reason for study: Assess left ventricular function, cardiac failure
Study quality: Good Satisfactory Poor

RV	13	(mm)	(N 10–26)
Sept.	8	(mm)	(N 7–11)
LVEDD	66	(mm)	(N 36–56)
LVESD	49	(mm)	(N 20–40)
LVPW	10	(mm)	(N 7–11)
Aorta	22	(mm)	(N 20–35)
LA	36	(mm)	(N 24–40)
FS	26	%	(N 27–40)
EF	50	%	(N 55–70)

Valves

Mitral Mild-to-moderate MR
Tricus. Mild TR
Aortic Thickened, not stenosed
Pulm. Appears normal

Doppler – 2-D

The left ventricle is dilated. There is extensive antero-apical hypokinesis. The aortic valve is slightly thickened and there is mitral annular calcification. The mitral valve is not stenosed and there is no mitral valve prolapse.

Doppler – colour flow mapping

There is no aortic gradient; mild-to-moderate MR is present. MR jet to two-thirds of LA. Mild TR. RV pressure = 38 mmHg.

Conclusions

Severe segmental LV dysfunction; moderate MR.

Comments

This echocardiography report demonstrates the typical findings when a patient has cardiac failure caused by previous anterior myocardial infarction. The left ventricular dysfunction is not global (typical of cardiomyopathy) but involves the infarcted area. There is overall LV dilatation with an increase of the LVEDD. The FS is the percentage change in LV size from diastole to systole measured at the base of the heart. It can be in the normal range despite the presence of LV dysfunction, if the base of the heart is not involved.

The ejection fraction can be estimated from the LVEDD and LVESD measurements. There are a number of formulas, which are applied automatically by the calculation software of the echocardiograph machine. It is difficult to obtain an accurate ejection fraction, which is a volume change measurement on the basis of two 2D-image measurements. These calculated ejection fractions tend to have a higher reference range than those obtained by nuclear heart pool scanning. MR is almost always detected when moderate LV dysfunction is present.

Mitral annular calcification is a common finding in elderly patients; it can be associated with MR, but not with mitral stenosis. The presence of left atrial enlargement suggests that the mitral regurgitation is not acute, but can also be associated with hypertension.

TR is commonly found in patients with heart failure, but may also be present in normal people. Interrogation of the regurgitant jet with continuous wave (CW) Doppler allows measurement of its velocity. This can be used to calculate the pressure difference across the valve. Since the pressure in the right atrium is usually close to 5 mmHg, the pressure in the RV can be calculated by adding 5 to the pressure difference. In this case the pressure difference across the valve is about 33 mmHg.

Key

EF = ejection fraction; FS = fractional shortening; LA = left atrium; LVEDD = left ventricular end-diastolic dimension; LVESD = left ventricular end-systolic dimension; LVPW = left ventricular posterior wall; MR = mitral regurgitation; Pulm. = pulmonary; RV = right ventricle; Sept. = septal thickness; TR = tricuspid regurgitation; Tricus. = tricuspid.

Figure 5.7 **Echocardiography report in a patient with cardiac failure caused by anterior myocardial infarction.**

2. Correct underlying causes if possible (e.g. angioplasty for an acute infarct or coronary artery bypass grafting or angioplasty for ischaemia) (Table 5.3). Restore sinus rhythm or control the heart rate. Ablate the VEB focus.
3. Control the failure.
   a. Decrease physical activity (e.g. bed rest for the acutely ill patient).
   b. Control fluid retention (e.g. by diuretics, low-salt diet, fluid restriction (1000–1500 mL for severe failure)).
      • Patients should be advised to weigh themselves daily. An increase in weight of 2 kg or more over a few days is usually an indication of significant fluid retention. A temporary increase in the diuretic dose will often prevent deterioration in symptoms.
   c. Oppose inappropriate activation of the renin–angiotensin system.
      • ACE inhibitors (ACEIs) are considered to be the drug class of choice for cardiac failure as they prolong life; symptomatic hypotension is the major side-effect in cardiac failure. ACEIs are indicated for all classes of heart failure, even for asymptomatic patients with left ventricular dysfunction. Every effort should be made to titrate the dose up to the maximum tolerated. The usual limitation is symptomatic hypotension.
      • AR blockers (ARBs) are indicated for patients intolerant (usually because of cough) of ACEIs. The most common reason for the cessation of ACEIs or ARBs is deterioration in renal function (usually in patients with renovascular disease). Some deterioration in renal function is usually acceptable.
      • The combination of an ARB and a neprilysin inhibitor (sacubitril/valsartan is the first one approved) has been shown more effective than an ACEI or ARB and may be used as first-line treatment for heart failure patients or as a replacement for an ACEI or ARB.

Table 5.3 Causes of ventricular failure

LEFT VENTRICULAR FAILURE

1. Volume overload
   a. Aortic regurgitation
   b. Mitral regurgitation
   c. Patent ductus arteriosus
2. Pressure overload
   a. Systemic hypertension
   b. Aortic stenosis
3. Myocardial disease
   a. Ischaemic heart disease
   b. Dilated cardiomyopathy – causes include:
      i.   idiopathic (most common)
      ii.   alcohol
      iii.   myocarditis
      iv.   familial (autosomal dominant)
      v.   tachycardia induced (usually AF) or very frequent VEBs
      vi.   peripartum
      vii.   neuromuscular disease (e.g. dystrophia myotonica)
      viii. connective tissue disease (e.g. scleroderma)
      ix.   haemochromatosis
      x.   sarcoidosis
      xi.   drugs (e.g. doxorubicin)
      xii.   radiation

Note: Restrictive cardiomyopathy and hypertrophic cardiomyopathy can be causes of heart failure.

RIGHT VENTRICULAR FAILURE

1. Volume overload
   a. Atrial septal defect
   b. Tricuspid regurgitation
2. Pressure overload
   a. Pulmonary stenosis
   b. Pulmonary hypertension
3. Myocardial disease
   a. Cardiomyopathy secondary to left ventricular failure
   b. Right ventricular infarction (rare)

- Renal function may improve again if the ACEI and diuretic doses are reduced and hypovolaemia is corrected. There is little therapeutic difference between the various ACEIs.
- Trials have also demonstrated some additional benefit when ACEIs and ARBs are combined. The treatment of cardiac failure involves polypharmacy. It is probably only a minority of patients who will be prepared to take an ARB, as well as all the other drugs usually prescribed. The combination also seems to increase the risk of acute renal failure and is rarely used.
- Add spironolactone. This aldosterone antagonist improves survival in class III or IV patients. It may be especially useful for the management of ascites and peripheral oedema. Hyperkalaemia may be a problem for patients with renal impairment. Start with 12.5 mg per day. Eplerenone is a newer aldosterone antagonist indicated for heart failure occurring soon after myocardial infarction.

- Asking the patient about the difficulties of adherence with a complicated drug regimen may be useful at this point.

d. Oppose inappropriate increases in catecholamine drive.
- Give beta-blockers. Trials with carvedilol, bisoprolol, nebivolol and extended-release metoprolol have shown improvements in symptoms and mortality for this drug used in patients with class II–IV heart failure.
- The drugs must be introduced at a low dose (e.g. 3.125 or 6.25 mg BD of carvedilol or 1.25 mg daily of bisoprolol) and titrated upwards as tolerated to 25 mg BD of carvedilol or 10 mg daily of bisoprolol.

e. Increase myocardial contractility (e.g. with digoxin).

   Note: The use of digoxin in cardiac failure is again controversial. Recent trials have suggested an increase in symptoms if cardiac failure patients who are in sinus rhythm and on treatment with digoxin, diuretics and ACEIs have their digoxin withdrawn. Re-assessment of digoxin mortality trials has suggested a possible increase in mortality for patients taking digoxin. Patients most likely to benefit symptomatically have more severe heart failure, an S3 gallop, impressive cardiomegaly and an ejection fraction < 20%.

f. Intravenous inotropes (e.g. dopamine or dobutamine) may have a place in the short-term treatment of severe cardiac failure. Patients may be admitted for a 'dobutamine holiday' (a course of treatment with intravenous dobutamine, usually for about 5 days) and have improved symptoms for some months. Levosimendan is an intravenous drug that works as a calcium channel activator. A 24-hour course may improve symptoms and possibly prognosis. No effective oral inotrope is available.

g. Control rhythm. Remember, severe cardiac failure has a poor prognosis. About 50% of these patients die suddenly of a ventricular arrhythmia. The detection of high-grade ventricular arrhythmias is an indication for an *implanted defibrillator*, which is associated with a proven improvement in prognosis. Routine use of these devices in patients with a low ejection fraction has been shown to improve survival, even when ventricular arrhythmias have not been recorded. There is controversy about the prophylactic use of these devices in elderly patients with non-ischaemic cardiomyopathy.

h. His bundle pacing in selected patients can resynchronise LV contraction.

i. Cardiac transplantation may now be offered to certain patients. The reduced availability of donor hearts and the improvement with beta-blockers of many patients who would otherwise be suitable for transplant have reduced the frequency of this procedure.

j. Biventricular pacing or cardiac resynchronisation therapy (CRT) is helpful for heart failure patients with very wide QRS complexes. The LV-pacing wire is placed via the coronary sinus into one of the left ventricular veins. This complicated procedure enables both ventricles to be paced and dyssynchronous contraction of the ventricles associated with a very wide QRS to be corrected. About 70% of patients improve with the treatment. Although echocardiographic measurements of dyssynchrony are available, they have not yet been able to predict a response to resynchronisation treatment and the current guidelines allow their use for symptomatic patients with LBBB who are in sinus rhythm.

k. Ventricular assist devices are sometimes used as a bridge to transplant in very ill patients. Survival for weeks or months is possible with these devices. Trials of entirely artificial hearts continue in small numbers of patients.

4. Correct iron deficiency. A number of studies have shown improvement in symptoms when patients who are iron deficient but not anaemic have their iron stores replenished with intravenous iron.

Possible lines of questioning

1. Would you recommend that *this* patient have an implanted defibrillator or resynchronisation pacemaker?

2. How would you help *this* patient manage his or her symptoms of cardiac failure from day to day?

3. How would you investigate *this* patient with a recent worsening of symptoms of heart failure?

Diastolic heart failure (heart failure with preserved ejection fraction)

Most breathless patients with heart failure have abnormal left ventricular systolic function, which is characterised by dilatation and hypokinesis. Some cases of cardiac failure, however, may be caused by diastolic dysfunction. In such cases, the myocardium is stiff, often because it is hypertrophied and does not relax normally. The condition seems to be more common in elderly patients. Hypertension is a common cause but infiltration of the heart with amyloid protein is common in elderly people and is an important cause. The diagnosis is difficult, but an echocardiogram will show preserved or increased systolic contraction without dilatation and there may be increased left ventricular thickness due to hypertrophy or infiltration and left atrial dilatation. Doppler echocardiography may show abnormalities of left ventricular filling caused by the stiffness of the ventricle. However, this is not easy to quantify and is dependent on variations in preload and afterload. Technetium scanning has been shown to be reliable in making the diagnosis of amyloid infiltration. The ECG typically shows low voltages in the chest leads where one would expect high voltages if the problem were left ventricular hypertrophy.

The condition may have a prognosis as bad as that of systolic heart failure. Treatment is similar, but beta-blockers are used early on and only small doses of diuretics should be required. Aldosterone antagonists reduce exacerbations and admissions, and the ARB-neprolysin inhibitors may subtly improve NYHA class and exacerbations. At least in theory, digoxin should be avoided if the patient is in sinus rhythm. Every effort should be made to control hypertension.

Hyperlipidaemia

Hyperlipidaemia may be present in patients under investigation for vascular disease, pancreatitis, hypothyroidism or diabetes mellitus. It often presents both diagnostic and management problems. It is not likely to be the major problem for a long-case patient.

The history

1. The patient should be able to indicate whether or not the main problem is vascular. If the problem is one of premature coronary artery disease, hypercholesterolaemia is the likely lipid problem. The most important inherited cause is *familial hypercholesterolaemia*, which is caused by a defective or absent low-density lipoprotein (LDL) receptor. The heterozygous form occurs in about 1 person in 500. As the transmission is autosomal dominant, the patient may know of first-degree relatives who have been

affected. There may even be family members with the homozygous form. These people usually present with a tenfold elevation in serum cholesterol levels as a result of an increase in plasma LDL levels and have a myocardial infarction before the age of 20 years. People with the heterozygous form typically have myocardial infarctions in their 30s and 40s and have a two- to threefold elevation in cholesterol level. More than 80% of affected men and nearly 60% of affected women have had myocardial infarcts by the age of 60 years. Find out whether the patient has already had a myocardial infarct and which relatives have been affected.

Familial combined hyperlipidaemia is associated with obesity or glucose intolerance and may be expressed as type IIa, IIb or IV hyperlipidaemia (Table 5.4). This is also an autosomal dominant trait. Patients develop hypercholesterolaemia and often hypertriglyceridaemia in puberty. Once again, there usually is a strong family history of premature coronary artery disease. There is no doubt that an elevated triglyceride level adds to the risk of hypercholesterolaemia.

Table 5.4 Hyperlipoproteinaemias

TYPE	LIPOPROTEIN ELEVATED	ELECTRO-PHORETIC MOBILITY	MECHANISM	SECONDARY CAUSES	CLINICAL FEATURES	ASSOCIATIONS
I	Chylomicrons	Origin	Deficiency; extrahepatic lipoprotein lipase or apo C-II deficiency	Rarely SLE	Eruptive xanthomata; lipaemia retinalis	Pancreatitis
IIa	LDL	β	Receptor defect	Cushing's; hypothyroidism	Xanthelasma; corneal arcus	CAD, PVD
IIb	LDL and VLDL	β and pre-β		Cholestasis; nephrotic syndrome	Tendon xanthomata (see Fig. 5.8)	
III	IDL	Broad β	Oversynthesis and / or abnormal apo E	Renal and liver disease	Palmar crease and tuboeruptive xanthomata; xanthelasma	CAD, PVD
IV	VLDL	Pre-β	Oversynthesis and / or under catabolism of VLDL	Diabetes mellitus; alcoholism; chronic renal failure	Usually no xanthomata	
V	VLDL and chylomicrons	Origin and pre-β	Saturation lipoprotein lipase by VLDL	As for IV	As for I	As for I

NOTES

- Apo A-I deficiency is associated with the absence of plasma HDL and severe premature CAD.
- Apo B deficiency is the defect in abetalipoproteinaemia (autosomal recessive), which is characterised by haemolytic anaemia (acanthocytosis), fat malabsorption and neurological defects (proprioceptive loss, retinitis pigmentosa).
- LCAT deficiency results in decreased HDL, cloudy corneas and progressive renal disease.

apo = apolipoprotein; CAD = coronary artery disease; HDL = high-density lipoprotein; IDL = intermediate-density lipoprotein; LCAT = lecithin cholesterol acyltransferase; LDL = low-density lipoprotein; PVD = peripheral vascular disease; SLE = systemic lupus erythematosus; VLDL = very-low-density lipoprotein.

Familial dysbetalipoproteinaemia is also associated with coronary artery disease. These patients have elevated cholesterol and triglyceride levels and are usually found to have obesity, hypothyroidism or diabetes mellitus. Find out whether there is any history of these and whether there has been atheromatous disease or vascular disease involving the internal carotid arteries and the abdominal aorta or its branches. Ask about claudication, which occurs in about one-third of patients.

2. The patient may be able to tell you his or her cholesterol and triglyceride levels and what they have been in the past. Some patients even know their LDL and high-density lipoprotein (HDL) levels.

3. If there is no history of coronary artery disease and the patient either knows the triglyceride level to have been very high or has a history of pancreatitis, the likely diagnosis is *familial hypertriglyceridaemia*. This is also a common autosomal dominant disorder and is associated with obesity, hyperglycaemia, hyperinsulinaemia, hypertension and hyperuricaemia. Although there is a slightly increased incidence of atherosclerosis, this is probably related to diabetes mellitus, obesity and hypertension rather than to the hypertriglyceridaemia itself.

4. Ask about the patient's alcohol consumption, any history of hypothyroidism or the ingestion of oestrogen-containing oral contraceptives. Any of these can precipitate a rapid rise in the triglyceride level, which may precipitate pancreatitis or the characteristic eruptive xanthomas. Between attacks, patients have moderate elevations of the plasma triglyceride level.

5. Next, find out about treatment. In familial hypercholesterolaemia, this will have been aimed at the cholesterol level itself and at any cardiovascular complications that have occurred. The patient should be well informed about a low-saturated-fat diet and may be aware of side-effects from medication usage.

6. The need for drug treatment of hyperlipidaemia depends on the lipid levels and on the patient's other vascular risk factors. Ask about a family history of premature coronary disease (first-degree relatives under the age of 60), previous vascular disease (coronary, cerebral or peripheral), smoking and diabetes mellitus.

7. Ask about any history of cutaneous xanthoma. These may have resolved with treatment or have been surgically removed.

The examination

1. Examine the cardiovascular system. There may be evidence of cardiac failure from previous myocardial infarcts or a sternotomy scar from previous coronary surgery. Occasionally one sees the scandalous situation of a patient with untreated hyperlipidaemia presenting with more angina after initially successful coronary surgery.

2. Look specifically for the interesting skin manifestations of these conditions.

   a. Patients with the heterozygous or homozygous form of familial hypercholesterolaemia may have *tendon xanthomas* (Fig. 5.8). These are nodular swellings that tend to involve the tendons of the knee, elbow and dorsum of the hand and the Achilles tendon. They consist of massive deposits of cholesterol, probably derived from the deposition of LDL particles. They contain both amorphous extracellular deposits and vacuoles within macrophages, and sometimes become inflamed and cause tendonitis.

   b. Cholesterol deposits in the soft tissue of the eyelid cause *xanthelasma* and those in the cornea produce *arcus cornea* (previously insensitively called *arcus senilis*). Xanthelasma occur in about 1% of the population and arcus cornea in 30% of people over 50. When corneal arcus is seen in younger people it is more often associated with hyperlipidaemia. Surveys of people with xanthelasma indicate a

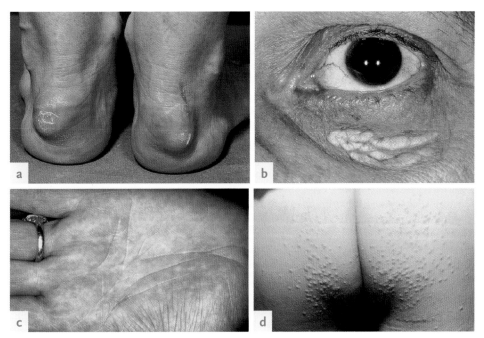

Figure 5.8 (a) Achilles tendon xanthoma. (b) Xanthelasma. (c) Palmar xanthoma. (d) Eruptive xanthomas.

(a) courtesy A F Lant, J Dequeker, London; (b) M Yanoff, J Duker. *Opthamology*. 3rd edn. Fig 12-9-18. Mosby, Elsevier, 2009, with permission; (c) and (d) courtesy R A Marsden, St George's Hospital, London.

slightly higher than average cholesterol level. Tendon xanthomas are diagnostic of familial hypercholesterolaemia, but the other signs are not as specific – only 50% of people affected have hyperlipidaemia.

The majority of patients with the homozygous form have even more interesting signs.

- Yellow xanthomas may occur at points of trauma and in the webs of the fingers.
- Cholesterol deposits in the aortic valve may be sufficient to cause aortic stenosis; occasionally mitral stenosis and mitral regurgitation can occur for the same reason.
- Painful swollen joints may also be present. Obesity is uncommon in these patients.

c. These skin manifestations may or may not resolve with treatment of the cholesterol level. Surgical treatment is sometimes indicated.

d. Eruptive xanthomas are a sign of hypertriglyceridaemia (levels often over 20 mmol/L). This is type V hyperlipoproteinaemia. Eruptive xanthomas occur on pressure areas, such as the elbows and buttocks, and resolve rapidly with treatment. The association here is with pancreatitis. The problem is often hereditary, but exacerbated with obesity, diabetes and alcohol consumption. It is a less definite risk factor for cardiovascular disease. Palmar xanthomata are a sign of dysbetalipoproteinaemia (type III hyperlipoproteinaemia). They also resolve with treatment.

3. If the history suggests combined hyperlipidaemia or hypertriglyceridaemia, obesity is likely to be present. Look also for signs of the complications of diabetes mellitus and for signs of hypothyroidism or the nephrotic syndrome (see Table 11.6, p. 315).

4. In sick patients with hypertriglyceridaemia, there may be signs of acute pancreatitis.

Investigations

1. A cholesterol level over 8 mmol / L with a normal triglyceride level suggests one of the familial hyperlipidaemias. This diagnosis can be confirmed by an assay of the number of LDL receptors on blood lymphocytes. The diagnosis is more often made from a combination of the lipid pattern, the history and the clinical examination (see Table 5.4). The other necessary investigations are those required for coronary artery disease.
2. Investigation of hypertriglyceridaemia includes tests to exclude possible underlying causes, such as hypothyroidism, diabetes mellitus and excessive alcohol intake. In familial hypertriglyceridaemia the plasma triglyceride level tends to be moderately elevated to 3–6 mmol / L (type IV lipoprotein pattern). The cholesterol level is normal. The triglyceride level may rise to values in excess of 12 mmol / L during exacerbations of the condition.
3. Familial combined hyperlipidaemia produces one of three different lipoprotein patterns – hypercholesterolaemia (type IIa), hypertriglyceridaemia (type IV), or both hypercholesterolaemia and hypertriglyceridaemia (type V).
4. Familial dysbetalipoproteinaemia (type III hyperlipoproteinaemia) results in the accumulation of large lipoprotein particles containing triglycerides and cholesterol. These particles resemble the remnants and intermediate-density lipoprotein (IDL) particles normally produced from the catabolism of chylomicrons and very-low-density lipoproteins (VLDLs). The patients are homozygous for the apolipoprotein E2 (apo E2) allele, which is unable to bind to hepatic lipoprotein receptors, thus preventing the rapid hepatic uptake of IDL and chylomicrons. The condition is usually expressed only in patients with hypothyroidism or diabetes mellitus and tests for these disorders are necessary. Apo E genotyping may sometimes be useful.

Management

1. A combination of diet and treatment of the underlying condition is usually required. Underlying diabetes mellitus and hypothyroidism must be treated.
2. Some patients with dysbetalipoproteinaemia respond dramatically to the introduction of thyroxine. Effective management of the condition tends to cause disappearance of the skin signs and improves the prognosis as far as vascular disease goes. Effective treatment of familial hyperlipidaemia from early adult life delays the onset of coronary artery disease.
3. Treatment is almost always begun with hydroxymethylglutaryl coenzyme A (HMG-CoA) reductase inhibitors (statins, e.g. pravastatin, lovastatin, atorvastatin, rosuvastatin). These drugs should be taken at night. Most cholesterol is manufactured at night. They work by inhibiting the synthesis of cholesterol in the liver by impeding the activity of the rate-limiting enzyme. Patients need to have their liver function checked after about a month. They are effective drugs; total cholesterol levels may be expected to fall at least 30%. The current indications for drug treatment of cholesterol allow a statin for patients with established symptomatic coronary artery disease at any total cholesterol level.
   a. The most frequent problem with these drugs is the occurrence of myalgias. Check the creatine kinase for rhabdomyolysis if there is muscle pain, but this is rare. The relatively long experience with statins suggests they are safe in quite large doses and current starting doses are two to four times those used in the past. Atorvastatin and rosuvastatin are the most potent statins and should be the drugs of choice for severe hypercholesterolaemia. Pravastatin and fluvastatin are alternative options for patients with myalgias, especially if on other CYP3A4 inhibitors. All the statins favourably affect the HDL:LDL ratio.

b. There is controversy about the need to treat levels that are already below 4 mmol/L. There is evidence that there are pleotrophic effects of the statins that reduce coronary risk separately from their effect on cholesterol. This also implies that, for secondary prevention, the use of statins may be beneficial for patients whose total cholesterol is below 4 mmol/L before drug treatment.

4. Ezetimibe reduces cholesterol absorption from the gut and thus interrupts its enterohepatic circulation. It does not seem to interfere with the absorption of fat-soluble vitamins. Its effect on cholesterol levels is substantial, although not as great as that of the statins. It is useful for patients who are intolerant of the statins or, when used in combination with a statin, for patients whose cholesterol level is not controlled on a statin alone.

5. Gemfibrozil increases the activity of lipoprotein lipase and is useful in hypertriglyceridaemia resulting from increased VLDL or IDL levels. Its main use is for patients with elevation of both cholesterol and triglyceride levels. Clofibrate is no longer in common use for lipid control.

6. A few patients may be taking one of the bile-sequestering resins – cholestyramine or colestipol. They are not absorbed, but can cause constipation and flatulence and can block the absorption of other drugs. Patients may need to take up to two sachets (8 g) three times daily.

7. If the cholesterol cannot be brought down to normal levels with diet and a resin, nicotinic acid (which blocks VLDL synthesis) can be added. This is an effective drug and may help block the compensating increase in hepatic cholesterol synthesis that occurs with bile-sequestering resins. It is also used to try to raise HDL levels. Side-effects include flushing, pruritus, abnormal liver function tests, hyperglycaemia and aggravation of peptic ulcer disease. The patient will probably have been begun on a small dose and had this gradually increased as tolerance improved. In practice it is a very difficult drug to use because of its side-effects.

8. A patient with one of the combined hyperlipidaemias is likely to need to lose weight, as well as to control the cholesterol and saturated fat intake, and with dysbetalipoproteinaemia may require treatment for hypothyroidism. All these patients need to avoid alcohol and oral contraceptives. Diet is the mainstay of treatment for reducing triglyceride levels; gemfibrozil or one of the newer fibrates may be used if diet fails.

9. The indications for treatment of hyperlipidaemia with drugs on the Pharmaceutical Benefits Scheme (PBS) are complicated. Total cholesterol, HDL, LDL and triglyceride levels, as well as the presence of other risk factors, are all part of the formula. Candidates should be familiar with the latest PBS rules.

10. A patient with familial hypertriglyceridaemia will have been managed in a similar way and may have required treatment for acute pancreatitis.

11. Patients with homozygous familial hypercholesterolaemia are unlikely to live long enough to be present in clinical examinations, but treatment can sometimes involve repeated plasma exchange and even liver transplantation.

12. When patients have muscle pains on statin treatment, reducing the dose or even giving the drug second daily may be worth trying. However, there are no trials showing that second-daily treatment is effective.

13. New classes of injectable cholesterol-lowering drugs such as the proprotein convertase subtilisin kexin (PCSK9) inhibitors are now available. Evolocumab is a monoclonal antibody that inhibits PCSK9 and reduces LDL lipoprotein a (Lp(a)) and apo B further when used with a statin. This drug is very expensive and is available on the PBS for patients with familial hyperlipidaemia, whose cholesterol is not controlled with maximum statin doses.

14. Drugs that specifically raise HDL have been disappointing.

:···:
: ## Possible line of questioning
:
: Does *this* patient need treatment for his or her lipid abnormalities?
:···:

Hypertension

Many long cases are likely to provide the examiners with an opportunity to ask about the management of hypertension. The examiners will want to hear sensible discussion from the candidate about a number of aspects of hypertension, including the diagnosis, appropriate investigations and approaches to treatment.

The history

1. Many patients are well informed about and very interested in their blood pressure. Find out when the diagnosis was made and what sorts of blood pressure readings were obtained before and after treatment. It is common for measurements to be made in a number of ways and in different settings. Apart from clinic measurements, the patient may have taken and continue to take his or her own blood pressure at home. There may have been ambulatory blood pressure (ABP) recordings made. It seems that hypertensive risk may be more closely related to non-clinic and ABP results than to those obtained in the outpatient clinic. ABP should, however, be lower than clinic readings to be considered normal. Measurements of < 135/85 mmHg during the day and < 120/75 mmHg at night are considered normal for automatic blood pressure recordings. See Table 5.5 for the current classification of clinic blood pressure levels.

   There is current controversy from the SPRINT trial, which used unattended automatic blood pressure measurements taken a number of times. Blood pressure readings were generally lower than home or surgery readings. The trial has led to a lowering of recommended blood pressure targets in the United States, but not in Australia or Europe, because of no evidence of greater benefits.

2. Ask about current and past antihypertensive treatment and about problems or side-effects caused by treatment. Next, find out about possible complications of hypertension. These include stroke, heart failure, peripheral vascular disease and renal failure.

Table 5.5 Classification of blood pressure by severity		
CATEGORY	**SYSTOLIC (mmHg)**	**DIASTOLIC (mmHg)**
Optimal	< 120 and	< 80
Normal	120–129 and/or	80–84
High normal	130–139 and/or	85–89
Mild hypertension (grade 1)	140–159 and/or	90–99
Moderate hypertension (grade 2)	160–179 and/or	100–109
Severe hypertension (grade 3)	≥ 180 and/or	≥ 110
Isolated systolic hypertension	≥ 140 and	< 90

Source: The Task Force for the management of arterial hypertension of the European Society of Hypertension (ESH) and of the European Society of Cardiology (ESC). 2018 ESH/ESC

3. Occasionally there may be symptoms that suggest a secondary cause of hypertension: paroxysmal sweating, palpitations and headache (phaeochromocytoma) or daytime sleepiness (sleep apnoea). Rarely, the patient may be aware of a diagnosis of renal artery stenosis, coarctation of the aorta or an adrenal tumour. Primary hyperaldosteronism is now more often recognised.

4. Ask about other risk factors for vascular disease, especially type 2 diabetes, but also hyperlipidaemia, a family history of premature coronary disease or stroke. The presence of any of these conditions, or of existing heart failure, coronary or cerebrovascular disease, is a strong indication for treatment.

5. There are often a number of factors that contribute to the problem. These include obesity, excess alcohol consumption, lack of physical exercise and a high salt intake. Other factors, such as cigarette smoking, add to the patient's overall risk. Ask what the patient knows about these factors and what efforts (if any) have been made to correct them. Some racial groups have a high risk of premature vascular disease and will benefit more from early and aggressive treatment. These include Aboriginal Australians, Torres Strait Islanders and Pacific Islanders.

The examination

See Chapter 16. Don't miss Cushing's syndrome. Feel for radiofemoral delay, but this is very rare.

Investigations

1. **Test the urine for protein**. Measure the serum electrolyte and creatinine, blood sugar, cholesterol and haemoglobin levels.

2. **Note the serum potassium**. The presence of hypokalaemia in patients who are not on diuretics should prompt investigations for primary aldosteronism. Measurement of plasma renin activity (PRA) and plasma aldosterone (PA) levels may be indicated. A high PA level and a low PRA level leading to a high aldosterone:renin ratio is consistent with primary hyperaldosteronism. The test is better performed off treatment. Other causes of hypokalaemia and hypertension include renovascular disease (both aldosterone and renin are elevated), Cushing's syndrome, chronic liquorice ingestion, Liddle's syndrome and, in the young, renin-secreting cancers (rarely).

3. **Ask about snoring**. A history of snoring and obesity should be investigated with sleep studies for sleep apnoea.

4. **Consider a CT angiogram or conventional renal angiogram for patients with intractable hypertension (especially young patients)**. These are the most sensitive tests for renal artery stenosis. Remember, however, that renal artery angioplasty has not been shown to improve blood pressure if the underlying problem is atheromatous disease.

5. **Ask about symptoms consistent with a phaeochromocytoma**. These need investigation with 24-hour urinary catecholamines.

6. **Investigate for Cushing's syndrome if there is any clinical suspicion**.

7. **Perform an ECG to look for evidence of ischaemic heart disease and for voltage changes that suggest left ventricular hypertrophy (LVH)** (Fig. 5.9). The presence of LVH on the ECG in hypertensives is associated with an adverse prognosis. Occasionally an echocardiogram is indicated if there is doubt about the presence of LVH.

Treatment

The decision to begin drug treatment is an important one because it is likely to be lifelong. The current recommendations are that a blood pressure of > 140 mmHg systolic

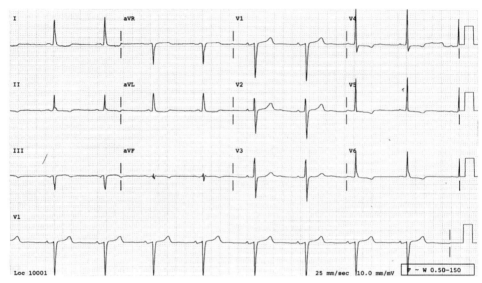

Figure 5.9 **Sinus rhythm. Left ventricular hypertrophy – the R waves are tall in the lateral leads and the S waves are deep in the septal leads. There are also lateral ST and T wave changes, called a strain pattern.**

or > 90 mmHg diastolic, or both, warrants a 'treatment plan'. It is now very clear that the aggressiveness of intervention depends very much on factors other than the blood pressure level. The whole gamut of cardiovascular risk factors must be taken into account.

Tables have been published by many cardiovascular societies that show the calculated risk of vascular events and the calculated reduction in number of events over time with treatment for patients with different risk factors. The decision to use drug treatment should be based on information of this kind. Typically, calculators of risk take into account age, sex, smoking status, level of blood pressure, cholesterol, race and existing cardiovascular disease.

Except for very severe hypertension, attempts should be made to bring the blood pressure down by modifying the factors that are known to increase it. Many patients, when faced with the threat of lifelong drug treatment, are amenable to suggestions to change the way they live.

Primary hyperaldosteronism can be treated effectively with spironolactone. Treatment of sleep apnoea with an appropriate continuous positive airways pressure (CPAP) mask can also make blood pressure control easier.

Patients with only a mild risk of cardiovascular problems and blood pressure < 150/95 mmHg should probably continue with conservative measures and be reassessed. However, at higher levels of blood pressure than this, drug treatment should be considered. Patients with very high risk (e.g. those with target organ disease or of Aboriginal race) should begin drug treatment if the blood pressure remains above 140/90 mmHg. Isolated systolic hypertension in the elderly (often defined as ≥ 160 mmHg) deserves therapy!

BLOOD PRESSURE REDUCTION WITHOUT DRUGS

1. **Weight reduction:** on average, 1 kg of weight loss will reduce systolic blood pressure by 2 mmHg. The goal should be reduction to a body mass index (BMI) of

$25 \text{ kg}/\text{m}^2$ and a waist circumference of < 94 cm for men and < 80 cm for women. Even lower BMIs should be recommended for some racial groups, such as Asians and Aboriginal Australians, whose cardiovascular risk increases at lower BMIs than does Europeans.

2. **Exercise:** 30 minutes of moderately intense exercise (e.g. brisk walking) at least 5 days a week can lower blood pressure by about 3–5 mmHg.
3. **Alcohol:** reductions of 4–5 mmHg can be achieved by alcohol restriction to two standard drinks per day for men and one per day for women.
4. **Salt:** reduction in salt consumption to 90 mmol/day can reduce blood pressure by more than 5 mmHg. Warn patients that prepared and snack foods are usually heavily salted.

The cumulative effect of these measures can be considerable, but repeated encouragement is likely to be required for patients to achieve them.

DRUG TREATMENT

Remember that all classes of drugs (Table 5.6) are fairly similar in their effect on blood pressure. The majority of patients will require more than one drug for effective blood pressure control.

There are many factors to be taken into account when a choice of antihypertensive drug is made (Table 5.7):

- previous intolerance to a class of drugs
- known contraindications to a class of drugs (e.g. renal artery stenosis and ACEIs)
- convenience of drug regimen (e.g. once-daily dosage)
- interaction with other medications (e.g. concerns about bradycardia with beta-blockers and verapamil)
- existing medical problems that favour the use of a class of drugs (e.g. cardiac failure and ACE inhibitors)
- cost
- possible additional protective effects of some antihypertensives (e.g. ACE inhibitors and patients who have had a stroke or have diabetes).

The current Heart Foundation recommendation is that treatment begin with a small dose of 2 drugs in a single tablet. An RAS inhibitor plus thiazide diuretic or calcium antagonist is a common choice. Some drugs are especially effective in combination:

- beta-blocker and dihydropyridine calcium channel antagonist
- ACE inhibitor or AR antagonist and thiazide
- ACE inhibitor or AR antagonist and calcium antagonist
- beta-blocker and alpha-blocker
- beta-blocker and thiazide.

Table 5.6 Classes of antihypertensive drugs
Thiazide diuretics
Angiotensin-converting enzyme (ACE) inhibitors
Beta-blockers
Non-dihydropyridine calcium channel blockers
Dihydropyridine calcium channel blockers
Angiotensin II receptor antagonists
Others: centrally acting (methyldopa), vasodilators (prazosin, hydralazine)
Aldosterone antagonists and potassium-sparing diuretics

Table 5.7 Factors affecting choice of antihypertensive drug	
CONDITION	**DRUG**
CONTRAINDICATION OR RELATIVE CONTRAINDICATION	
Asthma or COPD	Beta-blockers
Bradycardia or heart block	Beta-blockers, non-dihydropyridine calcium channel blockers (verapamil, diltiazem)
Cardiac failure	Calcium channel blockers
Diabetes mellitus	Thiazides, beta-blockers (relative contraindication)
Gout	Diuretics
Peripheral vascular disease	Beta-blockers
Pregnancy	Avoid most antihypertensives, especially ACE inhibitors; methyldopa, hydralazine and labetalol are safe
Renal vascular disease	ACE inhibitors, AR antagonists
POSSIBLE INDICATION OR BENEFICIAL EFFECT	
Angina	Beta-blockers, calcium channel blockers
Cardiac failure	ACE inhibitors, AR antagonists, diuretics, some beta-blockers
Myocardial infarction	ACE inhibitors, beta-blockers
Diabetes mellitus	ACE inhibitors, AR antagonists
COPD = chronic obstructive pulmonary disease; ACE = angiotensin-converting enzyme; AR = angiotensin receptor.	

Fixed-dose combinations of two or even three of these are available: ACEI and thiazide, calcium antagonist and ACEI or ARB +/− diuretic, beta-blocker and alpha-blocker (labetolol). These combinations are not approved for the initiation of treatment. Candidates should be familiar with the doses of the common antihypertensive drugs and their important side-effects.

UNCONTROLLED HYPERTENSION

Genuinely uncontrollable blood pressure is rare. It should not be diagnosed unless a thiazide is part of the treatment.

Consider:
1. poor adherence
2. hyperaldosteronism (investigate and add spironolactone[1]) or other rare primary cause (e.g. Cushing's syndrome, coarctation)

and recommend:
1. attempted weight loss
2. salt and alcohol restriction
3. exercise
4. sleep apnoea treatment (if indicated).

RENAL ARTERY DENERVATION

Catheter-based denervation of the renal artery can now be performed using radiofrequency energy or drug instillation. Early trials showed significant (up to 20 mmHg), sustained

---

[1]Spironolactone and potassium-sparing diuretics (e.g. amiloride) have recently been shown to be effective in difficult hypertension even in the absence of hyperaldosteronism.

blood pressure reduction for patients not controlled on four or five drugs, but more recent trials were much less impressive. The treatment is still experimental.

Possible lines of questioning

1. How would you manage *this* patient with uncontrolled hypertension despite prescription of three or four drugs?
2. How would you decide that *this* patient needs drug treatment for his hypertension?

Heart transplantation

Cardiac transplantation is now an accepted form of treatment for intractable cardiac failure. Numbers of patients who have either had a transplant or are on the waiting list for one are available for clinical examinations. Those awaiting transplantation are sick enough to require frequent admissions to hospital, and those who have had a transplant are often re-admitted for various routine investigations. Many patients who would once have required a transplant are now stable on treatment with beta-blockers and ACE inhibitors. Therefore, patients on a transplant list tend to have severe heart failure which has not responded to medical treatment or resynchronisation pacing. Patients are usually well informed about their condition and should be able to supply a lot of useful information to the candidate.

Although this fact should not be discussed with our surgical colleagues, heart transplantation is technically not a very difficult operation. Improvements in prognosis have followed medical advances, particularly in the area of the management of rejection. The 5-year survival rate is now slightly more than 75% for patients who have received a transplant since 1981 and the 1-year survival rate is about 90%. The average patient survives 15 years, but it is 20 years for a 30-year-old and 12 years for a 65-year-old.

As in all transplantation long cases, the examiners will expect the candidate to be familiar with the indications for and contraindications to the procedure. It is also important to know what investigations are required before a patient can be accepted for surgery and to understand the management problems that can occur in patients who have had the operation (Table 5.8).

The history

1. Try to establish the cause of the patient's cardiac failure. In younger patients, cardiomyopathy is more likely to be the problem, but nearly half the patients currently undergoing heart transplantation have ischaemic heart disease. Rheumatic valvular heart disease can also affect younger patients. Combined heart and lung transplantation is occasionally carried out for patients with primary pulmonary hypertension or cystic fibrosis. It may also be the treatment of choice for some forms of congenital heart disease, either in childhood or in adult life; if pulmonary hypertension is present, these patients have to be considered for combined heart and lung transplantation.

   Ask about previous myocardial infarction or angina and whether the patient knows the results of cardiac catheterisation. All patients undergoing a transplant are required to have cardiac catheterisation. There may have been a preoperative cardiac biopsy performed and the patient may be aware of the results of this test. Also ask about previous thoracotomies.

Table 5.8 Evaluation for heart transplantation

1. History and examination
2. Body weight
3. Cardiac assessment
   a. Ejection fraction: estimated by resting gated blood pool scan
   b. Echocardiogram: with measurement of left ventricular dimensions and assessment of the cardiac valves; examination for left ventricular thrombus
   c. Coronary angiography in patients with suspected ischaemic heart disease
   d. 24-hour Holter monitoring to evaluate for ventricular arrhythmias
   e. Right heart catheterisation to measure pulmonary vascular resistance and its response to vasodilators; fixed pulmonary hypertension is a contraindication to cardiac transplantation
4. HLA tissue typing
5. Chest X-ray and respiratory function tests, if indicated
6. FBC, ESR and coagulation studies
7. Biochemical profile, including liver function tests, electrolyte levels and estimation of creatinine clearance, serum cholesterol, triglycerides and blood sugar levels
8. Serology for antinuclear antibodies and immunoelectrophoresis
9. Bacteriology: swabs for methicillin-resistant *Staphylococcus aureus* and a Mantoux test if indicated; hepatitis A and B, toxoplasma, CMV, EBV, HIV and herpes simplex serology
10. Psychiatric, renal and dental consultations, if required
11. Social work report

If the cause of the cardiomyopathy is unknown, a myocardial biopsy, viral titres (including coxsackie A virus, echovirus, adenovirus and influenza titres) and iron studies (for haemochromatosis) are required.

Contraindications for heart transplantation: alcoholism, chronic renal disease, pulmonary parenchymal disease, continued tobacco use, advanced liver disease and advanced age. Diabetes mellitus is a relative contraindication.

CMV = cytomegalovirus; EBV = Epstein–Barr virus; ESR = erythrocyte sedimentation rate; FBC = full blood count; HIV = human immunodeficiency virus; HLA = human leukocyte antigen.

2. Ask about the patient's symptoms before surgery. Obtain an idea of the exercise tolerance and the severity of angina, if present. The patient may know the results of investigations of cardiac function, such as exercise tests and gated blood pool scans, before and after surgery.
3. Ask what treatment the patient was receiving before transplantation, particularly the doses of diuretics, ACE inhibitors and beta-blockers (e.g. carvedilol). Find out whether frequent admissions to hospital have been necessary and whether intravenous inotropes were required. There may have been recurrent ventricular arrhythmias before surgery. Treatment may have been with drugs, especially amiodarone, or an implanted defibrillator and antitachycardia pacemaker and resynchronisation device. Some patients have undergone previous surgery for arrhythmias. This may include resection of an aneurysm or myocardial resection following ventricular mapping. Occasionally, transplantation is used to treat intractable ventricular arrhythmias.
4. Find out how long it is since the transplant was performed. Ask whether there were any problems with the surgery – either technical or involving acute rejection. Find out how long the patient was in hospital and what further admissions to hospital have occurred since the operation. Ask whether a permanent pacemaker was inserted. Some patients awaiting transplant may have been given a ventricular assist device as a bridge to transplant; ask whether that was necessary.

5. Endomyocardial biopsies are fairly memorable events and the patient should be able to tell you how often these have been performed and when the last one was obtained. It is now routine to perform them at weekly intervals for the first 3 weeks after operation, every 2 weeks for the following month and every 6 months after that for patients whose condition is stable.

6. Find out what drugs the patient is taking currently. Transplant patients should not require anti-failure treatment, but will, of course, be taking immunosuppressive drugs. Almost all patients are now maintained on cyclosporin (ciclosporin); the dose is determined by its serum level. Cyclosporin and tacrolimus are nephrotoxic and cause hypertension and hyperlipidaemia. Newer immunosuppressive drugs include mycophenolate and rapamycin (sirolimus). Diltiazem is often used as a cyclosporin-sparing agent. It dramatically reduces cyclosporin metabolism and therefore the cost of treating patients. Often azathioprine is also prescribed and the dose is adjusted according to the white cell count.

7. Patients are often well informed about symptoms suggesting rejection – often these resemble an attack of pericarditis. The patient may know of boosts of prednisone that have been given for rejection episodes. Early episodes of rejection are often treated with 1 g of methylprednisolone IV for 3 days. Later rejection tends to be milder and may respond to an increase in oral steroids. Severe rejection is often treated with antithymocyte globulin or the murine monoclonal muromonab-CD3. Repetitive rejection may be treated with total lymphoid irradiation or methotrexate.

8. Enquire about complications of immunosuppression (Table 5.9). Many patients are also taking regular antibiotics to prevent *Pneumocystis jirovecii* (formerly *carinii*) infection. Cotrimoxazole twice daily 3 days a week is a common regimen.

9. Some general questions about the transplant patient's current life are very relevant. Find out how much difference has occurred in the patient's exercise tolerance and whether he or she has been able to go back to work. If the patient is currently an inpatient, find out why he or she has been admitted to hospital on this occasion. Ask about the patient's family and how it has coped with the illness and the transplant itself. Make some discreet enquiries about the patient's finances and whether there have been any problems returning to the transplant hospital for the various investigations required.

10. Ask about routine cardiac catheterisation. This is typically performed biannually in patients who have had transplants. Coronary artery intimal proliferation can cause ischaemic heart disease in the transplanted heart. Because the heart has been

Table 5.9 Commonly used immunosuppressants for heart transplant patients

DRUG	SIDE-EFFECTS	MONITORING / AVOIDANCE
Steroids	Cushingoid, diabetes, osteoporosis	Minimal dose
Cyclosporin	Renal impairment, hypertension, neurotoxicity	Blood levels, drug interactions
Mycophenolate	Mild marrow suppression, gastrointestinal upset	Reduce dose, check FBC
Methotrexate	Hepato- and marrow toxicity	FBC, liver function tests
Azathioprine	Hepato- and marrow toxicity, pancreatitis	FBC, liver function tests, TPMT
FBC = full blood count; TPMT = thiopurine methyltransferase.		

denervated there is not usually any pain. However, there are now patients in whom re-innervation seems to have occurred and led to symptoms of angina. This allograft arteriopathy is one of the most important problems after transplant. It represents a rejection phenomenon. The condition is usually diffuse, but once lesions causing 40% coronary stenosis have occurred, the prognosis is quite poor: the 2-year survival rate is only about 50%. The condition is present in 10% of recipients at 1-year post-transplant and in 50% at 5 years. Once myocardial infarction has occurred, the 2-year survival rate is only 10%–20%. Although the disease is a form of rejection, it is still considered important that the patient's cholesterol level be kept as low as possible. Find out whether the patient knows what his or her cholesterol level is and what treatment is being used to keep it low. Intravascular ultrasound is used increasingly to detect subclinical vasculopathy and to study the benefits of various antirejection regimens.

11. Hypertension is another important post-transplant problem. It is associated with the use of cyclosporin. Ask about blood pressure control and treatment.

12. Transplant patients have an increased risk of malignancy. Skin cancers (basal cell and squamous cell carcinomas) are common. There is also a higher incidence of lymphoproliferative disorders. Post-transplant lymphoproliferative disease (PTLD) is an increasingly recognised complication of the immunosuppression required for organ transplants. The incidence in heart transplant patients is less than that for those with liver transplants, but more than that for those with renal transplants. Primary or reactivated Epstein–Barr virus infection is thought to be the cause. The lesions tend to occur in unusual extranodal sites. Reduction in the amount of immunosuppression will sometimes help, but antiviral treatment with aciclovir or interferon may be necessary.

The examination

1. If the transplant has been successful, there should not be many signs. A median sternotomy scar will be present.
2. Look for signs of cardiac failure and pericarditis. Pericarditis can be an indication of rejection.
3. Note the small scars in the neck at the point of introduction of the endomyocardial biopsy forceps.
4. Look for any evidence of Cushing's syndrome from steroid therapy.
5. Examine the chest carefully for signs of infection, examine the mouth for candidiasis, look for infection at intravenous access sites and look at the temperature chart.

Investigations

These depend somewhat on the reason the patient has been admitted to hospital on this occasion.

1. Endomyocardial biopsies are performed routinely and at any suggestion of rejection. Ask about the results of these biopsies.
2. FBC may be indicated because of possible infection and to monitor the azathioprine dose.
3. Chest X-ray may show signs of cardiac enlargement, although this is a late sign of rejection. Changes of rejection on the ECG include a reduction in voltage caused by myocardial oedema or atrial arrhythmias. Sometimes the patient's ECG shows two sets of P waves: one comes from the transplanted heart and one arises from the residual atrium.

4. Recent assessments of myocardial function, including gated blood pool scans and resting or stress echocardiograms, may be available.
5. Routine coronary angiography may have been performed.
6. If there have been problems with possible infection, results of blood, urine and other cultures should be sought.

Management

The discussion should revolve around the patient's current problem or reason for admission. However, there is likely to be time to discuss the management of rejection, infection, cardiac failure or social problems.

1. Rejection may have been suspected because of pleuritic chest pain, deterioration in left ventricular function or ECG changes. It is diagnosed on the basis of a routine biopsy. The usual approach is to give the patient a boost of methylprednisolone – usually 1 g intravenously daily for 3 days – followed by a repeat biopsy.
2. Infections occurring as a result of immunosuppression are a major cause of death. Possible episodes of infection should be investigated thoroughly and treated aggressively with appropriate therapy. Opportunistic infections are relatively common as a late complication. Cytomegalovirus, herpes, *P. jirovecii*, fungal infection, and *Nocardia* and *Toxoplasma* are all more common than in non-immunosuppressed people.
3. Further cardiac failure may be an indication of rejection, which should be treated. Cardiac failure may also be an indication of silent myocardial infarction.
4. Hyperlipidaemia should be sought routinely and treated most vigorously with drugs and diet.
    There may be discussion about the patient's prognosis. The 1-year survival rate after transplant is about 90% and the 5-year survival rate is about 75%. The 10-year survival rate approaches 50%.
    The discussion of a patient awaiting cardiac transplantation will probably run along similar lines. However, it is important to know how well informed the patient is about what is likely to happen, whether he or she appears to fulfil the criteria for transplantation (see Table 5.8) and whether there appear to be any contraindications. Some patients awaiting transplantation are sick enough to require intravenous inotropes. There may even have been talk about the use of external circulatory assistance devices for use as a bridge to transplant.

Possible lines of questioning

1. How have *this* patient and his or her family dealt with this complicated illness?
2. What would make you suspect a rejection episode and how would you manage it?

Cardiac arrhythmias

The management of some cardiac rhythm disturbances is complicated. These patients may be in hospital while waiting for diagnostic tests or, in cases of serious arrhythmias, for treatment to become effective.

They sometimes represent diagnostic but more often management problems. Ventricular arrhythmias are a more common reason for admission than supraventricular arrhythmias, but patients with the latter may be awaiting diagnostic or therapeutic procedures. Atrial fibrillation (AF), the most common of the significant cardiac arrhythmias, is unlikely to be the patient's only problem if it appears in a long case.

The history

Ask why the patient is in hospital – all may be revealed without much further effort. Otherwise, the patient may know the name of the arrhythmia or be able to describe symptoms that make the diagnosis likely. If the rhythm problem is a serious and continuing one, the candidate may be fortunate enough to find the patient on an ECG monitor.

Possible presenting symptoms include:

1. rapid and irregular palpitations – suggest AF (Fig. 5.10)
2. rapid and regular palpitations, with or without dizziness and perhaps terminated by Valsalva manoeuvres – suggest supraventricular tachycardia (SVT) (Fig. 5.11)
3. rapid and regular palpitations with dizziness, syncope or near syncope – suggest ventricular tachycardia (VT), *particularly if there is a history of ischaemic heart disease*
4. syncope with bradycardia or no palpitations – suggests heart block (Fig. 5.12)
5. symptoms of AF and episodes of syncope – suggest sick sinus syndrome
6. a family history of sudden death – suggests the possibility of congenital long or short QT interval (Fig. 5.13), Brugada syndrome (channelopathy) or a structural cardiac problem such as hypertrophic cardiomyopathy
7. the occurrence of syncope in association with antiarrhythmic drug treatment – suggests the possibility of proarrhythmia; ask about class 1C drugs and sotalol, perhaps prescribed because of paroxysmal AF, as these drugs may also worsen bradyarrhythmias in patients with sick sinus syndrome.

Ask about previous known heart disease (e.g. ischaemic heart disease and VT, aortic stenosis and heart block) and recent cardiac, thoracic or abdominal surgery.

- Cardiac surgery may be complicated by heart block and all of the above may precipitate AF.

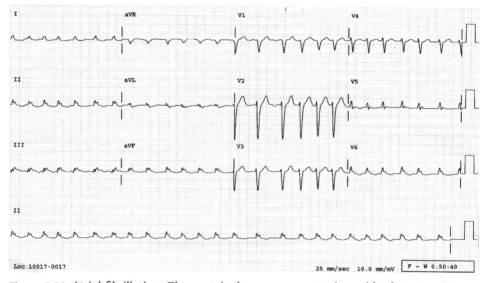

Figure 5.10 Atrial fibrillation. The ventricular response rate is rapid – between 95 and 160 beats / minute.

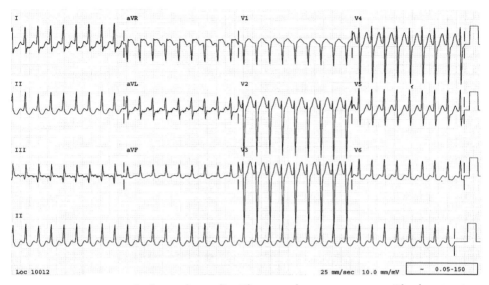

Figure 5.11 **Supraventricular tachycardia.** The complexes are narrow. The heart rate is about 200 beats / minute and the rhythm is regular.

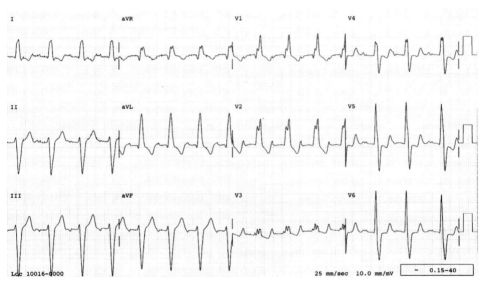

Figure 5.12 **Sinus rhythm. First-degree heart block, right bundle branch block (RBBB) and left anterior hemi-block (LAHB).** This combination of abnormalities is called *trifascicular block*. It is a sign of significant conduction system disease and, in a patient with recurrent syncope, suggests that intermittent complete heart block may be the cause of the symptoms.

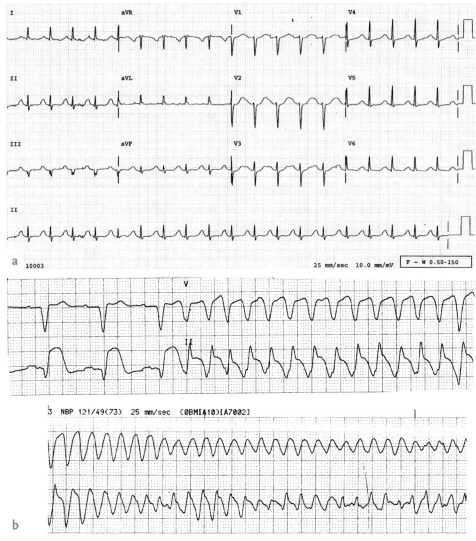

Figure 5.13 (a) Sinus rhythm. The QT interval is prolonged (423 ms) and the corrected QT (QTc) is 460 ms (normal < 440 ms). These patients are at risk of syncope or sudden death as a result of the development of polymorphic VT. (b) Polymorphic VT or *torsade de pointes*. This apparent twisting of the QRS complexes is named after the gold braid on French military uniforms.

- The 'grown-up' congenital heart disease patient may have persisting problems with atrial or ventricular arrhythmias following cardiac surgery in childhood.
- Atrial septal defects are often complicated by atrial arrhythmias even after they have been repaired.
- Consider the common causes and associations of AF:
  1. advancing age (3% of 65-year-olds, > 6% of people in their 80s)
  2. hypertension and obesity
  3. mitral valve disease

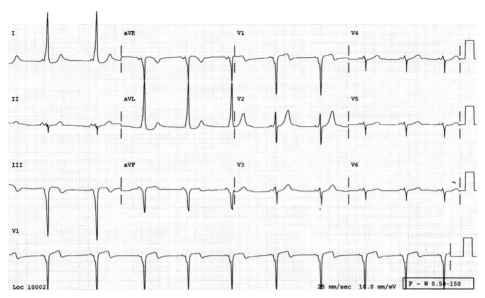

Figure 5.14 **Sinus rhythm. Wolff–Parkinson–White conduction. The PR interval is short and delta waves are visible. There are positive delta waves in lead I – seen as a slurred upstroke at the start of the R wave – and negative delta waves in lead III – seen as a slurred Q wave. These patients' ECGs are usually abnormal between their attacks of tachycardia but the *pre-excitation* (delta wave) may occur only intermittently. They are at risk of sudden death or syncope if atrial fibrillation or flutter occurs (they are often at increased risk of this arrhythmia) because very rapid ventricular rates may occur if the accessory pathway can conduct at high rates. Treat acute AF or flutter in this setting if unstable using electrical cardioversion (never use verapamil, adenosine or digoxin).**

4. ischaemic heart disease and myocardial infarction
5. recent thoracic or abdominal surgery
6. atrial septal defect
7. Wolff–Parkinson–White (WPW) syndrome (Figs 5.14 and 5.15)
8. alcohol excess and a recent alcoholic binge
9. pulmonary embolism
10. thyrotoxicosis
11. competitive exercise.

Ask whether the rhythm has been paroxysmal and self-limiting, persistent and requiring cardioversion, or permanent.

Find out about treatment.

1. Has the patient required intravenous drugs to control the heart? Have these been by infusion or by bolus injection? Intravenous adenosine is now the drug treatment of first choice for SVT. Patients may well remember its use. It causes a brief but distressing sensation of impending death.
2. Have physical manoeuvres been tried?
3. What oral drugs have been used in the past and during this admission? Make enquiries about the known side-effects of these drugs.

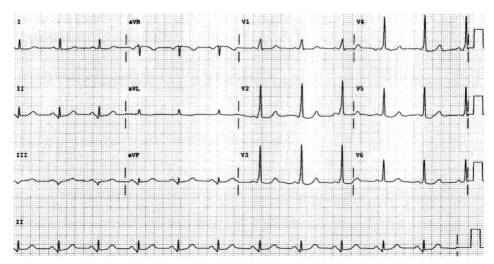

Figure 5.15 Sinus rhythm in WPW conduction. The delta waves and overall QRS are directed anteriorly in V1, superficially resembling RBBB. This is type A WPW where the bundle of Kent inserts into the left ventricular myocardium. Where the delta wave is initially isoelectric, the PR interval appears normal. Note also the close resemblance to an inferoposterior infarction.

4. The investigations the patient has undergone or may be about to undergo can help sort out the diagnosis.
   a. Certain tests, such as electrophysiological studies (EPSs), are more memorable than others. An EPS with induction of VT may mean that direct current (DC) cardioversion was required; despite sedation and reduced cardiac output, some memory of this may remain.
   b. A cardiac biopsy may have been performed to look for right ventricular cardiomyopathy (RV dysplasia), a cause of VT.
   c. Cardiac MRI, PET and CT scans are commonly used to look for the patchy changes of cardiac sarcoid or right ventricular cardiomyopathy (RV dysplasia).
   d. Other procedures may have been entirely therapeutic: for example, DC cardioversion performed electively under general anaesthesia suggests AF or atrial flutter; catheter ablation, often a fairly prolonged procedure, suggests SVT or VT; pacemaker insertion suggests bradycardia; antiarrhythmia surgery suggests VT or, less often now, SVT.
5. Catheter ablation is now a routine treatment for SVT that does not respond to simple drug treatment. Rarely there may be failure to suppress the arrhythmia, or a complication such as complete heart block or cardiac rupture can occur. Ablation is also very effective for many forms of VT. These include right, and the less common left, ventricular outflow tract tachycardias. These benign forms of VT can cause frequent recurrent episodes of self-limiting VT with LBBB or RBBB morphology, respectively. They may respond to treatment with verapamil, but are otherwise managed with catheter ablation. VT associated with previous infarction or a cardiomyopathy may also be treated with ablation, especially if episodes lead to more than occasional activation of the patient's defibrillator.
6. Patients with automatic implantable cardioverter-defibrillators (AICDs) can often provide vast amounts of useful information about their devices and about their arrhythmia.

The examination

Examine the cardiovascular system. Is the patient in sinus rhythm clinically? Look for thoracotomy scars, pacemakers and implanted defibrillators. Look for signs of cardiac failure, valvular heart disease and evidence of recent abdominal surgery or thyrotoxicosis.

Investigations

These depend on the actual rhythm problem.

1. **Resting ECG.** Look for:
   a. the current rhythm
   b. evidence of pre-excitation (Wolff–Parkinson–White conduction – see Fig. 5.15; Lown–Ganong–Levine syndrome)
   c. heart block
   d. old infarct
   e. paced rhythm (ventricular–ventricular inhibited (VVI) or dual-chamber atrial sensing and ventricular pacing or dual-chamber pacing)
   f. long QT interval (increased risk of polymorphic VT – *torsade de pointes*).
2. **The examiners may produce previous ECGs or parts of 24-hour Holter monitors.** Remember that a broad, complex tachycardia should be considered VT unless there is good reason to consider otherwise. There are a number of ECG criteria for distinguishing VT from SVT with aberrant conduction.
   Findings suggestive of VT include:
   a. a QRS > 0.14 seconds (if a RBBB pattern) or > 0.16 seconds (if a LBBB pattern)
   b. extreme axis deviation (between −90° and ±180°)
   c. atrioventricular (AV) dissociation (with P waves 'marching through' the QRS complexes)
   d. changes from the pre-existing QRS morphology in pre-existing bundle branch block (but note, these rules do not apply in SVT with aberration caused by WPW conduction).
      The presence of known ischaemic heart disease, or cardiac failure, is particularly useful. *Broad complex tachycardia in a patient with ischaemic heart disease is usually VT (95%).*
3. **EPS** may be used to assess inducibility of atrial and ventricular arrhythmias before and after treatment. It is now used in conjunction with catheter ablation as curative treatment for SVT caused by accessory pathways and for some types of VT. It can also be performed to ablate the AV node or the regions around the four pulmonary veins for patients with intractable and disabling AF. Ablation treatment has an increasing role for the management of ischaemic and non-ischaemic VT, usually in conjunction with an implanted cardioverter defibrillator.
4. **Routine investigations for patients with AF** include echocardiography, thyroid function testing and sometimes exercise testing. Echocardiography may reveal an underlying pathology that is responsible for the AF (e.g. mitral stenosis). It is important in helping to quantify embolic risk. Look at the echo for:
   a. valve abnormalities
   b. cardiomyopathy
   c. diastolic dysfunction of the left ventricle (especially important in hypertensive patients)
   d. left ventricular hypertrophy
   e. atrial size (consider atrial septal defect)
   f. mitral valve disease
   g. segmental wall abnormalities consistent with ischaemic heart disease.

Tests may be needed because of actual or potential drug side-effects (e.g. liver function or thyroid function tests for patients on amiodarone).

5. **Cardiac catheterisation** is often indicated for patients with ventricular arrhythmias, as they may have an ischaemic substrate. Patients whose VT has been stable but becomes unstable (often leading to more activity on the part of their cardioverter defibrillator) may have developed new ischaemia and should have this possibility investigated and treated.

Management

Much depends on the rhythm abnormality.

1. Arrhythmias that are not life-threatening are usually managed, at least at first, with drugs. Candidates will be expected to have a thorough working knowledge of the common antiarrhythmic drugs, their methods of action, indications and side-effects. Remember that many antiarrhythmic drugs have a potentially dangerous proarrhythmic effect.

2. The indications for permanent pacing (Table 5.10) and different uses for VVI, VVIR (rate-responsive) and DDD (dual-chamber) pacers (Figs 5.16 and 5.17) should be well understood. A basic understanding of antitachycardia devices and indications for their use (Table 5.11) is also important.

3. Automatic implanted cardioverter-defibrillators (AICDs) are increasingly used to manage recurrent VT.
   - They are often used in combination with antiarrhythmic drugs of some sort. They are becoming smaller, cheaper (between $25,000 and $40,000) and more complicated. It is now established that they improve mortality rates in selected patients.
   - They are usually the treatment of choice for hypotensive VT or missed sudden death from VF. Drug treatment of these conditions is not very effective.
   - The current models have leads that can be placed intravenously into the vena cava and for pacing purposes into the right ventricle.
   - They are small enough to be implanted like pacemakers in the chest wall, but are still noticeably larger than pacemakers (Fig. 5.18). Implantation takes place under local anaesthetic in the electrophysiology laboratory.

Table 5.10 Indications for permanent pacemaker insertion in adults

GENERALLY AGREED INDICATIONS

1. Intermittent or permanent complete heart block, with:
   a. symptomatic bradycardia
   b. cardiac failure
   c. arrhythmias that require treatment with drugs that slow conduction
   d. documented asystole of more than 3 seconds or escape rhythm with a rate < 40 beats / minute
   e. confusional states that improve with temporary pacing
2. Intermittent permanent second-degree AV block with symptomatic bradycardia
3. Sinus node dysfunction with symptomatic bradycardia

LESS CERTAIN INDICATIONS

1. Asymptomatic complete heart block; heart rate ≥ 40 beats / minute
2. Symptomatic type 2 second-degree heart block
3. Bifascicular or trifascicular block with syncope of unknown aetiology

NOT INDICATED

1. First-degree heart block
2. Asymptomatic type 1 second-degree heart block

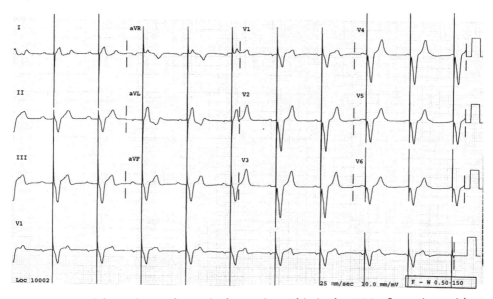

Figure 5.16 **Atrial sensing and ventricular pacing. This is the ECG of a patient with a dual-chamber pacemaker. Normal P waves are followed by an atrioventricular (PR) interval and then a pacing spike, which precedes a wide QRS complex with an LBBB pattern (pacing is from the right ventricular apex).**

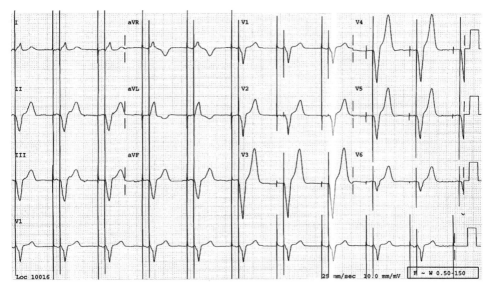

Figure 5.17 **Dual-chamber pacing. Pacing spikes precede both atrial and ventricular complexes.**

- The periprocedural mortality rate is less than 1%, compared with over 5% when surgical implantation was required.

The programming of these machines is complicated, but candidates should know that they are usually set to attempt reversion of VT by overdrive pacing (antitachycardia pacing, ATP) before administering a DC shock. Patients are usually, but not always,

Table 5.11 Indications for implanted cardioverter-defibrillators (ICDs)
GENERALLY AGREED INDICATIONS
1. Confirmed VF or hypotensive VT not related to acute infarct or severe electrolyte abnormality, but VF / VT not inducible at EPS – this means drug treatment cannot be tested by EPS
2. VF / VT with contraindications to drug treatment (intolerance)
3. Persistently inducible VT / VF despite drug treatment, ablation or surgery
4. Persistent spontaneous VT / VF despite drug treatment
5. Symptomatic long QT syndrome despite drug treatment
LESS CERTAIN INDICATIONS
1. Inducible but not spontaneous VT despite other treatment in high-risk patients
2. VT / VF apparently controlled, but in a high-risk patient
3. Serial drug testing possible, but defibrillator preferred
NOT GENERALLY INDICATED
1. Very frequent or incessant VT
2. Reversible cause
3. Recurrent syncope, VT / VF not inducible
4. Poor life expectancy (e.g. class IV cardiac failure, but not a transplant candidate)
Note: Increasingly proven VT or VF in a patient with poor LV function is considered an indication regardless of EPS findings. EPS = electrophysiological study; VF = ventricular fibrillation; VT = ventricular tachycardia.

Table 5.12 Assessment of patients experiencing frequent activations of a defibrillator
1. Check programming, e.g. false activations for AF or sinus tachycardia.
2. Exclude new ischaemia.
3. Introduce or increase antiarrhythmic treatment – usually amiodarone or beta-blocker.
4. Consider VT ablation.
AF = atrial fibrillation; VT = ventricular tachycardia.

aware of the onset of ATP and almost always aware of DC shock administration. Ask how the device has affected the patient's life and confidence, including how often it goes off and whether the box itself causes problems because of its size. Although AICDs can prevent sudden death, their presence is often associated with a feeling of insecurity. Patients may have clear memories of events leading up to activation of the device. They may avoid places where arrhythmias and activations have occurred. They often require repeated explanation and reassurance.

Patients who have begun to experience frequent episodes requiring ATP or DC shocks need to be assessed (Table 5.12).

Possible lines of questioning

1. How would you explain to *this* patient the risks and benefits of having an implanted defibrillator?

2. What would be your approach to a patient who has begun to receive frequent shocks from his or her device and has asked for it to be removed?

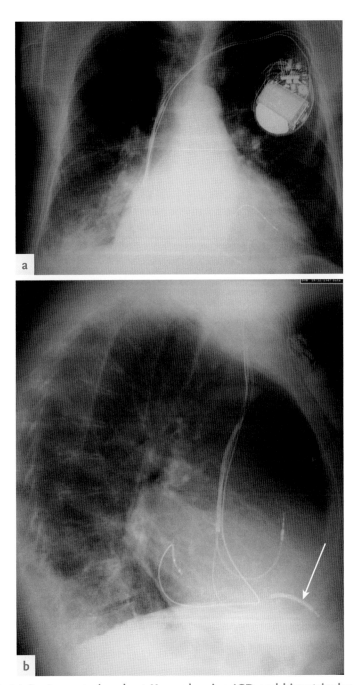

Figure 5.18 (a) Posteroanterior chest X-ray showing ICD and biventricular pacemaker. (b) Lateral view: the large defibrillation electrode (which also serves as an RV pacing electrode) (arrow) and the right atrial and left ventricular pacing leads are visible.

Figures reproduced courtesy of The Canberra Hospital.

The particular management problems of atrial fibrillation

Examiners require candidates to have a sensible approach to the management of AF and the opportunity for examiners to ask about this common condition will often arise. The principles of management are to:

- maintain sinus rhythm
- control the heart rate (if maintaining sinus rhythm proves difficult)
- protect from embolic events.

1. There is good evidence from recent trials that control of heart rate is at least as satisfactory an approach as that of trying aggressively to maintain sinus rhythm. Nevertheless, patients with paroxysmal AF often find the arrhythmia very disturbing. They should be told at the outset that it may not be possible to keep them in sinus rhythm, but that rate control and freedom from embolic episodes can be achieved. The prophylactic drug treatment of paroxysmal AF involves the use of a class III drug (sotalol or amiodarone) in most cases, but occasionally the class 1C drug flecainide can be used if the patient does not have ischaemic heart disease.

2. Rate control of persistent or paroxysmal AF can be achieved with less-toxic drugs. Digoxin is a common first-line treatment and is usually well tolerated. Some recent trials have suggested an increased mortality for patients treated with digoxin. It is not very effective on its own at controlling the heart rate during exercise. Many patients with chronic AF have persistent dyspnoea during exercise because of inadequate rate control. They benefit from the use of a beta-blocker or one of the non-dihydropyridine calcium channel blockers (diltiazem or verapamil). These can be used with or without digoxin. Control of the heart rate can prevent or reverse the impairment of left ventricular function that is associated with tachycardias (tachycardia-induced cardiomyopathy).

3. When patients remain unhappy with their symptoms despite rate control, further intervention should be considered.

4. DC cardioversion of AF can be a reasonable treatment for the first episode or for patients with infrequent episodes. DC cardioversion is safe in the absence of digoxin toxicity or hypokalaemia, but is associated with a risk of embolism if the patient's AF has been present for more than 48 hours. In this case, 1 month's therapeutic anticoagulation should be instituted before the procedure and continued for 4 weeks afterwards. An alternative is to perform a transoesophageal echocardiogram to look for left atrial appendage thrombus or spontaneous echocardiograph contrast (a sign of slow blood flow). The absence of these means that DC cardioversion is safe, but that warfarin must be given for 4 weeks afterwards because there is a persisting risk over this period.

5. Reversion of AF with drug treatment is difficult. Many episodes terminate spontaneously but drug treatment is given the credit. It is known that digoxin does not increase the reversion rate, but the class III drugs and flecainide do improve the chances somewhat. Sometimes control of the heart rate and awaiting spontaneous reversion can be an option. A decision to go on to DC cardioversion, however, should be made before 48 hours has passed.

6. Over many years attempts have been made to prevent AF by surgical or catheter ablation techniques. Pulmonary vein isolation is now commonly performed for intractable symptomatic AF. Radiofrequency energy is used to isolate the two pairs of pulmonary veins in the left atrium. The rationale for this approach is that almost all AF seems to be initiated by electrical activity arising from this part of the heart. Isolation of this area from the rest of the heart prevents the initiation of AF. The

Table 5.13 Major complications of atrial fibrillation ablation treatment
1. Cardiac perforation and pericardial tamponade
2. Complete heart block
3. Pulmonary vein stenosis
4. Atrio-oesophageal fistula
5. Constrictive pericarditis
The risk of a major complication is between 3% and 5%.

procedure is complicated and time-consuming (3–4 hours per case). It is not a practical solution for most cases of AF. Success rates of about 70% are usually quoted. Complications are not rare (Table 5.13). Success is more likely if:

- the AF is paroxysmal
- the left atrium is not very large
- the patient is not obese
- the patient does not drink much alcohol.

There is controversy over whether stopping anticoagulation is safe for patients with apparently successful ablation.

7. Protecting patients from embolic events is perhaps the most important aspect of the management of AF. Cerebral embolus is the most feared complication, but life-threatening peripheral embolisation (e.g. to the mesenteric bed) can occur. Patients should have this aspect of AF explained to them early on. The risk of embolism is low in people under the age of 60 and without any risk factors: < 0.5% a year. It can be as high as 30% for patients with mitral stenosis. The most recent advice has been to anticoagulate unless a patient seems at really low risk.

Use the CHA_2DS_2-VASc scoring (Birmingham 2009) system to help you decide whom to anticoagulate with AF:

CHA_2DS_2-VASc scoring system

Congestive heart failure (or LV systolic dysfunction): 1 point
Hypertension: 1 point
Age 75 and over: 2 points
Diabetes mellitus: 1 point
Stroke or TIA or thromboembolism: 2 points
Vascular disease (e.g. peripheral artery disease, myocardial infarction, aortic plaque): 1 point
Age 65–74: 1 point
Sc Sex category (i.e. female): 1 point

score = 0	no treatment
score = 1	male anticoagulant, female no treatment
score = 2 or more	anticoagulant

8. Patients with risk factors remain at risk of stroke even if sinus rhythm has been restored. Those with self-limiting paroxysmal AF are also at risk if episodes are more than a rare event. Antiplatelet drugs have no place in the current management of

Table 5.14 Novel oral anticoagulant (NOAC) doses for stroke prevention in atrial fibrillation		
DRUG	**DOSE**	**DOSE ADJUSTMENT**
Rivaroxaban	20 mg / day	15 mg if CrCl 30–49 mL / min
Apixaban	5 mg BD	2.5 mg BD if 2 of: age ≥ 80, weight ≤ 60 kg, creatinine ≥ 130 µmol / L
Dabigitran	150 mg BD	110 mg if age > 75 or CrCl 30–50 mL / min

AF. If anticoagulation is absolutely contraindicated, some physicians will pragmatically prescribe antiplatelet therapy (e.g. aspirin and clopidogrel) but any benefit is not evidence based.

9. Novel (non-vitamin-K antagonist) oral antithrombotic agents (NOACs) are the treatment of choice for these patients. They are at least as safe and effective as warfarin. They include: dabigatran, an oral antithrombin drug, and apixaban and rivaroxaban, which are activated factor X antagonists. The drugs are effective within a few hours of the first dose. The doses need to be reduced if renal function is impaired and the drugs are contraindicated for patients with severe chronic kidney disease (CKD) (CrCl < 30 mL / min). The current recommended dose regimens are shown in Table 5.14. In the United States and in some Australian renal units the drugs are being used for patients with very poor renal function and for dialysis patients. Gastrointestinal side-effects are common. The drugs cannot be monitored. They are not indicated for valvular AF (this means mitral stenosis or any type of mechanical valve replacement, but not other valve abnormalities). Dabigitran can be reversed and dialysed.

10. If warfarin is to be used, an assessment of the patient's ability to manage regular blood tests and dosage adjustments is necessary before treatment can begin. Patients are often reluctant to undertake the complexities of treatment but should be advised against declining therapy until all the risks of this approach versus alternatives have been carefully explained. The availability of home international normalised ratio (INR) testing machines that use a capillary blood sample has made the use of warfarin more acceptable to some patients (e.g. those who travel frequently). A number of studies have shown that this approach is safe for selected patients. The safe therapeutic range is an INR of between 2 and 2.5. Find out from the patient how the warfarin is managed and whether he or she knows the last few readings and dosage. Patients should be encouraged to keep a record of their INR results and warfarin doses. The examiners will expect considerable detail about the patient's warfarin management.

Remember that episodes of AF, for example, on a Holter monitor or at pacemaker interrogation, must last longer than 30 seconds to be considered significant. Trials are under way to determine the minimum length of an episode of AF that involves an embolic risk. It may be considerably longer than 30 seconds.

The management of patients who are anticoagulated and have an acute coronary syndrome is controversial (there are no definitive trials). Consider:

1. continuing warfarin or NOAC
2. reducing heparin dose during intervention
3. aspirin and clopidogrel or just clopidogrel (not ticagrelor)
4. a modern drug-eluting stent
5. discharge on clopidogrel and anticoagulant for 1–12 months, then anticoagulant alone.

Remember the aim is to balance bleeding and thrombotic risk.

THE PROBLEM OF AF AND RENAL FAILURE

Dialysis and severe CKD patients (eGFR < 30 mL/min) have both an increased thrombotic and an increased haemorrhagic risk. There is no clear evidence that they benefit from anticoagulation with warfarin. The decision should be individualised. For example, a young dialysis patient who has already had a stroke may benefit from treatment whereas an older patient with difficult-to-control hypertension and previous haemorrhagic problems may not.

Possible lines of questioning

1. How does *this* patient manage his or her warfarin treatment? Would you recommend changes?
2. Is *this* patient a candidate for a NOAC?
3. How would you advise *this* patient with CKD and AF with regard to anticoagulation?

Chapter 6

The respiratory long case

I here present the reader with a new sign, which I have discovered for detecting diseases of the chest. This consists in percussion ...

Leopold Auenbrugger (1760)

Bronchiectasis

Bronchiectasis is a reasonably common subject for a long case and usually poses a management problem. It is defined as pathological and permanent dilatation of the bronchi. There are associated destructive and inflammatory changes in the walls of the segmental and subsegmental bronchi. The diagnosis is not always straightforward because there are overlap syndromes (e.g. chronic obstructive pulmonary disease (COPD), asthma and chronic bronchitis) (Table 6.1).

The history

1. Find out when the patient's respiratory problems began. Cough and sputum production often begin in childhood, although adult onset is becoming more common.
   a. Ask about childhood whooping cough or measles.
   b. Lower respiratory tract infection with influenza and adenoviruses is an increasingly common cause of the disease.
   c. Potentially necrotising bacteria are also a cause if antibiotic treatment is inadequate – these include *Staphylococcus aureus* and *Klebsiella* organisms. The abnormal pulmonary defence mechanisms, or mucus clearance, associated with cystic fibrosis, tuberculosis (the most common cause worldwide), immunoglobulin deficiency, HIV infection and primary ciliary dyskinesia (immotile cilia syndrome), make these important causes of the condition.
   d. Localised bronchiectasis can occur in association with a space-occupying lesion, which can be endobronchial or a foreign body or longstanding lymphadenopathy. Symptoms include:
      - recurrent haemoptysis
      - dyspnoea and wheeze
      - chronic sinusitis (70%)

Table 6.1 Features suggesting predominant bronchiectasis
1. Clubbing (not present in chronic obstructive pulmonary disease or asthma)
2. Suspected chronic obstructive pulmonary disease, but smoking history less than 10 packet years
3. History of tuberculosis or recurrent pneumonia
4. Disadvantaged childhood
5. Unusual organisms in sputum (e.g. *Aspergillus*, atypical mycobacteria, *Escherichia coli*, *Klebsiella* spp.)

- recurrent pneumonia
- pleurisy
- systemic symptoms of weight loss
- fever
- anorexia
- symptoms of right heart failure – a late event.

2. Ask about recent precipitating causes of admissions to hospital (e.g. infection, haemoptysis).
3. Enquire about treatment – physiotherapy, postural drainage, antibiotics (as prophylaxis or treatment), bronchodilators, lung resection.
4. Determine whether the patient had childhood immunisations (e.g. MMR).
5. Ask about investigations in the past (e.g. CT scanning, ciliary function studies, sweat test).
6. Establish aetiology, such as childhood or early adult infections (e.g. pneumonia, measles, whooping cough) (Table 6.2). The majority of cases have no obvious cause if those due to cystic fibrosis are excluded.
7. Ask how the disease interferes with the patient's life (e.g. work). Infertility is usual in men with primary ciliary dyskinesia and is variable in affected women.

The examination

Examine the respiratory system carefully (see Table 16.10, p. 446).

1. Particularly note the unpleasant purulent sputum.
2. Examine carefully for clubbing, the yellow nail syndrome and localised crackles and wheezes.
3. Look for the position of the apex beat (don't miss dextrocardia – Kartagener's syndrome) and for the signs of right heart failure.
4. Consider the complications and look for them. These include:
   a. pneumonia
   b. pleurisy
   c. empyema
   d. lung abscess
   e. cor pulmonale
   f. cerebral abscess (very rare)
   g. amyloid (rare, but an important topic in the examination).

Investigations

Investigations should include:

- **chest X-ray film** (Fig. 6.1a) – which may be normal, or it may show 1–2 cm cystic lesions or, more often, streaky infiltration and thickened bronchial walls (tram tracking), especially in the lower lobes

Table 6.2 Causes of bronchiectasis

1. Congenital
   a. Cystic fibrosis
   b. Primary ciliary dyskinesia, including the immotile cilia syndrome (Young's syndrome)
   c. Congenital hypogammaglobulinaemia (especially IgA and IgG subclasses)
   d. Yellow nail syndrome
2. Acquired
   a. Infections in childhood (e.g. tuberculosis, pneumonia, measles, whooping cough)
   b. Localised disease (e.g. bronchial adenoma, tuberculosis, foreign body)
   c. Allergic bronchopulmonary aspergillosis (proximal bronchiectasis)
   d. Rheumatoid arthritis, Sjögren's syndrome
   e. Chronic obstructive pulmonary disease
   f. Recurrent aspiration
   g. Interstitial lung disease and pneumoconiosis
   h. Idiopathic (up to 50%)

Notes: Lung carcinoma rarely causes bronchiectasis as death tends to intervene first.
Aboriginal Australians who grew up in remote areas are at particular risk.

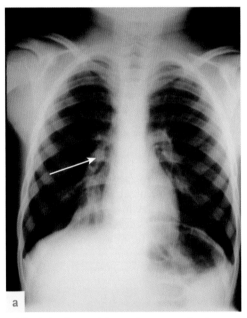

Figure 6.1 (a) **Right middle lobe bronchiectasis. Note the increased lung markings and the thickened bronchial walls (arrow).**

Figure reproduced courtesy of The Canberra Hospital.

- **sputum microscopy and culture** – the common organisms are *Haemophilus influenzae, Pseudomonas, E. coli,* pneumococcus, mycobacteria and *Staphylococcus aureus*
- **immunoglobulin (IgG, IgM, IgA) levels** (hypogammaglobulinaemia)
- **tests for cystic fibrosis and immotile cilia syndrome in young adults**
- **blood film for eosinophilia** – which may indicate allergic bronchopulmonary aspergillosis or asthma

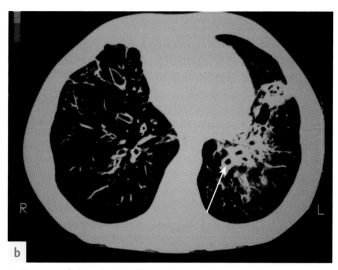

Figure 6.1 (b) **CT scan of the chest of a patient with bronchiectasis. Note the thickened bronchial walls (arrow).**

Figure reproduced courtesy of The Canberra Hospital.

- **ventilatory function tests** – which may show a restrictive defect or an obstructive pattern. They are therefore more useful in assessing severity than in making the diagnosis. A patient with bronchiectasis with a forced expiratory volume in 1 second (FEV_1) of < 40% predicted is said to have severe disease
- **arterial blood gas estimations** – which may show mild or moderate hypoxia and, later, respiratory failure – defined as an arterial oxygen tension (PaO_2) < 60 mmHg or an arterial carbon dioxide tension ($PaCO_2$) > 50 mmHg
- **high-resolution CT scanning (HRCT) of the chest** (Fig. 6.1b) – which is indicated in most patients to confirm the diagnosis. The typical findings are of airway dilatation (usually defined as a diameter greater than that of the accompanying branch of the pulmonary artery). Temporary dilatation can occur during acute infections so the scan should be performed when the patient is stable. Remember, the radiation dose of an HRCT is about 8 mSv and the test should be used sparingly, especially in children and young adults.

    The disease is usually generalised but if the scan shows it to be localised then resection may be indicated as long as the underlying cause is not systemic.

Treatment

The principles of treatment are as follows.

1. The facilitation (or maximisation) of clearance of sputum and the treatment of infection with antibiotics and of bronchoconstriction with bronchodilators.
2. Inhaled steroids may be of value if there is bronchial reactivity.
3. Twice-daily postural drainage (20 minutes morning and night) or newer physiotherapy techniques should be recommended (e.g. use of a flutter valve). Head-down drainage is now discouraged because of the risk of aspiration.
4. The use of antibiotics during exacerbations is routine, though of unproven benefit, and prednisone in tapered doses may be useful. The use of prophylactic nebulised antibiotics is a controversial treatment. Problem pathogens include *Mycobacterium*

avium complex (MAC), *Pseudomonas* and *Aspergillus*. Patients with frequent infections may benefit from long-term antibiotic treatment with macrolides. Recombinant deoxyribonuclease is useful for cystic fibrosis patients, but may be harmful for other patients with bronchiectasis.

5. Influenza and pneumococcal vaccines are advisable for all patients.
6. Treatment of heart failure should go *pari passu* with that of the lung disease.
7. Immunoglobulin deficiency can be treated with monthly IV injections of immuno-globulin, which decrease the incidence of infection and the need for hospitalisation.
8. Massive haemoptysis may occur as a result of bronchial wall erosion and the increased vascularity of the bronchial walls. It may respond to bronchial artery embolisation.
9. Smoking cessation (including of marijuana) is always essential.
10. Home oxygen is of unproven benefit but is often prescribed (to non-smoking patients) in severe disease ($FEV_1 < 40\%$). A screening test for eligibility is oxygen saturation of 93% or less on room air.
11. Surgery should be considered for localised disease to prevent progression, or as treatment of intractable haemorrhage.
12. Transplant is occasionally appropriate for end-stage disease.

Possible lines of questioning

1. How satisfactory do you think *this* patient's physiotherapy management has been?
2. Has *this* patient an effective plan to manage exacerbations of his or her disease at home?
3. How realistic is *this* patient's idea of the prognosis of the disease?
4. How much was *this* patient's childhood – education, sport and social activity – affected by the disease?

Lung carcinoma

Lung carcinoma is a common disease that candidates often encounter in the examination. It can pose a diagnostic and management problem, and remains a leading cause of cancer death in men and women. At diagnosis only 20% of patients will have local disease and half will have disseminated disease. The overall 5-year survival rate is less than 15%. The major cell types are set out in Table 6.3. Over the past 25 years, adeno-carcinoma has become more common than squamous cell carcinoma.

Table 6.3 Carcinoma of the lung – cell types

TYPE	FREQUENCY (%)	OVERALL 5-YEAR SURVIVAL RATE (%)
Adenocarcinoma	32	17
Squamous cell	29	15
Small (oat) cell	18	5
Large cell	9	11
Bronchioalveolar	3	42

The history

1. Find out how the diagnosis was made or suspected – a proportion of patients are asymptomatic and were diagnosed after a routine chest X-ray or scan. The most common early symptom is cough or change in the character of a smoker's cough.
2. Ask about the duration of illness and respiratory symptoms (e.g. haemoptysis, dyspnoea, increasing cough, chest pain), which may be very recent with a rapid growing tumour (e.g. small cell carcinoma). Dyspnoea may be due to associated COPD or to a pleural effusion, infection or bronchial obstruction. Pleural infiltration can cause chest pain.
3. Enquire about a history of unresolved pneumonia (a common reason for investigations to exclude carcinoma of the lung), pleural effusion or lung abscess.
4. Ask about systemic symptoms (e.g. weight loss, loss of appetite, lethargy).
5. Determine metastatic and non-metastatic symptoms (Table 6.4).
6. Ask about aetiology:
   a. smoking and exposure to the cigarette smoke of others (a dose–response relationship – long-term smokers have a 10- to 30-fold risk; discontinuation of smoking reduces the risk over 10–15 years, but the relative risk does not return to 1.0); women have a higher risk for a given level of exposure to cigarette smoke than men (1.5 : 1)
   b. genetics – there is a familial association, and *EGFR* and *ALK* mutations in adenocarcinoma
   c. occupational history (e.g. asbestos exposure, uranium miners); remember, the effect of asbestos plus smoking is synergistic, *not* additive: smoking and exposure to asbestos combined increase the risk 90-fold. Smoking, however, does not increase the risk of mesothelioma
   d. chronic scarring (e.g. tuberculosis, scleroderma, interstitial lung disease (ILD)) may be associated with adenocarcinoma.
7. Ask about investigations performed, such as chest X-ray changes (the only abnormal finding in 5% of cases), CT scans, bronchoscopy, sputum cytology, needle biopsy and thoracotomy. PET / CT scanning is used to assess for metastatic disease. It has been shown to detect metastases in up to 20% of patients previously thought suitable for surgery. The finding of a solitary nodule on a chest X-ray must be investigated, but benign causes include a post-infection granuloma or a hamartoma.
8. Enquire about the patient's work and home environments, including the number of dependants and the patient's ability to work.
9. Ask about treatment offered and begun.
10. Find out the patient's understanding of the condition and the likely prognosis.

The examination

1. Finger clubbing is a most important sign (see Table 16.11, p. 447). This is very rare in small cell carcinoma.
2. Chest signs will vary – listen carefully for a fixed inspiratory wheeze over a large bronchus – sign of bronchial obstruction by tumour.
3. Recurrent laryngeal nerve palsy may have caused hoarseness, and phrenic nerve paralysis may have caused an elevation of a hemidiaphragm.
4. An apical tumour may be responsible for Pancoast's syndrome (C8, T1 thoracic nerve destruction or compression, or Horner's syndrome, or both).
5. SVC obstruction can occur owing to central tumours (e.g. squamous cell, small cell). Test for Pemberton sign (facial congestion and cyanosis if patient elevates both arms).
6. Look for metastatic (e.g. supraclavicular lymphadenopathy and hepatomegaly) and non-metastatic manifestations, especially the neurological and endocrinological changes (see Table 6.4).

Table 6.4 Metastatic and non-metastatic manifestations of lung carcinoma

LOCAL EXTENSION
1. Pleural effusion
2. Rib involvement
3. Nerve involvement (e.g. Pancoast's tumour, Horner's syndrome, recurrent laryngeal nerve palsy, diaphragmatic paralysis)
4. Superior vena caval obstruction
5. Pericardial effusion
6. Oesophageal obstruction
7. Tracheal obstruction
8. Lymphangitis

DISTANT METASTASES
1. Cervical adenopathy
2. Cerebral, liver or bone metastases

NON-METASTATIC FEATURES
1. Anorexia, weight loss, cachexia, fever
2. Endocrine:
   a. Hypercalcaemia (increased parathyroid hormone occurs usually in squamous cell carcinoma)
   b. Hyponatraemia (antidiuretic hormone – small cell carcinoma)
   c. Ectopic adrenocorticotrophic hormone (ACTH) syndrome (usually small cell carcinoma)
   d. Gynaecomastia (all types – caused by ectopic gonadotrophin secretion)
   e. Carcinoid syndrome (small cell carcinoma)
   f. Insulin-like activity (squamous cell carcinoma)
3. Skeletal (very rare with small cell carcinoma):
   a. Clubbing
   b. Hypertrophic pulmonary osteoarthropathy (may be more common with adenocarcinoma)
4. Neurological:
   a. Eaton Lambert's syndrome (small cell carcinoma)
   b. Peripheral neuropathy or autonomic neuropathy
   c. Subacute cerebellar degeneration
   d. Polymyositis / dermatomyositis
   e. Cortical degeneration with dementia
   f. Acute transverse myelopathy
5. Haematological:
   a. Migrating venous thrombophlebitis, arterial thrombosis
   b. Diffuse intravascular coagulation
   c. Anaemia, leukoerythroblastosis, red cell aplasia, polycythaemia, eosinophilia
6. Skin: e.g. acanthosis nigricans, fibrinolytic purpura, scleroderma (alveolar cell carcinoma)
7. Renal: e.g. nephrotic syndrome (due to membranous glomerulonephritis)
8. Opportunistic infections (most often in those treated with chemotherapy)

Investigations

Screening of high-risk patients with chest X-ray or CT scanning may lead to an early diagnosis, but has not been shown to affect survival. The diagnosis may be difficult, even when suspected.

1. Sputum cytology may be helpful in centrally located lesions, but fibreoptic bronchoscopy is now more often done first.

2. The chest X-ray or CT may suggest the cell type: for example, peripheral nodule adenocarcinoma; central lesion with obstructive pneumonitis – squamous; mediastinal or hilar mass – small cell; or alveolar infiltrate – bronchoalveolar cell. Cavitation can occur, but not in small cell lung cancer.

3. A suspect shadow on the chest X-ray film should be investigated by fibreoptic bronchoscopy and biopsy or fine-needle aspiration (Fig. 6.2a and b). Bronchial brushings and washings, taken at bronchoscopy, should also be sent for cytological examination but have a lower yield than biopsy.

4. For peripheral lesions, especially those less than 2 cm in size, transthoracic fine-needle biopsy with CT guidance is very useful, but complications (e.g. pneumothorax, significant bleeding) can occur.

5. In patients with a malignant pleural effusion, thoracocentesis and pleural biopsy provide a high diagnostic yield (may need to be repeated if initially negative) (see Table 16.12, p. 449).

6. Other investigations may include bone marrow biopsy, mediastinoscopy and thoracotomy. Endobronchial ultrasound guided biopsy (EBUS) has replaced surgical biopsy in many centres.

7. Other possible causes (e.g. of a coin lesion) must be excluded. For this purpose, CT is helpful; demonstration of central or lamellar calcification usually indicates that a coin lesion is benign. Follow-up scans to confirm a lesion is unchanged are helpful. Positron emission tomography (PET) scans may be of value in cases when lesions are over 1 cm.

8. Once the diagnosis is made and the cell type identified, further investigations may be indicated to stage the disease.
   a. Symptoms and signs that suggest central nervous system, liver, bone, chest wall or mediastinal involvement need to be sought carefully.
   b. Full blood count (Table 6.5), serum calcium and liver function tests may suggest tumour spread.
   c. CT scanning of the chest and abdomen with contrast is an important aid in determining whether disease is localised.
   d. In small cell carcinoma, stage the disease into limited disease (lung primary, ipsilateral and contralateral hilar, mediastinal and supraclavicular nodes) or extensive disease – 70% of patients (contralateral lung, distant metastases).
   e. Non-small cell carcinoma is staged according to the tumour node metastases (TNM) international staging system (Table 6.6). In general, disease confined to one hemithorax and the ipsilateral cervical nodes is called *limited* and further involvement is described as *extensive* disease.

9. Assessment for resectability should include respiratory function tests. If the forced expiratory volume (FEV_1) is 1.5 L or more, this indicates that the patient could tolerate a pneumonectomy (a postoperative FEV_1 of 1 L or more is usually considered the minimum that will be tolerated). Otherwise, a patient who can climb three flights of stairs is usually considered well enough to tolerate surgery.

HINTS

- The size of a lesion is the most important factor in determining the likelihood of malignancy. Nodules < 8 mm in diameter have a 98% chance of being benign. Most lesions > 2 cm are malignant.
- A smooth border suggests a benign lesion; a spiculated border suggests malignancy.

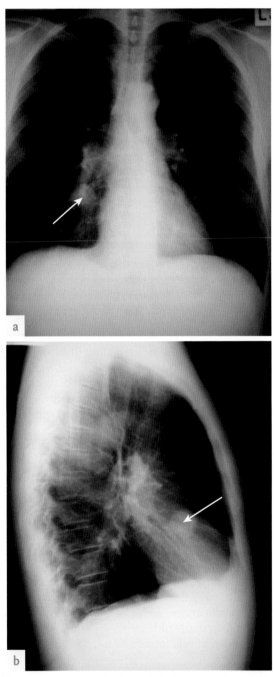

Figure 6.2 (a) PA film. A round opacity is visible in the right middle lobe (arrow). (b) Lateral film. A round opacity is visible in the right middle lobe (arrow).

Figures reproduced courtesy of The Canberra Hospital.

Table 6.5 Full blood count and liver function tests from a female patient with carcinoma of the lung

PARAMETER	VALUE	NORMAL VALUE
Haemoglobin	84 g/L	115–165 g/L (female)
Mean corpuscular volume (MCV)	95 fL	80–100 fL
White cell count (WCC)	$4.0 \times 10^9/L$	$4.5–13.5 \times 10^9/L$
Platelets	$95 \times 10^9/L$	$150–400 \times 10^9/L$
Erythrocyte sedimentation rate (ESR)	70 mm/h	3–19 mm/h (female < 50 years)
Bilirubin	84 mmol/L	< 20 mmol/L (total)
Aspartate aminotransferase (AST)	57 U/L	< 40 U/L
Alanine aminotransferase (ALT)	50 U/L	< 35 U/L
Lactate dehydrogenase (LDH)	780 U/L	110–230 U/L
Protein	60 g/L	62–80 g/L (total)
Albumin	33 g/L	32–45 g/L

Blood film: normochromic red cells, poikilocytosis, tear-drop cells. Some nucleated red cells (normoblasts) and myeloid cells (metamyelocytes and myelocytes). Some rouleaux formation. *Comment:* The combination of normochromic anaemia and the presence of marrow precursors in the peripheral blood is called a leukoerythroblastic reaction. It is typical of bone marrow infiltration by carcinoma or fibrosis. The abnormal liver function tests are non-specific, but suggest liver involvement in this setting. The elevated LDH level probably indicates liver damage, but can also occur when there is haemolysis.

Table 6.6 TNM international staging system for carcinoma of the lung (non-small cell)

STAGE	TNM			5-YEAR SURVIVAL RATE (%)	MANAGEMENT
IA	T1	N0	M0	61	Surgery
IB	T2	N0	M0	38	Surgery
IIA	T1	N1	M0	34	Surgery ± radiotherapy or chemotherapy
IIB	T2	N2	M0	24	Surgery ± radiotherapy or chemotherapy
IIIA	T3	N1	M0	9	Surgery + chemotherapy
	T1–3	N2	M0	13	Surgery and/or chemotherapy and/or radiotherapy
IIIB	T4	N0–2	M0	9	Surgery and/or chemotherapy and/or radiotherapy
	T1–4	N3	M0	3	Chemotherapy or palliation
IV			M1	1	Chemotherapy or palliation

M0 = no metastases; M1–M4 = ascending degrees of metastatic involvement; N0 = no lymph nodes; N1–N4 = ascending degrees of nodal involvement; T1–T4 = ascending degrees of increase in tumour size and involvement.

Treatment

The average 5-year survival rate for all types of carcinoma of the lung is about 15%.

SMALL CELL CARCINOMAS

1. These are only occasionally resected as they have usually metastasised at the time of diagnosis. They are, however, sensitive to chemotherapy and radiotherapy. Urgent therapy is needed if there is superior vena cava obstruction.
2. In patients with limited disease, chemotherapy and concurrent radiotherapy improve the prognosis. Untreated, the median survival is only about 4 months. Treatment often includes platinum-based drugs – etoposide and cisplatin or carboplatin.
3. Prophylactic cranial irradiation may be given to patients with complete responses. There is a risk of leukaemia, central nervous system metastases, dementia and second primary malignancies with treatment.

   Limited small cell carcinoma has a median survival with treatment of 11–18 months; 10%–20% are disease free at 2 years. Extensive small cell carcinoma has a median survival of 6–12 months with therapy.

NON-SMALL CELL CARCINOMAS

1. These may be resectable – unless tumour has spread to the contralateral lung or outside the thorax, or there is significant cardiopulmonary disease.
2. The most important prognostic factor is the stage of disease. Staging usually involves bronchoscopy and CT scanning of the chest, abdomen and brain (PET scanning is useful but not covered by Medicare for this indication), as well as a physiological assessment of the patient's fitness for surgery, from the point of view of both lung function and general health. One-third of patients have disease sufficiently localised for an attempt at resection.
3. Radiotherapy with 'curative intent' may be offered to patients if they refuse surgery or are unfit for surgery for other reasons. About 6% are alive after 5 years. Radiotherapy is not useful for patients who have had surgical resection of a peripheral tumour.
4. Adjuvant chemotherapy is not routine for surgical patients, but regimens including cisplatin may provide a small survival advantage (5% at 5 years). A common regimen involves four cycles over 12–16 weeks. Median survival is only a few months in patients with intracranial metastases or bone involvement.
5. Chemotherapy and radiotherapy are used for stage IV disease. Although these patients will succumb to the disease, there is evidence that this can prolong life and improve symptoms. Treatment is often guided by tumour characteristics – pemetrexed-based chemotherapy is preferred for non-squamous tumours. Some tumours have mutations at the tyrosine kinase domain, and the use of oral tyrosine kinase inhibitors (gefitinib and erlotinib) has been associated with an initial improved response. Resistance usually develops after about a year of treatment.

Possible lines of questioning

1. Has there been adequate pain relief?
2. How is the family coping? Does the patient plan to stay at home when things deteriorate?
3. How would you decide to recommend to *this* patient that palliative treatment is now preferable to further chemotherapy?

6. Airway obstruction as a result of carcinoma may be relieved by using Nd-YAG laser or brachytherapy for palliation.
7. Combination chemotherapy is sometimes appropriate (cyclophosphamide, doxorubicin, vincristine and cisplatin are commonly used). Survival benefit is only 1 or 2 months.

Chronic obstructive pulmonary disease (COPD)

This general term is usually applied to patients with persistent airflow limitation and a chronic inflammatory response in the airways and lung parenchyma to inhaled noxious particles and gases. Chronic bronchitis and emphysema are related diagnoses and, although these conditions are different, they usually occur together. COPD is common and presents major management problems. However, in the examination it is unusual for it to be the patient's only medical problem. The vast majority of patients with COPD (more than 95%) are or have been smokers. However, only about one-fifth of smokers experience a rapid enough decline in FEV_1 ever to develop COPD. The FEV_1/FVC (forced vital capacity) must usually be less than 70% for the diagnosis to be confirmed.

The history

1. Find out about symptoms, such as cough and sputum, dyspnoea, wheeze, impaired exercise tolerance, ankle oedema and weight loss. Remember that the diagnosis of chronic bronchitis is made largely from the history.
2. Work out the Medical Research Council (MRC) score for severity of dyspnoea (Table 6.7).
3. Ask about precipitating causes of disease exacerbation, such as an upper respiratory tract infection (this is most often viral), pneumonia, omission of drugs, symptoms of right ventricular failure, resumption of smoking, pneumothorax, sleep apnoea, oropharyngeal aspiration and gastro-oesophageal reflux disease.
4. Enquire about smoking habits. Ask about the number of cigarettes smoked per day and the length of use (10 packet years of smoking is usually a prerequisite), as well as exposure to other people's cigarette smoke – passive smoking. Absence of a smoking history weighs heavily against the diagnosis unless chronic asthma or alpha$_1$-antitrypsin deficiency is present, or exposure to dust or fumes (Box 6.1). Find out at what age the patient began to smoke. Commencement in adolescence when lung development is incomplete may lead to a more rapid decline in lung function.

Table 6.7 MRC dyspnoea score		
SEVERITY	**SCORE**	**LEVEL OF DYSPNOEA**
None	0	Only with strenuous exercise
Mild	1	Breathlessness when hurrying or walking up gentle hill
Moderate	2	Limited by breathlessness when walking compared with people of own age; has to stop for breath when walking at own pace
Severe	3	Stops for breath after 100 m
Very severe	4	Breathless undressing; too breathless to leave the house
Adapted from Fletcher CM. The clinical diagnosis of pulmonary emphysema – an experimental study. *Proc R Soc Med* 1952;45:577–84.		

Box 6.1 Exposures that increase risk of COPD

- Smoking
- Wood, charcoal, coal smoke[a]
- Grain dust
- Nitrogen dioxide
- Dust – coal mining, hard rock mining, tunnelling, brick manufacture, iron and steel making
- Organic dusts
- Plastic, textile and rubber manufacturing
- Leather and food manufacturing

[a]The indoor burning of wood, charcoal and animal dung for cooking is a major cause of COPD in developing countries.
COPD = chronic obstructive pulmonary disease.

5. Ask about occupational history. This may be important, particularly as an additive feature if the patient has pneumoconiosis or has been exposed to toluene in plastics factories. Exposure to the fumes of solid fuel fires and to air pollution is also a risk factor.
6. Ask about medications, especially steroids, home oxygen and bronchodilators.
7. Enquire about management at home and work and the social effects of the disease. Find out in detail how limited the patient is physically and whether ADLs are managed. Ask about financial problems associated with chronic illness and symptoms of depression caused by chronic disability and loss of self-esteem.
8. Ask about admissions to hospital with exacerbations of the disease. These are associated with a poor prognosis – over 8% 30-day mortality in some studies.
9. Ask about family history, such as alpha$_1$-antitrypsin deficiency causing emphysema (autosomal co-dominant inheritance; the most common variant associated with severe deficiency of alpha$_1$-antitrypsin (< 11 mmol/L) is the *ZZ* allele, which is responsible for 2% of cases of emphysema in smokers). The condition should be suspected when COPD develops early or after minimal smoking exposure.

The examination

Examine the respiratory system carefully (see Ch 16). The examination may be normal until airway obstruction is moderately severe. Look particularly for:

1. pursed-lip breathing (prolongs the expiratory time and may limit over-inflation) and use of accessory muscles
2. cyanosis and polycythaemia (*note:* clubbing does not occur unless another disease such as carcinoma has supervened)
3. intercostal recession
4. prolonged forced expiratory time (reduced in both obstructive and restrictive lung disease)
5. tracheal tug
6. reduced diaphragmatic movements, over-inflation, reduced chest wall movement and expansion; Hoover's sign (paradoxical inward movement of the lower costal margin during inspiration) is sensitive and specific for COPD
7. reduced breath sounds with or without wheezes (rhonchi) and early coarse inspiratory crackles
8. sputum

9. signs of right heart failure
10. signs of cachexia in patients with advanced disease (this is probably related to the increase in tumour necrosis factor alpha associated with chronic hypoxia rather than to the increased work of breathing)
11. side-effects of treatment (e.g. tremor as a result of the use of beta-agonists, or the various changes caused by steroids).

Investigations

1. **Spirometry** – by definition, spirometry will show airflow limitation and it can be used to grade severity (Table 6.8).
2. **Chest X-ray film** (Fig. 6.3) – look for signs of hyperinflation (flat diaphragms and a vertical heart shadow) and cor pulmonale and exclude pneumonia. Radiolucent bullae may be visible; they are very specific for emphysema. The X-ray may be normal if the patient has mild disease. High-resolution CT of the chest is more often performed and is more specific for emphysema. The percentage of low attenuation areas on lung CT correlates with disease severity and may predict prognosis especially in patients with acute exacerbations.
3. **Ventilatory function tests** – look for a considerable reduction of the FEV_1/FVC ratio (< 0.70). A normal FEV_1 excludes the condition. The amount of reversibility should be tested with bronchodilators. An increase in FEV_1 or FVC of more than 15% and of at least 200 mL is considered significant. Complete, or almost complete, reversibility means that the diagnosis is asthma rather than COPD. Some asthmatics smoke and have both conditions; many smokers claim to have asthma but have only COPD. Vital capacity or total lung capacity may be falsely decreased if measured by gas dilution techniques because of the non-homogeneity of ventilation in COPD. The diffusing capacity for carbon monoxide is reduced in emphysema – a value of $< 50\%$ is associated with exertion-induced hypoxia.
4. **Arterial blood gas levels** – look for respiratory failure at rest. The demonstration of significant hypoxia (usually a PaO_2 of < 55 mmHg, or < 59 mmHg if the patient has cor pulmonale) is required for the prescription of home oxygen treatment. Ventilatory failure is defined as $PaCO_2$ of > 45 mmHg.
5. **Haemoglobin value** – look for polycythaemia.
6. **Sputum culture** – will usually grow *Haemophilus influenzae*, *Streptococcus pneumoniae* or *Moraxella catarrhalis* during exacerbations *and* remissions.
7. **Electrocardiogram (ECG)** – look for signs of right ventricular hypertrophy and multifocal atrial tachycardia, which can complicate chronic lung disease (Figs 6.4 and 6.5).

Table 6.8 Severity of COPD based on post-bronchodilator FEV₁ – GOLDª classification		
GOLD 1	Mild	$FEV_1 > 80\%$ of predicted
GOLD 2	Moderate	FEV_1 50%–80% of predicted
GOLD 3	Severe	$FEV_1 < 50\%$
GOLD 4	Very severe	$FEV_1 < 30\%$

ªGOLD = Global initiative for Chronic Obstructive Lung Disease.
Global Initiative for Chronic Obstructive Lung Disease, a collaboration between the National Institutes of Health and the World Health Organization.

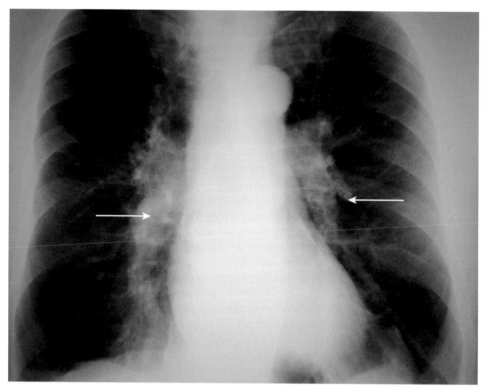

Figure 6.3 **COPD. Note the over-inflated lungs, flat hemi-diaphragms and prominent pulmonary arteries (arrows), a sign of pulmonary hypertension.**

Figure reproduced courtesy of The Canberra Hospital.

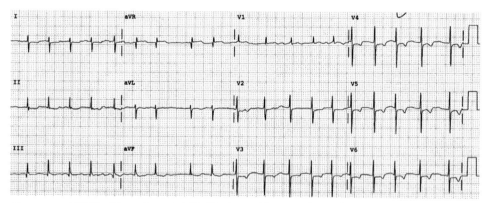

Figure 6.4 **COPD. There is atrial fibrillation with a moderately rapid ventricular response rate. There are prominent R waves in V1 and there is marked RAD (right axis deviation) (+110°). The right precordial T wave inversion suggests right ventricular 'strain'.**

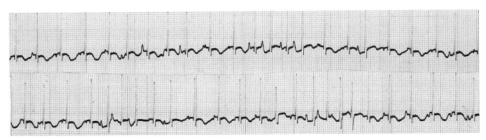

Figure 6.5 Multifocal atrial tachycardia L2 strip.

8. **Alpha$_1$-antitrypsin measurement** – this is now generally recommended. It should particularly be considered if the patient has never smoked or has associated cirrhosis or basilar emphysema, or rarely subcutaneous nodules from panniculitis.
9. **Assessment of nutrition** – body mass index (BMI = (weight in kg / height in cm)^2), grip strength, serum albumin, calcium and phosphate levels.
10. **Exercise testing** – to assess the need for ambulatory oxygen therapy and the degree of disability if there are discrepancies.

Differential diagnosis

1. Asthma
   Features suggesting asthma:
   a. non-smoker
   b. onset in childhood
   c. family history of allergy
   d. episodic attacks and also nocturnal symptoms
   e. a rapid response to treatment, especially steroids
   f. eosinophilia in the sputum
   g. atopic diathesis
   h. reversibility of obstruction.
2. Bronchiectasis
   Features suggesting bronchiectasis:
   a. daily sputum production with or without haemoptysis
   b. onset in childhood
   c. recurrent chest infection
   d. clubbing.

Treatment

1. The patient should stop smoking, as this decreases sputum production and bronchospasm and may reduce the rate of decline in lung function to that of a non-smoker (smoking cessation has been shown to prolong life). The candidate should have an approach to the treatment of nicotine addiction. This may involve the temporary use of nicotine substitutes, psychological counselling and encouragement, or the use of drugs such as bupropion.
2. Antibiotics can be used to shorten exacerbations (long-term chemoprophylaxis is indicated if there are four or more episodes a year), such as amoxicillin or doxycycline, given as a course at home at the first sign of purulent sputum. Remember that 25% of *H. influenzae* and 75% of *M. catarrhalis* infections are ampicillin resistant.
3. Regular bronchodilators are of value.
   a. Beta$_2$-agonists from metered-dose inhalers form the basis of treatment. A small change in FEV_1 and FVC may produce considerable subjective improvement. Some patients find the inhaler devices difficult to use.

Table 6.9 Inhaled medications for COPD
1. Begin with long-acting β_2-agonist, e.g. indacaterol, or long-acting antimuscarinic drug, e.g. tiotropium
2. Try combination of these different drug classes
3. Add inhaled corticosteroid, e.g. tiotropium and fluticasone proprionate / salmeterol

b. Inhaled long-acting anticholinergic drugs (Table 6.9), such as tiotropium bromide, provide symptomatic improvement and reduce exacerbations, but do not prolong life.

c. Inhaled steroids in high doses (e.g. 400 µg beclomethasone) reduce the rate of episodes of exacerbation, but should be discontinued if after a trial of 4–8 weeks of treatment there is no clinical or spirometric improvement.

d. Candidates should have a strategy to ensure effective use of the best device for a particular patient. Long-acting drugs, such as salmeterol, provide longer-acting bronchodilatation and are at least more convenient. Oral theophylline derivatives may have an additive effect with beta$_2$-agonists, perhaps because they improve respiratory muscle function. They are rarely used, however, partly because they cause oesophageal reflux, cardiac arrhythmias, nausea and insomnia, and partly because they are not very effective. Antitussives and mucolytics are controversial, but may be useful to prevent exacerbations.

e. When patients do not improve, consider problems with adherence or technique.

4. Pursed lip breathing and postural changes may be of value. Maintain adequate hydration.

5. Steroid use may be effective in an acute exacerbation and as a way of excluding asthma if there is persisting doubt. A trial of high doses for 2 weeks may be beneficial when bronchodilators are insufficient.

6. Maintenance steroid treatment should be given only if a short course has been shown objectively to be effective (i.e. improved respiratory function test results). Use the lowest dose possible. The associated weight gain, loss of muscle strength and osteoporosis may make the patient worse.

7. Annual influenza vaccine and 5-yearly pneumococcal vaccine are useful. Always know the immunisation status.

8. Pulmonary rehabilitation programs have been demonstrated in randomised controlled trials to improve symptoms and quality of life, but not to prolong life. Exercise and weight reduction increase patients' wellbeing, but not their lung function.

9. Domiciliary oxygen is indicated for patients with a PaO_2 of < 55 mmHg (SaO_2 < 88%) or cor pulmonale and a PaO_2 of < 59 mmHg. There is evidence that mortality rates are decreased by the use of domiciliary low-flow oxygen given for 15 hours per day or more (especially during sleep). This may work by reducing the progression of pulmonary hypertension. Find out what type of oxygen supplementation the patient uses (e.g. concentrator, cylinders) and how this is managed with regard to convenience and cost. Patients should not have home oxygen if they smoke.

10. Consider treatment of cor pulmonale. Heart failure is likely to improve with successful treatment of the lung disease. Spironolactone and diuretics may be useful. Patients with pulmonary hypertension secondary to COPD are not eligible for treatment with endothelin antagonists or sildenafil.

11. Alpha$_1$-antitrypsin deficiency can be treated by replenishing the missing antiprotease, which re-establishes antineutrophil elastase protection for the lower lung zones. An IV preparation can be administered weekly or monthly. This expensive treatment is

indicated only if alpha$_1$-antitrypsin levels are below 11 μmol/L. Only a small proportion of people with alpha$_1$-antitrypsin deficiency develop COPD and the treatment is not recommended unless there is demonstrated disease.

12. Lung transplantation is an option for younger (< 65 years) patients with end-stage disease and without serious co-morbidity who have not had previous thoracic surgery and have stopped smoking. The 1-year survival rate is more than 80% for this group.

13. The use of bi-level pressure ventilation (BiPAP) is a possible option for long-term management.

14. The management of severe exacerbations is difficult, particularly when these are associated with severe carbon dioxide retention and a reduced level of consciousness. Steroids and theophylline are both used commonly for these patients. Evidence for their effectiveness is not strong. Non-invasive ventilation (BiPAP) via a mask may improve symptoms and avoid the need for intubation. Intensive care units (ICUs) usually require some evidence of a potentially reversible problem before allowing intubation and mechanical ventilation. The patient's own wishes are important and should be obtained before he or she is too sick to make a decision.

15. Patients with COPD or other chronic lung diseases may ask about air travel. Commercial cabin pressures provide the equivalent of what would be 15% oxygen at sea level. If the patient's SaO_2 is < 95%, supplemental oxygen may be needed. An SaO_2 of < 88% is an indication for home oxygen and these patients should have their flow rate increased by 1 L/min when they fly. Patients with an SaO_2 between 88 and 95% should have an altitude simulation test before they fly.

Possible lines of questioning

1. How would you help *this* patient to stop smoking?
2. How would you manage an acute exacerbation – at home or in hospital?
3. When would home oxygen be appropriate for *this* patient?
4. Is *this* patient a candidate for lung transplant?

Sleep apnoea

Sleep apnoea should be suspected in patients who have:
- obesity
- hypertension
- fatigue and daytime sleepiness
- excessive snoring, or
- unexplained respiratory failure.

Obstructive sleep apnoea is a common cause of sleep disturbance (affects 2% of woman and 4% of men aged 30–60), but by no means the only explanation for it. Sleep apnoea patients commonly have some combination of these symptoms.

The history

Classically, in obstructive sleep apnoea, anyone else in the house will describe a history of loud snoring at night, associated with multiple periods of cessation of respiratory movement and waking and gasping for breath. Apnoeas of more than 10 seconds are

Table 6.10 The Epworth sleepiness scale
'How easily would you fall asleep in the following circumstances?' 0 = never, 1 = slight chance, 2 = moderate chance, 3 = high chance • Sitting reading • Watching television • At a meeting or at the theatre • As a passenger in a car on a drive of more than an hour • Lying down in the afternoon to rest • Sitting talking to someone • Sitting quietly after lunch (no alcohol) • When driving and stopped at traffic lights A normal score is between 3 and 8; a score of 11 to 20 indicates severe sleep apnoea.

considered significant, but for patients with this condition pauses of up to 2 or 3 minutes can occur and pauses of 30 seconds are common. Remember, though, that the majority of people who snore (40% of middle-aged men and 20% of middle-aged women) do not have sleep apnoea and brief apnoeas not associated with signs of arousal are normal for many people.

1. Ask the patient whether there have been problems with excessive daytime sleepiness and with working during the day.
2. Enquire whether the patient drinks alcohol and, if so, how much. Alcohol consumption is a common exacerbating factor.
3. Calculate the patient's Epworth sleepiness score (Table 6.10).
4. Ask whether there is a history of hypertension and whether this has been treated (50% of these patients have hypertension). Find out whether the patient has had angina or arrhythmias at night; both of these may be precipitated by the hypoxia associated with apnoea. Heartburn and non-cardiac chest pain caused by gastro-oesophageal reflux are also common.
5. Enquire about medications, such as hypnotics, that may have been prescribed for poor sleeping but actually aggravate sleep apnoea.
6. Ask about a previous diagnosis of COPD or symptoms of heart failure. The recurrent increase in afterload that occurs during apnoeic episodes can precipitate or exacerbate left ventricular failure. Fewer than 10% of patients develop right heart failure and significant pulmonary hypertension.
7. Ask about a history of tonsillar enlargement or throat surgery. In a few sleep apnoea patients there is a clear anatomical cause for the obstruction.
8. In the absence of excessive snoring, central sleep apnoea needs to be considered for a patient with the other symptoms.
9. Ask about symptoms suggestive of narcolepsy rather than sleep apnoea (Table 6.11). The sudden sleep attacks of narcolepsy can occur at any time, including during meals, conversation or driving. Patients may also report sudden loss of muscle tone from emotion (e.g. laughter). The result is an unexpected dropping of an object or a sudden buckling at the knees and falling down; cataplexy should be considered. Cataplexy is usually associated with narcolepsy, although it may precede narcolepsy by several years.
10. Ask about symptoms of the restless legs syndrome (RLS), which may also lead to daytime sleepiness (remember, RLS is associated with iron deficiency).
11. The use of diuretics or insulin may predispose patients to inadequate sleep and should not be confused with sleep apnoea.

Table 6.11 Differential diagnosis of daytime sleepiness
1. Not enough sleep (now sometimes considered related to 'poor sleep hygiene')
2. Poor adjustment to shift work
3. Use of sedative and stimulant drugs (e.g. sedatives, caffeine, narcotics)
4. Depression with or without early morning waking
5. Idiopathic hypersomnolence (sleepiness despite plenty of sleep without snoring)
6. Narcolepsy (uncommon, sudden, unexpected falling asleep)

12. Ask whether the patient drives a motor car and whether the risks of driving have been discussed. Also ask whether it has been recommended that the anaesthetist be informed of the patient's sleep apnoea before the administration of an anaesthetic.
13. Find out whether a CPAP mask has been prescribed and whether the patient finds it comfortable enough to use. Up to 50% of patients are unable to tolerate the device. If the treatment is tolerated, find out whether it has made a difference – many patients report a dramatic reduction in daytime sleepiness and improvement in wellbeing.
14. Find out how this chronic condition has affected the patient's family and work.

The examination

1. Assess the BMI, but remember that up to 50% of patients with obstructive sleep apnoea and most patients with central sleep apnoea are not obese.
2. Respiratory examination is usually normal.
3. Measure the blood pressure and look in the fundi for signs of hypertension.
4. The cardiovascular system should be examined carefully for evidence of pulmonary hypertension.
5. Inspect the head, neck and mouth for signs of uvular enlargement and macroglossia or tonsillar hypertrophy – 'pharyngeal crowding'. Look at and measure the neck circumference.
6. Perform a neurological examination to look for signs of autonomic neuropathy (e.g. diabetes mellitus, Shy–Drager syndrome), brain stem lesions or spinal cord disease (e.g. tumour, demyelination), which can cause central sleep apnoea.
7. Examine for neurological causes of obstructive sleep apnoea, such as myasthenia gravis or muscular dystrophy.
8. Look for signs of hypothyroidism or acromegaly.

Investigations

1. Consider sleep study monitoring (polysomnography) with the electroencephalogram, chin electromyogram, electro-ocular monitoring (to detect rapid eye movement (REM) sleep), oximetry, $PaCO_2$ monitoring and, if indicated, ECG monitoring (for arrhythmias).
2. For a definitive diagnosis, the apnoeic spells must be 10 seconds or longer in duration and at least five per hour must be recorded over several hours. The apnoea hypopnoea index (AHI) is the total number of episodes of apnoea or hypopnoea per night divided by the number of hours of sleep (mild 5–15, moderate 6–30, severe > 30). A value of 5 or greater is considered abnormal, but is probably not diagnostic in the absence of symptoms.
3. For patients with typical features of the condition, home PaO_2 monitoring overnight may be an option. A positive test (several significant desaturation episodes per hour) is enough evidence to justify treatment. A negative test, however, does not exclude the diagnosis.

4. Narcolepsy can also be diagnosed by a sleep study.
5. Hypothyroidism should be excluded with thyroid function tests if there is any clinical suspicion.
6. Check for proteinuria (uncommon, but may reach nephrotic levels in severe obesity).
7. Look at the ECG for arrhythmias. Echocardiography may be indicated to enable estimation of pulmonary artery pressures and to assess right ventricular function.

Treatment

1. If the patient has hypothyroidism, thyroid hormone replacement may reverse sleep apnoea.
2. Concomitant diseases such as cardiac failure, hypertension and asthma need to be treated vigorously. Nasal decongestants may be helpful. Weight loss is of value, but may be difficult to achieve. Respiratory depressants, such as tranquillisers, should be withdrawn.
3. CPAP is of value for long-term treatment of irreversible obstructive sleep apnoea (Table 6.12). CPAP devices are not always well tolerated, but the devices are improving steadily in comfort and portability. Nasal CPAP is effective in the majority of patients who can adjust to it. If there is residual sleepiness despite regular use of CPAP, modafinil may be a useful adjunct.
4. Surgical correction of upper airways narrowing caused by polyps, enlarged tonsils or macroglossia can lead to significant improvement, but may not fully reverse the problem. Excision of soft tissue in the oropharynx is of value for well-selected patients.
5. If there has been a recent stroke, observation may be all that is required, since respiratory function may improve with time. Patients with central sleep apnoea can often be successfully treated with bilevel positive airways pressure (BiPAP) ventilation.

Possible lines of questioning

1. When would you recommend a patient be tested for sleep apnoea?
2. What would you tell *this* patient what he or she might realistically expect from treatment for sleep apnoea?

Table 6.12 The effects of treatment for sleep apnoea from randomised clinical trials
EPWORTH SCORE > 11 AND > 15 APNOEAS / HOUR
• Reduced sleepiness
• Improved blood pressure
• Improved cognition
• Safer driving
• Improved mood and quality of life
EPWORTH SCORE > 11 AND 5–15 APNOEAS / HOUR
• Improved symptoms
• Improved daytime sleepiness
• Less evidence of quality of life or cognitive improvement
• No evidence of improved blood pressure
NORMAL EPWORTH SCORE WITH APNOEA
• No evidence of benefit of treatment

Table 6.13 Classification of interstitial lung disease (ILD)

1. ILD with known association
   - Drugs (methotrexate (Box 6.2), nitrofurantoin (Box 6.3))
   - Occupational exposure
   - Connective tissue disease
2. Granulomatous ILD
   - Hypersensitivity pneumonitis
   - Sarcoidosis
3. Idiopathic interstitial pneumonia (IIP)
   - Major IIP
     - idiopathic pulmonary fibrosis (IPF)
     - non-specific interstitial pneumonia (NSIP)
   - Respiratory bronchiolitis ILD (RBILD)
     - cryptogenic organising pneumonia (previously called bronchiolitis obliterans with organising pneumonia)
     - acute interstitial pneumonia
     - desquamative interstitial pneumonia (DIP)
4. Other ILD
   - Lymphangioleiomymatosis
   - Pulmonary Langerhans cell histiocytosis (PLCH) (histiocytosis X)

Interstitial lung disease, including idiopathic pulmonary fibrosis

Interstitial lung disease (ILD) may have a prolonged course for some patients, so patients can be available for the examinations. The pathological pattern on lung biopsy is often used to classify these as usual interstitial pneumonia (UIP) or non-specific-interstitial pneumonia (NSIP). The median survival time, however, is only 3–5 years. Discovering the aetiology may be difficult (see Tables 6.13 and 6.17).

The history

The diagnosis may not be obvious until you examine the patient, at which stage you may have to ask further questions about the following:

1. presenting respiratory symptoms (e.g. dry cough, dyspnoea, lethargy, malaise)
2. whether the patient knows the cause of the respiratory symptoms
3. the onset and duration of symptoms (these are clues) – pulmonary fibrosis has a very slow onset and patients are not acutely ill; if there is the insidious onset of cough, fever, malaise and myalgias over weeks to months, think about cryptogenic organising pneumonia (COP), which has a better prognosis and responds to steroids
4. the patient's gender and age (also clues) – for example, lymphangioleiomyomatosis (LAM) occurs essentially only in premenopausal women who often have a history of recurrent pneumothorax
5. the smoking history – respiratory bronchiolitis ILD (RBILD), desquamative interstitial pneumonia (DIP) and pulmonary Langerhans cell histiocytosis (PLCH) have a strong association with smoking, presumably via a smoking-induced immune response; patients with idiopathic pulmonary fibrosis (IPF) are often smokers[1]

---

[1]Smoking increases the risk of pulmonary bleeding in Goodpasture's syndrome. Hypersensitivity pneumonitis is more common in non-smokers.

6. systemic symptoms – for example, weight loss, fatigue, fever, rash and arthralgia, which may indicate a systemic disease, particularly a connective tissue disease (scleroderma, systemic lupus erythematosus, Sjögren's syndrome or rheumatoid arthritis) or sarcoidosis (Table 6.14)
7. pre-existing asthma – which may suggest Churg–Strauss syndrome (ask about renal disease)
8. any history of haemoptysis and renal disease – which may indicate Goodpasture's syndrome or SLE
9. drug use – cardiac (e.g. amiodarone (Box 6.4), hydralazine, procainamide), rheumatological (e.g. methotrexate (see Box 6.2), D-penicillamine), chemotherapeutic (e.g. busulphan, bleomycin, cyclophosphamide) and others (e.g. nitrofurantoin (see Box 6.3), bromocriptine)
10. any history of radiotherapy
11. a detailed lifetime occupational history, such as exposure to mineral dust (silicosis, asbestosis, coal worker's pneumoconiosis), chemical fumes (nitrogen dioxide, chlorine, ammonia) or organic dusts (Table 6.15)
12. any occupational history consistent with hypersensitivity pneumonitis (e.g. bird fancier's lung, farmer's lung from mouldy hay or grain dust in grain elevators); ask about recurrent Monday chest tightness (e.g. byssinosis from cotton, flax or hemp dust)

Table 6.14 Fibrotic and granulomatous lung disease

CONNECTIVE TISSUE DISEASES CAUSING FIBROSIS (ILD)
1. Rheumatoid arthritis (patients can also develop pleural disease, nodules, bronchiectasis, and acute lung injury)
2. Systemic lupus erythematosus (SLE)
3. Systemic sclerosis (ILD is the most common cause of death)
4. Polymyositis and dermatomyositis
5. Sjögren's syndrome
6. Polyarteritis nodosa (rare)

CAUSES OF GRANULOMATOUS LUNG DISEASE ON LUNG BIOPSY
1. Sarcoidosis
2. Tuberculosis
3. Chronic berylliosis
4. Extrinsic allergic alveolitis

ILD = interstitial lung disease.

Box 6.2 Methotrexate and the lungs

- Fewer than 5% of patients using methotrexate are affected.
- There is no correlation between the dose and the severity of the condition.
- The condition may occur at any time from the start of treatment.
- Patients present with fever, dyspnoea, cough and have diffuse pulmonary infiltrates.
- In severe cases there can be dense pulmonary infiltration.
- Mild eosinophilia is often present in the blood film.
- The prognosis is good with withdrawal of the drug, but a course of steroids is often indicated.

Box 6.3 Nitrofurantoin and the lungs

- Onset of symptoms may be acute or chronic.
- Problems can occur within days of starting treatment or even after previous uneventful use of the drug.
- Acute symptoms (20% of cases) include fever, chills, wheeze, myalgia, chest pain and rash.
- Chronic symptoms occur independently of acute ones and occur months or years after treatment has begun. They include cough and dyspnoea.
- CT scans and X-rays show reticular infiltrates, thickened peribronchial markings and later reduced lung volumes.
- Treatment means stopping the drug; steroids are not useful for the acute form, but may be for the chronic symptoms.

Box 6.4 Amiodarone and the lungs

- Subacute pneumonitis (patchy ground-glass appearance on CT)
- Pulmonary fibrosis (reticulonodular pattern on CT)
- Organising pneumonia (migrating alveolar opacities and nodules)
- Diffuse alveolar damage (diffuse bilateral opacities that look like pulmonary oedema)
- Alveolar haemorrhage (bilateral opacities – uncommon)
- Subpleural masses (cause chest pain and pleural rub)
- Subclinical pneumonitis (changes only on CT of ground-glass appearance)

Table 6.15 Asbestos and the lung

HEAVY EXPOSURE ASSOCIATED WITH:
1. Asbestosis
2. Bronchial carcinoma

TRIVIAL EXPOSURE ASSOCIATED WITH:
1. Pleural fibrosis and plaques
2. Mesothelioma after a latent period of 30–40 years

---

13. infections (e.g. aspiration pneumonia, miliary tuberculosis)
14. investigations (e.g. high-resolution CT of the thorax, lung biopsy or bronchial lavage)
15. treatment, if any
16. social problems as a result of the chronic disability.

The examination

1. Clubbing (consider idiopathic pulmonary fibrosis, but also asbestosis); cyanosis and lower lobe crackles (fine, late, inspiratory) make the diagnosis of idiopathic pulmonary fibrosis (IPF) likely.
2. If the signs suggest upper lobe pulmonary fibrosis, consider in your differential diagnosis silicosis, sarcoidosis, beryllium, cystic fibrosis, coal worker's pneumoconiosis, eosinophilic granuloma, ankylosing spondylitis and tuberculosis. Lower lobe pulmonary fibrosis may be due to IPF, scleroderma, asbestosis, aspiration or drugs.

3. Look for signs of associated systemic disease, as well as sarcoidosis and connective tissue disease that would rule out IPF. For example, erythema nodosum and anterior uveitis would suggest looking for evidence of sarcoidosis.
4. Assess the severity of the disease (signs of pulmonary hypertension).
5. Look for signs of drug side-effects (especially steroids).

Investigations

The goals of investigations are to find the aetiology, establish the severity of the disease and look for signs of active inflammation. If active inflammation is present, the condition may respond to immunotherapy (steroids or cyclophosphamide). If established fibrosis is present, such treatment is unlikely to help.

1. Chest radiography is the initial investigation, but may be normal (see Fig. 16.24, p. 453).
2. High-resolution CT of the thorax is the investigation of choice (Fig. 6.6). It is the most sensitive non-invasive test. The changes of ILD are characteristic. Note whether there is a localised or diffuse abnormality or progressive massive fibrosis (caused by silicosis and coal worker's pneumoconiosis). In two-thirds of patients with IPF, the CT scan may show the characteristic usual interstitial pneumonia (UIP) pattern – basal, subpleural reticular changes, honeycombing and traction bronchiectasis.
3. Cryptogenic organising pneumonia (COP) is a common idiopathic interstitial pneumonia (IIP). The CT and X-ray show single or multifocal airspace opacities in patients who have presented with cough, fever and malaise.

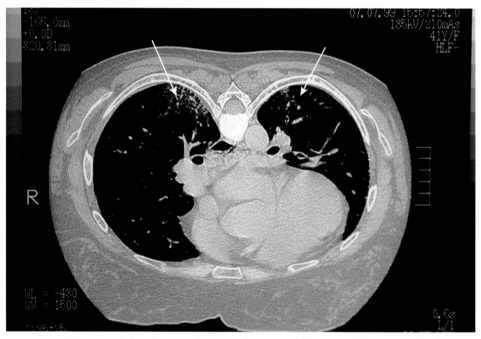

Figure 6.6 **CT scan of the thorax. There are increased lung markings posteriorly, more prominent on the right than on the left (arrows).**

Figure reproduced courtesy of The Canberra Hospital.

Table 6.16 Causes of pulmonary infiltrate and eosinophilia (PIE)

Prolonged pulmonary eosinophilia. This may be caused by: drugs (e.g. sulfonamides, sulfasalazine, salicylates, nitrofurantoin, penicillin, isoniazid, methotrexate, carbamazepine, imipramine, L-tryptophan); parasites (e.g. *Ascaris*); idiopathic
Loeffler's syndrome (benign and acute)
Allergic bronchopulmonary aspergillosis (always associated with asthma)
Tropical (e.g. microfilaria)
Eosinophilic pneumonia and vasculitis (e.g. polyarteritis nodosa, Wegener's granulomatosis)

4. Pulmonary function tests usually reveal a restrictive pattern, with reduction of lung volumes and reduced transfer factor. An obstructive pattern may be seen in sarcoidosis, histiocytosis X (typically found in men who smoke and have a history of pneumothorax) and LAM.
5. Blood gas levels will show hypoxia with a normal or low $PaCO_2$.
6. The erythrocyte sedimentation rate is often raised.
7. There may be hypergammaglobulinaemia and a raised lactate dehydrogenase (LDH) level. Eosinophilia may be a useful clue (Table 6.16). Serological testing for connective tissue diseases is routine.
8. A positive gallium-67 lung scan may indicate disease activity. Lung clearance studies using pertechnate may also be helpful (rapid clearance suggests active alveolitis).
9. Bronchoalveolar lavage can be performed and is most helpful if there is haemoptysis or an acute disease onset. It is suggested that fibrosis on a transbronchial biopsy associated with a lavage showing a predominance of polymorphonuclear cells is less responsive to treatment. Lymphocytosis on lavage suggests drug-induced or granulomatous disease.
10. Diagnoses likely to be made by transbronchial lung biopsy include sarcoidosis and lymphangitic spread of carcinoma; infection can be ruled out. Other specific diagnoses are not usually apparent.
11. Open lung biopsy or video-assisted thoracoscopic biopsy may be required to confirm the presence of idiopathic ILD, but only if there is clinical uncertainty and the test result could change treatment.

Treatment
This depends on the cause (Table 6.17).
1. Remove exposure, if appropriate. Stop smoking – this can stabilise or improve lung function in patients with a smoking-related ILD.
2. Treatment will not reverse established fibrosis.
3. Steroids may help in COP, chemical injuries, hypersensitivity pneumonias (acute disease only), sarcoidosis (severe disease), histiocytosis X (controversial) and connective tissue disease. However, there is no evidence that steroids improve survival in these conditions and they are of no value in dust diseases.
4. Treatment with prednisolone is usually begun at 1 mg/kg/day and reduced to half this dose after 4–12 weeks. Follow-up with measurement of spirometry, lung volumes and transfer factor is important to document response to treatment. Consider maintenance steroids in lower dosage for patients who are improving or stabilised.

Table 6.17 Causes of interstitial lung disease

SECONDARY ALVEOLITIS (PREVIOUSLY CALLED FIBROSING ALVEOLITIS)

1. Unknown cause
   - Idiopathic interstitial pneumonia (e.g. idiopathic pulmonary fibrosis; cryptogenic organising pneumonia, lymphangioleiomyomatosis)
   - Connective tissue disease (e.g. systemic lupus erythematosus, rheumatoid arthritis, ankylosing spondylitis, systemic sclerosis)
   - Pulmonary haemorrhage syndromes (e.g. Goodpasture's syndrome)
   - Graft versus host disease
   - Gastrointestinal or liver diseases (e.g. Crohn's disease, primary biliary cirrhosis)
2. Known cause
   - Asbestosis
   - Radiation injury (Box 6.5)
   - Aspiration pneumonia
   - Drugs (e.g. amiodarone, bleomycin, busulfan, nitrofurantoin, penicillamine, cocaine)
   - Exposure to gases or fumes

SECONDARY TO GRANULOMATOUS DISEASE

1. Unknown cause
   - Sarcoidosis
   - Granulomatosis with polyangiitis (GPA, previously Wegener's granulomatosis), Churg–Strauss disease (eosinophilic granulomatosis with polyangiitis)
2. Known cause
   - Hypersensitivity pneumonitis (extrinsic allergic alveolitis) to organic or inorganic dusts (silica, beryllium)

Box 6.5 Radiation and the lung

- Patients with radiation pneumonitis present 6 weeks after exposure with dyspnoea.
- CT shows hazy opacities and ground glass appearance.
- Areas outside the radiation field are sometimes involved.
- Changes may resolve after 6 months, or progress to a localised area of fibrosis of bronchiectasis.
- Severe disease may be treated with steroids but treatment is not always necessary.

5. Immunosuppressive agents are not effective for idiopathic pulmonary fibrosis but may be helpful in connective tissue disease-associated fibrosis, especially azathioprine, which can be used in combination with low-dose steroids. Antifibrotic agents are now available – pirfenidone and nintedanib (a tyrokinase inhibitor) reduce the decline in lung function. Pirfenidone causes skin sensitivity to sunlight and nintedanib causes diarrhoea.
6. Treat any associated gastro-oesophageal reflux as it may aggravate disease.
7. Consider general measures, e.g. administering pneumococcal and influenza vaccines.
8. Home oxygen therapy may provide symptomatic relief for hypoxaemic patients.
9. Unilateral lung transplantation may be considered for some patients in the final stage of their disease. This is potentially curative treatment. Younger patients with declining FVC and diffusion capacity for carbon monoxide (DLCO) measurements should be considered for transplant.
10. Treat any co-morbidities (Table 6.18).

Table 6.18 Common co-morbidities in ILD patients and management

1. Gastroesophageal reflux
   - Lung injury and increased fibrosis – proton pump inhibitor, assess for scleroderma
2. Infections
   - Worsen lung function – vaccinations against influenza and pneumococcus, antibiotics early
3. Osteoporosis
   - Rib and vertebral fractures can worsen breathing – vitamin D, etc.
4. Sleep apnoea
   - May make pulmonary hypertension worse – oxygen therapy, CPAP mask
5. Pulmonary hypertension
   - Increases mortality – oxygen therapy, vasodilators, endothelin antagonists

CPAP = continuous positive airways pressure; ILD = interstitial lung disease.

Possible lines of questioning

1. Do you think *this* patient's disease is active?
2. What lung function assessment would you make for *this* patient?
3. Is home oxygen indicated?
4. How would you assess *this* patient's prognosis?
5. Is lung transplant worth considering for *this* patient?

Pulmonary hypertension

Many patients with this chronic and often severe illness will have raised pulmonary artery pressures as a result of a cardiac or respiratory illness. The patient may or may not be aware of this complication of the underlying disease, but it is essential for the candidate to know when to look for it. Idiopathic pulmonary hypertension (IPH) is a rare but important condition, which is diagnosed when other causes of pulmonary hypertension have been excluded. By definition, pulmonary hypertension is present when the mean pulmonary artery pressure (PAP) exceeds 25 mmHg at rest or 30 mmHg during exercise.

Pre-capillary PH means a mean PAP of > 25 mmHg and a pulmonary capillary wedge pressure (PCWP) of < 15 mmHg. **Post-capillary PH** means a mean PAP > 25 mmHg and a PCWP of > 15 mmHg. Post-capillary PH is usually due to left heart failure or disease (e.g. mitral stenosis).

The classification of pulmonary hypertension was revised in 2008 and 2013. The Venice classification is now called the Dana Point classification. The term 'primary pulmonary hypertension' has been replaced with 'idiopathic pulmonary hypertension' (Table 6.19).

The history

1. Symptoms are usually non-specific but often severe. As usual, begin by asking whether the patient knows what is wrong and the reason for the admission, or visit, to hospital.
2. If pulmonary hypertension seems a possibility, ask about the possible causes (see Table 6.19). Remember to ask specifically about appetite-suppressing drugs. The use of fenfluramine and phentermine in combination and for long periods has been associated with the greatest risk.

Table 6.19 The Dana Point classification for pulmonary hypertension (2008, updated 2013)

1. PULMONARY ARTERIAL HYPERTENSION (PAH)

1.1 Idiopathic pulmonary hypertension (IPH)

1.2 Heritable PAH

    1.2.1 BMPR$_2$

    1.2.2 ALK$_1$, endoglin (with or without hereditary haemorrhagic telangiectasia)

    1.2.3 Unknown

1.3 Drug and toxin-induced

1.4 Associated with

    1.4.1 Connective tissue disease

    1.4.2 HIV infection

    1.4.3 Portal hypertension

    1.4.4 Congenital heart diseases

    1.4.5 Schistosomiasis

    1.4.6 Chronic haemolytic anaemia

1'. PULMONARY VENO-OCCLUSIVE DISEASE (PVOD) AND/OR PULMONARY CAPILLARY HAEMANGIOMATOSIS (PCH)

2. PULMONARY HYPERTENSION AS A RESULT OF LEFT HEART DISEASE

2.1 Systolic dysfunction

2.2 Diastolic dysfunction

2.3 Valvular disease

3. PULMONARY HYPERTENSION AS A RESULT OF LUNG DISEASES AND/OR HYPOXIA

3.1 Chronic obstructive pulmonary disease

3.2 Interstitial lung disease

3.3 Other pulmonary diseases with mixed restrictive and obstructive pattern

3.4 Sleep-disordered breathing

3.5 Alveolar hypoventilation disorders

3.6 Chronic exposure to high altitude

3.7 Developmental abnormalities

4. CHRONIC THROMBOEMBOLIC PULMONARY HYPERTENSION (CTEPH)

4.1 Chronic thromboembolic pulmonary disease

4.2 Other pulmonary artery obstructions

    4.2.1 Angiosarcoma

    4.2.2 Other intravascular tumours

    4.2.3 Arteritis

    4.2.4 Congenital pulmonary artery stenoses

    4.2.5 Parasites

5. MISCELLANEOUS

5.1 Haematological disorders: myeloproliferative disorders, splenectomy

5.2 Systemic disorders: sarcoidosis, pulmonary Langerhans cell histiocytosis, lymphangioleiomyomatosis, neurofibromatosis, vasculitis

5.3 Metabolic disorders: glycogen storage disease, Gaucher's disease, thyroid disorders

5.4 Others: tumour obstruction, fibrosing mediastinitis, chronic kidney disease on dialysis

ALK$_1$ = activin receptor-like kinase type I; BMPR$_2$ = bone morphogenetic protein receptor type 2; HIV = human immunodeficiency virus.

Adapted from G Simonneau, IM Robbins, M Beghetti, RN Channick et al. Updated clinical classification of pulmonary hypertension. *Journal of the American College of Cardiology* 2009; 54:S43–54.

3. If the patient has an illness that could be a cause, ask detailed questions about that condition, its severity and chronicity. There may be a family history in cases of IPH (6%; autosomal dominant condition with incomplete penetrance, 20%–80%). The majority of familial cases are associated with a mutation on the *BMPR2* gene.

4. Find out how symptomatic the patient is now. Idiopathic and secondary pulmonary hypertension cause dyspnoea. Almost all patients have dyspnoea at the time of diagnosis. Other less common symptoms include fatigue, chest pain, syncope and oedema. Cough and haemoptysis can be present. Ask about symptoms of connective tissue diseases and especially about scleroderma. Try to work out the patient's functional class (NYHA I–IV, often called the NYHA-WHO class when related to pulmonary hypertension).

5. Ask about previous or planned investigations. These may relate to the underlying condition – for example, respiratory function tests or scans, echocardiography (sometimes transoesophageal echocardiography) or cardiac catheterisation. A patient who presents with symptoms and signs of pulmonary hypertension needs a number of investigations before IPH can be diagnosed.

6. What general treatment has been recommended? This may be for the underlying cardiac or respiratory condition or for thrombosis. There may be a history of cardiac surgery in childhood for congenital heart disease. Oxygen supplementation is often prescribed. Find out how this is administered (e.g. via nasal prongs or a mask), for how many hours a day and whether it comes from a concentrator or oxygen tanks. Oxygen is very expensive unless subsidised. Ask about the cost and inconvenience of the treatment with regard to portability and noise (oxygen concentrators are noisy and use a lot of electricity). Has the treatment been helpful?

7. What drugs is the patient taking? Heparin and then warfarin are routine for pulmonary embolism, but warfarin is also used for some patients with IPH because of the risk of in situ thrombosis in the pulmonary arteries. Bronchodilators and steroids may have been prescribed for lung disease. The possibility of a heart or lung transplant, or both, may have been raised with the patient. The patient may be on a therapeutic trial or taking an agent, such as bosentan, ambrisentan, macitentan, sildenafil or the inhaled prostacyclin analogue iloprost. Patients involved in trials or taking new drugs are often very well informed about what is going on.

8. As with any chronic and possibly debilitating condition, questions about the patient's ability to work and manage the activities of daily living need to be detailed and comprehensive.

The examination

1. Try to assess the severity of the patient's dyspnoea as he or she undresses or by asking the patient to walk around the room.

2. Perform a thorough respiratory and cardiac examination (see Table 16.1, p. 413 and Table 16.10, p. 446). Look particularly for an elevated jugular venous pressure (JVP) with a large v wave. Feel for a parasternal impulse (right ventricular heave). Feel for a palpable P2 (and listen for tricuspid regurgitation).

3. Look for signs of chronic lung disease, congenital heart disease and connective tissue disease. Examine for signs of a deep venous thrombosis (DVT).

Investigations

Investigations are directed at finding an underlying reason for pulmonary hypertension – IPH is a diagnosis of exclusion – and at assessing its severity and potential reversibility. These investigations include those detailed below.

1. **Chest X-ray** – this will be abnormal in 90% of IPH patients. It may show ILD or an abnormal cardiac silhouette – right ventricular dilatation. There may be large

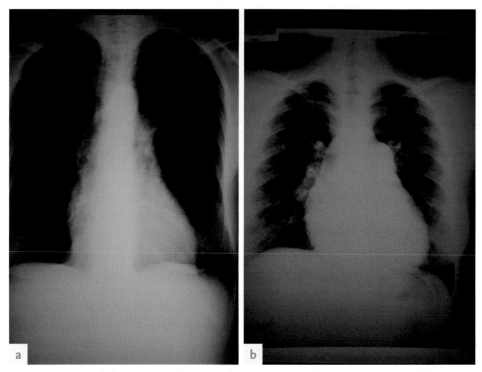

Figure 6.7 (a) and (b) Severe pulmonary hypertension. There is pruning of the
pulmonary arteries and right ventricular dilatation.

Figure reproduced courtesy of The Canberra Hospital.

proximal pulmonary arteries that appear 'pruned' in the periphery, and the right
ventricle may appear enlarged on the lateral film (Fig. 6.7a and b).

2. **Respiratory function tests** (normal, restrictive or obstructive pattern) – moderate
   pulmonary hypertension itself is associated with a reduction in the diffusion capacity
   for carbon monoxide (DLCO) to about 50% of predicted.

3. **ECG** – signs of right heart strain or hypertrophy are present in up to 90% of patients
   (Fig. 6.8).

4. **Blood gases** – hypercapnia in hypoventilation syndromes, but hypocapnia is more
   common in IPH because of increased alveolar ventilation. Mild hypoxia is seen in
   IPH, but is more severe when pulmonary hypertension is secondary to lung disease.

5. **CT pulmonary angiogram or ventilation–perfusion (V/Q) scan and Doppler
   venograms** – DVT and pulmonary embolism – assessment of extent of involvement
   of the pulmonary bed.

6. **High-resolution CT of the lungs** – looking for interstitial lung disease.

7. **Six-minute walking test** – predicts survival and correlates with NYHA-WHO class.
   Reduction in arterial oxygen concentration of > 10% during this test predicts almost
   threefold mortality risk over 29 months. Patients unable to manage 332 metres in 6
   minutes also have an adverse prognosis.

8. **Transthoracic or transoesophageal echocardiogram** (Fig. 6.9) – a transthoracic
   echocardiogram will usually enable left ventricular failure or severe mitral valve disease
   to be excluded. One or both will enable the assessment of known congenital heart

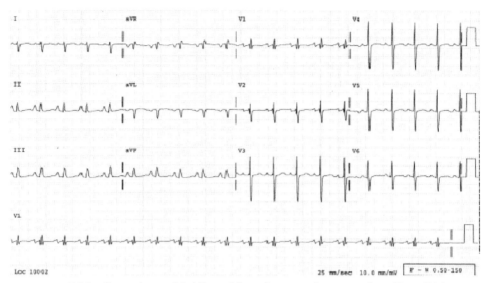

Figure 6.8 **ECG of a patient with idiopathic pulmonary hypertension. Note RAA (right atrial abnormality), 'P' pulmonale, right axis, right ventricular hypertrophy and strain pattern, and sinus tachycardia.**

disease, the detection of a left-to-right (or reversed) shunting (Eisenmenger's syndrome) and measurement, in many cases, of pulmonary artery pressures. The presence of tricuspid regurgitation (common in normal people and almost universal in the presence of raised right ventricular pressures) enables estimation of right ventricular and therefore pulmonary artery pressures in many patients.

The normal right ventricular and pulmonary artery systolic pressure is 20–25 mmHg. Assessment of pulmonary artery ejection characteristics can also be used to estimate pulmonary artery pressures. Right ventricular size and function can be assessed. Right ventricular dilatation and abnormal septal motion are useful signs of pulmonary hypertension. The right ventricle appears abnormal on echocardiograms in more than 90% of people with pulmonary hypertension.

9. **Catheterisation of the right heart** – this investigation is the gold standard and should also be performed if other tests have not been definitive. It is usually performed with a multiple-lumen flotation catheter and enables direct measurement of the right heart pressures. Left to right shunting can be detected by the collection of blood samples from the venae cavae, right atrium, right ventricle and pulmonary artery. A 'step-up' in the blood oxygen saturation indicates a shunt. The size of the shunt can be calculated if the cardiac output is measured by thermodilution. Measurement of the pulmonary artery wedge pressure enables the detection of mitral stenosis or the very rare pulmonary veno-occlusive disease. By definition, IPH means that the pulmonary capillary wedge pressure is < 18 mmHg (i.e. the raised pulmonary pressures are not secondary to left ventricular failure). Pulmonary vascular resistance can be calculated using the cardiac output, pulmonary artery pressure and pulmonary artery wedge pressure measurements. The formula is:

$$\text{pulmonary vascular resistance} = \frac{\text{pulmonary artery pressure} - \text{pulmonary artery wedge pressure}}{\text{cardiac output}}$$

This gives a result in mmHg/L/min or Wood units. The normal value is 1.7 mmHg/L/min.

Echocardiography Report

Reason for study: ?Pulmonary hypertension
Study quality: Good <u>Satisfactory</u> Poor

RV	32	(mm)	(N 10–26)
Sept.	8	(mm)	(N 7–11)
LVEDD	51	(mm)	(N 36–56)
LVESD	30	(mm)	(N 20–40)
LVPW	10	(mm)	(N 7–11)
Aorta	22	(mm)	(N 20–35)
LA	36	(mm)	(N 24–40)
FS	41	%	(N 27–40)
EF	72	%	(N 55–70)

Valves

Mitral   Mild MR
Tricus. Moderate TR
Aortic   Appears normal
Pulm.   Appears normal

Doppler – 2D

The right ventricle is dilated. There is paradoxical septal motion. The LV is not dilated. The cardiac valves appear normal. The main pulmonary artery was not dilated. No ASD was seen.

Doppler – colour flow mapping

Moderate tricuspid regurgitation was detected. The TR flow velocity was 4 m/s. Estimated RV pressure 70 mmHg. Mild MR is present. No ASD flow or intracardiac shunting was detected.

Conclusions

Severe pulmonary hypertension. RV dilated, abnormal septal motion. No intracardiac shunting detected.

Comment

The most important signs of pulmonary hypertension on 2D echocardiographs are RV dilatation and abnormal septal motion. The septum normally behaves as part of the left ventricle and contracts inwards, towards the lateral wall of the left ventricle. Significant increases in RV pressure cause the septum to move away from the left ventricle during systole. Measurement of the velocity of the regurgitant tricuspid valve jet enables estimation of RV pressures. It is difficult to exclude an ASD on a transthoracic echocardiogram unless it is of very good quality. A transoesophageal echocardiograph may be required if there is any doubt about the cause of pulmonary hypertension.

Key

ASD = atrial septal defect; EF = ejection fraction; FS = fractional shortening; LA = left atrium; LVEDD = left ventricular end-diastolic dimension; LVESD = left ventricular end-systolic dimension; LVPW = left ventricular posterior wall; MR = mitral regurgitation; Pulm. = pulmonary; RV = right ventricle; Sept. = septal thickness; TR = tricuspid regurgitation; Tricus. = tricuspid.

Figure 6.9 **Echocardiography report in a patient with pulmonary hypertension.**

Treatment

1. Treatment of pulmonary hypertension that is secondary to an underlying respiratory or cardiac condition begins with an attempt to optimise treatment or fix the underlying condition.
   a. **COPD:** bronchodilators, steroids, continuous oxygen.
   b. **ILD:** oxygen. Aggressive treatment of an underlying connective tissue disease may halt or slow progression of the pulmonary pressures.
   c. **Pulmonary embolus:** anticoagulation, vena caval filter and occasionally pulmonary embolectomy.
   d. **Mitral stenosis:** valvotomy or replacement.
   e. **Mitral regurgitation:** repair or replacement if left ventricular function remains reasonable.
   f. **Atrial septal defect:** surgery or, if suitable, closure in the catheter laboratory (e.g. with an Amplatzer closure device). There must be evidence of reversibility of the pulmonary pressure if it is close to systemic.
   g. **Eisenmenger's syndrome:** repair of the defect responsible for the shunt is not usually possible once reversal of shunting has occurred. Consider heart and lung transplant if conservative treatment (diuretics, digoxin and sometimes ACEIs) has failed.
2. General measures include continuous oxygen, diuretics, digoxin and spironolactone for problems with right heart failure. Use of the newer endothelin receptor antagonists (bosentan), prostaglandins (iloprost) or phosphodiesterase inhibitors (sildenafil) is generally indicated for IPH and pulmonary hypertension secondary to connective tissue disease and pulmonary embolism. Bosentan has also been approved for use in Eisenmenger's syndrome. Riociguat (guanylate cyclase stimulator) is effective for pulmonary hypertension secondary to pulmonary embolism.

IDIOPATHIC (PRIMARY) PULMONARY HYPERTENSION

Treatment of this progressive and debilitating condition involves the general measures outlined above. Untreated patients have a poor survival rate: 2–3 years median survival from the time of diagnosis.

1. Bosentan and ambrisentan have been approved for use for patients with IPH. These drugs are endothelin receptor antagonists. Endothelin-1 is a potent vasoconstrictor whose levels have been shown to be elevated in patients with IPH. Modest improvements in functional capacity and pulmonary artery pressures have been demonstrated after treatment of patients with IPH and those with underlying connective tissue disease. The drug is available only for patients with class III symptoms and a right atrial pressure of > 8 mmHg. Its side-effects include teratogenicity, an increase in liver enzyme levels and possibly male infertility. Prostacyclin analogues, such as iloprost, which are taken by inhalation, can also be effective. Continuous IV epoprostenol has been shown to improve symptoms and prognosis in a number of small randomised trials for IPH patients at least. Sildenafil (a phosphodiesterase inhibitor) is a vasodilator that must not be used in combination with nitrates because of the risk of severe and prolonged hypotension.
2. Combination treatment may be indicated if there is failure to respond to a single drug but this, in Australia, must generally be as part of a clinical trial and supervised in a specialist unit. Some of the drug manufacturers will provide sildenafil for patients already taking an endothelin antagonist. This means combination treatment is common but not subsidised by the PBS.
3. Suitable patients (severe unresponsive disease, right heart failure, young patient) should be considered for transplant. Successful outcomes have been shown with heart–lung,

double-lung or single-lung transplants. IPH has not been found to recur in the transplanted lung. The prognosis depends on the NYHA-WHO functional class: class I–II, 6 years; class III, 2.5 years; class IV, 6 months.

Possible lines of questioning

1. How would you decide whether *this* patient qualifies for an endothelin antagonist?
2. What alternative causes of *this* patient's dyspnoea would you consider? How would you investigate for them?

Sarcoidosis

This chronic, systemic, granulomatous disease is relatively common and patients occasionally require admission to hospital for investigation or treatment. It is an unusual lung disease in that it is less common in smokers. Although most patients present between the ages of 20 and 40 years, children and elderly people are sometimes affected. There are cases of familial sarcoidosis. At presentation, 90% of patients have pulmonary involvement and 40% have other organs affected. The disorder results from an exaggerated T-helper lymphocyte response that occurs for unknown reasons and is responsible for granuloma formation and fibrosis.

The history

1. Ask whether the patient has been admitted to hospital and, if so, why. The patient may already know the diagnosis and be an outpatient undergoing further investigations or treatment, or the diagnosis may be suspected because of lymphadenopathy or changes on chest X-ray (Fig. 6.10). Most patients present with asymptomatic hilar adenopathy (Table 6.20).
2. Ask about acute or subacute symptoms, as sarcoidosis develops in this way in about one-third of cases. The patient may have fever, weight loss, loss of appetite and malaise. The occurrence of erythema nodosum, joint symptoms and bilateral hilar adenopathy on the chest X-ray suggests an acute presentation. A combination of fever, facial nerve palsy, parotid enlargement and anterior uveitis may occur.
3. Symptoms suggesting a more insidious onset include persistent cough and dyspnoea. If the patient has chronic sarcoidosis, it is still important to find out how he or she originally presented, as the insidious onset is more often associated with chronic sarcoidosis and the development of damage to the lungs (up to 15% develop progressive pulmonary fibrosis – ILD) and other organs.

Table 6.20 **Clinical presentation of sarcoidosis**
• Abnormal chest X-ray (30%)
• Fever, weight loss, malaise, cough or dyspnoea (20%)
• Arthralgia and erythema nodosum (20%)
• Eye symptoms (25%)
• Palpable lymphadenopathy (5%)
• Skin abnormalities (5%)
• Rare: cardiac arrhythmias, hypercalcaemia or cranial nerve palsies

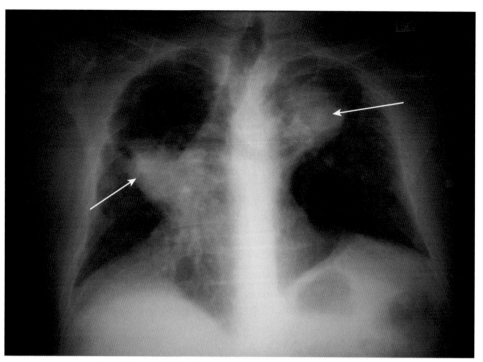

Figure 6.10 Massive bilateral hilar lymphadenopathy (arrows).

Figure reproduced courtesy of The Canberra Hospital.

4. Ask about skin eruptions (e.g. erythema nodosum, plaques, maculopapular lesions and subcutaneous nodules). Erythema nodosum, fever and migratory polyarthralgias, when found in combination with hilar lymphadenopathy, may indicate Lofgren's syndrome.

5. Eye symptoms occur in about one-quarter of patients. The patient may have noticed blurred vision, excess tears and light sensitivity due to uveitis. Involvement of the lacrimal glands can cause sicca syndrome, resulting in dry, sore eyes.

6. Ask about nasal stuffiness, as the nasal mucosa is involved in about one-fifth of patients. Occasionally, a hoarse voice or even stridor may result from sarcoid involving the larynx.

7. Renal involvement is uncommon but occasionally nephrolithiasis can result because of hypercalcaemia.

8. Ask about neurological symptoms – facial nerve palsy is the most common manifestation, but psychiatric disturbances and fits may occur.

9. Almost half the patients at some time in the course of the disease have arthralgia; even frank arthritis can occur.

10. The patient may be aware of cardiac abnormalities. Conduction problems, including complete heart block and ventricular arrhythmias, occur in about 5% of patients. Cardioverter-defibrillators are occasionally required. VT ablation treatment is difficult because of the diffuse nature of the cardiac involvement.

11. If the patient is female, ask about pregnancies. Sarcoidosis tends to abate in pregnancy but then flare up in the postpartum period.

12. Enquire about gastrointestinal symptoms (e.g. dysphagia from hilar adenopathy), although these are very rare. Liver involvement is common but rarely causes symptoms. The patient may know about abnormal liver function tests (usually a cholestatic picture).
13. Ask how the diagnosis was made. The CT scan has a characteristic appearance and may have been the only investigation performed, although in most cases the diagnosis is confirmed by biopsy. Specifically determine whether a lymph node biopsy or lung biopsy has been performed. Sometimes a skin or conjunctival biopsy may have been obtained to make the diagnosis. Bronchial or transbronchial lung biopsies are used to make the diagnosis in most cases. Occasionally, mediastinoscopy with lymph node biopsy is needed to make the diagnosis.
14. Ask about treatment. Find out whether the patient has been receiving steroids and what dose is currently being taken. Various other treatments may have been tried, including NSAIDs, cyclosporin and cyclophosphamide.
15. Ask about the disease impact on the patient and his or her family.

The examination

1. Begin with an examination of the skin.
   a. You might be lucky enough to find erythema nodosum. These raised red or purple lesions are most commonly found on the lower limbs. They resolve spontaneously after 3 or 4 weeks.
   b. Look at the face, back and extremities for maculopapular eruptions. These are elevated spots less than 1 cm in diameter that have a waxy, flat top. There may also be lupus pernio on the face (Fig. 6.11). These are purple swollen nodules with

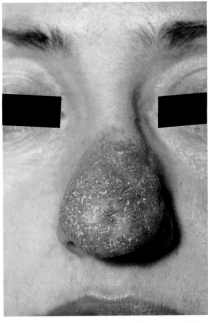

Figure 6.11 **Lupus pernio. The nose shows typical scaly violaceous swelling.**

F Ferri, Sarcoidosi-lupus perni. *Ferri's color atlas and text of clinical medicine.* Fig 11.4. Elsevier, 2009, with permission.

a shiny surface, which particularly affect the nose, cheeks, eyelids and ears. They may make the nose appear bulbous; occasionally the mucosa of the nose may be involved and the underlying bone can be destroyed. Lupus pernio sometimes also involves the fingers and knees. Pink nodules may be found in old scars.

2. Examine the eyes for signs of uveitis. Yellow conjunctival nodules may be present. Examine the fundi for papilloedema. Feel the parotids. Uveoparotid fever presents with uveitis, parotid swelling and seventh cranial nerve palsy.

3. Next, examine the respiratory system. Most commonly, physical examination of the chest reveals no abnormality. Look particularly for signs of interstitial lung disease; basal end-inspiratory crackles may be present. Pleural effusions occur rarely.

4. Next, examine all the lymph nodes. Lymphadenopathy is sometimes generalised.

5. Now examine the abdomen for hepatomegaly (20%) and splenomegaly (up to 40%).

6. Examine the joints for signs of arthritis, which is almost always non-deforming.

7. Examine the nervous system. Look particularly for facial nerve palsy.

8. Feel the pulse (heart block or arrhythmia) and look for signs of right ventricular failure or cardiomyopathy. Note the presence of a pacemaker or defibrillator box.

Investigations

1. A full blood count may reveal lymphocytopenia and sometimes eosinophilia.

2. The ESR is often raised. There may be hyperglobulinaemia.

3. The ACE level is raised in about two-thirds of patients with active sarcoidosis but unfortunately is not diagnostic; ACE is also sometimes elevated (5%) in healthy persons or those with primary biliary cholangitis, leprosy, atypical mycobacterial infection, miliary tuberculosis, silicosis, acute histoplasmosis and hyperparathyroidism. ACE is not elevated in patients with malignancies (e.g. lymphoma). Hypercalcaemia and, more commonly, hypercalciuria may be present.

4. The chest X-ray is usually abnormal (Table 6.21) and the changes can be classified into four stages:
   - *Stage 1* Bilateral hilar lymphadenopathy alone
   - *Stage 2* Bilateral hilar lymphadenopathy and pulmonary infiltration
   - *Stage 3* Pulmonary infiltration without hilar lymphadenopathy
   - *Stage 4* Pulmonary fibrosis.

   Patients with stage 1 X-rays are considered to have an acute reversible form of the disease, whereas the other stages tend to be more chronic. The chest X-ray may show paratracheal lymphadenopathy; cavitation and pleural effusions are rare. Cavities may become colonised with *Aspergillus*. CT scans of the chest may show a ground-glass appearance when active alveolitis is present. Always think about excluding tuberculosis and histoplasmosis.

Table 6.21 Chest X-ray changes in sarcoidosis

1. Hilar lymphadenopathy – up to 90%
2. Paratracheal lymphadenopathy – less than 80%
3. Reticulonodular changes – 70%
4. Peripheral nodules – less than 5%
5. Cavitation – less than 5%
6. Pleural effusion – less than 5%
7. Linear atelectasis – less than 1%

5. If there is parenchymal granulomatous involvement, respiratory function tests reveal the changes that are typical of interstitial lung disease, with reduced lung volumes and diffusing capacity, but a normal FEV_1/FVC ratio. Occasionally, a mixed pattern of obstruction and restriction is seen.

6. Blood gas estimations may show mild hypoxaemia.

7. A gallium-67 lung scan usually shows a pattern of diffuse uptake, but increased uptake in the lacrimal and parotid glands (panda sign) or in the right paratracheal and left hilar areas (lambda sign) is more specific for sarcoidosis. Enlarged nodes also tend to show up on the scans.

8. Bronchoscopy with transbronchial biopsy will usually establish the pathological diagnosis. Bronchioalveolar lavage will show an increase in the number of $CD4^+$ T-helper lymphocytes. However, this is not diagnostic of the condition.

9. Biopsy of lymph nodes, skin or liver may be diagnostic. The non-caseating granulomas found in sarcoidosis are non-specific; they are also found in berylliosis, leprosy, hypersensitivity pneumonitis and granulomatous infection, and in lymph nodes that drain adjacent carcinomas.

10. If cardiac involvement is suspected then an MRI or PET scan is the best way of delineating the extent of cardiac involvement and the risk of significant arrhythmias.

Treatment

Indications for treatment are lack of resolution of active pulmonary sarcoidosis with increasing symptoms or worsening lung function; neurological, renal or cardiac complications; major eye disease; and occasionally severe systemic symptoms (e.g. fever and weight loss).

1. The drug of choice is prednisolone. This is begun in high dose (1 mg/kg) for up to 6 weeks and then tapered over the following few months. Treatment is continued for 12 months. The prognosis is good. About 50% of patients develop some permanent organ damage but, in most, this is mild.

2. Patients who require longer treatment may be offered steroid-sparing drugs, including chlorambucil, methotrexate or azathioprine.

3. Hydroxychloroquine may be useful for skin disease.

4. Infliximab (a monoclonal antibody directed at tumour necrosis factor (TNF)) has been shown to improve lung function for patients already being treated with steroids and cytotoxics.

Possible lines of questioning

1. Does *this* patient have treatment for his or her sarcoidosis?
2. What follow-up regimen – reviews and investigations – would you recommend for *this* patient?

Cystic fibrosis

The survival of children with cystic fibrosis (CF) into adult life is now common. Over 50% of patients reach the age of 30 years and the prognosis is improving all the time. Although paediatricians are often reluctant to give up these patients, there are more surviving patients under adult physicians' care than with paediatricians. A small number of cases are diagnosed in adult life.

Cystic fibrosis is a common, serious, congenital inherited defect in Caucasian people. It has an autosomal recessive inheritance and the gene has been identified. The mutation is in the cystic fibrosis transmembrane conductance regulator protein gene on chromosome 7. The mutation causes increased sodium and chloride excretion in sweat and increased resorption of sodium and water from respiratory mucosa. The trait is present in about 1 in 25 Caucasians and 1 in 3000 has the condition. It is rare in other races. It is a chronic disease that can affect the lungs, pancreas, bowel, liver and sweat glands.

The history

1. Ask about presentation:
   a. Age at diagnosis – 90% of patients are diagnosed at 4–6 weeks of age by screening tests.
   b. Presenting symptoms – the patient may have been told that he or she had meconium ileus as a baby or recurrent respiratory infections in early life; failure to thrive may suggest the diagnosis. Many patients, however, are asymptomatic at the time of diagnosis.
   c. Pulmonary symptoms – these include cough and sputum, haemoptysis, wheeze, dyspnoea.
   d. Nasal polyps and sinusitis – are relatively common.
   e. Gastrointestinal symptoms – include problems maintaining weight; diarrhoea and steatorrhoea (malabsorption secondary to pancreatic insufficiency – 90% of patients); constipation, rectal prolapse, abdominal distension and bowel obstruction (defective water excretion into the bowel).
   f. Heat exhaustion in hot weather – patients with cystic fibrosis can lose large amounts of salt in their sweat, which sometimes causes problems, particularly in the tropics.
   g. Cardiac symptoms – the patient may know of cardiac involvement (cor pulmonale is a very late development).
   h. Jaundice and variceal bleeding – focal biliary cirrhosis and portal hypertension occur occasionally.
   i. Diabetes mellitus – cystic-fibrosis-related diabetes is different from typical type 1 diabetes and occurs in up to 20% of 18-year-olds with CF and upwards of 50% of 30-year-olds.
2. Ask about diagnosis. The patient may know whether a sweat test was performed. Collection of sweat and measurement of the chloride concentration is still the accepted method of diagnosing the condition. A sweat chloride concentration of more than 70 mmol/L suggests cystic fibrosis in an adult. Otherwise, a combination of respiratory and malabsorptive problems may be considered enough to make the diagnosis. A list of the major and minor diagnostic criteria is presented in Table 6.22. DNA markers are likely to be used increasingly in the diagnosis. At the moment this is difficult because there are a large number of abnormal genotypes (over 2000) that can result in the disease. Screening for the commonest mutations is the basis for the two-stage newborn screening testing conducted in all states. If two mutations are recognised the diagnosis is made, while if only one is found the child is referred back for sweat testing.
3. Ask about family history – the autosomal recessive inheritance means siblings and other close relatives may be affected.
4. Ask about treatment. Pulmonary disease is the main determinant of mortality. Aggressive treatment of the pulmonary complications has had the greatest effect on the improvement in life expectancy. The patients are usually well aware of this and are largely responsible for their own treatment. The condition is a chronic suppurative progressive

Table 6.22 The diagnosis of cystic fibrosis
SWEAT TEST
• Elevated chloride sweat test (98%) – pilocarpine iontophoresis on 100 mg of sweat
> 70 mmol / L diagnostic in adults
> 60 mmol / L diagnostic in children
40–60 mmol / L suggestive
< 40 mmol / L normal
OTHER FEATURES SUGGESTING THE DIAGNOSIS
• Azoospermia in males (95%)
• Family history of cystic fibrosis (70%)
• Nasal polyps
• Meconium ileus equivalent (distal bowel obstruction from inspissated secretions)
• Rectal prolapse
• Focal biliary cirrhosis
• Diabetes mellitus

one causing bronchiolitis, bronchitis, pneumonia (uncommon in children) and eventually bronchiectasis. The pathology is probably the result of the formation of viscous mucous plugs, which lead to distal infection and lung damage.

a. The mainstay of treatment is physiotherapy, which the patient, with help from family and a physiotherapist, performs. Ask about deep breathing, percussion, postural drainage, the use of the positive end-expiratory pressure (PEP) techniques such as the PEP mask, and the forced expiratory technique called 'huffing'.

b. Ask about inhaled therapies. This may include nebulised hypertonic saline, then inhaled DNAase (once daily).

c. The patient should also know what antibiotics have been used and whether continuously or intermittently. Nebulised bronchodilators and antibiotics are commonly prescribed. *Staphylococcus aureus* and *Pseudomonas aeruginosa* are common pathogens because of their ability to grow on the abnormal bronchial mucus of cystic fibrotic lungs. The patient may know if the *Pseudomonas* is antibiotic resistant. Macrolide antibiotics, especially azithromycin, are being used because of their anti-inflammatory properties. Ask whether he or she has had pneumococcal or influenza vaccination.

d. Ask whether treatment for complications, such as haemoptysis, cor pulmonale or pneumothorax, has been required. Minor haemoptysis, where less than 250 mL of blood is lost, occurs in about 60% of patients. Major haemoptysis occurs in about 7% of patients and bronchial artery embolisation may be required. Cor pulmonale may require treatment with diuretics, spironolactone and possibly vasodilators, but aggressive treatment of the lung disease and supplementary oxygen are more important in the long term. Pleurodesis used to be the treatment of choice for recurrent pneumothorax, but this may result in a contraindication to lung transplantation.

5. Enquire about gastrointestinal symptoms. These tend to be less of a problem, but malabsorption may make weight gain very difficult for these patients. Ask what pancreatic enzyme replacement the patient uses and how often. Enzyme therapy is based on the fat content of each meal ingested. Enquire about food intolerances, adherence to enzymes and presence of abdominal symptoms such as abdominal pain.

6. Ask about the number of admissions to hospital over the past 12 months and the length of each stay. Routine admission to hospital three or four times a year for

intensive physiotherapy and intravenous antibiotics and bronchodilators (a tune-up) can be advantageous.

7. Enquire about social support. Ask whether the patient knows about or belongs to the local cystic fibrosis association and whether he or she has been in touch with other affected patients. However, patients in direct contact with other patients with CF increase the risk of cross-infection. It is recommended that no patient with CF comes in contact with another CF patient.

8. Try to find out tactfully whether the patient understands the inheritance of the disease; male patients may know that azoospermia is usually present owing to destruction of the vas deferens by abnormal secretions (95%). Sperm aspiration and in vitro fertilisation are possible. Eighty per cent of women are fertile, and pregnancy and breastfeeding are often successful. Find out in some detail how a young adult copes with this debilitating and life-shortening disease.

The examination

1. Looking at the patient's chest shape is beneficial, and at overall nutritional status – malnourished patients often have a protuberant abdomen. Muscle bulk is considered a good indicator of the severity and prognosis in a particular patient. Measure the patient's height and weight.

2. Ask the patient to cough. Listen for a loose cough and examine any sputum for the degree of purulence.

3. Now examine the respiratory system carefully. Note clubbing, which is present in the majority of patients. Look for abnormal chest wall development. Look for signs of past treatment for pneumothorax or transplant (scars).

4. Estimate forced expiratory time and examine the chest, listening particularly for crackles, wheezes and reduced breath sounds.

5. Examine the heart for signs of cor pulmonale and right ventricular failure.

6. Examine the abdomen for signs of faecal loading, especially in the right iliac fossa, organomegaly, such as hepatomegaly, or hard liver edge, as in cirrhosis, splenomegaly and other signs of portal hypertension as well as sites of insulin injections in the abdominal wall, also scars of previous surgery including those for meconium ileus at birth.

Investigations

1. Sputum culture: colonisation with *H. influenzae* and *S. aureus* tends to occur in young patients and this is sometimes followed by nosocomial *E. coli* and *Proteus* spp. By the age of 10 years, *Pseudomonas* is the main pathogen in most patients, but usually it does not cause systemic infection.

2. A full blood count: to look for anaemia, which may be caused by malabsorption or chronic disease; the white cell count may indicate acute infection. Polycythaemia is rare, despite chronic hypoxia.

3. The electrolyte levels and liver function tests: there may be evidence of deficiencies of fat-soluble vitamins (A, D, E and K). The creatinine level should be known before aminoglycosides are used.

4. The chest X-ray (Fig. 6.12a and b): should be compared with previous films if these are available. Increased lung markings are present in 98% of patients. These occur particularly in the upper lobes. Cystic bronchiectatic changes occur in more than 60% of patients. Mucous plugs may be seen in one-third and atelectasis occurs in just over 10% of patients. Look also for pneumothorax and pleural changes at the site of previous pneumothoraces or pleurodesis.

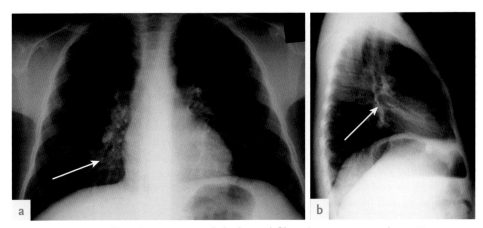

Figure 6.12 Cystic fibrosis. (a) PA and (b) lateral films in a young patient. Note increased lung markings in the right middle lobe with 'tram tracking' – increased bronchial wall thickness (arrows).

Figures reproduced courtesy of The Canberra Hospital.

5. Chest CT is not routine, but may help define focal areas of bronchiectasis that are occasionally amenable to resection.
6. Spirometry readings may fluctuate because of airway inflammation. An FEV_1 that is persistently less than 40% indicates a poor prognosis.

Management

Try to form an idea of the patient's ability to cope with the illness, as so much of the management depends on this.

1. Intensive and repetitive physiotherapy is the mainstay of treatment. Inactivated influenza vaccine and the pneumococcal vaccine should be routine.
2. Intravenous antibiotics may be indicated for acute exacerbations of pulmonary disease if these are severe or fail to respond to oral antibiotic treatment. In most cases, dual IV antibiotics including one of the aminoglycosides and a semisynthetic penicillin are used.
3. Nebulised and dry-powder tobramycin are both approved after extensive trials as being beneficial in treating *Pseudomonas* lung disease in CF. Nebulised anti-*Pseudomonas* antibiotics improve lung function and prognosis.
4. Malabsorption may require aggressive treatment with pancreatic enzyme supplements, including lipase, and frequent small meals as well as vitamin supplements.
5. Double-lung transplantation is now an accepted, although still uncommon, treatment in patients with advanced disease. Cystic fibrosis does not recur in the transplanted lung. The 5-year survival rate is only about 65%.
6. Human recombinant DNAase seems effective in degrading the concentration of DNA in sputum, reducing sputum viscosity and improving the patient's ability to clear pulmonary secretions. DNAase has been proven to be effective both in those with established CF lung disease and in preventing decline in lung function when commenced in patients who have well-preserved lung function.
7. Small molecules are able to correct the CF conductance regulator. Ivacaftor is an oral treatment for patients with the G55 1D mutation. For those with the F508 deletion, elexacaftor and tezacaftor are added (triple therapy).

Tuberculosis

The increased incidence of pulmonary tuberculosis (TB) over the past 10 years or so and its association with HIV infection have made it a possible long case. Protection from *Mycobacterium tuberculosis* is via cell-mediated immunity involving CD4+ T-helper lymphocytes. The defects of these cells in number and effectiveness, which is characteristic of HIV infection, explain this susceptibility. It may be a difficult diagnostic or management problem, or both. It also has important social and public health implications.

The history
The patient is likely to know that the diagnosis has been made or is suspected.
1. Find out whether the patient is a recent immigrant and, if so, from where.
2. Ask whether there has been a previous diagnosis of any other serious medical problem that might interfere with cell-mediated immunity, such as malnutrition, alcoholism or HIV infection.
3. Establish how the diagnosis was made and how long ago.
4. Ask about some of the important symptoms – weight loss, sweats and fever, cough with purulent and blood-stained sputum, and pleuritic chest pain from pleural lesions or uncontrolled coughing.
5. Ask what investigations have been performed or are planned. TB may have been suspected after a chest X-ray was performed because of respiratory symptoms or as a routine screening test. The patient may remember having to give early morning sputum specimens on a number of occasions or having had a bronchocospy with washings, if sputum was not being produced. Bronchoscopy may have been performed to exclude other causes of an abnormal chest X-ray, such as carcinoma of the lung.

    A tuberculin (Mantoux) skin test may have been performed as a screening test or to support the diagnosis where cultures have been negative. A positive tuberculin test is still significant, even if the patient has received a bacille Calmette–Guérin (BCG) vaccination in the past. Remember, if the patient is in a high-risk group (HIV positive, immunosuppressed, in close contact with a clear-cut case of TB or has evidence of prior TB on chest X-ray), the Mantoux test is considered positive with just 5 mm of induration (vs 15 mm in low-risk patients).
6. Find out what treatment regimen the patient is receiving. Considerable detail must be sought about the drugs themselves – doses (if known), how long treatment will continue, how the drugs are administered (supervised or unsupervised) and what side-effects have occurred (Table 6.23). Remember that rifampicin and rifabutin colour body fluids, including urine, orange.

Table 6.23 Common antituberculous drugs and their side-effects		
DRUG	**MAIN SIDE-EFFECTS**	**USUAL DOSE / DAY**
Rifampicin	Hepatitis, flu-like illness	600 mg
Isoniazid	Hepatitis, fever, peripheral neuropathy	300 mg (reduced to 2 or 3 doses a week in chronic kidney disease)
Streptomycin	Ototoxicity, renal impairment	1 g (not safe in pregnancy)
Ethambutol	Optic neuritis	15 mg / kg
Pyrazinamide	Hepatitis	1.5–2 g
PAS	Hepatitis, diarrhoea, hypersensitivity	12 g
PAS = para-aminosalicylic acid.		

7. Ask whether there has been a trigger for reactivation of previous infection (diabetes mellitus, old age, HIV infection).
8. Find out what effect this serious and chronic disease has had on the patient's life. Has the patient been able to work or go to school? Do friends and workmates know the diagnosis? Does the patient's occupation involve a public health risk?
9. Establish how the problem has been handled from a public health aspect. What screening has been done on the patient's family and friends? Are any of the family also being treated?

The examination

Early in the course of the illness there may be no specific signs. Of those patients without HIV infection who have TB, 80% have only pulmonary disease. However, the majority of patients with HIV and TB have both extrapulmonary and pulmonary disease.

1. Note the patient's general appearance. Look for wasting and cachexia that may be associated with the risk factors for TB (HIV, alcoholism) or may be a result of the disease (which is also known as consumption for this reason).
2. Examine the lungs for signs of the aggressive primary infection that can occur in immunocompromised patients. These include a pleural effusion or tuberculous empyema and lobar collapse (as a result of lymphadenopathy and bronchial obstruction).
3. Post-primary disease is more common in adults. There is almost always a loose cough and often haemoptysis. There may be no abnormal findings, but you should look especially for upper lobe signs, including coarse crackles and wheezes due to partial bronchial obstruction caused by lymphadenopathy, and the rare amphoric breath sounds that occur over a cavity.
4. Extrapulmonary disease most commonly involves the lymph nodes (especially in HIV patients). Examine all the palpable lymph node groups. The most often affected are the cervical and supraclavicular nodes. There is usually painless swelling.
5. Involvement of the genitourinary tract can be associated with haematuria and tenderness over the flanks.
6. The bones are involved in a small number of cases. The lumbar spine (Pott's disease), hips and knees are most affected. Collapse of the vertebral bodies may cause kyphosis and even paraplegia.
7. Tuberculous pericarditis can cause symptoms and signs of pericarditis and occasionally tamponade.

8. Abdominal TB can cause various gastrointestinal signs. There may be a palpable abdominal mass. Severe abdominal tenderness suggests tuberculous peritonitis.

Investigations

1. The diagnosis of active disease depends on microscopy of a specimen that shows mycobacteria (e.g. send three morning sputum specimens on separate days, followed by confirmation by culture of the organism). Traditionally, specimens of sputum or gastric or bronchial washings (often useful for children), or a lymph node biopsy, are stained with the Ziehl–Neelsen stain. Modern laboratories are more likely to use auramine–rhodamine stains and fluorescence microscopy. Only about 60% of patients with eventually proven TB have positive microscopy. Culture of the organism takes about 6 weeks, but is needed for the definitive diagnosis. These organisms should then be tested for sensitivity to the main antituberculous drugs. This takes up to 8 more weeks. If multidrug resistance (MDRTB) is suspected, the *rpo* gene can be tested: it is responsible for 95% of rifampicin resistance. Polymerase chain reaction (PCR) testing can now provide rapid identification of *M. tuberculosis*, but is not available everywhere and does not distinguish between viable and non-viable organisms.

2. A QuantiFERON-TB Gold–interferon-gamma (IFN-γ) assay is sensitive for the diagnosis of mycobacterial infection with some false positives for atypical mycobacteria.

3. A chest X-ray showing the typical pattern of infiltrates and cavities in the upper lobe strongly suggests the diagnosis, but many other patterns are consistent with TB (Figs 6.13–6.15).

4. The Mantoux (purified protein derivative, PPD) test needs to be carefully interpreted (Table 6.24). A positive test depends on the patient's risk of having TB. Tuberculin skin testing is useful for screening for latent TB. The test may be negative in severe disease (e.g. in up to 50% of cases of miliary TB), in those who are immunosuppressed, including the elderly, or if exposure is only recent (repeat in 3 months). IFN-γ release assays use a specific tuberculosis antigen to stimulate release of IFN-γ from T cells

Table 6.24 Tuberculin (Mantoux) skin testing[a]

CRITERIA FOR A POSITIVE TEST[b]

A. ≥ 5 mm (HIGH RISK)
1. Abnormal chest X-ray consistent with prior TB
2. Close contact with a documented case
3. Immunosuppressed: HIV, transplant patient or on ≥ 15 mg / day prednisone

B. ≥ 10 mm (INTERMEDIATE RISK)
1. Healthcare workers, nursing home patients
2. Recent immigrants from high-prevalence regions
3. Prisoners, IV drug users
4. Diabetic patients
5. Prednisone (< 15 mg / day)

C. ≥ 15 mm (LOW RISK)
Everyone else

If positive and no active disease on chest X-ray and by sputum for acid-fast bacteria: treat for latent TB (isoniazid for 9 months).

[a]Contraindicated if a history of necrotic skin reaction to previous testing. Prior BCG vaccination does not invalidate the results.
[b]False negatives occur in anergy or with recent exposure (recheck after 12 weeks) or in the elderly (recheck after 3 weeks).

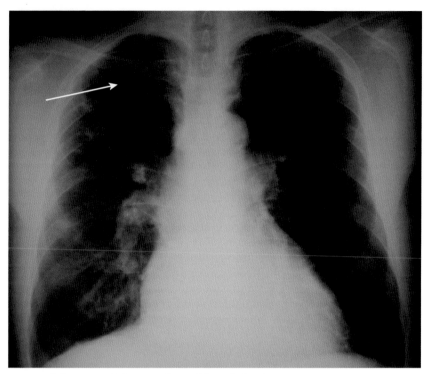

Figure 6.13 Right upper lobe scarring; old TB infection (arrow).

Figure reproduced courtesy of The Canberra Hospital.

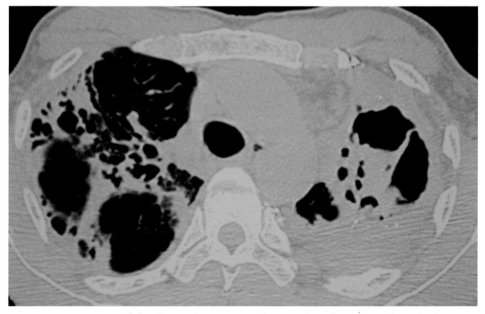

Figure 6.14 CT scan of the thorax in TB; note destructive changes and cavitation from TB.

Figure reproduced courtesy of The Canberra Hospital.

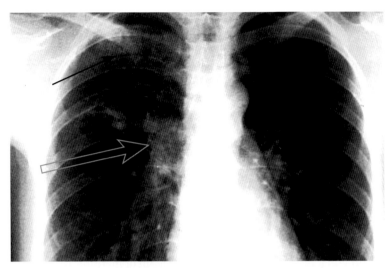

Figure 6.15 **Pulmonary TB. Two small round areas of shadowing are seen in the right upper zone (black arrow). The right hilum is enlarged by the enlarged draining lymph nodes (open arrow). This combination of focal shadowing and enlarged lymph nodes is the primary (Ghon) complex of TB. With healing, calcification may occur in the parenchymal and nodal lesions. In contrast, in TB reactivation or re-infection, cavitation may occur and there is no lymphadenopathy.**

The Canberra Hospital X-Ray Library, reproduced with permission.

in vitro. These tests are more specific than tuberculin testing and may be useful where rates of TB are low. They are not affected by previous BCG vaccination. A positive screening test should be followed by a chest X-ray to look for active disease.
5. Biopsies of the pleura, lymph nodes or bone marrow may be needed. Bronchoscopy is sometimes necessary to exclude other causes of X-ray changes.
6. The fasting blood sugar level should be taken to rule out diabetes mellitus.
7. HIV patients may have TB despite a completely normal chest X-ray. They may also have less typical chest X-ray findings – often lower lobe changes without cavities. They are more likely to have infection with other mycobacteria, such as MAC. Remember that the diagnosis can be made even when the organism is not isolated. All patients with TB should be tested for HIV infection.

Treatment

There are four first-line drugs for the treatment of TB: isoniazid, rifampicin, ethambutol and pyrazinamide. These are all given orally. Second-line drugs tend to be more toxic and are used only for organisms resistant to the first-line drugs. They include moxifloxacin, streptomycin, quinolone, kanamycin and amikacin (parenteral), and cycloserine, ethionamide and PAS (para-aminosalicylic acid). The initial isolate should undergo drug susceptibility testing, especially if treatment seems to have failed or there is a relapse of symptoms.

Treatment of latent TB reduces the risk of transmission and the risk of progression to active disease by up to 90%. Nine months of treatment with isoniazid is commonly recommended.
1. Treatment begins with a combination regimen of three drugs (usually isoniazid, rifampicin and pyrazinamide) for 2 months. A fourth drug (usually ethambutol) is

often given until the organism's sensitivities are available. The aim here is to kill the majority of the organisms, improve the patient's symptoms and render him or her non-infectious. This is followed by 4 months of treatment with two drugs (isoniazid and rifampicin).

2. Adherence to the full course of treatment is very important, but difficult to ensure. Complicated public health arrangements, with monitoring of compliance, may be needed to enforce treatment. Direct observed treatment (DOT) is insisted on by public health authorities if compliance seems doubtful. These patients present as required to be observed taking their treatment.

3. The response to treatment is monitored by repeat sputum cultures until they become negative. Persisting positive cultures after 3 months suggest resistance of the organism or non-adherence on the part of the patient. Patients are probably not an infectious risk if no sputum is produced or if the sputum is consistently acid-fast bacilli (AFB) negative.

4. Patients need to be aware of the most important side-effects of treatment, which include hepatitis (up to 5% in the general population and 30% in HIV patients), deafness and visual disturbance (see Table 6.23). Small increases in the transaminases (to three times normal) are no cause for alarm and are poor predictors of significant hepatotoxicity. Treatment should be reviewed immediately if jaundice develops.

5. Multiple drug resistance is becoming increasingly common and should be expected if the infection was acquired from a patient with a known resistant organism or if the infection was acquired in parts of Asia or South America. The addition of a fluoroquinolone to the regimen should be considered while resistance studies are under way.

6. Prevention of infection by vaccination with BCG is not widely practised in Australia; its effectiveness is uncertain. In high-risk areas, vaccination of children has been shown to reduce the risk of cerebral TB. The Mantoux test should be interpreted as usual regardless of previous BCG vaccination (15 mm is a positive skin test for low-risk individuals). If the Mantoux test is positive (≥ 5 mm) in a high-risk group (patients with exposure to TB (especially household contacts), or who are HIV infected, on prolonged steroid treatment (≥ 15 mg ≥ 1 month) or have undergone organ transplant), prescribe treatment with isoniazid for latent TB (5 mg/kg/day for 9 months). If close (e.g. household) contacts are negative on the tuberculin test, treat for 12 weeks and repeat the skin test: this reduces the chance of the development of open TB by 90%. If the test is ≥ 10 mm in an intermediate-risk group (IV drug abusers, prisoners, healthcare workers, nursing-home patients, homeless people or those with diabetes), also treat with isoniazid. Screening of contacts and high-risk patients with tuberculin testing is an important public health measure.

7. Patients starting on biological agents for inflammatory disease should be screened for possible TB with QuantiFERON-TB Gold serology and, if positive, a chest X-ray.

Possible lines of questioning

1. How would you decide whether *this* patient's antituberculous treatment is adequate and when it might be stopped?

2. How would you screen a patient about to start a biological agent for TB?

Lung transplantation

Although lung transplantation is an uncommon procedure, transplant patients have chronic management problems that make them very suitable long cases. Fifty percent 10-year survival is now achieved in experienced centres. The examiners will have the opportunity to ask questions about the patient's underlying pulmonary problem, the general indications for lung transplant, management of the complications of transplant and, of course, the types of social problems associated with a severe chronic illness. Occasionally, patients who are being assessed for possible transplant may be suitable for the clinical examinations.

The history

1. Find out why the patient is in hospital (it is probably just for the clinical examinations).
2. Obtain some basic information about the transplant: how long ago, how many lungs were transplanted and whether the patient's heart was also originally someone else's.
3. Enquire what the original lung disease was. Emphysema (including that caused by alpha$_1$-antitrypsin deficiency) is the most common indication, accounting for about half of the unilateral transplants and one-third of the bilateral transplants. Idiopathic pulmonary hypertension, cystic fibrosis and Eisenmenger's syndrome are the main indications for heart/lung transplants.
4. Ask how successful the procedure has been from the patient's point of view. Lung function tests should be normal after bilateral transplant and nearly so after unilateral transplant. A decline in lung function test measurements of more than 10% usually is important. Patients are often aware of their results.
5. Find out what complications the patient can remember. Ask about known rejection episodes and how they were managed. Have there been difficult infections? The patient may know what organisms have been detected. Stenosis of a bronchial anastomosis site is an occasional early problem. This is often treated with dilatation and stenting.
6. Review what medications the patient is taking. If necessary, prompt for prednisolone, cyclosporin, mycophenolate, azathioprine and tacrolimus. Find out whether blood levels of tacrolimus and cyclosporin are measured regularly. Remember that these two drugs are metabolised via the cytochrome P450 pathway in the liver and blood levels may be affected by other medications (so make sure you review all of the drugs being taken).
7. If the patient is being assessed for transplant, try to find out whether the patient fits the current guidelines for transplant (Tables 6.25 and 6.26). In general, suitable patients are sick enough to require the operation but not too sick to present an intolerable operative risk.
8. Establish how the patient has coped with the procedure, its complications and the immunosuppressants. What regular follow-up is carried out? Many transplant units have a transplant nurse available after hours whom the patient can contact directly if there are problems.

Table 6.25 Age criteria for lung transplant			
	UNILATERAL	**BILATERAL**	**HEART/LUNG**
AGE (YEARS)	< 65	< 60	< 55

Table 6.26 Indications and contraindications for lung transplant	
INDICATIONS	**CONTRAINDICATIONS**
COPD – FEV_1 < 25% predicted, $PaCO_2$ > 55 mmHg **Cystic fibrosis, bronchiectasis** – FEV_1 < 30% or complications (e.g. cachexia, severe haemoptysis) or $PaCO_2$ > 50 mmHg, PaO_2 < 55 mmHg **ILD** – progressive symptoms, VC, DLCO < 60% **Pulmonary hypertension** – NYHA class III or IV, pulmonary artery pressure > 55 mmHg, cardiac index < 2 L/min **Eisenmenger's syndrome** – severe symptomatic impairment. The 2-year prognosis is not improved for these patients	**Relative** Diabetes Osteoporosis Alcohol excess Still smoking Likely compliance problems Atypical mycobacterial colonisation of lungs Weight > 130% of ideal or < 70% of ideal **Absolute** HIV, hepatitis B, hepatitis C and liver disease, malignancy, other organ failure
COPD = chronic obstructive pulmonary disease; DLCO = diffusion capacity for carbon monoxide; FEV_1 = forced expiratory volume; ILD = interstitial lung disease; NYHA = New York Heart Association; VC = vital capacity.	

The examination

Perform a thorough respiratory examination.

1. Look especially for thoracotomy scars and attempt an assessment of the patient's functional capacity (e.g. look for signs of breathlessness while the patient is undressing and, if the room is big enough, get the patient to walk backwards and forwards). An anterior submammary scar is often present. Patients with unilateral transplants will often have a normal lung examination on the side with the scar and signs of the original disease on the other side (e.g. the crackles of interstitial disease).
2. Listen for end-inspiratory pops and squeaks (bronchiolitis obliterans at an advanced stage can be associated with the development of bronchiectasis).
3. Note signs of infection – fever and areas of bronchial breathing or crackles.
4. Look for sputum and assess the cough.
5. Is the patient Cushingoid?

Management

The detection of complications and their management is likely to dominate the discussion.

1. **Rejection:** early rejection episodes are common and are treated with boost doses of prednisone. Symptoms of acute rejection include malaise, fever, dyspnoea and cough. Clinical assessment may reveal crackles, decreasing FEV_1, hypoxia and a raised white cell count. The chest X-ray may show infiltrates and pleural effusions. A transbronchial biopsy tends to be performed if there is any suspicion of rejection and allows an accurate diagnosis. In some places, routine biopsies are performed to detect asymptomatic rejection. It is not clear, however, whether these should be treated.
2. **Infection:** most lung transplant patients develop infections requiring treatment. Infection is the most common cause of death. A combination of immunosuppression and local problems, such as impaired ciliary activity, are relevant. Infections with cytomegalovirus (CMV), adenovirus, influenza A and paramyxovirus are common and associated with a significant mortality. Invasive fungal organisms, such as *Aspergillus*, result in an even worse prognosis. Patients now receive at least 3 months of routine prophylactic antibiotic, antiviral and antifungal treatment. This approach has improved the early postoperative prognosis.

3. **Immunosuppression:** the usual problems with immunosuppressive drugs occur in lung transplant patients. Renal impairment, hypertension and hyperlipidaemia are frequent problems. Osteoporosis and peripheral neuropathy are also seen. Five per cent of lung transplant patients develop lymphoproliferative disorders.

4. **Bronchiolitis obliterans:** the gradual onset of small airways obstruction is a manifestation of chronic rejection. It does not usually begin until 2 or more years after transplant, but is detectable in at least half of transplant patients within 5 years. It may occur more often in those who have had more frequent acute rejection episodes and in those with a human leukocyte antigen (HLA) mismatch with the donor. There tends to be a very gradual onset of dyspnoea, fatigue and cough. Patients have a slowly decreasing FEV_1 but chest X-rays are often normal. CT scans may show a central mottling opacity. Biopsy will establish the diagnosis. The prognosis is not good. Sometimes an aggressive increase in immunosuppression may stabilise the condition, but it cannot be reversed and often the patient deteriorates rapidly.

5. **Disease recurrence:** sarcoidosis and some forms of idiopathic ILD can recur in the transplanted lungs.

Possible lines of questioning

1. What happened to *this* patient during the period after the transplant? Were there complications, extended stays in an ICU, etc.?
2. What would make you suspect a rejection episode; how would you manage it?

Coronavirus disease 2019 (COVID-19)

Although candidates will not encounter active COVID-19 in the long-case examination, patients who have been infected may be encountered. The examiners will then have the opportunity to ask you about the presentation, diagnosis, treatment (and complications), disease course and long-term outcome. The discussion about issues may range from respiratory failure (acute respiratory distress syndrome) to cardiac and thrombolitic complications, and inflammatory complications such as Guillain–Barré syndrome or multisystem inflammatory syndrome (Kawasaki-like disease). The physical and psychological complications will be important to understand and manage. Many patients have prolonged symptoms after infection and may be disabled, and you will need to know and describe the details.

Chapter 7

The gastrointestinal long case

One finger in the throat and one in the rectum makes
a good diagnostician.

Sir William Osler (1849–1919)

Irritable bowel syndrome (IBS)

This common condition (prevalence 10% of people, 1.5 : 1 women:men) may emerge
as the history is taken but would be an unusual main problem. The whims of the
examiners might, however, turn this into a health issue they wish to talk about.

The history

The patient may have been told the diagnosis.

1. Ask about longstanding, intermittent symptoms that began usually before age 50.
   They include (by definition):
   a. abdominal pain (usually mid or lower abdomen), plus
   b. diarrhoea or constipation, or a mixed pattern
   c. bloating or even visible abdominal distension (there may be a picture on the
      patient's phone for you to look at).
   d. no alarm features – IBS does not cause rectal bleeding or anaemia, weight loss,
      vomiting or dysphagia
   e. no structural cause found.
2. Ask about risk factors including:
   a. history of infection causing gastroenteritis – most accepted risk factor; up to 20%
      of people develop IBS after an attack of gastroenteritis
   b. family history of IBS
   c. food intolerances (symptoms are often postprandial)
   d. history of physical or sexual abuse
   e. previous or current somatisation disorder, anxiety or depression.
   The pathophysiology of the condition is not well understood. The intestinal tract is
usually hypersensitive to distension. IBS is associated with bacterial dysbiosis (an alteration
of the microbiome) and, in a subset, low-grade inflammation (with increased numbers

---

Box 7.1 Definition of irritable bowel syndrome (based on Rome IV criteria)

1. Abdominal pain associated with a change in bowel habit[a]
2. Two of the following for the abdominal pain:
   - pain relieved (or aggravated) by defaecation, and / or
   - pain associated with more frequent or less frequent stools, and / or
   - pain associated with looser or harder stools.
3. Occurs over a period of at least 3 months and began 6 months or more ago
4. No alarm symptoms or signs (anaemia, iron deficiency, weight loss, nocturnal symptoms, onset > 50 years of age, family history of inflammatory bowel disease / coeliac)

---

[a]May be diarrhoea, constipation, or mixed (alternating).

Box 7.2 Alarm features

- Onset at age > 50
- Anaemia or iron deficiency
- Weight loss
- Rectal bleeding
- Family history of inflammatory bowel disease or coeliac disease
- Nocturnal symptoms, e.g. diarrhoea

---

of mast cells). Intestinal transit may be increased or decreased, with some evidence of abnormal serotonin signalling.

The diagnosis

If the presentation is typical (Box 7.1) and there are NO alarm features (Box 7.2) then IBS can be positively diagnosed clinically with no further investigations.

The examination

The gastrointestinal examination is usually normal. There may be scars from previous surgery (e.g. misdiagnosed acute appendix or gallbladder disease). Mild tenderness may be present – always exclude abdominal wall pain (Carnett's test should be negative – i.e. no increased tenderness on tensing the abdominal wall muscles).

Investigations

1. Coeliac disease can be confused with IBS and serological testing is recommended on a gluten-containing diet, especially if there is diarrhoea.
2. A blood count to rule out anaemia and a C-reactive protein (CRP) or stool calprotectin to look for evidence of inflammatory bowel disease (IBD) is helpful.
3. Routine testing for thyroid function, raised erythrocyte sedimentation rate (ESR), and stool for ova and parasites is not recommended. A food diary may help to identify lactose intolerance as the problem. Food allergy testing is not recommended. Colonoscopy should generally be performed only if alarm symptoms (e.g. recent symptoms in an older patient) are present.

Management

Begin with explanation and reassurance.

1. A diet high in insoluble fibre (psyllium, ispaghula) is somewhat effective, especially for constipation, but soluble-fibre diets (corn and wheat bran) are no better than placebo.

2. A low FODMAP diet (fermentable oligosaccharides, disaccharides, monosaccharides and polyols) followed by slowly reintroducing excluded food groups to identify the poorly tolerated foods can help over 50%, but compliance can be an issue.
3. Osmotic laxatives help constipation but not abdominal discomfort.
4. Loperamide can improve diarrhoea (stool consistency and frequency), but not other symptoms. A bile salt binder can help diarrhoea in a subset with IBS and bile salt overflow into the colon, inducing secretion.
5. Mebeverine or peppermint oil may help reduce abdominal pain.
6. Low-dose tricyclic antidepressants improve pain and other symptoms (number needed to treat = 4). They can be more helpful for IBS diarrhoea because of their anticholinergic effects.
7. Selective serotonin reuptake inhibitors (SSRIs) are at best modestly effective, but may help constipation more than diarrhoea (by increasing gut serotonin).
8. Narcotics should be avoided (because of dependency and constipation, plus they can paradoxically exacerbate pain).
9. These patients are at risk of having their gallbladder and appendix unnecessarily removed, and these surgical interventions should be discouraged unless there is a very clear indication.
10. Life expectancy is not altered, and a minority with IBS will spontaneously resolve over time, but any change in symptoms should be taken seriously.

Possible lines of questioning

1. Do you think any further investigations are indicated for *this* patient?
2. If *this* patient asked to try a series of exclusion diets, what would you recommend?

Peptic ulceration

This long case is usually a straightforward management problem. The most important causes of chronic peptic ulcer disease are *Helicobacter pylori* infection and traditional non-steroidal anti-inflammatory drugs (NSAIDs), including low-dose aspirin. The COX-2-specific NSAIDs have a lower incidence of peptic ulceration. Idiopathic ulcers (*H. pylori* negative, NSAID negative) are increasingly being reported. The Zollinger–Ellison syndrome (gastrinoma) is a very rare but important cause. Patients are usually admitted to hospital with peptic ulcer disease because of complications – typically haemorrhage, but more rarely perforation.

The history
1. Determine whether the patient currently has dyspepsia or a past history of dyspepsia (i.e. epigastric pain or discomfort, early satiety or postprandial fullness; bloating and heartburn are not considered dyspepsia symptoms). Typical ulcer symptoms include burning or sharp epigastric pain related to meals, or may wake the patient from sleep at night, and are relieved by antacids or antisecretory drugs. However, many patients with these symptoms do *not* have peptic ulcer disease, and ulcers are often associated with atypical symptoms. Duodenal and gastric ulcers cannot be distinguished from one another on the basis of symptoms. The differential diagnosis of dyspepsia includes functional dyspepsia (a gastroduodenal motility disorder), gastro-oesophageal reflux

disease (usually also causing heartburn or acid regurgitation), gastric cancer (especially in older patients with new onset of symptoms or with alarm features such as weight loss), biliary pain (typically severe, constant pain in the right upper quadrant or epigastrium that occurs episodically and unpredictably and lasts at least 20 minutes, but usually hours), chronic pancreatitis, pancreatic cancer or intestinal angina (chronic mesenteric ischaemia, which causes severe postprandial pain such that the patient is afraid to eat and loses weight).

2. Diabetes mellitus, thyroid dysfunction, hyperparathyroidism and connective tissue diseases can also cause dyspepsia.

3. Ask about the course of the symptoms and, if intermittent, the number of recurrences and treatments given. Ask about other alarm symptoms, such as recurrent vomiting (e.g. gastric outlet obstruction) or weight loss. Gastroparesis is rare and usually presents with recurrent vomiting, weight loss and abdominal pain.

4. Ask about the types of investigations the patient has had in the past. If an ulcer was apparently documented, determine whether this was by endoscopy (the most sensitive and specific test), or just by symptoms alone (which is not enough for a definite diagnosis). Determine whether the patient knows if *H. pylori* status was determined from gastric biopsies or by non-invasive tests, such as urea breath testing, stool antigen testing or serology (can remain positive after successful eradication so serology is not a gold standard test).

5. A history of past ulcer or other gastric surgery is important because of the associated complications (e.g. pain or bloating owing to bile reflux gastritis or an afferent loop syndrome, recurrent ulceration, early or late dumping, post-vagotomy diarrhoea, anaemia as a result of iron, vitamin B_{12} or folate deficiency, and osteomalacia or osteoporosis).

6. Ask about the family history: a strong family history of peptic ulcer may reflect the multiple endocrine neoplasia (MEN) 1 syndrome.

7. Enquire carefully about medication use – medications (e.g. digoxin, potassium, iron, oral antibiotics) can induce dyspepsia, which can be confused with peptic ulcer. *All* NSAIDs are an important cause of dyspepsia with or without chronic ulceration. Alcohol can also induce acute dyspepsia (but not chronic ulcers). Patients with an ulcer history may be taking maintenance acid suppression. First-line treatment for *H. pylori* usually includes a proton pump inhibitor (PPI) plus two antibiotics (amoxicillin and clarithromycin) for 7 days, but 30%–40% now fail, and should progress to second-line treatment.

8. Ask about anticoagulation, including NOACs (novel (non-vitamin-K) oral antico-agulants). Anticoagulation increases the risk of gastrointestinal bleeding.

9. If relevant, determine why the patient is in hospital on this occasion. If the admission is because of acute gastrointestinal bleeding, then the treatment applied needs to be documented. Bleeding can be the only symptom of peptic ulcer, and older (> 70) patients and those at a higher dose of NSAIDs are at a higher risk. Urgent endoscopy is done to treat current severe bleeding or to prevent rebleeding. Remember that morbidity (e.g. need for transfusion, rebleeding rates) but not mortality is improved with oral or intravenous PPIs. A conservative transfusion strategy (transfusing if Hb < 70 g/L, in stable patients) is associated with improved survival.

The examination

Physical examination in patients with suspected peptic ulcer disease is usually unhelpful. Epigastric tenderness is not a specific sign. An upper abdominal scar may indicate past ulcer surgery. Look for alarm signs, including evidence of anaemia (e.g. from bleeding) or current bleeding (melaena, tachycardia, postural hypotension), or an abdominal mass or lymphadenopathy (e.g. gastric or pancreatic carcinoma).

Investigations

1. **Endoscopy:** this is the standard test for determining that an active peptic ulcer is present. It is also the key test in a patient with upper gastrointestinal bleeding to determine whether the patient is at high risk of rebleeding and also to provide endoscopic therapy where required. Patients with active bleeding or a visible vessel at endoscopy need endoscopic therapy (e.g. injection with adrenaline (epinephrine) followed by coagulation with a heater probe). Patients with a low risk of rebleeding (i.e. a clean ulcer base) can be discharged immediately, if stable. Those at higher risk for rebleeding require admission for PPI therapy and observation. For patients with upper gastrointestinal tract bleeding, it is important to exclude other causes by endoscopy, including variceal bleeding, erosions, angiodysplasia, a Mallory–Weiss tear or a Dieulafoy's lesion (rupture of a large submucosal artery). Alternative causes of dyspepsia may be found at endoscopy including occasionally gastric cancer or MALT lymphoma. Where possible, biopsies should be obtained at a diagnostic endoscopy in ulcer patients to determine the *H. pylori* status (but false-negative results can occur in the setting of upper GI bleeding).
2. **Abdominal imaging:** in the patient with unexplained severe dyspepsia where endoscopy is normal, ultrasound can be useful in certain clinical circumstances to investigate for biliary tract pathology. CT scanning is more sensitive for pancreatic disease.
3. **Atypical peptic ulcer:** peptic ulceration in an unusual location, peptic ulcers resistant to therapy, an ulcer relapse after operation, or frequent or early ulcer recurrence can occur in the Zollinger–Ellison syndrome. This syndrome can also be associated with enlarged duodenal or gastric folds, or diarrhoea or steatorrhoea. The diagnosis is made by measuring the fasting serum gastrin level: > 300 pg/mL is suggestive and > 1000 pg/mL is almost diagnostic (remember on a PPI the gastrin level will often be raised, but usually not above 300 pg/mL). Acid secretion can be confirmed by testing the pH of gastric juice obtained at endoscopy. Preoperative localisation of the tumour is then attempted by CT or MRI scanning, and somatostatin receptor-based imaging (e.g. dotatate PET scan). If unable to locate the tumour, endoscopic ultrasound can be utilised, or, if necessary, angiographic venous sampling. In patients with metastatic or multifocal disease, surgery is avoided, but all other cases require surgical exploration. High-dose PPIs are used to control the disease medically.

   Remember that hypergastrinaemia also occurs in hypochlorhydria (gastric pH is not acidic; e.g. in atrophic gastritis and pernicious anaemia, following vagotomy, on a PPI, or with chronic kidney disease). Other causes of hypergastrinaemia with acid hypersecretion include a retained gastric antrum after peptic ulcer surgery, massive small bowel resection, gastric outlet obstruction and thyrotoxicosis. If hypercalcaemia is present in patients with ulcer disease, this may suggest MEN1 (with hyperplasia, adenoma or carcinoma of the parathyroid, pituitary and pancreatic islets; hyperparathyroidism and pituitary adenoma are most often associated with the Zollinger–Ellison syndrome in MEN1). In MEN1 (autosomal dominant with variable penetrance), there is often a strong family history of peptic ulcer disease.

Treatment

1. There is consensus that, if peptic ulcer disease is documented and *H. pylori* is present, this infection should be treated. Most duodenal ulcers will be cured by this approach, as will most gastric ulcers unless associated with NSAID use.

2. The optimal approach for curative treatment of *H. pylori* is currently three drugs (e.g. PPI plus amoxicillin plus clarithromycin), which give cure rates of approximately 60%–70%. Side-effects occur with such treatment in up to 20% of cases.

3. Patients with gastric ulcers may be advised to have a repeat gastroscopy to confirm healing and exclude carcinoma. However, 98% of cancers will be detected at the initial gastroscopy and biopsy. Therefore, repeat endoscopy is usually recommended only if symptoms have not been relieved or no initial biopsies were obtained. Duodenal ulcers do not require follow-up endoscopy.

4. In peptic ulcer disease, confirm that *H. pylori* infection has been cured (e.g. by repeat endoscopic biopsy, or urea breath testing or stool antigen testing, at least 1 month after completing treatment).

5. NSAID ulcers should initially be treated with a PPI, which is effective even if the NSAID is continued (although this does delay healing).

6. PPIs are more effective than histamine H_2-receptor antagonists in promoting ulcer healing. NSAID use is an independent risk factor for peptic ulcer and therefore eradication of *H. pylori* in this situation may not prevent ulcer disease if NSAIDs are continued.

7. Certain patients taking traditional NSAIDs have a higher risk of ulcer complications. These include elderly patients, those having their first 3 months of treatment, those on higher doses, those with a past history of peptic ulcer, those taking concomitant corticosteroid therapy or anticoagulants, and those with other serious medical illnesses. NSAID ulcers often present with complications without a history of dyspepsia because these drugs are analgesic agents that may mask symptoms. The prostaglandin E_1 analogue misoprostol and PPIs both substantially reduce the risk of NSAID-induced gastric and duodenal ulcers; histamine H_2-receptor antagonists in standard doses do not prevent NSAID-induced gastric ulcers. *H. pylori* eradication before treatment reduces, but does not eliminate, the risk of aspirin-induced ulcer development. *H. pylori* eradication alone provides insufficient protection from gastroduodenal complications arising from non-selective NSAID use in high-risk patients, who will still require a PPI.

8. Long-term PPI use is generally safe, but PPIs can rarely cause hypomagnesaemia, and vitamin B_{12} and iron malabsorption, possibly an increased risk of fractures from calcium malabsorption, microscopic colitis (diarrhoea), acute interstitial nephritis and drug-induced lupus. The risk of *Clostridium difficile* infection is increased. It is unclear whether PPI users are at an increased risk of pneumonia or dementia.

Possible lines of questioning

1. Should *this* patient continue on a PPI?
2. Should *this* patient with atrial fibrillation be anticoagulated? How would you explain the risks and benefits to the patient?
3. Should *this* patient who is taking antiplatelet treatment be protected with a PPI?

Malabsorption and chronic diarrhoea

This can be a difficult long case. It is usually a diagnostic problem. Coeliac disease (Table 7.1), chronic pancreatitis and previous gastric surgery account for 60% of cases of malabsorption.

Table 7.1 Coeliac disease

DIAGNOSTIC CRITERIA FOR COELIAC DISEASE

1. Positive serology by tissue transglutaminase (tTG) on a gluten-containing diet
2. Abnormal duodenal biopsy consistent with coeliac disease
3. Clinical, biochemical and histological improvement on a gluten-free diet (no wheat, rye or barley) (histological retesting not routine)

Notes: Requiring relapse on reinstitution of gluten is rarely considered necessary today.

Splenomegaly in coeliac disease usually indicates that lymphoma has complicated the disease because otherwise splenic atrophy is characteristic and manifests with Howell–Jolly bodies in the peripheral blood smear.

CAUSES OF LACK OF RESPONSE TO A GLUTEN-FREE DIET

1. Incorrect diagnosis
2. Patient not adhering to the diet
3. Collagenous sprue
4. Refractory coeliac disease (may have no response initially or relapse after a period of remission on a gluten-free diet – type I does not progress to lymphoma while type II has an abnormal clone of intraepithelial lymphocytes and can progress to T-cell lymphoma)
5. Intestinal lymphoma
6. Diffuse ulceration
7. Other intercurrent disease, e.g. lactose intolerance, pancreatic insufficiency, microscopic colitis, small intestinal bacterial overgrowth

COMPLICATIONS OF COELIAC DISEASE

1. T cell lymphoma
2. Ulceration of the small bowel
3. Incidence of carcinoma of the gastrointestinal tract is generally slightly increased
4. Osteoporosis

The history

1. Ask about presenting symptoms including:
   a. pale, bulky, offensive stools (steatorrhoea)
   b. weight loss
   c. weakness (e.g. from potassium deficiency)
   d. anaemia (megaloblastic, iron deficiency, etc.)
   e. bone pain (osteomalacia)
   f. glossitis and angular stomatitis (due to vitamin B group deficiency) (Fig. 7.1)
   g. bruising (vitamin K deficiency)
   h. oedema (a due to protein deficiency)
   i. peripheral neuropathy (due to vitamin B_{12} or B_1 deficiency)
   j. skin rash (eczema, dermatitis herpetiformis) (Fig. 7.2)
   k. amenorrhoea (due to protein depletion)
   l. cognitive impairment in deficiencies of B vitamins, e.g. B_{12}.
2. Ask about the time of onset of symptoms and their duration.
3. Ask aetiological questions concerning:
   a. gastrectomy, other bowel surgery
   b. history of liver or pancreatic disease
   c. drugs, e.g. alcohol, neomycin, cholestyramine, isoniazid (niacin deficiency), PPIs (hypomagnesaemia)
   d. history of Crohn's disease including previous terminal ileum resection (vitamin B_{12} deficiency)
   e. previous radiotherapy

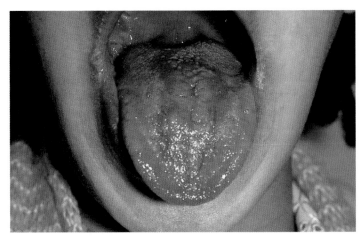

Figure 7.1 Glossitis in the mouth.

From J J Kanski. *Clinical diagnosis in ophthalmology*, 1st edn. Maryland Heights, MO: Mosby, 2006, with permission.

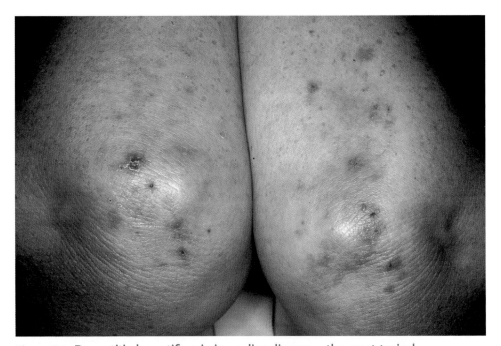

Figure 7.2 Dermatitis herpetiformis in coeliac disease – the most typical manifestation is polymorphic eruption above the elbows.

S Kárpáti. Dermatitis herpetiformis. *Clinics in Dermatology* 2012; 30(1):56–9, with permission.

    f. gluten-free diet treatment at any stage
    g. history of diabetes mellitus
    h. risk factors for HIV infection.
4. Ask about current treatment (e.g. diet, pancreatic supplements, vitamin supplements, cholestyramine, antibiotics).

5. Enquire about family history (e.g. coeliac disease, inflammatory bowel disease).
6. Ask about faecal incontinence secondary to diarrhoea, the impact of symptoms, and social problems related to the chronic illness.

The examination

Pay particular attention to the current weight and nutritional status (e.g. BMI), the presence of abdominal scars, skin lesions (e.g. bruising, dermatitis herpetiformis (see Fig. 7.2), pigmentation (Fig. 7.3), erythema nodosum (see Fig. 7.6), pyoderma gangrenosum (see Fig. 7.5), stomatitis, perianal lesions), signs of anaemia, oedema, signs of chronic liver disease, signs of peripheral neuropathy and lymphadenopathy.

Investigations (Table 7.2)

1. Demonstrate malabsorption:
   a. **the 'big six' laboratory screen tests** – look for a low serum iron, prolonged international normalised ratio (INR), low calcium, low cholesterol, low carotene and a positive Sudan stain of the stool for fat (which is a good screening test for steatorrhoea)
   b. **faecal fat estimation over 3 days** – more than 7 g per day is abnormal; note that patients with severe small bowel diarrhoea of any cause without fat malabsorption may lose up to 14 g per day; this gold standard test is very useful if you strongly

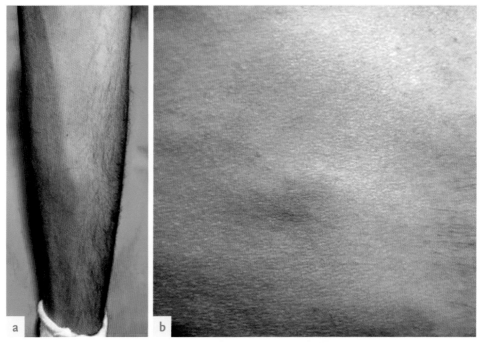

Figure 7.3 **Whipple's disease and skin pigmentation. Erythema nodosum-like subcutaneous, slightly erythematous nodules affecting (a) the lower legs and (b) the abdomen. Clinical features may include weight loss, diarrhoea, abdominal pain, arthralgias and continuous rhythmic eye movements of eye convergence with masticatory muscle contractions.**

J Schaller. Erythema nodosum-like lesions in treated Whipple's disease: Signs of immune reconstitution inflammatory syndrome. *Journal of the American Academy of Dermatology* 2008; 60(2):277–8, with permission.

Table 7.2 Typical results of investigations in malabsorption

INVESTIGATION	COELIAC DISEASE	BACTERIAL OVERGROWTH	WHIPPLE'S DISEASE	TERMINAL ILEAL DISEASE	CHRONIC PANCREATITIS
Stool fat	High	High	High	High	Very high
Folate (serum)	Low (in > 50%)	High to normal	Low	Normal	Normal
Small bowel biopsy (proximal)	Subtotal or total villous atrophy	Abnormal culture (> 10^5 organisms on quantitative jejunal fluid culture); histology often normal	Clubbing and flattening of villi, PAS-positive macrophages	Normal	Normal

PAS = periodic acid–Schiff technique.

suspect fat malabsorption based on the screening evaluation, but this test is now not widely available; if chronic pancreatitis is possible (e.g. history of alcohol abuse), order a faecal elastase

c. **glucose (or the less accurate lactulose) breath hydrogen test** – for small intestinal bacterial overgrowth (SIBO); think about this possibility in the setting of macrocytosis with a high folate and low B_{12} level, or in patients with structural, motility or immunoglobulin deficiency disorders that predispose to bacterial overgrowth.

2. Evaluate the consequences:
   a. blood count with particular attention to red cell indices
   b. serum iron and ferritin, serum and red cell folate, and vitamin B_{12} studies
   c. serum albumin estimation
   d. vitamin D level (25-OH vitamin D), serum calcium, phosphate and alkaline phosphatase estimations
   e. clotting profile – INR
   f. cholesterol and carotene.
3. Find the cause.
   a. Check small bowel X-ray films for localised disease (e.g. Crohn's disease or anatomical causes of bacterial overgrowth such as diverticula or blind loops).
   b. Check gastroscopy and small bowel biopsy (the optimal number for diagnosis of coeliac disease is four duodenal biopsies from the second portion of duodenum and two from the first portion of duodenum as disease can be patchy); note if multiple duodenal ulcers (e.g. as a result of Zollinger–Ellison syndrome, lymphoma, jejunoileitis).

   Subtotal villous atrophy may be present histologically in:
   • coeliac disease
   • collagenous sprue
   • SIBO
   • tropical sprue
   • giardiasis
   • lymphoma
   • hypogammaglobulinaemia
   • Whipple's disease
   • medications including olmesartan, ipilimumab or methotrexate.

   Note that tissue transglutaminase (tTG) is the most useful screening test for coeliac disease as long as the patient is still eating a gluten-containing diet. Remember that 2% of the population is IgA deficient and will have negative serology, so check IgA levels if testing is negative and your suspicion is high. Do not rely on antigliadin antibodies. HLA genotyping has a good negative predictive value, and is particularly useful (if negative) in symptomatic individuals with a family history of coeliac disease or those who are self-treating with a gluten free diet.

Serology is not a substitute for small bowel biopsy, which remains the gold standard test if coeliac disease is suspected in adults.

c. Vitamin B_{12} absorption may be abnormal in ileal disease, bacterial overgrowth, pernicious anaemia or pancreatic disease.

d. Greatly raised faecal fat levels (> 40 g per day) strongly suggest pancreatic disease, but this test is now uncommonly available. An alternative is faecal elastase testing (note that watery diarrhoea can cause a false-positive result). Suspected pancreatic disease is investigated by plain abdominal X-ray films (for calcification), CT scan (pancreatic protocol) and, if needed, magnetic resonance cholangiopancreatography (MRCP) or endoscopic ultrasound; pancreatic function testing is not performed routinely.

Treatment

Treatment depends on the cause and also involves the replacement of essential nutrients (Table 7.3).

Management of coeliac disease

Coeliac disease is a commonly missed diagnosis! Have a low threshold for ordering serology; patients may present with no gastrointestinal symptoms. Remember to consider the possibility of coeliac disease in a patient with no abdominal symptoms who has osteoporosis or osteomalacia, abnormal transaminases, new neuropsychiatric symptoms or unexplained iron deficiency. In IgA deficiency, the IgA and tTG may be falsely negative, and the serum IgG deamidated gliadin peptide (DGP) is the most sensitive and specific serology test. Small bowel biopsy on a gluten-containing diet (e.g. at least two slices of bread daily for 2 weeks) will confirm the diagnosis.

1. The management of coeliac disease includes a gluten-free diet (exclusion of wheat, rye and barley; there is controversy about oats). Symptoms usually improve in weeks and histology in several months; tTG antibody normalises in 3–6 months.
2. A strict diet does reduce disease complications.
3. Lack of response to a gluten-free diet may be caused by inadvertent gluten exposure, the presence of another problem (e.g. lactose intolerance, pancreatic insufficiency, bacterial overgrowth), refractory sprue (which may respond to corticosteroids) or lymphoma (T cell enteropathy: unresponsive to steroids).
4. Pneumococcal vaccine is recommended because of the hyposplenism of coeliac disease.
5. Osteoporosis is a complication to consider testing for and managing.
6. IBD, microscopic colitis, thyroid dysregulation and adrenal insufficiency not only mimic clinical features of coeliac disease but can also coexist with it.
7. Latent coeliac disease can be diagnosed if the small bowel biopsy appears normal but there is positive tTG serology. For these patients, a gluten-free diet is not usually recommended, but follow-up with repeat biopsy is indicated if the symptoms recur.

Possible lines of questioning

1. How would you investigate *this* patient for malnutrition?
2. How would you reassess *this* patient's diagnosis of coeliac disease?

Table 7.3 Causes and treatment of malabsorption

1. LIPOLYTIC PHASE DEFECTS
POSSIBLE CAUSES
a. Chronic pancreatitis
b. Cystic fibrosis

TREATMENT
a. Reverse causes
b. Pancreatic enzyme supplements
c. Medium-chain triglycerides

2. MICELLAR PHASE DEFECTS
POSSIBLE CAUSES
a. Extrahepatic biliary obstruction
b. Chronic liver disease
c. Bacterial overgrowth (e.g. as a result of small bowel blind loops)
d. Terminal ileal disease (e.g. Crohn's disease or resection)

TREATMENT
a. Reverse causes (e.g. antibiotics for bacterial overgrowth)
b. Cholestyramine if bile acid cathartic effect is important (e.g. < 100 cm of ileum resected)
c. Medium-chain triglycerides (MCTs) for steatorrhoea (e.g. > 100 cm of ileum resected in Crohn's disease; MCTs do not require bile salts for absorption)
d. Fat-soluble vitamin supplements

3. MUCOSAL AND DELIVERY PHASE DEFECTS
POSSIBLE CAUSES
a. Coeliac disease (see Table 7.1)
b. Tropical sprue
c. Lymphoma, intestinal lymphangiectasia
d. Whipple's disease
e. Small bowel ischaemia, resection
f. Amyloidosis
g. Hypogammaglobulinaemia
h. HIV infection (Kaposi's sarcoma, idiopathic)

TREATMENT
a. Reverse causes – gluten-free diet (coeliac disease), antibiotics (Whipple's disease)
b. Fat-soluble vitamin supplements

Inflammatory bowel disease

Both ulcerative colitis and Crohn's disease are common conditions in hospitals and outpatient clinics. They present both diagnostic and treatment problems. The patient will usually know the diagnosis, but you may have to decide which type of IBD is present.

The history

1. Start by establishing the current symptoms and detailing the impact of the disease on the patient. Proceed to establishing the chronological plot of the disease activity and its correlation with the treatment provided. Find out about symptoms at presentation and, if relevant, the current reason for admission. Ulcerative colitis (UC) typically presents in young adults with relapsing bloody diarrhoea, malaise, fever and weight

loss. Crohn's disease can present like UC or can have a variable presentation, including an insidious onset of pain, diarrhoea, weight loss, malabsorption, intestinal obstruction or symptoms suggestive of 'appendicitis'.

2. Ask about local complications and extracolonic manifestations (Table 7.4).

3. Enquire about sexual orientation if relevant (infective proctitis in men who have sex with men must be considered in the differential diagnosis).

Table 7.4 Complications of inflammatory bowel disease

ULCERATIVE COLITIS

LOCAL

1. Toxic megacolon (diameter of colon > 6 cm on plain abdominal X-ray film)
2. Perforation
3. Massive haemorrhage
4. Strictures
5. Carcinoma of the colon – often multicentric and related to disease extent and duration

EXTRACOLONIC

1. Liver disease
   a. Fatty liver
   b. Primary sclerosing cholangitis (large duct or small duct (pericholangitis))
   c. Cirrhosis
   d. Carcinoma of the bile duct
   e. Amyloidosis
2. Blood disorders
   a. Anaemia (owing to chronic disease, medications, iron deficiency, ileal involvement, haemolysis from sulfasalazine or microangiopathy)
   b. Thromboembolism (as a result of antithrombin III deficiency, stasis, dehydration)
3. Arthropathy
   a. Peripheral (large joints)
   b. Ankylosing spondylitis
4. Skin and mucous membranes
   a. Ulcers (Fig. 7.4)
   b. Pyoderma gangrenosum (independent of disease activity) (Fig. 7.5)
   c. Erythema nodosum (coincides with active disease) (Fig. 7.6)
5. Ocular – uveitis, conjunctivitis, episcleritis

CROHN'S DISEASE

LOCAL

1. Anorectal disease (including anal fissures or fistulas, pararectal abscess or rectovaginal fistula)
2. Obstruction (usually terminal ileum)
3. Fistula
4. Toxic megacolon and perforation (rare)
5. Carcinoma of the small and large bowel

EXTRACOLONIC

Similar to ulcerative colitis, except for the following:

1. Liver disease – primary sclerosing cholangitis is less common
2. Gallstones are more common (owing to decreased bile salt pool)
3. Renal disease includes urate and calcium oxalate stones, pyelonephritis (owing to fistulas), hydronephrosis (ureteric obstruction), amyloidosis
4. Malabsorption as a result of small bowel involvement (or resection)
5. Osteomalacia

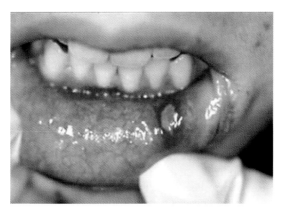

Figure 7.4 **Aphthous ulcers.**

S O Akintoye, M S Greenberg. Oral soft tissue lesions: recurrent aphthous stomatitis. *Dental Clinics of North America* 2005; 49(1):31–47, Fig 2, with permission.

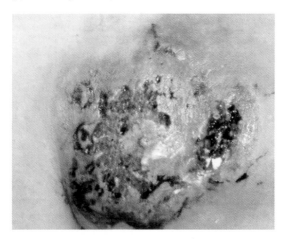

Figure 7.5 **Pyoderma gangrenosum.**

Reproduced from E Wierzbicka-Hainaut et al. Pyoderma gangrenosum récidivant lors des grossesses. Recurring pyoderma gangrenosum in pregnancy. *Anales de Dermatologie et de Venereologie* 137(3):225–9. © 2010 Elsevier Masson SAS. All rights reserved.

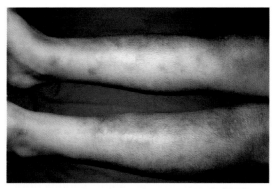

Figure 7.6 **Erythema nodosum. The differential diagnosis includes inflammatory bowel disease, Behçet's disease, a recent streptococcal throat, sarcoid and TB.**

J Mana, J Marcoval. Erythema nodosum. *Clinics in Dermatology* 2007; 25(3):288–94. Elsevier, with permission.

4. Ask about medications – NSAIDs, retinoic acid and possibly oral contraceptives can cause a similar picture.
5. Determine the investigations at the time of presentation and subsequently (and particularly whether infectious causes were considered).
6. Ask about the number of hospital admissions and a detailed surgical history (you must establish the full disease course).
7. Ask whether regular follow-up colonoscopy has been performed in patients with longstanding colitis to demonstrate adequate control on current treatment and for colorectal cancer surveillance.
8. Find out about treatment, including medications and any side-effects – such as sulfasalazine / 5-aminosalicylic acid preparations (mesalazine, olsalazine), local or systemic steroids (e.g. budesonide, prednisone), antibiotics (ciprofloxacin, metronidazole or others that may cause pseudomembranous colitis), immunomodulators (e.g. azathioprine, mercaptopurine), and biologicals (anti-tumour necrosis factor (TNF) antibody drugs such as, for example, infliximab or adalimumab, or anti-integrin vedolizumab, or anti IL12/23 antibody ustekinimab, etc.).
9. Enquire about family history of IBD or bowel carcinoma.
10. Ask about smoking – a greater proportion than average of Crohn's disease patients are smokers and the risk of developing UC rises when people give up smoking.
11. Ask about incontinence episodes, establish the current stoma care (if present) and enquire about the impact of the disease on their quality of life, including employment.
12. Enquire about malnourishment symptoms and weight loss; find out if they see a dietitian.
13. Ask your patient about fertility and survivorship aspects, including screening of other malignancies (relevant in immunosuppression), bone mineral density and vaccinations.

The examination

A thorough gastrointestinal system examination is important. Evaluate the general state of nutrition and hydration. Examine any stoma if present: site, surrounding skin, number of lumens, spout, effluent (look and feel the bag – e.g. hard or soft stool), and ask about output (high or low) and complications. Feel for any tenderness or abdominal masses. Look for anal lesions externally (Fig. 7.7). Always ask for the results of a rectal examination. Look for the signs of Cushing's syndrome if the patient is taking steroids (often present!). Search for the other extracolonic manifestations, being guided by the history (e.g. arthropathy, skin lesions (see p. 158), uveitis, anaemia, liver disease).

Investigations

It is important to exclude other causes of colitis (Table 7.5). For the investigation of inflammatory bowel disease, the following should be considered.

1. **Infection must be excluded:** the causes include amoebiasis (especially if a travel history – diagnosed by rectal mucosal scraping or warm stool examination), *Yersinia* (if terminal ileitis), *Shigella, Salmonella, Campylobacter, Escherichia coli* 0157:H7 and, if recent use of antibiotics or hospital admission, pseudomembranous colitis (*Clostridium difficile* toxin). Lymphogranuloma venereum (a chlamydial disease that is sexually transmitted), gonorrhoea and syphilis (particularly in men who have sex with men), and other infections in immunocompromised hosts (e.g. herpes, cytomegalovirus (CMV), cryptosporidium, *Isospora belli*) should be considered in patients at risk.
   Remember that TB can, uncommonly, mimic Crohn's disease. Also, reactivation of TB is a major risk with anti-TNF therapy; a chest X-ray and tuberculin skin test are mandatory before starting this therapy.

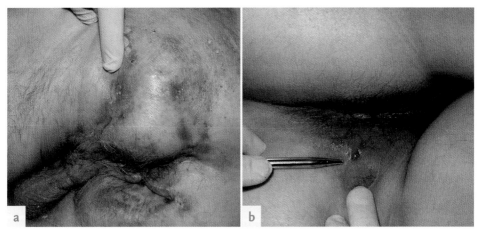

Figure 7.7 (a and b) External anal fistula in Crohn's disease.

Courtesy Dr Lawrence J Brandt, Bronx, New York.

Table 7.5 **Causes of colitis**
1. Inflammatory bowel disease
2. Infections, including pseudomembranous colitis
3. Microscopic or collagenous colitis
4. Radiation
5. Ischaemic colitis
6. Diversion colitis (colonic loops excluded from the faecal stream)
7. Toxic exposure (e.g. peroxide or soapsud enemas, gold-induced colitis)
8. Diverticular disease – segmental colitis

2. **Plain abdominal X-ray film:** it is important to look for bowel wall thickening (oedema), gaseous distension and evidence of toxic megacolon in UC. In Crohn's disease, also look for loops of matted bowel and small bowel obstruction.

3. **Blood count:** check for anaemia (caused by chronic disease, blood loss, medications, macrocytic anaemia in ileal disease, or haemolytic anaemia from an autoimmune process, microangiopathic disease or sulfasalazine). Check the white cell count (e.g. leukopenia from azathioprine). Look at the ESR (or CRP) for evidence of active disease.

4. **Liver function tests and blood levels of electrolytes, urea and creatinine:** these patients may develop liver disease, or it may be a complication of treatment (think primary sclerosing cholangitis in patients with UC and cholestatic liver function derangement). Crohn's disease may lead to renal stones, pyelonephritis, hydronephrosis or amyloidosis. Remember that hypoalbuminaemia is a sign of severe disease.

5. **Faecal calprotectin:** this is a useful test, looking for active colonic (+/− small bowel) inflammation. It is not specific for IBD, however, and can be elevated by other causes, e.g. infection.

6. **Colonoscopy:** this is a very useful investigation to assess whether or not disease is patchy and, if so, to assess its extent. Note any decreased mucosal translucency, loss of vascular pattern, granular and friable mucosa, hyperaemia, ulceration and pseudopolyps in the report. Ulcerative colitis always begins in the rectum and extends

proximally without skip lesions. Mucosal biopsies may not differentiate UC from Crohn's disease or other causes of colitis, but mucus depletion and prominent crypt abscess formation are more suggestive of UC. Granulomas (in 25%) or focal inflammation are found in Crohn's colitis (but note that granulomas also occur in biopsies from *Chlamydia trachomatis* and syphilitic proctitis or in cases of tuberculosis). Surveillance colonoscopy (looking for dysplasia / malignancy) should occur every 1–3 years (depending on risk), beginning 8 years after diagnosis of at least distal UC, or Crohn's colitis involving at least one-third of the colon. If severe inflammation is present, assessment for dysplasia may be misleading. If high-grade dysplasia is found, endoscopic resection can be considered. Colectomy is another therapeutic option.

7. **Antibody testing:** the presence of perinuclear antineutrophil cytoplasmic antibodies (p-ANCA) and anti-*Saccharomyces cerevisiae* antibodies (ASCA) does not make the diagnosis, but p-ANCA-negative and ASCA-positive patients are more likely to have Crohn's disease than UC (the test is specific but not sensitive, and is not helpful in the initial assessment of suspected IBD).

Treatment

ULCERATIVE COLITIS

In UC, grade the severity of the disease:

- **mild** – fewer than four bowel motions per day, minimal bleeding, normal temperature and pulse
- **acute severe** – more than six bloody bowel motions per day, plus at least one of: temperature > 37.8°C, pulse > 90 beats / min, haemoglobin < 105 g / L, elevated ESR or CRP and raised inflammatory markers
- **fulminant** – as per the criteria for acute severe, plus 10 or more bloody bowel motions per day, usually accompanied by abdominal tenderness and/or distension.

  1. In an acute attack of colitis, remember to correct hypokalaemia and obtain a plain abdominal X-ray to assess for toxic megacolon (risk of perforation). Do not prescribe opiates or anticholinergic agents to prevent megacolon.
  2. Arrange DVT prophylaxis.
  3. Send off a stool sample looking for *Clostridium difficile* (which can still occur without recent antibiotics!) and other bacterial or viral infections that could mimic an exacerbation.
  4. Oral prednisone is usually utilised in the first instance to gain disease control. In acute severe UC, intravenous steroids are the mainstay of treatment. In those who fail to respond (assessed after 3 days), both infliximab (more common) and cyclosporin are considered as rescue therapies to try and avoid acute colectomy. In fulminant colitis, broad-spectrum IV antibiotics may be considered. Close cooperation with a surgeon who is interested in this field and with a stoma therapist is important early on in severe disease; these consultations provide information and psychological support to the patient.
  5. In mild-to-moderate ulcerative colitis, sulfasalazine or other 5-ASA agents are useful (induction doses are around 4 g daily) to both achieve and maintain remission. Sulfasalazine is 5-ASA linked with sulfapyridine, which is the cause of most intolerance (allergic reactions such as skin rash – including Stevens–Johnson syndrome – and Heinz body haemolytic anaemia; and side-effects such as nausea, headache, folate deficiency and reversible male infertility). The other 5-ASA agents (e.g. mesalazine, olsalazine, balsalazide) tend to be better tolerated. Steroids may be required to allow a patient to enter remission, but do NOT maintain remission, nor prevent relapse. Remember to correct iron and folate deficiency if necessary.

6. If proctitis is the problem, first-line treatment is topical / rectal 5-ASAs, +/− oral 5-ASAs (topical is superior to oral in proctitis, but the combination is more effective than either alone). Topical steroids can help, but do not maintain remission.

7. Azathioprine or 6-mercaptopurine (6MP) is useful if there are repeated episodes of UC. Side-effects include pancreatitis in 3% of patients and reversible bone marrow suppression in < 10% of patients. Avoid methotrexate. Biological therapy can be considered if the disease is not responding to the above measures.

8. Colectomy is 'curative' (though not without complications). This is partly why it is important to try and distinguish UC from Crohn's disease (though a distinction cannot be made in up to 10% of patients). Indications for surgery include chronic ill-health and severe disease, complications (e.g. perforation, massive bleeding) and severe disease not responding to optimal medical treatment in 7–10 days. Patients with UC (especially if extensive disease) are also at high risk for colorectal cancer. If high-grade dysplasia is found on colonoscopy and biopsy, if not amenable to endoscopic resection then a colectomy is recommended. Although the standard Brooke ileostomy is the simplest procedure, the ileal pouch anal anastomosis is increasingly being used as it maintains intestinal continuity, although it does leave the patient with four to eight bowel movements daily, and sometimes with minor incontinence (20%), and is often complicated by pouchitis (in up to 50% of patients). The latter usually responds to treatment with metronidazole or probiotics.

CROHN'S DISEASE

You are more likely to encounter Crohn's disease in the clinic and exam than ulcerative colitis. A rectal exam for fistula is routine (the results will be provided for you). Small bowel imaging modalities (used to help diagnosis and / or assess disease extent) include CT enteroclysis or magnetic resonance (MR) enteroclysis or enterography. Capsule endoscopy is widely available, but remember the capsule may obstruct the small intestine in Crohn's disease. Fistula can be evaluated by radiology (e.g. CT, MR and fistulography) and examination under anaesthesia.

Always advise the patient to stop smoking. Always try to taper off and stop steroids once the patient is in remission. Remember, disease always recurs after surgical resection and the risk increases with time. The goals of therapy are to control symptoms and try to achieve deep remission (endoscopy and histology returns to normal), so many clinicians are now more aggressive in introducing biological therapy early. A multidisciplinary team approach is needed to manage what can be a devastating disease in the long term.

1. 5-ASA is not effective in Crohn's disease, although it is sometimes tried in mild disease (not recommended).

2. Steroids are effective for inducing remission but never for maintenance of remission. Budenoside (a steroid derivative that acts locally and is 90% inactivated by the liver) is useful in ileocolonic disease.

3. Azathioprine (or 6-mercaptopurine) is useful for those who cannot cease steroids and to reduce risk of relapse (including post-resection surgery). Methotrexate is an alternative if azathioprine fails (Table 7.6).

4. With extensive ileal disease or resection, diarrhoea may respond to a bile-salt-sequestering drug (cholestyramine or colestipol).

5. Biological therapy is used in moderate to severe disease, or disease not responding to other treatment. Options include anti-TNF agents (e.g. infliximab, adalimumab), anti-integrin agents (e.g. vedolizumab) and anti-interleukin agents (e.g. ustekinumab) (see Table 7.6). These agents are used for both induction of remission and maintenance of remission. An anti-TNF (or ustekinumab) is preferred in fistulising disease.

Table 7.6 Immunosuppression in inflammatory bowel disease

AZATHIOPRINE OR 6MP	METHOTREXATE	BIOLOGICALS
BEFORE STARTING		
• Genetic testing for TPMT polymorphism • Rule out hepatitis B and C • Update immunisations	• Start folic acid • Baseline LFTs • Counsel to avoid alcohol • Rule out hepatitis B and C • Update immunisations	• Update immunisations • Pap smear • Rule out hepatitis B and C • QuantiFERON-TB Gold test (or Mantoux) • Chest X-ray (for TB) • Consider: HIV, varicella zoster antibody, ANA, Anti-ds DNA testing
MONITORING PROGRAM		
• FBC/LFTs weekly in 1st month, then 2-weekly in 2nd month, then monthly to 3-monthly • Consider metabolite levels (6-TGN/MMP) to assess efficacy/compliance	• LFTs monthly for 3 months, then 3-monthly (AST, ALT, albumin) • Consider liver biopsy if ≥ 50% of LFTs over a year abnormal	• 6-monthly review • Both infliximab and adalimumab trough levels +/− anti-drug antibody levels can be requested
MAJOR SIDE-EFFECTS		
• Leukopenia (dose dependent) • Pancreatitis (idiosyncratic) • Allergy (fever/rash/arthritis) • Lymphoma • Can be continued in pregnancy if cannot use other therapy	• Hepatotoxic • Bone marrow depression • Interstitial pneumonitis • Contraindicated in pregnancy/conception (women and men)	• Infusion/injection site reactions (acute, delayed) • Neutropenia • Infections • Hepatosplenic T cell lymphoma (combined with azathioprine) • Demyelinating disease • Heart failure • Skin rashes (psoriatic-like) • Most safe in pregnancy – check the specific product

ALT = alanine aminotransferase; ANA = antinuclear antibody; AST = aspartate aminotransferase; FBC = full blood count; LFTs = liver function tests; 6MP = 6-mercaptopurine; Pap = Papanicolaou; TPMT = thiopurine methyltransferase.

6. Metronidazole and/or ciprofloxacin is modestly useful for severe perianal disease and fistulae, which tend to recur once treatment is stopped; azathioprine or anti-TNF therapy may be tried in difficult or severe cases.

7. Surgery is reserved for the complications of Crohn's disease (e.g. internal fistula with abscess, intestinal obstruction not responding to medical management). The best operation is resection. Strictureplasty may allow relief of localised obstruction without the deleterious effects of multiple resections. Surgical resection is sometimes considered in preference to medical management in isolated, short-segment disease of the terminal ileum.

8. When a total colectomy is needed, a standard ileostomy is the procedure of choice. The recurrence rate of the disease is unchanged by surgery.

9. The extra-intestinal manifestations (EIMs) of IBD that respond to treatment of active disease include: oral ulcers, erythema nodosum, large joint arthritis and episcleritis. EIMs that are *independent* of active disease include: primary sclerosing cholangitis, ankylosing spondylitis, uveitis, pyoderma gangrenosum, and renal stones and gallstones.

Possible lines of questioning

1. How active is *this* patient's inflammatory bowel disease?
2. What workup would you do before starting on an anti-TNF drug?
3. What is your assessment of *this* patient's nutritional state?
4. What are your recommendations for screening for colon cancer for *this* patient?

Colon cancer

This is a particularly common tumour that usually develops in patients aged 50 years or more, although those at risk with hereditary syndromes will present at a younger age. Because early disease is curable, there has been increased interest in colon cancer screening. Hence, a history of polyps or colon cancer is increasingly likely to be encountered in the examination.

The history

1. The patient may have been diagnosed recently as having a colon cancer. In this case, ascertain the reasons for diagnostic testing:
   a. a recent change in bowel habit or bright red blood per rectum (from a rectal or left-sided colon cancer)
   b. symptoms of anaemia
   c. new-onset abdominal pain
   d. symptoms suggestive of small bowel obstruction (with a slow-growing caecal cancer)
   e. symptoms from involvement of the bladder or female genital tract owing to local invasion
   f. sacral plexus pain, which is a very late manifestation
   g. a positive faecal occult blood test on screening (note: if unexplained iron deficiency is also present it is a particularly worrying result).
2. If colon cancer was identified, ask whether the patient knows what staging tests (e.g. CT scans, PET scans) have been done and what treatment has been undertaken. If radiotherapy was given to the pelvis, enquire about any ongoing symptoms of proctitis or cystitis.
3. Determine whether the patient understands the prognosis and ascertain the social support network. Ask whether stoma therapy has been discussed.
4. If the patient has a history of polyps, try to find out from the patient whether these were adenomatous, hyperplastic or sessile serrated polyps, and their approximate size and number. If they do not know, request information from the medical record. Adenomatous polyps may be tubular or villous (or tubulovillous); invasive cancer is more likely in larger polyps (10% of those > 2.5 cm are malignant). If polyps were detected, ask the patient whether surveillance colonoscopy has been conducted in the past, and if so when this began and how often. Surveillance colonoscopies generally occur every 1–5 years (depending on polyp type, number and size, plus taking into account other risk factors, such as family history).
5. The family history needs to be carefully obtained for any patient with a history of polyps or colon cancer. If the patient describes having had hundreds or thousands

of adenomatous polyps throughout the large bowel, then familial adenomatous polyposis (FAP) is the diagnosis (until proven otherwise). These polyps usually occur after puberty and most individuals are affected by the age of 25 years. If the colon is not removed, almost all will have colon cancer before the age of 40. In this type of clinical case, ask about the presence of any soft-tissue or bony tumours (Gardiner's syndrome), or tumours in the central nervous system (Turkot's syndrome), which are variants of FAP.

Most patients with FAP will have undergone a total colectomy with ileoanal anastomosis. Ask about continence and stool frequency if this operation has been performed. Screening for duodenal and periampullary cancers every 1–3 years by endoscopy is generally recommended.

Ask whether any offspring of a patient with this condition have been screened. Flexible sigmoidoscopy on an annual basis is recommended (and colonoscopy once adenomas start to be detected). DNA testing of peripheral blood mononuclear cells for the presence of the mutated *APC* gene at puberty is also useful (after first testing affected relatives to validate the presence of the *APC* mutation) in screening offspring.

The MuTYH-associated polyposis (MAP) syndrome (autosomal recessive) can present just like FAP.

If there is a strong family history of colon cancer, consider the possibility of Lynch syndrome (see below). There is a 70% lifetime risk of colon cancer in this autosomal dominant disease. There is often also a family history of either ovarian or endometrial carcinoma. Members of such families are typically screened by colonoscopy every 1–2 years, beginning at the age of 25 years, as well as undergoing pelvic ultrasonography and endometrial biopsies.

6. Enquire about any history of documented inflammatory bowel disease. The risk of colorectal cancer in a patient with UC is small during the initial 7–10 years after development of pancolonic disease, but then increases approximately 1% per year. Ask whether or not colonoscopic surveillance has been undertaken. Patients with Crohn's colitis should now also be offered similar surveillance.

7. Ask whether there has been any history of possible septicaemia or endocarditis (fever, malaise, etc.). *Streptococcus bovis*, *Clostridium septicus* or *Enterococcus faecalis* bacteraemia indicates an underlying high risk of occult colon cancer and requires aggressive investigation.

8. Hamartomas of the gastrointestinal tract with mucocutaneous pigmentation (Peutz–Jeghers syndrome) increase the risk of both large and small bowel cancer, as well as breast, uterine and ovarian cancers. Affected patients should undergo surveillance by colonoscopy and gastroscopy every 3 years from 18 years of age.

9. Determine whether there is any history of a ureterosigmoidostomy for correction of congenital exstrophy of the bladder, which increases the risk of colon cancer 15–30 years later.

10. Diabetes mellitus, renal transplant and acromegaly may be associated with an increased risk of colorectal malignancy; regular full-dose aspirin use may reduce the risk of colon cancer.

The examination

1. Look for evidence of jaundice or anaemia.
2. If the patient is currently undergoing 5-fluorouracil-derived chemotherapy, look at the palms and soles for evidence of hand–foot syndrome (very tender, symmetrical erythema) (Fig. 7.8).

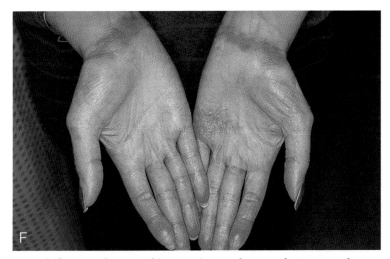

Figure 7.8 Hand–foot syndrome. Skin reaction to docetaxel. Note erythema and oedema of the palms in this patient.

A T Skarin. *Atlas of diagnostic oncology*, 4th edn, Fig 21.4F. Mosby, Elsevier, 2010, with permission.

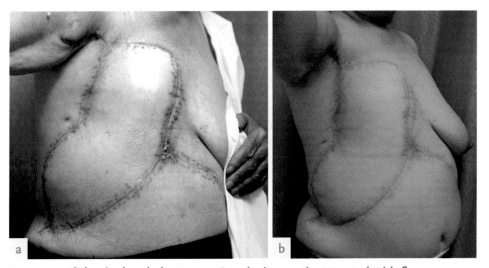

Figure 7.9 Abdominal and chest scars / marks in a patient treated with flap surgery and radiotherapy. (a) Appearance during radiotherapy showing healing of the T-junction despite irradiation. (b) Appearance at 3 months after chemotherapy.

From F Behan, M Findlay, C H Lo. *The keystone perforator island flap concept*. Elsevier Australia, 2012, Fig 6.6, with permission.

3. Carefully examine the abdomen, in particular looking for any evidence of malignant deposits in the liver or other intraperitoneal masses, or skin changes that are consistent with radiotherapy. Record any scars on the abdomen (Fig. 7.9).
4. Results of a rectal examination need to be obtained.
5. Other lymph node groups should be examined and evidence of metastatic malignancy elsewhere (e.g. the lungs, bones or brain) should be sought.

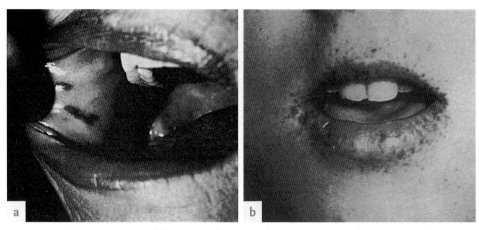

Figure 7.10 **Pigmentation of Peutz–Jeghers syndrome. (a) Buccal mucus in the mouth. (b) Discreet brown–black lesion of lips.**

(a) F S McDonald (ed.). *Mayo Clinic images in internal medicine*, with permission. © Mayo Clinic Scientific Press and CRC Press. (b) D V Jones et al., in M Feldman et al., *Sleisenger and Fordtran's gastrointestinal disease*, 6th edn, Ch 112. Saunders, Elsevier, 1998, with permission.

6. Look for the pigmentation of Peutz–Jeghers syndrome, in which there is an increased risk of colon and other cancers (Fig. 7.10).
7. Multiple skin lesions (e.g. sebaceous adenomas and carcinomas, basal cell and squamous cell carcinomas, keratoacanthomas) occur in a variant of hereditary non-polyposis colorectal cancer (Torres syndrome).

Investigations

1. **Screening:** faecal occult blood testing is a common screening tool utilised in the community for colorectal cancer. The possibility of hereditary non-polyposis colon cancer (HNPCC, or Lynch syndrome) should be considered for certain patients. This includes the '3–2–1' rule (Amsterdam II criteria): patients who have *three or more relatives* with a history of Lynch syndrome-associated cancer (colorectal, endometrial, small bowel, ureteric or renal pelvis cancer), where one of these is a first-degree relative of the other two; at least *two generations* of the family have been affected; and at least *one* member was affected younger than 50. Screening starts at age 25 in affected families. In most patients with HNPCC, germ-line mutations have occurred in one of six DNA mismatch repair genes. Commercial testing is available for *hMSH2* and *hMLH1* mutations and these have a high sensitivity. 'Microsatellite instability' (MSI) is the expansion or contraction of short repeated DNA sequences. MSI has been observed in more than 90% of samples of tumour tissue from patients with HNPCC who fulfil the clinical (Amsterdam) criteria for this disease and also in up to 15% of tumours from patients with sporadic colorectal cancer. The presence of MSI may indicate a better prognosis and better response to adjuvant chemotherapy. Testing for the presence of MSI in a tumour or adenoma should be an initial screening test for patients suspected of having HNPCC, and positive cases should undergo genetic screening.
2. **Symptomatic patients:** most will have had the cancer identified by colonoscopy. With the increasing introduction of screening measures in asymptomatic patients (e.g. faecal occult blood testing), earlier-stage colon cancers will be detected in average-risk patients. The prognosis depends on the stage of disease. Survival is decreased if the bowel wall is penetrated (Dukes' B2 stage) or with lymph node involvement (Dukes' C stage).

Treatment

1. For colon cancer, total tumour resection in local disease is the treatment of choice, undertaken either endoscopically or surgically. Before surgery, patients should be evaluated for the possibility of metastatic disease, including a careful physical examination. Many physicians would also order a CT chest / abdomen / pelvis +/− MRI pelvis, liver function tests and measure the baseline carcinoembryonic antigen (CEA) level. If possible, a complete colonoscopy should be undertaken to look for evidence of synchronous cancers or polyps. If colonoscopy was not performed before the operation, it should be carried out as soon as practicable after the operation.

2. Following a resection, patients are often followed up for 5 years with annual physical examinations and surveillance colonoscopy every 1 year after resection, then 3–5-yearly depending upon the previous colonoscopy. Measuring CEA levels every 3 months for 2 years after surgery for Dukes' B or C stage disease, as a test for tumour recurrence, is often recommended but remains controversial.

3. If metastatic disease is present, resection of the primary colorectal tumour does not change prognosis and should be done only for symptomatic reasons. The exception is limited metastases to the liver only, where 25% may be cured by resection.

4. Determine whether the patient has had radiation therapy to the pelvis, which may have been offered with a rectal cancer. Some patients may have received chemotherapy; in particular, patients with Dukes' C stage have often had adjuvant leucovorin-modulated 5-fluorouracil for 6 months. Oxaliplatin may be added.

Possible lines of questioning

1. What would you tell *this* patient about his or her prognosis?
2. For which patients would you recommend chemotherapy after bowel resection?
3. When might surgery for metastases be useful?

Chronic liver disease (CLD)

Cirrhosis alone or in combination with other disease will often crop up. It is a pathological diagnosis. This discussion will be limited to those aspects of cirrhosis and chronic hepatitis which tend to be most frequent in the examination.

The history

Cirrhosis can present with ascites (see Fig. 7.12), jaundice (see Fig. 7.13), abdominal pain, acute bleeding or encephalopathy. Patients occasionally present with only weakness, lassitude or loss of libido. There may be no symptoms (incidental cirrhosis).

1. Ask about length of history of liver disease including:
   a. known abnormal liver function tests, a past history of hepatitis or jaundice, including contacts, or a history of obesity (non-alcoholic fatty liver disease)
   b. alcohol intake (in men, 80 g per day for more than 10 years is usually necessary; women need less exposure)
   c. history of drug addiction (intravenous), sexual orientation, transfusions, tattoos, etc.
   d. drug history (e.g. for chronic hepatitis: methyldopa, isoniazid, nitrofurantoin)
   e. history of diabetes mellitus, cardiac failure or arthropathy (haemochromatosis)
   f. overseas travel (e.g. acute hepatitis).

2. Ask about treatment (e.g. dietary supplements, diuretics, beta-blockers, salt or fluid restriction, alcohol or other drug abstinence, steroids, lactulose, neomycin, rifaximin). Is the patient a transplant candidate?

3. Ask about complications, such as any history of encephalopathy. An early sign of this is reversal of the sleep cycle. Is there any history of portal hypertension (ascites or bleeding from varices), or recent abdominal pain (gallstones – usually pigment stones, acute alcoholic hepatitis, etc.)?

4. Ask about recent fever, abdominal pain or tenderness, or evidence of altered mental status – in the setting of ascites this suggests spontaneous bacterial peritonitis (SBP) and it is important to start antibiotic treatment as soon as ascitic fluid, blood and urine have been obtained for culture and analysis. Determine whether there have been one or more previous episodes of SBP – an indication for long-term prophylactic antibiotic therapy. In the setting of cirrhosis, an admission for gastrointestinal (GI) bleeding is an indication for short-term antibiotic cover as mortality is reduced.

5. Ask about investigations (e.g. liver biopsy, endoscopy for varices, surveillance ultrasound).

6. Ask about operations (e.g. transjugular intrahepatic portosystemic shunt (TIPS), transplant).

7. Enquire about erectile dysfunction, loss of libido.

8. Enquire about social problems (e.g. employment, family).

The examination

1. Note nutritional status (including obesity) and the patient's racial origin. Hepatitis B and C viruses are endemic in South East Asia, Italy and Egypt. Look for tattoos – tattoo needles are a source of infection. Examine carefully for the signs of chronic liver disease (Figs 7.11–7.13). Also, note any hepatic encephalopathy, signs of portal hypertension, including splenomegaly, ascites, oedema and signs of bleeding (e.g. melaena).

2. Consider hepatocellular carcinoma (particularly in haemochromatosis, and cirrhosis as a result of hepatitis B or C virus infection, or non-alcoholic steatohepatitis (NASH)). In patients with decompensated cirrhosis, examine for a hard mass and liver bruit (hepatoma).

3. Look for the signs of haemochromatosis (now rare) (Fig. 7.14). In young patients, consider Wilson's disease and look carefully for Kayser–Fleischer rings (Fig. 7.15). If there is deep jaundice with scratch marks and xanthelasma (see Fig. 16.3, p. 415), particularly in a woman, consider end-stage primary biliary cholangitis.

4. Exclude severe right heart failure, tricuspid regurgitation or constrictive pericarditis clinically in all patients. Search for other causes and sequelae (Tables 7.7 and 7.8).

Investigations

Management of cirrhosis depends on the aetiology, morphology and hepatic function. It is important to make a diagnosis and exclude potentially reversible causes of further liver deterioration.

1. **Liver function tests:** these should be used to confirm abnormalities, follow progress and give an idea of prognosis (particularly a low albumin level and prolonged INR). An aspartate aminotransferase (AST) to alanine aminotransferase (ALT) ratio of > 2.0 suggests alcoholic liver disease.

2. **Full blood count:** this is helpful because anaemia may be caused by chronic disease, blood loss, folate deficiency, bone marrow depression, hypersplenism, haemolysis or sideroblastic anaemia. Round macrocytes are common in alcoholics. Remember that

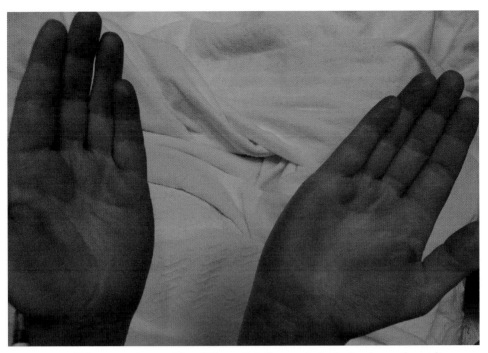

Figure 7.11 **Palmar erythema. The differential diagnosis includes hyperthyroidism, rheumatoid arthritis, polycythaemia and pregnancy (normal).**

A Nautiyal, K B Chopra. Liver palms – palmar erythema. *American Journal of Medicine* 2010; 123(7): 596–7, Fig 1, with permission.

Table 7.7 Causes of cirrhosis in adults
1. Alcohol
2. Postviral (hepatitis C, B, D)
3. Non-alcoholic steatohepatitis
4. Drugs (e.g. methyldopa, chlorpromazine, isoniazid, nitrofurantoin, propylthiouracil, methotrexate, amiodarone)
5. Autoimmune chronic hepatitis
6. Haemochromatosis
7. Wilson's disease
8. Primary sclerosing cholangitis
9. Primary biliary cholangitis
10. Secondary biliary cirrhosis
11. Alpha$_1$-antitrypsin deficiency
12. Cystic fibrosis
13. Budd–Chiari syndrome
14. Cardiac failure, chronic constrictive pericarditis
15. Cryptogenic (idiopathic)

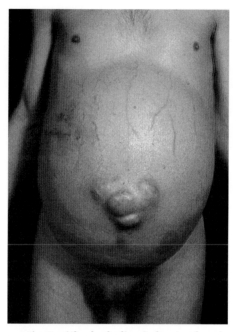

Figure 7.12 Ascites in a patient with alcoholic cirrhosis showing distended abdomen, dilated superficial collateral veins, haemorrhagic scratch marks due to pruritus and coagulopathy, umbilical varices, and plaster in left iliac fossa indicating diagnostic paracentesis.

A Forbes, J J Misiewicz, C C Crompton, M Levine et al. (eds). *Atlas of clinical gastroenterology*, 3rd edn. 2005, in F Ferri. *Ferri's clinical advisor 2012*. Fig 1-300, Mosby, Elsevier, 2012, with permission.

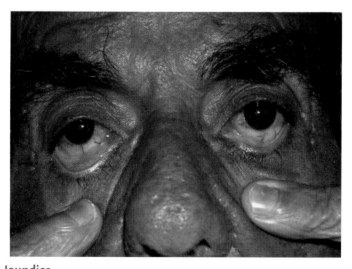

Figure 7.13 Jaundice.

Tyring S, Lupi O and Hengge U *Tropical dermatology* 2006; Fig 12.15, with permission.

Table 7.8 Sequelae of cirrhosis
1. Portal hypertension (ascites, varices)
2. Portal vein thrombosis
3. Spontaneous bacterial peritonitis
4. Hepatic encephalopathy
5. Hepatorenal syndrome
6. Hepatocellular carcinoma
7. Osteoporosis or osteomalacia (particularly cholestatic liver disease)

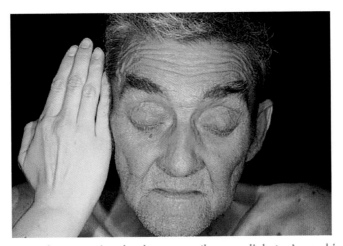

Figure 7.14 Haemochromatosis, also known as 'bronze diabetes', combines diabetes mellitus, cirrhosis and generalised hyperpigmentation. These patients have iron overload.

J P Callen, K E Greer, A S Paller, L J Swinyer. *Color atlas of dermatology*, 2nd edn. Philadelphia, WB Saunders, 2000, with permission.

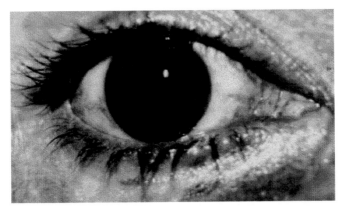

Figure 7.15 Kayser–Fleischer ring.

M M Deguti, J F Uwe Tietge, E R Barbosa, E L R Cancado. The eye in Wilson's disease: sunflower cataract associated with Kayser–Fleischer ring. *Journal of Hepatology* 2002; 7(5), with permission.

leukopenia and thrombocytopenia occur in hypersplenism. A low platelet count in the setting of chronic liver disease suggests portal hypertension.

3. **Biochemistry/renal function tests:** these are important to exclude the hepatorenal syndrome. Hyponatraemia is common in cirrhosis.
4. **Ascitic tap** (Tables 7.9 and 7.10): rule out spontaneous bacterial peritonitis if ascites is present (> 250/mm³ polymorphs).

Table 7.9 Causes of ascites and interpretation of ascitic fluid studies
CAUSES
1. Related to portal hypertension (serum-to-ascites albumin gradient (SAAG) > 11 g/L):
a. Cirrhosis (most important – 97% accurate for portal hypertension)
b. Alcoholic hepatitis
c. Cardiac ascites (right heart failure or constrictive pericarditis)
d. Budd–Chiari syndrome (hepatic vein thrombosis) or inferior vena caval obstruction (see Table 7.10)
2. Not related to portal hypertension (SAAG < 11 g/L):
a. Peritoneal carcinomatosis
b. Peritoneal tuberculosis
c. Pancreatitis
d. Nephrotic syndrome (see Table 11.6, p. 315)
EXAMINATION OF ASCITIC FLUID FOLLOWING A DIAGNOSTIC PARACENTESIS
1. *SAAG* – ≥ 11 g/L in portal hypertension (e.g. cirrhosis)
2. *Blood* – suggests traumatic tap, malignancy or a recent invasive test
3. *Turbid or white fluid* – suggests infection or chylous ascites
4. *Cell count* – 0–300 × 10⁶/L mononuclear cells is normal; > 500 cells or > 250 polymorphs × 10⁶/L suggests spontaneous bacterial peritonitis
5. *Lactate* – increased in spontaneous bacterial peritonitis
6. *Amylase* – elevated in pancreatic ascites
7. *Cytology* – for malignant cells
8. *Culture* – for spontaneous bacterial peritonitis

Table 7.10 Budd–Chiari syndrome
Typically young adults who have pain (owing to hepatic congestion), hepatomegaly and ascites
CAUSES
1. Idiopathic (thrombosis or fibrous obliteration of hepatic vein)
2. Myeloproliferative disease, especially polycythaemia rubra vera
3. Malignant disease (e.g. renal, pancreatic, hepatocellular carcinoma, adrenal, testicular, thyroid)
4. Oral contraceptives or pregnancy
5. Paroxysmal nocturnal haemoglobinuria (PNH)
6. Drugs (e.g. azathioprine, adriamycin)
7. Fibrous membrane, trauma, schistosomiasis, amoebiasis
DIAGNOSIS
1. *Liver function tests* – non-specific, but serum alkaline phosphatase level may be high
2. *Ascitic tap*
3. *Ultrasonography with Doppler flow studies* – less sensitive than angiography but diagnostic in > 85% of cases
4. *Technetium sulfur colloid liver scan (increased caudate lobe uptake)* – less useful
5. *Magnetic resonance angiography (and venography)* – diagnostic
6. *Liver biopsy* – highly suggestive ('nutmeg' liver)

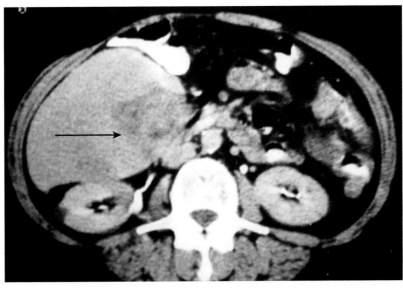

Figure 7.16 CT scan of abdomen showing a hepatocellular carcinoma (arrow), confirmed on biopsy.

Figure reproduced courtesy of The Canberra Hospital.

5. **Ultrasound or abdominal CT scan** (Fig. 7.16)**:** this may help exclude biliary obstruction and infiltration. The texture of the liver may suggest infiltration (e.g. fat) or nodularity (cirrhosis).
6. **Fibro-scanning:** this can be used in place of biopsy to help diagnose cirrhosis.
7. In the setting of dyspnoea, consider **hepatopulmonary syndrome**. Platypnoea (dyspnoea that is worse when the patient sits up and is relieved by lying down) and orthodexia (arterial desaturation when upright) are strongly suggestive; a diagnosis of intrapulmonary vascular dilatation may be possible by contrast echocardiography.
8. Always assess for possible causative factors (see Table 7.7).
   - Obtain hepatitis B and C serologies.
   - Screen for antimitochondrial antibody (AMA) if primary biliary cholangitis is suspected. In suspected chronic hepatitis (e.g. in a young woman with raised globulins) test for antinuclear antibody (ANA), smooth muscle antibody (SMA), and anti-liver and kidney microsomes type 1 (anti-LKM1) antibody. In type I autoimmune chronic hepatitis there is marked hyperglobulinaemia, and ANA and SMA are present. In type II, ANA is negative, but anti-LKM1 is present in high titre and liver cytosol antigen may be present (this antibody also occurs in low titre in hepatitis C). In the rare overlap syndromes, the only serological abnormality may be AMA, but the histology shows autoimmune hepatitis, or the patient is ANA or SMA (but not AMA) positive and has primary biliary cholangitis (autoimmune cholangiopathy) on histology.
   - Order iron studies and, in a young patient, serum copper and caeruloplasmin levels. Alpha$_1$-antitrypsin deficiency should be considered; absence of the alpha$_1$ fraction on a protein electrophoresis is a useful clue.
   - Evaluate for evidence of inflammatory bowel disease if there are colonic symptoms. Perinuclear antineutrophil cytoplasmic antibodies (p-ANCAs) occur in up to 80%

Table 7.11 **Child's classification of patients with cirrhosis in terms of hepatic functional reserve**

Score	1	2	3
Serum bilirubin (µmol/L)	< 35	35–50	> 50
Serum albumin (g/L)	> 35	28–35	< 28
Ascites (see Fig. 7.12)	None	Mild–moderate, diuretic responsive	Poorly controlled
Encephalopathy	None	Mild/moderate	Severe
INR	< 1.7	1.7–2.3	> 2.3
Child–Pugh (CP) A: 5–6 points (1-year survival 100%), CP B 7–9 points (1-year survival 80%), CP C 10–15 points (1-year survival 45%).			

of patients with ulcerative colitis and are a marker for primary sclerosing cholangitis (60% of cases).

- Screening for hepatocellular carcinoma (HCC) is recommended for any patient with cirrhosis. Screening is now by 6-monthly liver ultrasound.
- Assess the hepatic functional reserve of patients with known or suspected cirrhosis (see Table 7.11).

9. **Liver biopsy:** this is a definitive test and probably should be done if the diagnosis is uncertain, unless there are specific contraindications (e.g. coagulopathy).

HINT

The Child–Pugh score (Table 7.11) can be used as an *aide memoire* for the complications of chronic liver disease viz. jaundice, coagulopathy, poor nutrition, ascites and encephalopathy.

Treatment

Decide whether the patient has acute or acute-on-chronic disease and whether the disease is compensated or decompensated. Management includes treating hepatocellular failure (synthetic function) and portal hypertension (plumbing). Cirrhosis is irreversible. However, removing causative factors, such as alcohol, iron overload and drugs, or treating viral infection is of value.

HEPATOCELLULAR FAILURE

Acute hepatic encephalopathy can be precipitated by bleeding into the GI tract or electrolyte disturbances (e.g. alkalosis increases the ammonia crossing the blood–brain barrier, or hypokalaemia, which increases renal ammonia production). Hypokalaemia may be caused by recent diuretic use. Infection (e.g. spontaneous bacterial peritonitis), drugs (e.g. sedatives), a high-protein diet, constipation, deteriorating liver function (e.g. alcoholic binge, hepatocellular carcinoma) and rarely metabolic disturbances (e.g. hypoglycaemia, hypoxia) may also precipitate encephalopathy.

Management

1. Management consists of removing the precipitating factors. This can include medications and endoscopic treatment to stop bleeding, giving a low-protein high-energy diet,

treating infection, correcting electrolyte disturbances, avoiding sedatives/other contributing medications, and the use of lactulose (lowers colonic pH and thus ammonia absorption) or rifaximin (thought to decrease the number of ammonia-producing colonic bacteria), or both.

2. Chronic hepatocellular failure should be managed by treating the cause where possible.
3. Control encephalopathy and ascites (e.g. lactulose or rifaximin, salt restriction, diuretics).
4. Watch for gastrointestinal bleeding and kidney disease.
5. In autoimmune chronic hepatitis, steroids help in patients without viral markers.

PORTAL HYPERTENSION

Clinical features include splenomegaly, the presence of collaterals, ascites and fetor hepaticus. Low platelets on the blood count are a clue. Investigations include endoscopy for oesophageal varices, ascitic tap and abdominal ultrasound with Doppler arterial and venous flow studies.

Management

1. An attempt should be made to assess the bleeding risk for a patient with varices. High-risk patients (75% risk of haemorrhage over 1 year) are those with Child's class C cirrhosis, gross ascites and large varices. All patients with large varices should be recommended prophylactic treatment – usually with beta-blockers or variceal band ligation.
2. Bleeding varices should be managed acutely by replacing intravascular volume (transfuse only if the haemoglobin is less than 70 g/L or bleeding is massive) and correcting coagulation abnormalities. Intravenous octreotide or terlipressin (triglycyl lysine vasopressin), or alternatively vasopressin combined with glyceryl trinitrate, is a first-line therapy, but only a temporary measure. Also give antibiotic cover for a maximum of 7 days (e.g. IV ceftriaxone or oral norfloxacin). Oesophageal variceal banding therapy is effective (and superior to sclerotherapy) in stopping acute bleeding. Balloon tamponade at the gastro-oesophageal junction with a gastric balloon is rarely required; oesophageal balloon tamponade may worsen the prognosis. To prevent recurrent variceal bleeding, elective endoscopic banding to obliterate varices may be effective. Non-selective beta-blockers (e.g. propranolol, carvedilol) can reduce portal pressure and may be useful in patients with good liver function. TIPS is preferable to shunt surgery. Mortality is high for 'crash' portacaval shunts.
3. Treatment of ascites consists of gentle diuresis (maximum weight loss of 500 g per day). Begin with salt restriction and spironolactone but increase the dose slowly. If the urinary sodium to potassium ratio is > 1, a dose of 150 mg/day is usually adequate; if the ratio is less than 1, higher doses are needed. Frusemide is given if necessary. A combination of frusemide 40 mg daily and spironolactone 100 mg daily may be the most helpful, although there is evidence that spironolactone alone may be as effective. Therapeutic paracentesis is a safe alternative in patients with tense ascites, especially when there is also peripheral oedema. Intravenous salt-poor albumin is given to replace the protein lost in ascitic fluid and 5–10 L can be removed; the procedure can be repeated as necessary. Therapeutic paracentesis is contraindicated in renal failure or severe coagulopathy. These patients are at risk of spontaneous bacterial peritonitis. Antibiotic treatment (e.g. ceftriaxone) is indicated if SBP is suspected (advanced cirrhotic patient presenting with fever, abdominal tenderness or encephalopathy) or the ascitic fluid has a polymorph cell count > $250/mm^3$. Usually there is a dramatic clinical response (within 5 days); otherwise repeat the

parecentesis. Lifelong antibiotic prophylaxis (e.g. norfloxacin) is subsequently required unless the liver is transplanted. SBP is associated with a poor 6-month survival. Short-term antibiotic prophylaxis is also indicated in an upper GI bleeder with cirrhosis.

4. In resistant ascites, an alternative to regular paracentesis is TIPS. Remember, though, that this is contraindicated in encephalopathic patients.

5. Nutrition is important for these decompensated patients. Nasogastric feeding has been shown to be helpful if oral intake is inadequate.

6. Liver transplantation is the definitive treatment in suitable patients.

RENAL DISEASE AND CIRRHOSIS

Renal impairment in cirrhosis is not always due to hepatorenal syndrome, and first you must look for and cease any nephrotoxic drugs if possible (especially NSAIDs and diuretics), exclude infection (e.g. SBP), ensure hypovolaemia is identified and corrected, and consider other causes of renal disease (e.g. hepatitis C or B glomerulonephritis – look for proteinuria, casts, etc.).

Hepatorenal syndrome (HRS) occurs in those with advanced chronic liver disease or liver failure and can be acute and rapidly progressive (type I) or subacute (type II). It is associated with high mortality rates. The diagnosis of HRS is based on excluding the risk factors above and lack of improvement over 48 hours during volume expansion with albumin. Diuretics should have been stopped. If the diagnosis of HRS is made, albumin plus a vasoconstrictor is utilised (a vasopressin analogue, e.g. terlipressin, or alpha-adrenergic agonist, e.g. noradrenaline), and listing for transplant should be considered. Without transplant, HRS is often a preterminal event.

HEPATITIS B

Hepatitis B virus (HBV) may be transmitted parenterally (intravenous drug users, infected blood products, etc.) or sexually. Intermediate to high prevalence populations include New Zealand Māoris and people from South East Asia, the Middle East and Western Africa. Most infected adult individuals seroconvert and develop immunity; however, a small proportion become chronic carriers or progress to chronic hepatitis and ultimately cirrhosis. Children younger than 6 years who are acutely infected also have high rates of chronic infection. The risk of developing HCC in HBV cirrhosis is high.

The diagnosis of hepatitis B is made by positive serology (hepatitis B surface antigen (HBsAg) positive) and active disease is usually associated with the hepatitis B e-antigen (HBeAg)-positive state, as well as elevated serum transaminase levels, particularly the serum ALT level (Table 7.12).

Measuring for HBV DNA provides a more accurate assessment of viral load. Precore mutants of HBV are usually diagnosed in patients who are HBeAg negative and HBeAb positive, but have elevated transaminase and HBV DNA levels.

The most accurate method of staging the disease is by means of a liver biopsy. The liver biopsy is important to assess the extent of the inflammation and fibrosis in those with chronic hepatitis. However, fibroscanning is increasingly used as a non-invasive method of assessing fibrosis.

Management

1. The aim of antiviral therapy is to stop viral replication (i.e. seroconversion from positive HBsAg and HBeAg to negative HBsAg and HBeAg, and lower HBV DNA levels), as well as to normalise ALT levels and histology. Loss of HBsAg is ideal

Table 7.12 Interpreting hepatitis (hep) B serological testing			
HBsAg	**ANTI-HBc**	**ANTI-HBs**	**DIFFERENTIAL DIAGNOSIS (MOST LIKELY)**
+	−	−	Acute hepatitis B
−	+	+	Previous infection
−	−	+	Immunised
+	+	−	Acute or chronic hepatitis B[a] (or inactive carrier)
−	+	−	One of: recovering from acute infection; false positive; chronic infection with undetectable HBsAg; past infection with immunity but anti-HBs not detected
+	+	+	Two different hepatitis B infection strains

[a]High ALT and AST indicates infection (versus carrier).
HBsAg = hepatitis B surface antigen; HBc = hepatitis B core antibody; HBs = hepatitis B surface antibody.

(a functional cure), but current therapy is ineffective with regards this endpoint. Those with elevated ALT levels and high levels of HBV DNA should be treated, as well as those with cirrhosis regardless of their serology. 'Inactive carriers' (normal transaminases, HBV DNA $< 10^5$ copies/mL and normal biopsy) usually do not require antiviral therapy unless undergoing, for example, bone marrow transplant for another indication.

2. Treatment options include peginterferon or nucleoside/nucleotide analogues (e.g. entecavir, tenofovir). Peginterferon can be considered in those with well-compensated disease who do not want long-term treatment (treatment is limited to 48 weeks), but has many side-effects. Entecavir and tenofovir are the preferred nucleoside/nucleotide analogues and are well tolerated, with low rates of resistance. Treatment is usually 5 years to lifelong. Lamivudine is not recommended owing to high rates of drug resistance.

3. Liver transplantation can be considered in patients with decompensated HBV liver disease, but without proper preparation HBV infection recurs in the transplanted liver and may cause very aggressive liver disease. Fortunately, strategies are available to overcome this problem. Currently, antiviral drugs are used prior to transplantation to lower HBV-DNA levels and then large doses of hepatitis B immunoglobulin are used in the peritransplantation period. This strategy is extremely effective in preventing recurrence after liver transplantation.

HEPATITIS C

Hepatitis C virus (HCV) is predominantly parenterally transmitted and is particularly common in intravenous drug users. The virus is also commonly found in migrants from endemic regions, including South East Asia, Egypt and Italy. The majority of patients are incidentally found to be infected and are usually asymptomatic, although fatigue is a common symptom. If the patient is HCV antibody positive, confirm the diagnosis with HCV RNA.

Extrahepatic manifestations are listed in Table 7.13. The disease process is insidious in onset. Approximately 80% of infected individuals go on to develop chronic hepatitis over a 20-year period. It is estimated that 20%–30% of patients with chronic hepatitis C eventually develop cirrhosis. Once cirrhosis develops, symptoms are more common and the signs of end-stage liver disease can appear, with jaundice, weakness, wasting

Table 7.13 Extrahepatic manifestations of hepatitis C
• Mixed cryoglobulinaemia (Fig. 7.17)
• Porphyria cutanea tarda (Fig. 7.18)
• Leukocytoclastic vasculitis (Fig. 7.19)
• Membranoproliferative glomerulonephritis
• Lichen planus (Fig. 7.20)
• Hashimoto's thyroiditis
• Sjögren's / sicca syndrome
• Autoimmune hepatitis
• B cell lymphoma
• Immune thrombocytopenia / autoimmune haemolytic anaemia
• Polyarthralgias and polyarthritis
• Diabetes mellitus

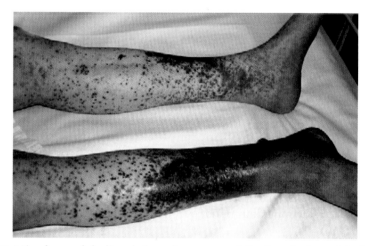

Figure 7.17 Mixed cryoglobulinaemia and purpura of the legs in hepatitis C.

M Ramos-Casals. The cryoglobulinaemias. Reprinted with permission from Elsevier (*The Lancet*, 2012, vol no 379(9813):348–60).

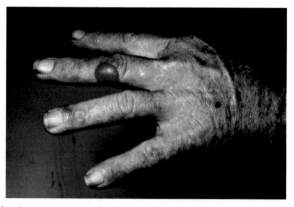

Figure 7.18 Porphyria cutanea tarda.

N Talley, S O'Connor. *Clinical examination*, vol 1, Fig 14.8. Elsevier Australia, 2018, with permission.

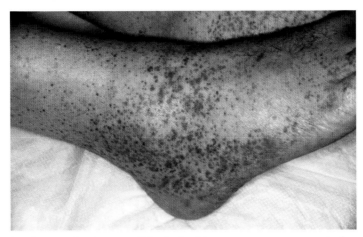

Figure 7.19 Leukocytoclastic vasculitis (palpable purpura: can occur in hepatitis C or B, mixed cryoglobulinaemia, Henoch–Schönlein purpura or cancer (or be idiopathic); differential diagnosis is cutaneous emboli especially in meningococcus infection).

D M Elston, P J McMahon, W D James. *Andrews' diseases of the skin clinical atlas*, Fig. 35.49. Elsevier, 2018, with permission.

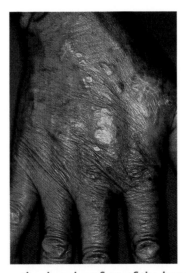

Figure 7.20 Lichen planus on the dorsal surface of the hand. Wickham's striae can be easily identified in the upper right lesion. Note the flat-topped lesions.

J L Bolognia, J L Jorizzo, J V Schaffer. *Dermatology*, 3rd edn. Elsevier, 2012, with permission.

and gastrointestinal bleeding. After 25 years of infection, about 4% of patients with cirrhosis develop HCC.

Diagnosis is based on a positive HCV antibody enzyme-linked immunosorbent assay (ELISA) test and then the active virus is checked with HCV-polymerase chain reaction (PCR) testing.

Quantitative HCV-PCR is useful in monitoring the response to treatment. A liver biopsy is helpful to stage the disease and estimate the extent of fibrosis, although the non-invasive fibroscan is replacing liver biopsy in practice.

Management

1. Management needs to take a holistic approach (Table 7.14). Curative therapy is now available for hepatitis C with a number of pan-genotypic direct-acting antiviral agent regimens, and achieves a high, sustained virological response (cure) rates in over 90% of patients.
2. Patients who develop end-stage liver disease may be transplant candidates.

Screen for hepatocellular carcinoma

Surveillance for HCC (hepatoma) is necessary if there is cirrhosis from any cause, and especially hepatitis C or B.

It is recommended that patients have an ultrasound every 6 months; alpha-fetoprotein can also be requested (in addition to ultrasound) – the combination increases detection rates but also false-positive rates. Small tumours can be resected if the patient does not have significant portal hypertension. Otherwise transplant is sometimes possible (if advanced liver disease with a solitary tumour ≤ 5 cm, or up to three tumours all ≤ 3 cm) and can be curative. Palliative approaches (or as a bridge to transplant) include radiofrequency or microwave ablation (RFA/MWA), transarterial chemoembolisation (TACE) and stereotactic body radiation therapy (SBRT). Those with advanced disease (including advanced cirrhosis) can be offered systemic therapies, such as sorafenib, regorafenib or lenvatinib (multitargeted tyrosine kinase inhibitors), which modestly improve survival.

HAEMOCHROMATOSIS

This is an autosomal recessive disease marked by increased intestinal absorption of iron and progressive iron loading of parenchymal cells of the liver, pancreas, heart and other organs. The diagnosis is now most often made before symptoms develop (from routine iron studies or genetic testing of relatives of affected patients) and is much commoner in men (menses protect women). Classic symptoms, when present, include fatigue/lethargy, skin hyperpigmentation, diabetes mellitus, arthralgia/arthropathy (especially hands) and impotence. The classic triad of cirrhosis with skin hyperpigmentation and diabetes ('bronzed diabetes' (see Fig. 7.14)) is a late manifestation of the disease. HCC occurs in up to 30% of patients with cirrhosis.

Hereditary haemochromatosis is a common genetic disorder in Caucasians, with a prevalence of at least 1 in 250. Diagnosis is suggested by an increased transferrin saturation (≥ 45%) and a raised ferritin level (> 300 µg/L in men and > 200 µg/L in premenopausal women is suggestive). The serum ferritin level is an acute-phase reactant and may be elevated in other chronic inflammatory conditions, notably those involving the liver, including NASH, alcoholic liver disease and chronic viral hepatitis.

Diagnosis is made by identifying the genetic defects. In difficult cases, liver biopsy is useful to measure the amount of iron overload and the extent of liver disease (fibrosis, cirrhosis, etc.). A liver biopsy is also indicated if the ferritin is over 1000 µg/L, or liver enzymes are elevated. There are specific features on biopsy: a Perls' Prussian blue stain visually demonstrates the extent of iron overload. It is important to determine the hepatic iron concentration and index (usually > 1.9) on liver biopsy specimens.

The genetic defect has been localised to the short arm of chromosome 6. The gene has been termed *HFE*. Two common mutations have been described: *C282Y* and *H63D*. Patients with phenotypic haemochromatosis are usually homozygous for the *C282Y* mutation; very few are compound heterozygotes (*C282Y* and *H63D* mutation). Homozygotes for *H63D* may not be at risk; 5% of those with haemochromatosis have none of these mutations. Genetic testing is recommended for all first-degree relatives of the proband. In those cases homozygous for *C282Y*, there is a one in four chance of the

Table 7.14 Principles of management of hepatitis C virus

GENERAL

- Rule out coexistent HIV and hepatitis B. Newly diagnosed patients should be tested for hepatitis A and B antibodies – if negative, vaccinate.
- Counsel about the routes of HCV transmission – do not donate blood; ensure wounds are covered and blood-contaminated surfaces are cleaned with diluted household bleach; avoid sharing toothbrushes, razors or needles; note the risk of sexual transmission is low.
- There should be a discussion about pregnancy. The rates of vertical transmission are approximately 5%, and currently there are few data about the safety of the oral antivirals in pregnancy.
- Screen and counsel for depression (depression is relevant to interferon-based therapies).
- Manage alcohol, obesity, cigarette smoking and marijuana exposure (can promote hepatic fibrosis), and recommend ceasing all illicit drugs (none of these are now a contraindication to antiviral therapy).
- Review hepatotoxic drugs – avoid NSAIDs in advanced liver disease, remember the dose of paracetamol should not exceed 2 g per 24 hours (and know that the use of statins is safe for patients with stable HCV infection).
- Coffee consumption (more than two cups per day) may be beneficial (but is not an established recommendation).
- If cirrhosis is present – manage as previously discussed in this chapter.

ANTIVIRAL THERAPY

- After acute infection, up to 80% of HCV patients become chronically infected. If HCV is chronic (i.e. detectable HCV viral level at 6 months), consider therapy.
- With the advent of oral antiviral therapy, the use of peginterferon / ribavirin has almost become obsolete. Cure / SVR is attained in up to 95% of patients. The oral drug combinations tend to be well tolerated. Optimal treatment regimens depend on genotype, drug availability (know current drug availability), any prior exposure to HCV antivirals and the presence of cirrhosis.
- Glomerulonephritis, cryoglobulinaemia and porphyria cutanea tarda may respond to antiviral therapy. In those with HCV and severe vasculitis, consider additional therapy (e.g. plasmapheresis; remember drug interactions with HCV regimens).
- Before beginning treatment in any patient – assess renal function, order a full blood count and differential, and liver function tests.
- Assess for any severe co-morbidity (e.g. cardiac disease).
- Assess disease stage – review non-invasive markers of liver fibrosis (AST / ALT ratio, AST to platelet ratio index (APRI)), and the ultrasound-based transient elastography (do not routinely ask for a liver biopsy).
- With non-interferon-based therapies, generally sustained virological response (SVR) to treatment should be assessed by measuring the viral load at 12 weeks after stopping therapy.
- Assess safety and potential drug interactions if planning to start anti-viral therapy.

SPECIFIC EXAMPLES OF INTERFERON-FREE ANTIVIRAL OPTIONS

Pan-genotypic (1, 2, 3, 4, 5, 6)

- Sofosbuvir + velpatasvir – 12 week treatment regimen for non-cirrhotics and cirrhotics (the addition of ribavirin can be considered for those with compensated cirrhosis and HCV genotype 3). Nausea is a common side-effect. Sofosbuvir is not recommended if eGFR is < 30 mL / min / 1.73 m^2.
- Glecaprevir + pibrentasvir – 8-week treatment regimen for non-cirrhotics, 12–16 for those with cirrhosis. Headache, fatigue, nausea, diarrhoea and an unconjugated hyperbilirubinaemia are reported side-effects.
- Ledipasvir-sofosbuvir – genotype 1 (can also be used for 4, 5, 6); 8–12-week treatment regimen for non-cirrhotics, 12–24 weeks for cirrhotics. Ribavirin may be added in certain circumstances. Nausea is a common side-effect. Sofosbuvir is not recommended if eGFR is < 30 mL / min / 1.73 m^2.
- Elbasvir-grazoprevir – genotype 1 and 4; 12-week treatment regimen for both non-cirrhotics and cirrhotics. Headache is commonly reported, and can cause an increase in ALT and bilirubin.
- Daclatasvir + sofosbuvir – genotype 1 or 3; 12–24-week treatment regimen, ribavirin may be added for those with cirrhosis. Fatigue, headache, insomnia, nausea and diarrhoea are reported side-effects.
- Daily fixed-dose combination of glecaprevir (300 mg) / pibrentasvir (120 mg) for 8 weeks (or 12 weeks if cirrhosis present) and sofosbuvir (400 mg) / velpatasvir (100 mg) for 12 weeks are other alternatives.
- Daily fixed dose of glecaprevir (300 mg) / pibrentasvir (120 mg) for 8 weeks (or 12 weeks in compensated cirrhosis).
- Daily fixed dose of sofosbuvir (400 mg) / velpatasvir (100 mg) for 12 weeks.

ALT = alanine aminotransferase; APRI = aspartate aminotransferase to platelet ratio index; AST = aspartate aminotransferase; eGFR = estimated glomerular filtration rate; HCV = hepatitis C virus; SVR = sustained virological response.

siblings being homozygous. The children's chance of developing haemochromatosis depends on the other parent (homozygous normal indicates no risk).

Management

1. Phlebotomy is indicated if the patient is a *C282Y* homozygote or *C282Y/H63D* compound heterozygote and has raised ferritin (>200 μg/L in females, > 300 μg/L in males; some guidelines suggest phlebotomy only if > 500 μg/L in asymptomatic individuals), or if symptomatic or cirrhotic.
2. Treatment is through regular venesection (once to twice weekly, may be decreased to monthly if elderly or frail) until ferritin is 20–50 μg/L (also aiming to maintain Hb > 120 g/L) – this may take up to 2 years. Maintenance phlebotomy regimens (targeting ferritin 50–100 μg/L) may be once every 3–6 months. Fifty units of blood removed per year equals about 12.5 g of iron withdrawn. However, patients with iron overload as a result of mutations of the iron export protein ferroportin may not tolerate this rate of removal.
3. The avoidance of alcohol is important.
4. Manifestations that respond to phlebotomy include malaise, fatigue, skin hyperpigmentation, insulin requirements and abdominal pain. Less responsive are arthropathy, hypogonadism and advanced cirrhosis.
5. Hepatocellular carcinoma is *not* prevented by venesection in patients with established cirrhosis, but life expectancy is normal in those without end-organ damage whose iron stores are reduced.

NON-ALCOHOLIC STEATOHEPATITIS (NON-ALCOHOLIC FATTY LIVER DISEASE)

Non-alcoholic fatty liver disease is divided into non-alcoholic fatty liver (NAFL) and non-alcoholic steatohepatitis (NASH). NAFL patients have hepatic steatosis without inflammation, whereas NASH patients have associated inflammation. A proportion of patients with NASH will progress to cirrhosis. NASH is defined by histological features, resembling those of alcoholic hepatitis, which are present in patients who have not consumed excessive quantities of alcohol. The majority of patients present because they are inadvertently found to have abnormal liver function tests or steatosis detected on imaging. Even though clinical findings are uncommon, hepatomegaly is the most frequent sign detected. The typical liver function abnormalities are a two- to threefold elevation of the serum aminotransferase levels, with the serum ALT greater than the serum AST level (the opposite of alcoholic liver disease). The serum alkaline phosphatase and gamma-glutamyl transferase (GGT) levels may be similarly elevated. Viral markers are absent.

NASH is more common in women and the most frequently associated underlying clinical conditions are obesity, hypertension, insulin resistance or type 2 diabetes mellitus, and hyperlipidaemia, particularly hypertriglyceridaemia. Look for evidence of the metabolic syndrome (including hypertension, increased waist circumference and high lipids). Nevertheless, studies have documented lean Asian men with NASH. Although the peak age of presentation is the fifth and sixth decades of life, NASH is now the most common cause of liver disease in adolescents.

Exclude drug causes such as use of steroids, tamoxifen and amiodarone. The definitive diagnostic test is a liver biopsy but it is *not* usually required. Other liver disease must be excluded by a liver screen (e.g. haemochromatosis, chronic viral hepatitis) (Table 7.15). The typical histological features are macrovesicular steatosis with an associated necroinflammatory infiltrate (usually mononuclear) and a variable degree of fibrosis.

Studies have documented elevations in both cardiovascular and hepatic mortality.

Table 7.15 **Causes of hepatic steatosis**	
METABOLIC DISORDERS	**DRUGS AND TOXINS**
Obesity	Alcohol
Diabetes mellitus	Methotrexate
Hyperlipidaemia	Organic solvents
Jejunoileal bypass	Amiodarone
Total parenteral nutrition	Glucocorticoids
Hepatitis C	HIV antiretrovirals

Management

Management options are limited to treating the underlying clinical condition, with slow weight loss and exercise recommended for obese patients and strict control of hyperlipidaemia and hyperglycaemia. Statin therapy is safe for patients with hypercholesterolaemia. Bariatric surgery can be considered. Alcohol should be avoided. Vaccination and modification of cardiovascular risk factors should occur. Vitamin E supplementation can be considered in the absence of diabetes and if there is fibrosis. Pioglitazone can be considered in type 2 diabetics. If cirrhosis is present, this should be managed as previously outlined.

Possible lines of questioning

1. Has *this* patient developed portal hypertension?
2. From your history, what do you think is the likely aetiology of *this* patient's liver disease?
3. Is *this* patient a candidate for antiviral treatment?
4. You have said *this* patient has non-alcoholic fatty liver disease. What other causes of liver disease would you recommend be excluded?

Liver transplantation

Liver transplantation is now an important therapeutic option in patients with irreversible, progressive liver disease for which there is no acceptable alternative therapy and no absolute contraindication. The 1-year survival rate overall is 75%. In the examination setting, a patient will either have chronic liver disease and be a candidate for transplantation or be a transplant recipient who has a problem.

The history

1. Obtain details of the patient's liver disease, including diagnosis and duration. Candidates for liver transplantation include patients with cirrhosis (MELD > 12) (complicated by, for example, portal hypertension, HRS or HCC), primary sclerosing cholangitis, autoimmune chronic hepatitis, chronic portal–systemic encephalopathy, Budd–Chiari syndrome, inherited metabolic diseases (e.g. Wilson's disease, alpha$_1$-antitrypsin deficiency), highly selected patients with cholangiocarcinoma, and acute or subacute hepatic failure refractory ascites or encephalopathy.
2. The timing of the transplantation is crucial. This should be considered when the patient is in end stage but before complications have occurred that may preclude proceeding (e.g. preterminal variceal bleeding, irreversible hepatorenal syndrome,

development of a catabolic state, irreversible coagulopathy, vascular instability with ascites or incapacitating osteopenic bone disease). Those with end-stage liver disease who have had a life-threatening episode of decompensation or whose quality of life has become unbearably reduced are potential candidates. Accepted criteria include a Child–Pugh score > 6, an episode of variceal bleeding or spontaneous bacterial peritonitis, or stage II encephalopathy in acute liver failure. A model for end-stage liver disease (MELD), which has been developed at the Mayo Clinic and is based on three parameters (serum bilirubin, INR and creatinine), helps predict survival and is widely used (transplant candidates usually have a score > 12–14).

3. If the patient may be a candidate for liver transplantation, enquire about potential contraindications. Relative contraindications include:
   - active sepsis / infection
   - metastatic malignancy
   - cholangiocarcinoma
   - continuing alcohol consumption
   - AIDS (HIV is not a contraindication if suppressed)
   - diffuse portal vein thrombosis and advanced cardiopulmonary or renal disease
   - a prior portacaval shunt (TIPS is not a contraindication) / other anatomical abnormalities that preclude liver surgery
   - poor social support.

   Severe hypoxaemia as a result of intrapulmonary shunting is another potential contraindication (patients with the hepatopulmonary syndrome and hypoxia can benefit, but a PaO_2 of < 50 mmHg is a relative contraindication; severe portopulmonary hypertension not responsive to treatment is a contraindication).

4. Ask about tests that have been done in preparation for transplant and the results. These typically include cardiac and pulmonary tests (electrocardiogram, echocardiogram, stress test, chest X-ray, pulmonary function tests), renal tests (urine protein and creatinine, and glomerular filtration rate estimation) and liver tests (imaging to exclude HCC and to define the vascular anatomy).

5. Enquire about complications of the patient's liver disease (e.g. previous variceal haemorrhages, ascites, encephalopathy / pre-coma, hypoxaemia caused by hepatopulmonary syndrome, HCC, etc.).

6. If the patient has had a transplant, enquire about the postoperative course, including whether further surgery was carried out (e.g. drainage of abscesses, reconstruction of the biliary tract for control of bleeding, re-transplantation for graft failure and for hepatic arterial thrombosis). Also ask about postoperative infections.

   a. Ask about complications of liver transplantation. Early on (in the first 5 days) these include:
      - primary graft failure
      - technical problems (e.g. bleeding, hepatic arterial thrombosis, bile leaks, portal vein thrombosis)
      - kidney disease
      - pulmonary complications (atelectasis, pleural effusion, infection).

   b. Major problems after discharge from hospital include:
      - rejection
      - infection
      - biliary complications
      - hypotension
      - diabetes mellitus
      - renal disease

- coronary artery disease
- recurrent disease
- bone disease
- nutrition
- de-novo cancer.

c. Infections occur in most patients, largely related to immunosuppression. Those that occur in the first month tend to be similar to those in immunocompetent patients (e.g. line-related infections). From 1 to 6 months post-transplant, opportunistic infections can be seen (e.g. *Pneumocystis jirovecii*, CMV, fungal). The patient may know the donor and recipient CMV status. Beyond 6 months, if there is good graft function, infections tend to be community acquired. However, if there is poor graft function, or high levels of immunosuppression, opportunistic infections remain a consideration. Ask about prophylactic antibiotic therapy.

d. Biliary strictures may also occur from 4 weeks after transplantation.

e. Acute liver rejection is rarely seen after the initial 6 months. Chronic rejection usually occurs 6 weeks to 9 months after transplantation; there is progressive cholestasis and diagnosis is best made by liver biopsy. Bone disease and ectopic calcification may occur some months after transplantation.

7. Ask about current medications and related complications with their use.

   a. Cyclosporin or tacrolimus may induce:
   - cholestasis (dose-dependent)
   - hypertension
   - nephrotoxicity
   - gum hypertrophy
   - seizures (controlled by phenytoin, which induces cyclosporin metabolism)
   - CNS effects, including tremor and central pontine myelinolysis. Patients with a low serum cholesterol level are at increased risk of central nervous system toxicity.

   b. Steroids in high doses may induce a number of problems, including aseptic necrosis of long bones, cataracts and psychosis. Enquire about drug adherence.

   c. Mycophenolate may cause bone marrow suppression or GI side-effects.

8. Try to find out tactfully whether there have been any concerns about malignancy. The incidence of skin cancers and lymphomas (especially in the CNS) is increased with immunosuppression.

The examination

1. The pre-transplant patient should be examined for signs of chronic liver disease and complications of liver disease. Note clubbing (which occurs in cirrhosis and might indicate hepatopulmonary syndrome in this setting).

2. The post-transplant patient should be examined for liver tenderness (e.g. acute rejection) and jaundice (e.g. vanishing bile ducts in chronic rejection, biliary stricture). Examine the chest for infection and the mouth for candidiasis. The temperature must be taken (Table 7.16). Examine the central nervous system (e.g. cyclosporin toxicity or cerebral infarction from perioperative hypotension or air embolism). Tap the spine for tenderness (e.g. vertebral collapse). Take the blood pressure (hypertension may occur at any time after transplantation; it is often caused by cyclosporin).

Investigations

Pre-transplant patients need tests to confirm the diagnosis, determine current liver synthetic function (e.g. serum albumin, INR) and rule out contraindications. Ultrasound

Table 7.16 **Causes of fever in the outpatient with a liver transplant**
• Biliary tract (stricture and cholangitis)
• Pneumonia (e.g. *Pneumocystis*, bacterial, fungal)
• Urinary tract sepsis
• Hepatitis (acute or recurrent)
• Central nervous system infection (especially fungal)
• Viral infection (e.g. cytomegalovirus, herpes, varicella-zoster)

and CT scanning are routine. In patients with possible or definite malignancy, metastases must be sought. Assess bone density; osteopenia is common in liver disease and increases following transplant. Cardiopulmonary and psychiatric evaluations are important.

Management

Routine outpatient monitoring after transplantation should include a full blood count, electrolyte levels, renal and liver profile, and drug levels (e.g. trough cyclosporin / tacrolimus levels). Remember drug interactions with cyclosporin. Diabetes mellitus may supervene as a result of treatment with tacrolimus or steroids. Hypertension should be treated. Diseases that can recur in the graft include hepatitis B and C, Budd–Chiari syndrome, primary biliary cholangitis, primary sclerosing cholangitis and autoimmune hepatitis, amongst others.

Possible lines of questioning

1. Is *this* patient with liver failure a candidate for liver transplant?
2. What complications of immune suppression has *this* patient experienced?
3. Were there complications related to the transplant procedure?

Chapter 8

The haematological long case

The modern haematologist, instead of describing in
English what he can see, prefers to describe in Greek
what he can't.

Richard Allan John Asher (1912–69)

Haemolytic anaemia

This is an uncommon but important long case. It is usually a diagnostic problem.
Coombs' positive haemolytic anaemia is most often encountered in the examination.

The history

1. Ask about the symptoms of anaemia (e.g. fatigue, shortness of breath on exertion)
   and whether the patient has noticed or been told about jaundice.
2. Determine whether there is a history of known haemolytic episodes. Onset at an
   early age or a family history suggests an intrinsic red cell defect (e.g. hereditary
   spherocytosis or elliptocytosis (both autosomal dominant), sickle cell anaemia).
3. Ask about symptoms of connective tissue disease:
   a. Joint pain or swelling may also occur in acute sickle cell crisis and especially affect
      the knees and elbows.
   b. Refractory leg ulcers occur in hereditary spherocytosis and sickle cell
      syndromes.
   c. Systemic lupus erythematosus (SLE) and other connective tissue disorders may
      be associated with warm antibody immunohaemolytic anaemia.
4. Lymphoma is associated with both warm and cold antibodies and anaemia.
5. A history of pain in the abdomen, back and elsewhere suggests sickle cell anaemia
   or paroxysmal nocturnal haemoglobinuria. Congenital haemolytic anaemias can
   result in pigment gallstones that can cause symptomatic cholelithiasis and even acute
   cholecystitis; these episodes can be confused with acute crises.
6. Ask about neurological problems:
   a. Spinal cord lesions can occur with hereditary spherocytosis.
   b. Paraspinal masses (extramedullary haemopoiesis) are a rare complication of any
      hereditary haemolytic anaemia or lymphoma.

    c. Acute sickle cell crisis can also result in neurological impairment, particularly stroke.

    d. Tertiary syphilis may cause paroxysmal cold haemoglobinuria.

    e. In thrombotic thrombocytopenic purpura (TTP) there are often fluctuating neurological abnormalities. For other features of TTP, remember the mnemonic FAT RN:

    Fever

    Anaemia (microangiopathic haemolytic)

    Thrombocytopenia

    Renal failure

    Neurological abnormalities.

7. List all drugs that have been taken, for example:

    a. Methyldopa, penicillin and quinidine can cause warm antibody immunohaemolytic anaemia (WAIHA).

    b. Antimalarials, sulfonamides and nitrofurantoin cause haemolysis in subjects deficient in glucose-6-phosphate dehydrogenase (G6PD).

    Note: Between 10% and 20% of people taking methyldopa have a positive direct Coombs' test, but only a small minority of these develop haemolysis. The drug alters Rh antigens so that antibodies are produced against them, which then cross-react with normal Rh antigens. The indirect Coombs' test is therefore positive, even when the drug is not added to the test. The other drugs produce an indirect Coombs' test result only when the drug is added to the mixture, because in that case the antibodies are directed against a combination of drug and cell membrane.

    c. Fludarabine, which is often increasingly used as first-line treatment of chronic lymphocytic leukaemia in patients under the age of 65 and non-Hodgkin lymphoma, may cause exacerbation of warm autoimmune haemolytic anaemia (AIHA). When fludarabine is combined with the anti-CD20 monoclonal rituximab, as is current practice, AIHA is mitigated.

8. Enquire about any operations, particularly mechanical heart valve replacement (10% of those with aortic valve prostheses have significant haemolysis; this percentage is lower with mitral valve prostheses unless a paravalvular leak is present, as the pressure gradient is lower). Severe haemolysis in these patients suggests a paravalvular leak.

9. Consider the other occasional cause of haemolysis within the circulation – external trauma, such as occurs in joggers who wear thin-soled shoes, and the traditional group, bongo drummers. In these cases, haemolysis is intravascular and haemosiderinuria is characteristic.

10. Determine the patient's ethnic background (e.g. Greeks or Italians may inherit the beta-thalassaemia trait; both thalassaemias are common on the subcontinent and alpha-thalassaemia is common in China and South East Asia; males of African, Mediterranean or Asian descent may have G6PD deficiency).

11. The patient may have an underlying medical problem associated with the risk of developing microvascular fragmentation of red cells. These conditions include: disseminated intravascular coagulation (DIC), which is usually caused by vessel wall changes related to an underlying disease, such as disseminated malignancy, renal graft rejection or malignant hypertension; TTP, which is of unknown aetiology; and haemolytic uraemic syndrome (HUS, with similar features to TTP), which can follow gastroenteritis caused by *E. coli 0157:H7* infection (do not treat these cases with an antibiotic, as this increases the risk of HUS!).

The examination

1. A careful haemopoietic system examination is required. The characteristic 'chipmunk' facies in a young person with thalassaemia is caused by maxillary marrow hyperplasia and frontal bossing.
2. Look for pallor and icterus.
3. Examine the heart for a valve prosthesis or severe aortic stenosis (traumatic haemolysis). Profound anaemia may be associated with high-output cardiac failure. An iron overload state in thalassaemia major from repeated transfusions may cause skin pigmentation, cardiac failure and hepatomegaly.
4. Carefully palpate for the spleen; splenomegaly from any cause (see Table 16.21, p. 463) may result in haemolysis. Lymphadenopathy may indicate lymphoma (associated with warm or cold antibody haemolysis), chronic lymphocytic leukaemia or, in practice, glandular fever (cold agglutinin haemolysis).
5. Signs of chronic liver disease should be noted – in severe cirrhosis, spur cell (acanthocyte) anaemia is occasionally observed.
6. Examine for focal neurological signs. Look in the fundi – retinal detachment, retinal infarcts and vitreous haemorrhages can be manifestations of sickle cell anaemia; Kayser–Fleischer rings (see Fig. 7.15, p. 177) may be present in the cornea when haemolysis is caused by Wilson's disease.
7. Joint swelling and tenderness, and occasionally aseptic necrosis of bone (e.g. neck of femur), also occur in sickle cell anaemia; bony infarcts may become infected (e.g. *Salmonella* osteomyelitis).
8. Look for leg ulceration. Note any signs of connective tissue disease.
9. Test the urine – urobilinogen may be present with haemolysis; it may be dark from the presence of free haemoglobin as a result of intravascular haemolysis and the sediment may be abnormal (e.g. TTP).
10. Fever may occur with septicaemia or malaria-associated haemolysis, with acute crises in sickle cell anaemia and in TTP.

Investigations

It is important to confirm that haemolysis is present, exclude intravascular haemolysis and perform tests to determine the aetiology. The history and physical examination may have provided hints about the likely aetiology.

1. Ask for the results of a:
   * blood count
   * reticulocyte count
   * serum bilirubin
   * lactate dehydrogenase.

   Haemolysis is likely to be present if there is a normochromic normocytic anaemia with an increased reticulocyte count (but reticulocytosis also occurs with blood loss or partially treated anaemia) and release of red blood cell components (increased unconjugated bilirubin and, more variably, lactate dehydrogenase).
2. Usually serum haptoglobin is absent and haemosiderin is present in the urine. Intravascular haemolysis is documented by the presence of methaemalbumin in the plasma and, less often, of haemoglobin in the urine.
3. The presence of fragmented red cells (schistocytes) suggests valve haemolysis, DIC and TTP (or HUS). TTP (or HUS) is very likely when fragmented red cells occur in association with thrombocytopenia and normal coagulation studies. Test for renal and neurological impairment.

4. The blood film usually shows polychromasia; it may show other red cell changes (Tables 8.1 and 8.2). In thalassaemia, the anaemia is often hypochromic and always significantly microcytic.

5. If a congenital intracorpuscular defect seems unlikely, ask for a Coombs' test to determine whether the anaemia is immunohaemolytic. The polyspecific direct Coombs' test measures the ability of anti-IgG and anti-C3 to agglutinate the patient's red blood cells. Warm antibodies (80% of cases) react at body temperature and may occur with lymphoma (usually non-Hodgkin), chronic lymphocytic leukaemia, solid tumours (lung, colon, kidney and ovary), SLE and drugs, or may be idiopathic. They are usually IgG antibodies directed at the Rh antigens. Cold-reactive antibodies (cold autoimmune haemolytic anaemia – CAIHA) are precipitated by exposure to room temperature ('cold') – cold agglutinin disease (IgM antibodies) may occur acutely with Epstein–Barr infection, glandular fever, mycoplasma infection or hepatitis C, and chronically may be caused by lymphoma or may be idiopathic; paroxysmal cold haemoglobinuria (IgG antibodies) is rare.

Table 8.1 Full blood count and liver function tests from a female patient with autoimmune haemolytic anaemia (AIHA)

PARAMETER	VALUE	NORMAL RANGE
Haemoglobin	63 g/L	115–165 g/L (female)
Mean corpuscular volume (MCV)	100 fL	80–100 fL
White cell count (WCC)	15.0×10^9/L	$4.5–13.5 \times 10^9$/L
Platelet count	350×10^9/L	$150–400 \times 10^9$/L
Erythrocyte sedimentation rate (ESR)	58 mm/h	3–19 mm/h (female < 50 years)
Reticulocyte count	18%	0.2%–2.0% of red cell count
Bilirubin (total)	45 mmol/L	< 20 mmol/L
Aspartate aminotransferase (AST)	30 U/L	< 45 U/L
Alanine aminotransferase (ALT)	40 U/L	< 40 U/L
Lactate dehydrogenase (LDH)	451 U/L	110–230 U/L
Protein (total)	72 g/L	62–80 g/L
Albumin	42 g/L	32–45 g/L
Haptoglobin	< 0.2 g/L	0.3–2.0 g/L

- *Blood film:* moderate anisocytosis, numerous spherocytes, prominent polychromasia; nucleated red cells, neutrophilia and band forms.
- *Direct Coombs' test positive:* reaction grade 0–4.

COMMENT

The patient has severe normochromic anaemia with marked reticulocytosis. The very high reticulocyte count suggests haemolysis rather than blood loss. The polychromasia, nucleated red cells and reticulocytosis are signs of increased marrow erythroid activity. The raised bilirubin and reduced haptoglobin levels are consistent with haemolysis. The classical triad suggesting haemolysis is a raised LDH level, reduced haptoglobin level and unconjugated hyperbilirubinaemia. The presence of spherocytes suggests hereditary spherocytosis or immune haemolysis. If there were fragmented red cells, mechanical haemolysis or microangiopathic haemolysis would be likely. Normal red cell morphology would suggest hypersplenism or paroxysmal nocturnal haemoglobinuria. The presence of 'bite' cells would suggest G6PD deficiency.

In this case the candidate should ask for a Coombs' test to distinguish autoimmune haemolytic anaemia from hereditary spherocytosis.

Table 8.2 Haemolytic anaemia

CLASSIFICATION	PERIPHERAL BLOOD MORPHOLOGY	DIAGNOSTIC TEST	TREATMENT

1. Immune haemolysis
  a. 'Warm' antibody
    i. autoimmune (lymphoma, connective tissue disease, idiopathic)
    ii. drug-induced
	Spherocytes	Coombs' (antiglobulin) test; differential Coombs' test (IgG, complement)	Clinically significant haemolysis – steroids; if steroids not tolerated or do not control disease – splenectomy; if still refractory – azathioprine, cyclophosphamide or rituximab
			Discontinue drugs

b. 'Cold' antibody i. cold agglutinin (post-infection, lymphoma, idiopathic)	Red cell agglutination in cold	Cold agglutinins Coombs' test – C3 on red cell surface Anti-I (e.g. mycoplasma) or anti-i (e.g. glandular fever)	Maintain warm environment; treat any precipitating cause (e.g. mycoplasma, CLL); immunosuppressives only if severe disease Rituximab plus chemotherapy plus fludarabine if severe Transfusions given through a blood warmer
2. Mechanical haemolysis a. Microangiopathic (DIC, TTP, vasculitis, etc.)	Schizocytes, microspherocytes	Evidence of intravascular haemolysis; evidence of underlying disease state	TTP: plasmapheresis (immunosuppression may also be required) DIC: treat the underlying cause
b. Heart valve	Urinary haemosiderin often positive; schizocytes		Correct iron deficiency; replace valve if indicated; folate
c. March haemoglobinuria (rare as for e.g. marathon runners)			Avoid marathons

3. Infection
  a. Septicaemia
  b. Parasitic (e.g. malaria)
	Spherocytes, fragments, intraerythrocyte parasites	Blood cultures, thin and thick smears	Treat infection

4. Acquired membrane abnormalities a. Cirrhosis	Spur cells (acanthocytes)	Liver function tests	Splenectomy is controversial
b. Chronic kidney disease	Burr cells (echinocytes)	Renal function tests	Treat renal failure Correct iron deficiency
c. Paroxysmal nocturnal haemoglobinuria	Spherocytes, microcytes	Flow cytometry (CD55, CD59)	Steroid or androgen therapy may reduce haemolysis; transfuse with washed red cells Eculuzimab (anti-C5) reduces transfusion requirements and thrombotic episodes

Continued

Table 8.2 **Continued**			
CLASSIFICATION	**PERIPHERAL BLOOD MORPHOLOGY**	**DIAGNOSTIC TEST**	**TREATMENT**
INTRACORPUSCULAR			
1. Haemoglobinopathies a. Amino acid substitutions (e.g. sickle cell)	Sickle forms, hypochromic	Sickle preparation, Hb electrophoresis, family study of HbS	Detect infection early and treat; maintain adequate folic acid levels; acute crises – analgesia, oxygen if hypoxic, erythrocyte exchange (for priapism, stroke, acute chest syndrome) Hydroxyurea may be used to increase HbF proportional to HbS
b. Thalassaemias – beta-thalassaemia	Microcytic, target cells, tear drops	HbA$_2$ and HbF levels, globin synthesis study, gene mapping, family studies	Beta-thalassaemia major – supportive: transfusion, iron-chelating therapy, bone marrow transplant for major thalassaemic syndromes
c. Thalassaemias – alpha-thalassaemia variants; HbH disease (3-gene deletion alpha-thal)	Heinz bodies on incubation	Hb electrophoresis, brilliant cresyl blue preparation	Folic acid; avoid oxidant drugs; treat underlying disease
2. Inherited membrane abnormalities (e.g. spherocytosis)	Spherocytes	Osmotic fragility (increased) – but test is rarely performed, red cell membrane protein (5-EMA) study	Splenectomy corrects the anaemia; it should be considered when recurrent episodes of transfusion requiring anaemia occur Try to avoid during childhood owing to risks of post-splenectomy overwhelming sepsis
3. Metabolic abnormalities (e.g. G6PD deficiency)	'Bite and blister' cells, spherocytes	G6PD assay, G6PD electrophoresis	Prevent haemolytic episodes (avoid oxidant drugs, broad beans)
CLL = chronic lymphocytic leukaemia; DIC = disseminated intravascular coagulation; G6PD = glucose-6-phosphate dehydrogenase; Hb = haemoglobin; TTP = thrombotic thrombocytopenic purpura.			

6. If the haemoglobinuria usually occurs at night and there is pancytopenia and venous thrombosis, paroxysmal nocturnal haemoglobinuria (PNH) should be strongly suspected (an acquired stem cell disease secondary to a defective *PIG-A* gene). The disease may also be associated with aplastic anaemia, in which the neutrophil alkaline phosphatase score is low (but this test is now rarely performed). The most reliable test is analysis by flow cytometry for glycosylphosphatidylinositol (GPI)-linked proteins (e.g. CD55 or decay-accelerating factors (DAFs) on the red cell surface, and CD59 or homologous restriction factor). PNH, which is an acquired clonal disease, is a result of a mutation that causes faulty or absent production of the GPI anchor molecule. Various linked proteins are missing from the red cell surface and, as a result, the cells are not protected from lysis by complement. Tests for other causes of haemolysis are presented in Table 8.2.

Treatment

This depends on the underlying disease process, which should be reversed if possible (e.g. drug withdrawal, treatment of transplant rejection, adoption of another sport or musical instrument) (see Table 8.2).

1. a. Steroids are useful in immunohaemolytic anaemia caused by warm-reactive antibodies. The usual approach is to commence at a starting dose of 1 mg/kg/day of prednisolone. The haemoglobin level will usually rise within the first week. Concurrent use of folate is often recommended. Once a normal haemoglobin level has been achieved, the steroid dose must be tapered slowly. There is an 80% early remission rate, but only 20% of patients achieve long-term remission with steroids.
   b. Splenectomy works as well as steroids, and is indicated in poorly responsive or resistant disease.
   c. Immunosuppressive treatment is reserved for those who do not respond to steroids and splenectomy. Azathioprine and cyclophosphamide have each been used with some benefit. Response takes 2–3 months.
   d. Normal human immunoglobulin is often effective.
   e. There is increasing evidence of the efficacy of rituximab in very refractory cases, but AIHA remains an 'off-label' indication.
2. Transfusion is not usually indicated unless there is symptomatic anaemia with a haemoglobin level < 80 g/L as it may exacerbate haemolysis. The antibody in immunohaemolytic anaemia is likely to react with all normal donor cells so that standard cross-matching is not possible.

   Laboratory testing in such cases most often reveals a 'pan agglutinin' autoantibody. Occasionally the autoantibody has Rh antigen specificity and donor red cells lacking the antigen can be safely transfused under close observation.
3. When cold-reactive antibodies are responsible, steroid treatment is less effective. Avoidance of cold can be helpful. The disease tends to progress unless the underlying cause can be treated.
4. The chimeric antibody, rituximab, which attaches to the CD20-binding site on B lymphocytes and induces their destruction, may be useful in severe cases of resistant autoimmune haemolytic anaemia.
5. The acute haemolytic episodes of patients with G6PD deficiency are self-limiting (only older red blood cells are affected) and require no specific treatment. Hydration should be maintained to protect renal function. Patients should be warned to avoid precipitating factors (e.g. broad beans, antimalarials and sulfonamides).
6. Valve haemolysis may be improved by iron supplements and an increase in haemoglobin (reduced cardiac output). Paravalvular leaks often need to be repaired and occasionally the prosthetic valve may have to be replaced with a larger one.
7. TTP is usually treated with plasmapheresis; early treatment improves the mortality rate from almost 100% to 10%. Twice-daily treatment is combined at first with high-dose steroids. Even severe neurological deficit, including coma, may be reversible. Immunosuppression may be required in cases with autoimmune aetiology. Antiplatelet drugs are of uncertain benefit. Rituximab may be used early as immunosuppression, with cyclophosphamide and vincristine used when refractory. Relapses (10%) can usually be treated successfully. Platelet transfusions must be avoided as they exacerbate thrombosis.
8. Splenectomy is virtually curative for patients with hereditary spherocytosis and elliptocytosis (only 10% have severe haemolysis), and may be useful in selected patients with massive splenomegaly, immunohaemolytic anaemia, certain haemoglobinopathies and enzymopathies. All patients undergoing splenectomy should receive pneumococcal

Table 8.3 Treatment advice for patients having a splenectomy
1. Vaccinate for pneumococcus, *Haemophilus influenzae* type B, group C meningococcus and influenza 2–3 weeks before splenectomy if possible. Booster doses every 5 years (annually for 'flu').
2. Consider continuous prophylactic penicillin V 250 mg BD.
3. Patients should wear an alert bracelet. Overwhelming sepsis may present as obtundation and antibiotics should be given immediately.
4. Animal bites should be treated aggressively with local disinfection and systemic antibiotics.
5. Patients with possible septicaemia should have antibiotics to cover encapsulated organisms (pneumococcus, meningococcus and *H. influenzae*).

vaccine preoperatively if possible. Sometimes, prophylactic treatment with penicillin is recommended for 2 years following splenectomy (Table 8.3). Failure of splenectomy to control haemolysis may be caused by an accessory spleen (which can be detected by a liver–spleen scan).

9. PNH can be treated with washed red cell transfusions and steroids.
   a. Heparin and warfarin should be used for thrombotic episodes.
   b. Bone marrow transplant may be curative.
   c. Trials of the monoclonal antibody eculizimab, which blocks the complement cascade below C5, have shown major benefits, with a reduction in transfusion requirements and reduced incidence of thrombosis; the drug prevents the complement-driven haemolysis in PNH. The Commonwealth Department of Health has a specific eculizimab access program for Australian patients.

Possible lines of questioning

1. What tests are likely to help you most in investigating *this* patient's anaemia?
2. How would you manage *this* patient's forthcoming splenectomy?

Thrombophilia

The discovery of new thrombophilic factors has made the patient with recurrent or even a single thrombotic episode a very suitable long case. Suspect this possibility if the patient is under 50 or has a family history of recurrent thromboses (Table 8.4). Apart from those with homozygous Factor V Leiden or antithrombin deficiency, most patients with these conditions will never have a thrombotic event unless there is an associated temporary risk factor.

The history

1. Ask about the reasons for any recent admissions to hospital. There may have been a recent episode of venous or rarely arterial thrombosis, or the patient may have been admitted for a procedure that has a high risk of thrombosis. Acquired thrombophilia is more likely in patients over age 50 years.
2. Ask about the nature of thrombotic episodes. These may have been arterial or venous, or both. Find out how often the problem has occurred and what part of the body was involved.
3. Ask whether a thrombotic tendency has been identified and how this was done (the patient may know).

Table 8.4 Occurrence of and risk associated with the thrombophilic factors

	DEEP VENOUS THROMBOSIS	NORMAL POPULATION	RELATIVE RISK	ARTERIAL THROMBOSIS
APC resistance (heterozygous)	50%	4%	8 times	–
Antiphospholipid antibodies	Common	Sometimes – at low titre	8 times	+
AT III, protein C and S	10%	1%	20 times	–
Prothrombin gene mutation	15%	3%	4 times	–
High homocysteine	15%	5%	3 times	+
Factor V Leiden	20%	3%–7%	5–10 times	–
APC = activated protein C; AT = antithrombin.				

4. Ask what anticoagulation therapy is currently being used. The possibilities include:
   • unfractionated heparin
   • fractionated heparin given subcutaneously
   • low-molecular-weight heparin
   • warfarin
   • aspirin or (less likely) clopidogrel or dipyridamole
   • novel (non-vitamin-K antagonist, or direct) oral anticoagulant: NOAC (DOAC).
      In Australia, anti-Xa agents apixaban and rivaroxaban are approved for both prevention and treatment of venous thromboembolism (VTE), whereas the direct thrombin inhibitor dabigatran is approved only for VTE prevention. They are fixed-dose oral agents, compared with warfarin, and do not require routine monitoring. Adjustments are made to the dose for elderly patients and those with severe chronic kidney disease. These agents are similar to conventional therapy (enoxaparin followed by warfarin), with similar rates of recurrence of DVT or pulmonary embolism (PE) and bleeding events. Antidotes for anti-Xa and direct thrombin inhibitors are not widely available as yet. The NOACs are not recommended for patients with mechanical heart valves or malignancy-related thrombosis.

5. If the patient is or has been on treatment with warfarin, find out how much he or she understands about the drug, including the importance and necessary frequency of international normalised ratio (INR) testing and the target INR. The patient should probably know the most recent INR result and have some understanding of food and drug interactions with warfarin. For a patient on warfarin, ask about the usual frequency of blood tests and whether practical difficulties have been encountered in getting to the pathology laboratory. Ask who usually relays INR results and dosage changes to the patient, and whether the patient has ever used a home INR tester.

6. Enquire about a family history of thrombosis and whether the patient's own problem has led to the testing of other family members. In general, 50% of first-degree relatives will inherit the mutation if there is an identified autosomal dominant hereditary factor (e.g. protein C, protein S and antithrombin deficiency). Remember, a family history of thrombosis greatly increases a patient's risk. Patients with a thrombophilic defect, but without a family history of thrombosis, have only a slightly increased risk. The absence of a family history may make thrombophilia testing irrelevant, as positive tests will probably not change management.

7. Ask about other factors that may increase thrombotic risk, including smoking, oestrogen-containing oral contraceptives, pregnancy, malignancy, recent surgery and immobility. Long aeroplane flights are controversial as a risk factor, but have received extensive discussion in the popular press.

8. If the event has followed a surgical operation, ask what prophylaxis was used to try to prevent thrombosis.

9. In women, ask about previous unexplained miscarriages. This can be associated with the presence of antiphospholipid antibodies, which are autoantibodies against various platelet surface molecules, including phospholipids. These include lupus anticoagulant (which prolongs the aPTT), anticardiolipin and anti-β_2 glycoprotein antibodies. Consider this possibility too if there is a history of unusual thromboses or eclampsia and pre-eclampsia.

10. Specifically ask about previous myocardial infarction. The occurrence of myocardial infarction in young women with normal coronary arteries has been associated with factor V Leiden mutation.

11. Ask whether there have been chronic venous problems in the legs. Damage to the venous system can cause chronic oedema and ulceration that can be quite disabling (post-thrombotic syndrome). If there have been chronic problems, asking detailed questions about their effect on the patient's life is essential.

12. Ask about the congenital abnormality, homocysteinuria, which is associated with a Marfanoid habitus and premature strokes and coronary artery disease. Homocysteine is a thrombophilic agent.

13. Ask about features of PNH – recurrent episodes of dark urine, anaemia and pancytopenia.

14. Ask about malignancy – cancer is a major risk factor for the development of VTE especially in the elderly. Ask about past and family history of malignancy and previous screening tests performed. Perform a systems review to find systems that may warrant further investigations.

The examination

1. Note the presence or absence of an intravenous heparin infusion. If present, look at the infusion rate.

2. Note the presence of obesity and look for signs of venous insufficiency from previous venous thromboses.

3. Examine the legs for oedema, venous ulceration and venous valvular insufficiency.

4. Check the peripheral pulses for evidence of arterial obstruction.

5. Note the presence of abdominal wall bruising from subcutaneous low-molecular-weight heparin injections.

6. There may be evidence of a myeloproliferative disorder, SLE, nephrotic syndrome (oedema) or a malignancy.

Investigations

There is a case now for testing anyone with a significant arterial or venous thrombosis for thrombophilic factors (Tables 8.4 and 8.5), especially those with a family history of thromboembolic disease. Certainly, unusual or repeated thromboses should be investigated, as set out below. The currently available routine screening tests are listed in Table 8.6.

1. **Factor V Leiden** is an abnormal factor V molecule. The abnormality is caused by a point mutation that affects the cleavage site on the activated molecule. The abnormal factor V is resistant to neutralisation by APC, which forms part of the natural anti-coagulation pathway. The condition is also called APC resistance, along with other

Table 8.5 Indications for thrombophilia investigations

1. Recurrent venous thrombosis
2. Venous thrombosis before the age of 45
3. Thrombosis at an unusual site:
   - portal vein
   - cavernous sinus
   - hepatic vein
4. Adverse family history of venous thrombosis
5. In young women prior to commencing hormonal contraception – this is controversial

Table 8.6 Tests for thrombophilia

1. Full blood count and ESR (and tests for myeloproliferative disorders and possibly malignancy)
2. Factor V Leiden (APC resistance)
3. Antiphospholipid antibodies, including lupus anticoagulant
4. Antithrombin
5. Protein C and S (off warfarin for 2 weeks)
6. Prothrombin gene mutation
7. Plasma homocysteine
8. Occasionally PNH testing by flow cytometry
9. Occasionally factor VIII and von Willebrand factor levels

APC = activated protein C; ESR = erythrocyte sedimentation rate; PNH = paroxysmal nocturnal haemoglobinuria.

rare mutations that lead to the same functional defect. The mutation occurs in 4% of the general population in Australia and in up to 50% of people with a family history of recurrent venous thrombosis. The condition is autosomal dominant. The heterozygous state is associated with an eightfold increase in venous thrombotic risk; the homozygous state also occurs and these people have 100 times the average risk.

The thrombotic risk is higher for women with this condition because of the additional risk associated with pregnancy and the use of oral contraceptives containing oestrogen. Use of these drugs causes a 35 times increased risk of a thrombotic event (approximately a 3% risk over 10 years). The mechanism is probably that of lowering antithrombin levels.

2. **Antithrombin deficiency** is present in a mild form in about 1 in 2000 of the population. The thrombotic risk is somewhat unpredictable, but the occurrence of a first thrombotic event in these patients is a relative indication for lifelong anticoagulation therapy with warfarin.

3. **Proteins C and S** are natural anticoagulants. Their deficiency is associated with recurrent venous thrombosis and pulmonary embolism, but the level of increased risk is less clear than that for the abnormalities above. There is overlap between the serum levels in people with, and apparently those without, an increased risk of thrombosis. Testing must occur after at least 2 weeks without warfarin treatment. In homozygotes with protein C deficiency, warfarin may induce skin necrosis.

4. **Prothrombin gene mutation** is present in about 3% of the Australian population. This point mutation leads to an increased plasma level of prothrombin. Its detection requires DNA PCR analysis. It is an autosomal dominant trait and leads to a fourfold increase in the risk of venous thrombosis.

5. **Homocysteine level** is an independent risk factor for coronary artery disease and may play a role in venous thrombosis in certain patients with inherited enzyme deficiencies in homocysteine metabolism. The test for genetic mutation is available, but usually not indicated for venous thrombosis alone.

6. **Combined thrombophilic abnormalities** are relatively common and further increase the thrombotic risk.

7. **Antiphospholipid syndrome** is diagnosed if there is clinical evidence of thrombosis or a suggestive history of miscarriage plus an abnormal antiphospholipid antibody test on two occasions. *Anticardiolipin* antibodies and *lupus anticoagulant (IgG or IgM antiphospholipid)* antibodies are associated with an increased risk of venous thrombus and arterial embolus. In most cases, both are abnormal. The transient presence of these antibodies at low titres is common, is often associated with infection and is probably not of clinical significance. They may be present as part of SLE or occur alone (primary antiphospholipid syndrome).

8. Consider investigations for other diseases that are 'prothrombotic'. These include malignancy, cardiac failure, nephrotic syndrome and haematological conditions such as PNH, polycythaemia and thrombocythaemia. A limited screening for occult malignancy may be warranted.

Management

Try to identify transient and continuing risk factors.

1. In general, an initial episode of thrombosis is treated in the usual way, with low-molecular-weight heparin or intravenous non-fractionated heparin or NOACs. This should be followed by at least 6 months of anticoagulation for idiopathic above-knee DVTs or for PE, with discussion on risks and benefits of long-term anticoagulation. The use of a NOAC, which offers the convenience of a fixed dose, should be discussed. Initial treatment with heparin is not always necessary because of the rapid onset of action of these drugs; heparin is still preferred for initial therapy in certain circumstances, such as initial treatment in patients with unstable VTE such as massive PEs or in pregnancy-related VTE.

2. Patients with antithrombin deficiency will still respond to treatment with heparin because of the presence of small amounts of antithrombin III. Tests for the vitamin-K-dependent proteins C and S should be performed before the patient is begun on warfarin.

3. Patients with protein C and S deficiency or heterozygous APC resistance do not need long-term anticoagulation until after their second thrombotic event. Homozygous APC deficiency is an indication for long-term warfarin treatment.

4. All patients with thrombophilia and their affected asymptomatic relatives need aggressive prophylaxis before surgery or during periods of immobilisation. Surgical prophylactic treatment should include heparin, compressive stockings and foot pumps, and early mobilisation. Aspirin is of proven benefit for the secondary prevention of venous thrombosis. Individuals who are at risk during air travel, such as those with hereditary thrombophilia and a history of VTE, need consideration for prophylaxis (NOAC or subcutaneous fractionated heparin) if travelling for > 6 hours. They may benefit from general measures (frequent ambulation, hydration and calf exercises) as well as graduated compression stockings. Pharmacological prophylaxis needs to be individually assessed.

5. Pregnant women with a history of DVT require prophylaxis (with heparin) throughout pregnancy and until the puerperium. Warfarin and NOACs are contraindicated in pregnancy.

6. The detection of antiphospholipid antibodies in women with miscarriages is an indication for treatment with low-molecular-weight heparin with or without low-dose

aspirin during pregnancy. Patients should be advised strongly against smoking and should avoid oestrogen-containing oral contraceptives. Progesterone-only preparations appear to be safe.

7. There is still controversy about the long-term treatment of patients with antiphospholipid syndrome, but recurrent unexpected thrombosis is an indication for long-term anticoagulation with warfarin maintaining an INR between 2 and 3.

Possible lines of questioning

1. Would you recommend that *this* patient change from warfarin to a NOAC?
2. How would you advise *this* woman with a history of pulmonary embolism about the management of her pregnancy?

Polycythaemia

The myeloproliferative disorders (Table 8.7) often occur in the clinical examination. They present a diagnostic and management problem. Primary polycythaemia vera, or polycythaemia rubra vera (erythraemia or increased red cell mass), is the commonest myeloproliferative disease. It occurs in late middle life and is slightly commoner in males. Secondary causes of polycythaemia (erythrocytosis) must be excluded (Table 8.8).

The history
The patient will probably know the diagnosis. If you suspect polycythaemia, ask about:
1. symptoms of polycythaemia or polycythaemia vera:
   a. vascular problems, such as:
      - transient ischaemic episodes
      - angina
      - peripheral vascular disease (thrombosis and digital ischaemia)
      - intra-abdominal venous thrombosis, including the Budd–Chiari syndrome
   b. bleeding from the nose and bruising
   c. symptoms of peptic ulceration (increased four to five times in polycythaemia rubra vera)
   d. abdominal pain or discomfort from gross splenomegaly or urate stones
   e. pruritus after showering ('aquagenic pruritis')[1]
   f. gout

Table 8.7 **Myeloproliferative disorders**
1. Polycythaemia rubra vera
2. Myelofibrosis
3. Essential thrombocythaemia
4. Chronic myeloid leukaemia
5. Chronic eosinophilic leukaemia, chronic neutrophilic leukaemia
6. Systemic mastocytosis

---

[1] A term likely to impress the examiners

Table 8.8 Causes of polycythaemia
ABSOLUTE POLYCYTHAEMIA (INCREASED RED CELL MASS)
1. Primary – polycythaemia rubra vera (*JAK2* V617F mutation positive)
2. Secondary polycythaemia
a. increased erythropoietin:
i. renal disease (e.g. polycystic disease, hydronephrosis, tumour)
ii. hepatoma
iii. cerebellar haemangioma
iv. uterine myoma
v. virilising syndromes
vi. Cushing's syndrome
vii. phaeochromocytoma
viii. self-injection of erythropoietin (e.g. athletes)
b. hypoxic states (erythropoietin secondarily increased):
i. chronic lung disease
ii. pulmonary arteriovenous malformations
iii. sleep apnoea
iv. cyanotic congenital heart disease
v. abnormal haemoglobins (high-affinity variants)
vi. carbon monoxide poisoning
RELATIVE POLYCYTHAEMIA (DECREASED PLASMA VOLUME)
1. Dehydration
2. Smokers' polycythaemia – carboxyhaemoglobinaemia (erythrocyte mass also increased)
3. Stress polycythaemia

   g. symptoms of hyperviscosity:
- fatigue
- dizziness
- headache
- syncope
- difficulty concentrating

2. symptoms of a disease causing secondary polycythaemia (see Table 8.8), such as:
  a. chronic respiratory diseases
  b. sleep disorders and obstructive sleep apnoea (OSA)
  c. chronic cardiac or congenital heart diseases
  d. renal diseases (especially polycystic kidneys, hydronephrosis or erythropoietin secretion from a tumour including renal cell cancer and hepatic cell cancer)
  e. the use of coal tar derivatives, which can cause the production of abnormal haemoglobin such as methaemoglobin, as secondary polycythaemia may occur as a result of methaemoglinaemia

3. investigations performed and how the diagnosis was made, e.g.:
  a. blood counts
  b. abdominal imaging
  c. renal, pulmonary and cardiac investigations
  d. whether the erythropoietin level and JAK2 kinase mutation have been measured

4. the treatment initiated (e.g. phlebotomy – how often and for how long; radioactive phosphorus; treatment of renal, pulmonary or cardiac disease)
5. resolution of symptoms with treatment
6. social problems related to chronic disease.

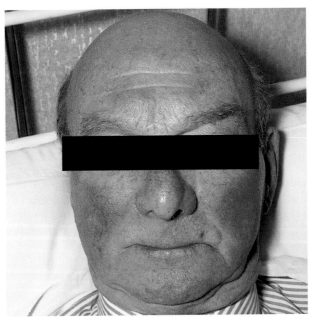

Figure 8.1 This face is a diagnostic clue for polycythaemia vera. Patients are frequently plethoric and may have rosacea.

M R Howard, *Haematology: an illustrated colour text*, 32:64–5, Elsevier, 2013, with permission.

The examination

1. Stand back and look at the patient. Note plethora (Fig. 8.1), the state of hydration, cyanosis and any Cushingoid features.
2. Examine the patient's hands for nicotine stains, clubbing and signs of peripheral vascular disease. Note any gouty tophi.
3. Look for scratch marks and bruising on the arms and take the blood pressure (systolic hypertension accompanies an increased red cell mass and phaeochromocytoma is associated with increased erythropoietin).
4. Look at the eyes for injected conjunctivae and examine the fundi for hyperviscosity changes.
5. Examine the tongue for central cyanosis.
6. Examine the cardiovascular system for signs of cyanotic congenital heart disease, if appropriate, and the respiratory system for signs of chronic lung disease.
7. Examine the abdomen for hepatomegaly (hepatoma must be excluded) and more importantly splenomegaly, which occurs in 80% of cases of polycythaemia rubra vera, but not in secondary polycythaemia. Palpate for renal masses (polycystic kidneys, hydronephrosis, carcinoma). Rarely, uterine fibromas may be found, or very rarely virilisation may be noted.
8. Look at the legs for scratch marks (pruritus may be secondary to elevated plasma histamine levels), gout and evidence of peripheral vascular disease.
9. Auscultate over the cerebellar regions for a bruit (cerebellar haemangioblastoma). Note any upper motor neurone signs (cerebrovascular disease due to thrombosis or the hyperviscosity syndrome).
10. Check the urine for evidence of renal disease.

Table 8.9 An approach to the diagnosis of polycythaemia vera
1. *JAK2* mutation present (up to 95% of cases)
2. Splenomegaly
3. Normal *PaO₂*
4. Splenomegaly, or leukocytosis and thrombocytosis
5. Low or normal erythropoietin level
6. Rule out secondary causes (e.g. smoking, chronic lung disease, tumours)

Investigations

Confirm the presence of polycythaemia (haematocrit > 60% for men or > 56% for women) and establish whether this is primary or secondary. Remember that erythrocytosis is an increase in the absolute red cell mass, which occurs as a result of some stimulus (usually hypoxia), and erythraemia (polycythaemia vera) is an increase in red cell mass of unknown aetiology (Table 8.9).

Note: Red cell mass and plasma volume are no longer routinely measured.

1. In polycythaemia vera the following are increased:
   a. haemoglobin value
   b. haematocrit value
   c. red cell count, white cell count (including the absolute basophil count)
   d. platelet count and more variably the neutrophil alkaline phosphatase (NAP) score. Check the mean corpuscular volume and red cell distribution width (RDW). Microcytic erythrocytosis can be caused only by polycythaemia vera or hypoxic erythrocytosis (RDW usually elevated), or haemoglobinopathies (RDW normal).
2. The ESR is very low in both primary and secondary polycythaemia.
3. Assess for splenomegaly (and renal disease) with an abdominal ultrasound or CT scan.
4. Check the arterial blood gases (in polycythaemia vera, 80% of patients have an arterial oxygen saturation > 92% and in almost all it is > 88%).
5. Serum erythropoietin level is usually substantially reduced or absent in polycythaemia vera and elevated in secondary polycythaemia. Remember, however, that certain tumours (haemangioblastoma, renal cell carcinoma, renal sarcoma and carcinoma of the liver) cause polycythaemia by excreting erythropoietin.
6. The total vitamin B_{12} level is elevated in 75% of cases of polycythaemia vera. The vitamin B_{12} level is raised owing to increased transcobalamin I and III, made by neutrophils which have an increased turnover.
7. Rule out renal disease, if indicated.
8. In polycythaemia vera there is significant panhyperplasia and iron stores are often reduced, but in secondary polycythaemia the bone marrow usually shows only an erythroid hyperplasia. There are no consistent cytogenetic markers. Bone marrow biopsy is not essential for the diagnosis: it is necessary only if another myeloproliferative disorder is suspected. Fibrosis may be seen in the advanced stages of polycythaemia vera.
9. Genetic testing is very useful. The *JAK2* mutation is present in most patients with polycythaemia vera.

Treatment

1. The aim is to lower the haematocrit value to < 0.42 in women and < 0.45 in men and maintain it at this level. Patients may die of thrombosis, which seems related entirely to the elevated red cell mass. Thrombotic risk can usually be reduced with

phlebotomy alone, but aspirin is usually thought to give additional protection. Untreated cases have a median survival of 2 years because of the thrombotic risk. This is extended to more than 10 years with phlebotomy alone.

Polycythaemia rubra vera should be treated by phlebotomy.

Frequent venesection is required until a state of iron deficiency has been produced. This will then limit red cell production and the frequency may be reduced.

In patients at high risk for thrombosis (i.e. age > 60 years, prior thrombosis), venesection should be supplemented with a myelosuppressive agent. Hydroxyurea is usually first line but it increases the risk of leukaemia; interferon alpha (IFN-α) may be a safer option in high-risk women of child-bearing age or a JAK2 inhibitor (ruxolitinib) in the setting of major constitutional symptoms.

2. Radioactive phosphorus (phosphorus-32) irradiates the bone marrow and was easy to use and effective, but it increases the incidence of acute myeloid leukaemia and is no longer available.

3. Alkylating agents (e.g. busulfan) must be monitored closely for the same reason and should not be given routinely. Both P32 and busulfan substantially increase the risk of secondary acute leukaemia (6–10 fold).

4. Pruritus may not respond to antihistamines, and IFN-α or psoralen with ultraviolet light (PUVA) therapy may be required.

5. Hyperuricaemia should be treated with allopurinol.

6. IFN-α may help reduce the problem of symptomatic splenomegaly.

7. Secondary polycythaemia is treated by removal of the cause. Consider phlebotomy if the haematocrit exceeds 0.55 or there is a high thrombotic risk, or a high degree of hyperviscosity symptoms.

Median survival is more than 10 years for treated patients

Possible line of questioning

What would you tell *this* patient about the likely course of his or her polycythaemia?

Idiopathic myelofibrosis

This is a rare form of chronic myeloproliferative clonal disorder. Patients are often asymptomatic at the time of diagnosis. The condition is frequently diagnosed following a routine full blood count or the discovery of splenomegaly. Some patients present with tiredness, night sweats and weight loss. Occasionally a painful splenic infarct may be the presenting symptom. Myelofibrosis may also be the result of a number of malignant and non-malignant conditions (Table 8.10).

Median survival is 4–5 years, but patients with severe anaemia (< 100 g/L), and those of older age, with constitutional symptoms or leukocytosis have a worse prognosis (median survival about 2 years).

The examination
There may be occasional signs of aggressive extramedullary haematopoiesis, e.g.:
- bowel or urethral obstruction
- ascites
- pericardial effusion

Table 8.10 Causes of myelofibrosis	
NON-MALIGNANT	**MALIGNANT**
1. Systemic lupus erythematosus 2. HIV infection 3. Renal osteodystrophy 4. Tuberculosis 5. Hyperparathyroidism	1. Chronic myeloid leukaemia (CML) and other myeloproliferative disorders 2. Acute leukaemia 3. Lymphoma (Hodgkin and non-Hodgkin) 4. Multiple myeloma 5. Metastatic carcinoma

- skin masses
- spinal cord compression.

Rapid splenic enlargement can cause splenic infarction (with the sudden onset of left upper quadrant pain and tenderness). The typical patient is over 50 years of age and has marked splenomegaly (> 10 cm) and mild-to-moderate hepatomegaly.

Investigations

1. The white cell counts may be normal, increased or decreased. The blood film will show teardrop poikilocytes and a leukoerythroblastic picture (i.e. presence of myelocytes, metamyelocytes and nucleated red blood cells). Any process that infiltrates the bone marrow may cause this picture (e.g. malignancy, TB, fungi).
2. Bone marrow biopsy (aspiration is usually impossible) may reveal karyotypic abnormalities on cytogenetic examination. This finding is associated with a worse prognosis. The *JAK2* V617F mutation is seen in up to 50% of cases.
3. The condition must be distinguished from myelofibrosis secondary to other conditions that may be amenable to specific treatment, such as:
   - lymphoma
   - leukaemia
   - myeloma
   - polycythaemia
   - chronic myeloid leukaemia (CML)
   - systemic lupus erythematosus.

Treatment

Treatment is primarily supportive. Most patients are treated with repeated blood transfusions.

1. Hydroxyurea is helpful for symptomatic patients with organomegaly or marked thrombocytosis.
2. Folate and vitamin B_{12} may help if these are deficient; erythropoietin has not been particularly effective. Allopurinol is used when there is hyperuricaemia.
3. Splenectomy may be indicated if massive splenomegaly has occurred.
4. Alkylating agents are contraindicated.
5. Cure is possible only with allogenic bone marrow transplantation for the few patients who are young enough and for whom a suitable donor can be found.
6. Leukaemic transformation may occur in 10% of patients.
7. The JAK2 kinase inhibitor ruxolitinib is effective at ameliorating the natural history and reducing splenic volume; the effect is seen even in those patients who do not harbour the *JAK2* mutation.

Possible lines of questioning

1. Would you consider any other diagnosis as a possible cause of *this* patient's myelofibrosis?
2. How would you discuss the prognosis with him or her?

Essential thrombocythaemia

This is a relatively common form of chronic myeloproliferative clonal disorder. Many patients are asymptomatic and the diagnosis is made on a routine platelet count.

Patients may present with symptoms related to a high platelet count ($> 800 \times 10^9/L$; some patients with even higher counts are 'platelet millionaires') – especially thrombo-embolism, but also poor memory, erythromelalgia (painful, red extremities) and migraine. Patients may have haemorrhagic problems, especially from the gut, and easy bruising due to abnormal platelet aggregation at very high platelet counts. An acquired deficiency of von Willebrand factor (VWF) may occur when platelet numbers are very high. This may be due to increased numbers of circulating platelets resulting in increased binding and removal of large VWF multimers from plasma.

Modest splenomegaly (< 5 cm) is seen in 50% of patients.

Investigations

1. A definitive diagnosis requires exclusion of reactive thrombocytosis secondary to infection, polycythaemia, malignancy, inflammation, bleeding, recent surgery or an asplenic state.
2. Cytogenetic studies may be necessary to exclude CML (Philadelphia (Ph) chromosome t(9;22) or its products: BCR–ABL fusion mRNA or BCR–ABL protein).
3. The *JAK 2* V617F mutation is seen in 50% of cases.

Treatment

1. Asymptomatic patients, even if they have a platelet count of more than one million, often need no treatment. Unexpectedly, bleeding tends to be more of a problem when the platelet count is over one million and thrombosis when it is less than one million.
2. Neurological symptoms and erythromelalgia should first be treated with aspirin. Failure of response is an indication to reduce platelet numbers, usually with hydroxyurea or IFN-α. Anagrelide is a more specific antimegakaryocyte agent that can be useful for symptomatic patients, but hydroxyurea and aspirin may be more effective in preventing vascular events.
3. Transformation to acute leukaemia is uncommon ($< 10\%$) and often the result of prior alkylating chemotherapy.
4. The condition usually runs an indolent and benign course and the continuing temptation to treat asymptomatic patients should be strongly resisted. A small percentage of cases transform to acute leukaemia or myelofibrosis.

Possible line of questioning

Does *this* patient with thrombocythaemia require treatment?

NOTES ON HAEMATOLOGICAL MALIGNANCIES

1. Survival has improved, e.g.:
   - Hodgkin's long-term survival – 85%
   - childhood acute lymphocytic leukaemia (ALL) – 78%
   - diffuse large cell lymphoma treated with rituximab and chemotherapy – 60%.
2. Many treated patients may have late effects of treatment:
   - secondary malignancies: acute myeloid leukaemia (AML), breast cancer, skin malignancies
   - osteoporosis
   - cardiac disease: early coronary disease, left ventricular dysfunction – anthracyclines
   - neurocognitive defects
   - pulmonary disease: interstitial lung disease, bronchiolitis obliterans (cryptogenic organising pneumonia)
   - endocrine disease: early menopause, infertility – ask about ovum or sperm harvesting and storage. Patients may be on hormone replacement treatment (men and women).

Chronic myeloid leukaemia

Many patients with CML are diagnosed from routine blood tests – symptoms tend not to be specific (Table 8.11). Patients are between 30 and 80 years old with a peak incidence at 55. It is rare, but accounts for about 20% of leukaemias.

Investigations

1. Patients may have moderate splenomegaly (6–8 cm) and a white cell count > 50 × 10^9/L. The white cell differential count will show two peaks: one at the neutrophil stage and the other at the myelocyte stage.
2. Basophilia and eosinophilia are common.
3. In the blast phase over 20% of white cells are blasts.
4. Diagnosis depends on finding the Ph chromosome (> 90%) – a shortened chromosome 22. Translocation of part of chromosome 22 to chromosome 9 results in a hybrid gene *BCR–ABL* rearrangement on chromosome 9. This *BCR–ABL* fusion gene is an oncogene coding for a protein with tyrosine kinase activity which affects cell proliferation, differentiation and survival.

Table 8.11 CML symptoms
SYMPTOMS AT PRESENTATION
1. Fatigue
2. Malaise
3. Loss of weight
4. Abdominal discomfort and fullness from splenomegaly
5. Infection
6. Thrombotic episodes (e.g. stroke, myocardial infarction, venous thrombosis)
SYMPTOMS OF PROGRESSION OF DISEASE
1. Fever
2. Infections
3. Bone pain
4. Joint pain
5. Haemorrhage or thrombosis

5. The platelet count is usually elevated and there is mild normochromic anaemia.
6. There is no association with alkylating agents and no evidence of a viral cause.

Treatment

Untreated, the disease will eventually undergo blastic transformation.

1. A cure or long-term remission can be achieved with allogenic bone marrow transplantation from a compatible donor in those who fail to respond or are intolerant of tyrosine kinase inhibitor therapy (see below).
2. Imatinib (a tyrosine kinase inhibitor – TKI) has revolutionised treatment of CML. This drug causes apoptosis of cells expressing *BCR–ABL*. It is now the first-line treatment for all patients. Its use can be associated with:
   * hepatotoxicity
   * myalgia
   * fluid retention.

   The therapeutic target of all TKI treatment is the achievement of a major molecular response, which is defined as a ≥ 3 log reduction of the baseline quantitative *BCR–ABL* assay, preferably before 12 months from the point of commencing treatment (i.e. ≤ 0.1% *BCR–ABL* transcript to housekeeping genes is a major response; non-detectable on two consecutive samples is a complete response). Some patients will develop mutations in the *BCR–ABL* transcript that confer resistance to imatinib. Second-generation TKIs, dasatinib and nilotinib, are available and are active in these cases – they are also available as first-line therapy. The choice of the agent in first-line therapy is dependent on matching the side-effect profile with co-morbidity. It is possible to switch between agents if there is a suboptimal molecular response. Side-effects include oedema, GI intolerance and rash (imatinib); pleural effusion (dasatinib); and increased risk of vascular complications (nilotinib).
3. IFN-α therapy is sometimes helpful in the chronic phase. It may induce differentiation of the immature cells and be synergistic with imatinib in achieving a major molecular response.

Possible line of questioning

How would you discuss the treatment options and side-effects with *this* patient with newly diagnosed CML?

Lymphomas

These diseases provide complicated diagnostic and management problems. Treatment in expert units is important, because many patients can be cured. Cure should be possible in more than 85% of patients with Hodgkin disease and in up to 40% of those with non-Hodgkin lymphomas.

Remember that the cell lineage is uncertain for Hodgkin disease (although probably mostly B cell), but 80% of non-Hodgkin lymphomas in Australia are of B cell origin. There are a number of slightly different classification systems. Some are based on the cell type (Table 8.12), some on histopathology (Table 8.13) and others on clinical staging (Table 8.14).

Note: Fortunately only four types of lymphoma are common: diffuse large cell and follicular cell in people over 40, Hodgkin's lymphoma in people under 40 and small lymphocytic lymphoma (SLL) / chronic lymphocytic leukaemia (CLL) in the elderly.

Table 8.12 World Health Organization classification of lymphomas (lymphoid malignancies) – more common types		
B CELL	**T CELL**	**HODGKIN'S DISEASE**
Precursor B cell neoplasm	**Precursor T cell neoplasm**	**Nodular lymphocyte predominant**
Precursor B cell lymphoblastic leukaemia / lymphoma	Precursor T cell lymphoblastic lymphoma / leukaemia	
Mature (peripheral) B cell neoplasms	**Mature (peripheral) T cell neoplasms**	**Classic Hodgkin disease**
B cell chronic lymphocytic leukaemia / small lymphocytic lymphoma	Adult T cell lymphoma / leukaemia	Nodular sclerosis Hodgkin disease
Plasma cell myeloma / plasmacytoma	Mycosis fungoides	Lymphocyte-rich Hodgkin disease
MALT lymphoma, mantle cell lymphoma	Peripheral T cell lymphoma	Mixed cellularity Hodgkin disease
Follicular lymphoma	Angioimmunoblastic T cell lymphoma	Lymphocyte-depleted Hodgkin disease
Diffuse large B cell lymphoma	Anaplastic large cell lymphoma	
Burkitt lymphoma		
Note: There is an overlap of cell types between leukaemias and lymphomas. Leukaemia is diagnosed when the malignant cells are primarily found in the blood and bone marrow, and lymphoma when there are solid tumours of the immune system.		
MALT = mucosa-associated lymphoid tissue.		

Hodgkin lymphoma (see Table 8.13) presents either with discrete, rubbery, painless nodes or with generalised symptoms (fever, night sweats, weight loss and sometimes pruritus). Mediastinal adenopathy usually occurs in young people with nodular sclerosing disease. Older people with generalised symptoms, in whom the only enlarged nodes may be in the abdomen, often have lymphocyte-depleted Hodgkin disease.

The majority of cases of non-Hodgkin lymphomas (see Table 8.13) present with painless enlargement of peripheral lymph nodes (a lymph node of > 1 cm diameter that has been present for 6 weeks or more for no obvious reason should be biopsied). The great majority of patients with peripheral lymph node enlargement do not have a malignancy. Localised or generalised painless adenopathy with or without hepatosplenomegaly may also occur. It may present with just an abdominal mass. Presentation with mediastinal adenopathy is much less common than in patients with Hodgkin disease (except in T lymphoblastic lymphoma and primary mediastinal B large cell lymphoma where mediastinal disease is always present). In some patients the disease may arise at an extranodal site (e.g. the gastrointestinal tract – 5%). These patients may present with abdominal pain, obstruction or haemorrhage.

Waldeyer's ring, mesenteric and epitrochlear node involvement are more common in non-Hodgkin than in Hodgkin disease. In low-grade non-Hodgkin lymphoma, lymphadenopathy has often been present for a long time.

Other uncommon presentations include skin infiltration and direct renal infiltration. Primary neurological infiltration is also uncommon. Low-grade gastrointestinal lymphomas (e.g. mucosa-associated lymphoid tissue (MALT) lymphomas) are less common.

Table 8.13 Histopathological classification of lymphoma

HODGKIN LYMPHOMA

1. Lymphocyte predominant (5%)
2. Classical Hodgkin lymphoma (95%) – subtypes:
   - nodular sclerosing (70%),
   - mixed cellularity (20%),
   - lymphocyte rich (5%),
   - lymphocyte depleted (rare)

NON-HODGKIN LYMPHOMA

The Rappaport classification has largely been replaced. There are a number of new classifications, including the International Working Formulation (this classification translates into the clinical setting better than the others).

International working formulation

I. Low-grade lymphoma
   1. Small lymphocytic cell
   2. Follicular, mixed cleaved cell
   3. Follicular, mixed small cleaved and large cell
II. Intermediate-grade lymphoma
   1. Follicular large cell
   2. Diffuse small cleaved cell
   3. Diffuse mixed small cleaved cell
   4. Diffuse large cell
III. High-grade lymphoma
   1. Large cell immunoblastic
   2. Lymphoblastic cell
   3. Small non-cleaved cell (Burkitt and non-Burkitt)

Table 8.14 Staging of lymphoma – Ann Arbor classification

STAGE I	Disease confined to a single lymph node region or a single extralymphatic site (Ie)
STAGE II	Disease confined to two or more lymph node regions on the same side of the diaphragm, plus or minus splenic involvement
STAGE III	Disease confined to lymph node regions on both sides of the diaphragm (III1 = upper abdomen; III2 = lower abdomen), with or without localised involvement of the spleen (IIIs), other extralymphatic organ or site (IIIe), or both
STAGE IV	Diffuse disease of one or more extralymphatic organs (with or without lymph node disease)

For any stage:

a. no symptoms

b. fever, weight loss > 10% in 6 months or night sweats.

The history

1. Ask about the presenting symptoms and causes of symptoms, such as palpable nodes, cough as a result of mediastinal node involvement, systemic symptoms, bone pain due to marrow infiltration or pathological fractures, spinal cord compression, splenic pain and alcohol-induced pain (rare).
2. Is there a history of infection (as a result of decreased cell-mediated immunity in Hodgkin disease or depressed humoral immunity from chemotherapy or radiotherapy)?

3. Ask about the history of the predisposing condition, such as Klinefelter's syndrome, HIV infection, congenital or acquired immune deficiency, use of immunosuppressive drugs or autoimmune disease (e.g. Sjögren's syndrome). Ask also about the use of phenytoin (pseudo-lymphoma).

4. Find out the investigations performed – particularly lymph node biopsy and PET or CT scans. MRI scanning may have been used for suspected spinal cord, brain or bone marrow involvement. Lymphangiography and staging laparotomy are now rarely indicated. Lumbar puncture is important in high-grade lymphoma investigation if central nervous system involvement is suspected. PET scans are replacing other modalities for staging and bone marrow biopsy for staging is required only in certain lymphomas (usually NHL).

5. Ask about the treatment undertaken, as this gives an indication of the stage and type of disease. Ask about the side-effects of any treatment; for example, a radiation field such as mantle radiation can result in:
   - pneumonitis
   - hypothyroidism
   - pericarditis
   - myocardial fibrosis
   - spinal cord injury.
   Ask whether the patient has been informed about possible long-term complications of treatment.

6. Determine the prognosis given and what the patient's understanding of this seems to be.

7. Find out about the patient's social situation – dependent family members, social support, ability to work, reactions to disease (e.g. depression, coping mechanisms), etc. As for other malignancies, work out the Eastern Co-operative Oncology Group (ECOG) performance status (Table 8.15).

The examination

1. Examine the haemopoietic system thoroughly. Particularly note any lymph nodes (Fig. 8.2) and assess carefully for splenomegaly.

2. Attempt to stage the disease clinically (see Table 8.14). Remember that staging is much less relevant for non-Hodgkin lymphomas because spread is haematogenous and not contiguous. Fewer than 10% of even nodular non-Hodgkin lymphomas are localised and suitable for local irradiation at the time of presentation.

3. Note any radiotherapy marks (and the field covered).

4. Look for evidence of infection (e.g. herpes zoster).

Table 8.15 ECOG performance status	
GRADE	**ECOG PERFORMANCE STATUS**
0	Fully active; no restriction on activities compared with before the disease
1	Restricted, but only from strenuous activity. Able to perform light or sedentary work
2	Able to look after self; mobile but not able to work
3	Only partly able to look after self; in bed or chair for more than 50% of waking hours
4	Completely confined to bed or chair; unable to look after self at all

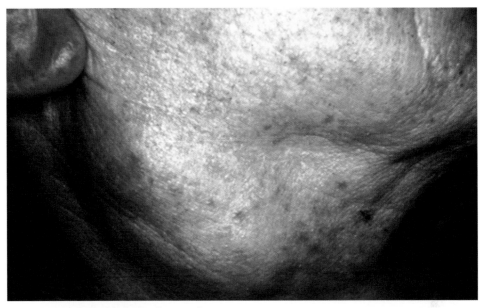

Figure 8.2 **Cervical lymphadenopathy.**

J W Little, D A Falace, C S Miller, N L Rhodus, *Dental management of the medically compromised patient*, 7th edn. Fig 24-6. Mosby, Elsevier, 2008, with permission.

5. If the patient is clinically anaemic, consider a Coombs' positive autoimmune process in your differential.
6. Assess for any evidence of the hyperviscosity syndrome (Waldenström's macroglobulinaemia secondary to a monoclonal gammaglobulin); look in the fundi.

Investigations

Investigations are aimed at determining the grade and stage of the disease.

1. The first step is to obtain histological confirmation of disease. Ask to see the pathology report if excision lymph node biopsies have already been performed. Fine-needle biopsy is not good enough to define lymph node architecture. Reed–Sternberg cells are *not* pathognomonic of Hodgkin disease, but may occur in cases of glandular fever, other viral diseases and with other malignancies.
2. The next step is to stage the disease further.
   a. Ask for:
      • LDH
      • neck, abdominal, pelvic and chest imaging – usually a PET or CT scan (but do look at the chest X-ray (Fig. 8.3) as it may provide some initial evidence for hilar adenopathy).
   b. A bone marrow biopsy is often indicated for NHL patients.
   c. If there is a major leukaemic component, order flow cytometry of the peripheral lymphocytes to aid in the diagnosis.
3. a. In Hodgkin disease there may be:
      • agranulocytosis (sometimes with marked eosinophilia or a leukemoid reaction)
      • an elevated ESR
      • a reversed CD4:CD8 ratio.

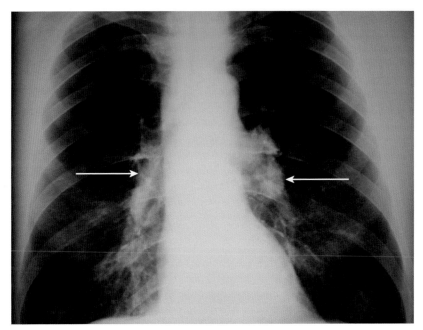

Figure 8.3 **Chest X-ray showing bilateral hilar lymphadenopathy (arrows).**
Figure reproduced courtesy of The Canberra Hospital.

b. PET scanning is more sensitive than gallium scanning in staging the disease at diagnosis and in monitoring residual disease – a combined PET/CT scan is currently widely available and is used for staging lymphomas.

c. Staging laparotomies are now only rarely performed, but previously treated patients may bear the scar. Staging in this invasive way is less relevant now that systemic treatment is more often used for all patients. Always re-stage after treatment.

Treatment

HODGKIN LYMPHOMA (85% OF PATIENTS ARE CURABLE)

Treatment depends on the stage of the disease (see Table 8.14) and presence of risk factors. Histological type is less important.

- Stages I, IIA and IIB – radiotherapy or abbreviated course of chemotherapy followed by radiotherapy (20 Gy to affected sites).
- Stages III and IV – full course of standard chemotherapy (e.g. ABVD – adriamycin, bleomycin, vinblastine and dacarbazine) or escalated chemotherapy. Consolidation radiotherapy may be considered in those with bulky disease (up to 30 Gy).

Salvage treatment

Relapse less than 1 year after initial treatment or failure to achieve complete remission is an indication for second-line therapy. For relapse after more than 1 year, retreatment can be given using the original regimen. Further radiotherapy can be used for relapse outside the radiation field if the patient has early-stage disease. Autologous stem cell transplant after high-dose chemotherapy is an alternative.

Table 8.16 Routine annual tests for patients treated for Hodgkin lymphoma
1. Thyroid function tests (TFTs) and clinical examination of the thyroid
2. Full blood count – looking for leukaemia and myelodysplastic syndromes (maximum risk at 3–12 years)
3. Mammography and breast examination – increased risk of breast cancer from 10 years after treatment

Brentuximab vedotin is an antibody–drug conjugate directed against CD30 on the Reed–Sternberg cell. It can produce good responses for patients who have failed standard treatment and may be a bridge to allogenic transplant.

Prognosis

This depends on the stage, disease bulk, age and performance status. In general, in:
- stage I, expect 85%–95% 10 years disease-free survival
- stage II, expect 80%–90% 10 years disease-free survival
- stages III and IV, expect 60% 10 years disease-free survival.

Complications of treatment

1. The improvement in survival achieved with current treatment means that complications of treatment are more likely to cause death in long-term survivors. Routine annual testing and review are recommended (Table 8.16).
2. Secondary malignancies, including leukaemia and carcinomas, are associated with the use of alkylating agents.
3. Breast cancer risk is associated with chest irradiation.
4. Chest radiotherapy also increases the risk of coronary artery disease after 10 years or more, and of hypothyroidism.
5. Radiotherapy and chemotherapy increase the risk of carcinoma of the lung, which is significantly greater again for smokers.
6. Infertility can occur in men and women treated with chemotherapy. The chance of recovery of fertility is much greater for young patients. Sperm or ovarian tissue banking and fertility preservation may be offered to patients.

NON-HODGKIN LYMPHOMA

Prognosis and treatment depend mainly on the histological type (particularly whether it is nodular or diffuse and based on the International Working Formulation – see Table 8.13); most cases (80%) of low-grade lymphomas are stage III or IV at presentation and require only observation if the patient is asymptomatic (Table 8.17). Symptoms suggesting a need for treatment include:
- systemic symptoms (weight loss, malaise, etc.)
- bulky, uncomfortable lymph nodes
- bone marrow failure
- compression symptoms.

The International Prognostic Index (Table 8.18) has proved a useful way of assessing the patient's likely course. More recently, treatment decisions have been based on the WHO classification (see Table 8.12).

Treatment protocols: WHO classification

1. **Precursor B cell neoplasms:** precursor B cell lymphoblastic leukaemia / lymphoma is usually the childhood malignancy acute lymphocytic leukaemia. The lymphoma is rare in adults and rapidly progresses to become leukaemia. Combination chemotherapy

Table 8.17 Recommendations for screening of NHL survivors

CANCER – PATIENTS SHOULD BE ADVISED OF THEIR RISK
1. Breast cancer – from age of 40 or if chest was irradiated 8 years after irradiation:
  • annual mammogram
  • consider annual MRI if radiation treatment was given between the ages of 10 and 35
  • consider referral for chemoprevention
2. Lung cancer:
  • smoking cessation
3. Skin cancer:
  • annual complete skin examination
  • sun screen

CARDIOVASCULAR HEALTH 1. Referral to cardiologist for evaluation after treatment 2. Resting and stress echocardiograms; frequency depending on risk factors 3. Risk factor control
ENDOCRINE 1. Infertility – refer to reproductive endocrinologist 2. Hypothyroidism – annual thyroid examination and thyroid function tests if treatment included neck irradiation
NEUROLOGICAL AND PSYCHIATRIC EVALUATION 1. Annual review to include assessment of psychiatric health including problems with depression 2. Screening for neurocognitive impairment if cranial irradiation or intrathecal therapy was received
NHL = non-Hodgkin lymphoma.

Table 8.18 International Prognostic Index – clinical risk factors for a poor outcome
1. Age > 60 2. Lactate dehydrogenase (LDH) level elevated 3. Ann Arbor stage III or IV 4. > 1 extranodal site 5. Physical performance, e.g. Karnosky score > 70 (self-caring, mobile, etc.)
• 0–1 risk factors = low risk • 2 risk factors = low-to-intermediate risk • 3 risk factors = intermediate-to-high risk • 4–5 risk factors = high risk

is used to induce remission and continuing treatment to attempt cure. The cure rate in adults is about 50%.

2. **Mature B cell neoplasms:** B cell CLL/SLL is the most common lymphoid leukaemia and represents about 75% of non-Hodgkin lymphomas. Patients with only bone marrow involvement and lymphocytosis are not usually treated. They have a median survival of more than 10 years. Once liver and splenic involvement have occurred, treatment is likely to be required at some stage, but may not be recommended until bone marrow failure is present. Oral chlorambucil or the more potent intravenous drug fludarabine, often combined with rituximab, is most often recommended. Young

patients may benefit from bone marrow transplant. Newer CD20 antibodies such as ofatumumab and obinutuzumab may be used in combination with chlorambucil in first-line therapy for the elderly or patients with multiple co-morbidities. Ibrutinib, a Bruton's tyrosine kinase inhibitor that works through the B cell receptor signalling pathways, may be used for relapsed disease. Side-effects of ibrutinib include platelet dysfunction resulting in an increased bleeding risk and increased risk of atrial fibrillation. Idelalisib, an oral inhibitor of the PI3K signalling pathway, is also used in relapsed CLL. Side-effects include colitis and pneumonitis.

3. **MALT-type lymphoma (extranodal marginal zone B cell lymphoma) (8%):** these gastric mucosal lymphomas are curable when localised. MALT is associated with *Helicobacter pylori* infection. Eradication of the infection will usually induce remission (75%). Otherwise, radiation treatment is used and, for more widespread or resistant disease, rituximab-based therapy may be used. Endoscopic follow-up is important. Splenic marginal zone lymphoma (SMZL) may follow hepatitis C infection, which should be treated; if symptomatic without hepatitis C, rituximab or splenectomy can induce a long remission.

4. **Mantle cell lymphoma (6%):** the majority of these present as a systemic disease. Treatment is not very successful. The usual approach is combination chemotherapy followed by radiotherapy. Chemotherapy may be used with rituximab (the anti-CD20 antibody). Bone marrow transplant is offered to younger patients.

5. **Follicular lymphoma (22%):** asymptomatic patients may require no treatment. Combination treatment (rituximab, cyclophosphamide, vincristine and prednisone (RCVP) or rituximab, cyclophosphamide, hydroxydaunorubicin (doxorubicin), oncovin (vincristine) and prednisone (R-CHOP)) can achieve a 75% remission rate. Maintenance rituximab treatment continued for up to 2 years is helpful to improve progression-free survival. Relapses are common and retreatment with multiple chemotherapy regimens is the usual clinical course. Between 5% and 7% of patients per year develop histological transformation into diffuse large B cell lymphoma. Follicular lymphoma (low-grade) prognosis can be further estimated from Table 8.19.

6. **Diffuse large B cell lymphoma (30%):** treatment is usually begun with combination chemotherapy (often R-CHOP). This may be followed by radiotherapy if there is bulky stage I or stage II disease. Six cycles of treatment will produce a cure in up to 70% of patients. Monoclonal antibody treatment with rituximab is used for most patients. Bone marrow transplant is more effective than further chemotherapy for

Table 8.19 Follicular lymphoma survival rates

RISK FACTORS
1. Age > 60 years
2. Haemoglobin < 12 g/dL
3. Ann Arbor stage III or IV disease
4. > 4 lymph nodes or other sites of disease
5. Increased lactate dehydrogenase (LDH)

NUMBER OF RISK FACTORS	5-YEAR SURVIVAL (%)	10-YEAR SURVIVAL (%)
0–1 (36% of patients)	91	71
2 (37% of patients)	78	51
≥ 3 (27% of patients)	53	27

Table 8.20 Cure rates and 5-year survival rates for diffuse large B cell lymphoma based on the International Prognostic Index

PRE-TREATMENT CHARACTERISTICS (RISK FACTORS)
1. Age > 60
2. Stage III or IV
3. > 1 extranodal site involved
4. ECOG status $\geq$ 2
5. Serum LDH normal

NUMBER OF RISK FACTORS	CURE RATE (%)	5-YEAR SURVIVAL (%)
0–1 (35% of patients)	87	73
2 (27%)	66	51
3 (22%)	53	27

patients who relapse: it can achieve up to 40% long-term disease-free survival. The International Prognostic Index (IPI), which is based on five pretreatment characteristics (see Table 8.20), predicts survival.

7. **Burkitt lymphoma:** this is a rare disease in Australia, but is more common in Africa. Intensive combination chemotherapy with attention to the central nervous system will produce a cure in about 70% of patients.
8. **Hairy cell leukaemia:** this is an indolent lymphoma with leukaemic features. The peripheral smear shows lymphocytes with hairy projections. Look for splenomegaly and cytopenia. It responds well to chemotherapy with cladribine.
9. **Immunodeficiency-associated lymphoma:** the WHO classifies these lymphomas into four groups:
   a. lymphoproliferative diseases associated with primary immune disorders
   b. HIV-associated lymphomas
   c. post-transplant lymphomas
   d. methotrexate-associated lymphoproliferative disorders.

These are usually aggressive B cell, CNS and Hodgkin lymphomas, and treatment is as for the type of lymphoma.

Bone marrow (haematopoietic stem cell) transplant

Disease resistant to standard-dose chemotherapy can be treated with bone marrow 'conditioning'. This means ablation or partial ablation of the bone marrow using chemotherapy or radiotherapy, or both. Bone marrow transplant is then performed with autologous stem cells (from bone marrow or peripheral blood) or, less often, cells from a compatible donor. The mortality rate associated with this procedure (now < 5% in low-risk autologous transplants) and the success of engraftment have improved with the use of haematopoietic growth factors. Long-term outcomes are uncertain, as are the indications for the use of this treatment in patients with less aggressive disease. Follow-up of treated non-Hodgkin lymphomas is similar to that for Hodgkin lymphoma patients. Allogenic bone marrow transplant is less well established in the treatment of lymphomas. It is also used for aplastic anaemia and some inherited diseases of blood cell production (e.g. immunodeficiencies and thalassaemia).

Ask a transplant patient about complications of the procedure (see Table 8.24).

Possible lines of questioning

1. What is your assessment of the stage of *this* patient's lymphoma?
2. Are further investigations indicated for staging?
3. Is *this* patient a candidate for bone marrow transplant? Physically? Psychologically?
4. What do you think *this* patient's current ECOG score is?

Multiple myeloma (myeloma)

This is a disseminated malignant disease of plasma cells. It can present as a diagnostic or a management problem. Myeloma occurs more commonly in the elderly – the median age is 60 years – and more often in men. It is more common in people whose occupations involve exposure to petroleum and in those exposed to nuclear radiation. Chronic antigenic stimulation may play a role in B cell clonal transformation. A number of chromosomal deletions and translocations have been identified in myeloma patients that have prognostic implications. Some myelomas begin as monoclonal gammopathies of uncertain significance (MGUS). MGUS are much more common than myeloma – they are found in up to 10% of 80-year-olds – and they evolve to myeloma at a rate of 1% a year ('smouldering myeloma').

The history

1. Ask about presenting symptoms:
   a. bone pain or pain with movement affects more than half of the patients, which occurs particularly in the ribs or axial skeleton and may cause pathological fractures. Malignant plasma cells in the bone marrow produce cytokines that stimulate osteoclast activity and cause lytic lesions in bone.
   b. bacterial infection is the presenting problem in one-quarter of patients, particularly pneumonia and urinary tract infections (total immunoglobulins are increased, but the level of normal functional immunoglobulins is reduced as a result of reduced production and increased destruction; in advanced marrow disease there is white cell depletion); the CD4 count is low and there is hypogammaglobulinaemia; the most common organisms are *Streptococcus pneumoniae*, *Staphylococcus aureus* and *Klebsiella pneumoniae* in the lungs, and *E. coli* in the urinary tract
   c. symptoms of anaemia (normochromic and normocytic) – as a result of bone marrow depression from infiltration, chronic disease, renal failure or treatment
   d. bleeding tendency – caused by paraprotein inactivation of plasma procoagulants and reduced platelet function (coating of platelets with antibodies) and thrombo-cytopenia as a result of bone marrow suppression
   e. renal disease symptoms (due to stone formation secondary to hypercalcaemia, hyperuricaemia, tubular damage by light chains, therapy, urinary tract infection, contrast studies, plasma cell infiltration or amyloid) – renal failure affects one-quarter of patients and half develop renal impairment; renal impairment at the time of diagnosis means a poor prognosis
   f. hypercalcaemic symptoms due to bone lysis
   g. hyperviscosity symptoms once plasma viscosity exceeds 5 (normal is about 1.8)
   h. spinal cord compression or, rarely, diffuse sensorimotor neuropathy
   i. skin changes, such as pruritus, purpura, yellow skin, hypertrichosis (rare), erythema annulare (rare)
   j. systemic amyloid deposition (10%–15%).

2. Find out how the diagnosis was made. This nearly always requires biopsy of the marrow or an extramedullary plasmacytoma.
3. Ask about treatment – ask about drugs (e.g. bisphosphonates, thalidomide) and their side-effects, radiotherapy and bone marrow transplant (actual or planned).
4. Enquire about the patient's social history, including dependants, work, ADLs, etc.
5. Determine the patient's understanding of this life-threatening condition and its prognosis – how much information he or she has about possible further problems and treatment.

The examination

1. Inspect the patient for signs of:
   a. weight loss
   b. anaemia
   c. general debility.
2. Examine the haemopoietic system. Pay particular attention to a search for bony tenderness. Kyphosis may be caused by compression fractures. Splenomegaly and lymphadenopathy occur only very rarely.
3. Note signs of anaemia and purpura. Look for skin rash.
4. Look for signs of infection (e.g. pulmonary consolidation).
5. Check carefully for any signs of spinal cord compression.
6. Check the urine analysis and temperature chart.

Investigations

1. Once the diagnosis is suspected, check the full blood count (and film) for anaemia (and rouleaux) and a raised ESR. Obtain a serum protein electrophoretogram (SPEP or EPG) of serum and urine and an immunoelectrophoretogram (IEPG). An 'M' component (monoclonal globulin peak) is found in 95% of cases (any immunoglobulin class may appear as the 'M' component). Light chains are present in the urine in 50%–75% of patients (Bence–Jones proteinuria cannot be detected by dipstick urine analysis).
2. Analysis of circulating light chains in the serum is a more sensitive way of detecting light chain myeloma as an abnormal $\kappa{:}\lambda$ ratio is seen. It is helpful in monitoring the response to treatment of such patients.
3. The bone marrow must be examined for plasma cells (> 10% in myeloma). Check the beta$_2$-microglobulin level (see below). Also check the serum calcium, urate levels and the renal function.
4. Look at X-ray films of the skull (Fig. 8.4), chest, pelvis (Fig. 8.5) and proximal long bones for fractures, osteoporosis and lytic lesions. As there is little osteoblastic activity, bone scans are much less sensitive than plain X-rays.
5. MRI scans may be the best way to investigate pain and possible nerve root or spinal cord compression.
   The diagnostic features of multiple myeloma, in order of importance, are:
   - clonal plasma cells in the bone marrow (≥ 10% involvement is consistent with the diagnosis) or soft tissue plasmacytoma
   - CRAB (hyper**C**alcaemia, **R**enal disease, **A**naemia and **B**one lytic lesions)
   - production of serum and/or urine paraprotein (50% are IgG, 33% are IgA, 5% are IgM, 10% are only light chains, 2% are nil).
   The disease can be staged according to certain criteria (Table 8.21).
   An elevated serum beta$_2$-microglobulin level (which reflects the myeloma cell burden and renal functional impairment) indicates a reduced median survival. Other poor prognostic features include advanced age and certain high-risk cytogenetic abnormalities. With the use of newer anti-myeloma therapies, survival for multiple myeloma is improving.

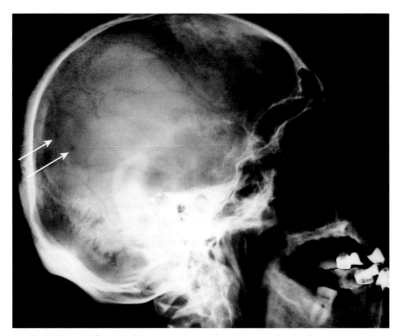

Figure 8.4 **Skull X-ray of a myeloma patient showing multiple lucent areas – 'pepper-pot skull' (arrows).**

Figure reproduced courtesy of The Canberra Hospital.

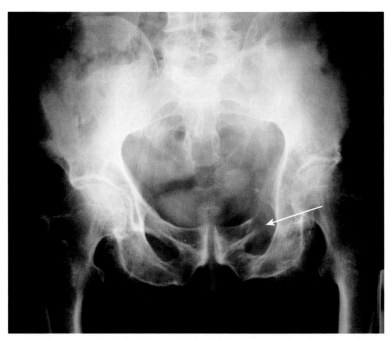

Figure 8.5 **Pelvic X-ray of the pelvis: destruction of left superior ramus of ischium (arrow).**

Figure reproduced courtesy of The Canberra Hospital.

Table 8.21 International staging system	
	MEDIAN SURVIVAL (MONTHS)
• **Stage 1** – beta$_2$-microglobulin < 3.5 mg/L and serum albumin ≥ 3.5 g/dL	62
• **Stage II** – neither I nor II	44
• **Stage III** – beta$_2$-microglobulin ≥ 5.5 mg/L	29
Source: The International Myeloma Foundation.	

Treatment

1. Irradiation is helpful for localised bone pain and spinal cord compression. Patients with a single bone plasmacytoma will often get prolonged disease-free survival after treatment with local radiotherapy.
   a. Zolendronate or one of the other bisphosphonates should be given to patients with more than stage I disease.
   b. Bisphosphonates reduce bone pain, fracture rates and episodes of hypercalcaemia. There is evidence that they improve the prognosis.
2. For those with more diffuse disease:
   a. General measures, such as adequate hydration and use of bicarbonate for Bence–Jones proteinuria, are important to prevent renal failure. Intravenous contrast material must be used cautiously and only with excellent hydration.
   b. Allopurinol may protect renal function from urate nephropathy related to treatment.
   c. Treat hypercalcaemia and bacterial infection.
   d. Avoid live vaccines.
   e. Erythropoietin may improve the anaemia.
3. Is the patient a candidate for transplant (usually an autograft) (Fig. 8.6a)? Suitable patients:
   • have a low ECOG score
   • are < 70 years old
   • have few co-morbidities.
   Transplant-related mortality is now < 1%.
4. Systemic therapy is indicated for patients who are symptomatic or have evidence of end-organ damage. Treatment is begun with high-dose steroids in combination with thalidomide or cyclophosphamide. An alternative is bortezomib, a proteosome inhibitor, as upfront therapy in combination with dexamethasone and cyclophosphamide. The latter option is preferred in those suitable for autologous transplant or who have renal impairment at diagnosis.
   The most important side-effect of thalidomide and bortezomib, and to a lesser extent of lenalidomide, is peripheral neuropathy. Patients being initiated with anti-myeloma therapy, particularly with thalidomide, should be considered for VTE prophylaxis as their risk of venous thrombosis is high.
5. Alkylating agents should be avoided if the patient may be a candidate for haematopoietic stem cell transplant. Such drugs may prevent stem cell harvesting by damaging these cells. Melphalan and prednisone were standard treatment; other alkylating agents (e.g. cyclophosphamide) are probably equally effective for patients unsuitable for bone marrow transplant. Resistance to one alkylating agent is often, but not always, associated with resistance to the others.

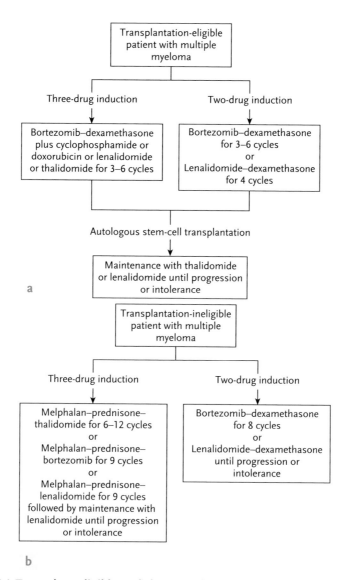

Figure 8.6 **(a) Transplant-eligible and (b) transplant-ineligible patients with multiple myeloma: management options.**

Older patients (ineligible for autologous transplant, see Fig. 8.6b) typically receive melphalan, thalidomide and prednisone (MTP) orally. A combination of bortezomib, melphalan and prednisone (VMP) is an alternative. Typically, treatment is given intermittently until it is no longer tolerated or there is a loss of response. The patient's progress must be monitored with regular protein EPG studies.

6. Relapse is treated for suitable patients with autologous stem cell bone marrow transplant. Novel agents such as carfilzomib and pomalidomide are available through clinical trials or special access programs.

7. Smoldering myeloma (asymptomatic myeloma) is defined by the presence of a monoclonal peak (> 30 g/L), or the presence of more than 10% plasma cells in the

bone marrow, in the absence of end-organ damage. This does not require treatment but serial monitoring is needed, as there is a significant risk of progression into symptomatic myeloma

DIFFERENTIAL DIAGNOSIS

Monoclonal gammopathy of undetermined significance

A smaller monoclonal peak (< 30 g/L), fewer than 10% plasma cells in the bone marrow and absence of lytic bone lesions suggest this diagnosis. Urinary light chains are absent. Infection, renal failure and anaemia are not increased. No therapy is required.

Waldenström's macroglobulinaemia

The EPG has a peak consisting of monoclonal IgM. These patients are generally older than those with myeloma. The hyperviscosity syndrome is often present. Symptoms and signs include:
- lassitude and confusion
- bleeding
- anaemia
- infection
- lymphadenopathy and splenomegaly
- dilated retinal veins
- perivenous haemorrhages
- (rarely) chronic kidney disease.

Lymphadenopathy and splenomegaly do not usually occur in patients with myeloma, whereas lytic bone destruction and hypercalcaemia are rare in Waldenström's. Ten per cent of the macroglobulins are cryoglobulins. An underlying lymphoproliferative disorder may be present. Treatment with plasmapheresis is effective in removing IgM paraprotein. Prednisone, fludarabine and chlorambucil are useful. Rituximab (anti-CD20 monoclonal antibody) and thalidomide have also been used successfully. Median survival is 4 years.

Localised myeloma

Only one plasma cell tumour is present. Solitary plasmacytomas often occur in the nasopharynx or paranasal sinuses. The major complications of myeloma are absent. Only 50% of cases show a monoclonal peak. Local radiotherapy is the usual treatment.

POEMS syndrome

This is an atypical form of myeloma. The features include:

Polyneuropathy

Organomegaly

Endocrinopathy

Monoclonal gammopathy (osteosclerotic myeloma, or IgA or IgG M proteins with lambda light chains)

Skin changes.
- There is a progressive sensorimotor polyneuropathy associated with myeloma-like bone lesions.
- Unlike multiple myeloma patients, over half these patients have hepatomegaly and lymphadenopathy and some have splenomegaly.
- Male erectile dysfunction and gynaecomastia and female amenorrhoea occur as a result of hyperprolactinaemia.
- A few patients have hypothyroidism and one-third have type 2 diabetes.
- Skin changes include clubbing, hypertrichosis, thickening and increased pigmentation.

- Elevated vascular endothelial growth factor (VGEF) occurs in two-thirds of patients.
   Treatment of the myeloma component in the usual way often helps the other manifestations. Local bone lesions often respond to radiotherapy. The natural history is of progression of peripheral neuropathy to respiratory failure over some years.

Possible lines of questioning

1. Is there a differential diagnosis for *this* patient with a diagnosis of myeloma?
2. Is local treatment or systemic treatment indicated for *this* patient with myeloma?
3. Should alkylating agents be used for *this* patient?

Bone marrow (haematopoietic cell) transplantation

Bone marrow transplantation is being performed for an increasing number of indications. Patients are chronically ill and often available for examinations. Two groups of patients are treated in this way: first, those with a malignant condition (Table 8.22), who have had their bone marrow conditioned by irradiation or chemotherapy given in marrow-toxic doses to treat a malignancy. Partial marrow ablation is increasingly used especially in older patients. The other indication is for patients with a defective bone marrow, often the result of an inherited disease (Table 8.23). Autologous transplants (when the patient's own marrow or stem cells are stored and then re-infused) are now more common than allogenic transplants (when another person is used as the donor of marrow or stem cells).

The history

As with all transplant long cases, you may find it most efficient to start with asking about current management including medications and follow-up, then work your way to establish an understanding of the previous events occurring around or after transplant

Table 8.22 Malignant indications for bone marrow transplant		
CONDITION	AUTOLOGOUS	ALLOGENIC
Acute leukaemia	Yes (uncommon)	Yes
Chronic myeloid leukaemia	Yes (rare)	Yes (uncommon now except in TKI failure)
Lymphoma	Yes (common)	Yes
Hodgkin disease	Yes (common)	Yes
Carcinoma of the breast	No	No
Carcinoma of the testis	Yes	No
Multiple myeloma	Yes	Yes
Wilms' tumour	Yes	No
TKI = tyrosine kinase inhibitor.		

Table 8.23 Non-malignant indications for bone marrow transplant		
CONDITION	AUTOLOGOUS	ALLOGENIC
Aplastic anaemia	No	Yes
Sickle cell disease	No	Yes
Thalassaemia	No	Yes
Gaucher disease	No	Yes
Severe combined immunodeficiency	No	Yes
Fanconi anaemia	No	Yes
Autoimmune disease (RhA, multiple sclerosis)	Yes	No
Rh = Rhesus.		

(primarily infection and rejection-related complications) and then focus on the points mentioned below:

1. Ask what the indication for the transplant was.
2. Find out whether there has been a problem leading to the current admission to hospital (if the patient is an inpatient).
3. Ask whether other treatment has been tried unsuccessfully. (For example, bone marrow transplant is often the treatment of choice for relapse after treatment for leukaemia or lymphoma.)
4. Find out whether the bone marrow transplant was autologous or allogenic. How was the marrow conditioned before transplant (radiotherapy, chemotherapy, or both) and, if the transplant was autologous, how were the stem cells harvested (from peripheral blood or by bone marrow aspiration)?
5. If the transplant was allogenic, does the patient know the donor? Only about 30% of people have an HLA-compatible relative. For the rest, a volunteer unrelated donor is used. HLA antigens are inherited together and rarely cross over. The patient may know how close the match was.
6. Ask for how long the patient was in hospital after transplantation. (Engraftment is usually quicker and complications are fewer after autologous transplant.) Ask specifically about problems with infection in the early period and how complications were managed.
7. Find out what effects this complicated illness and treatment have had on the patient's life and ability to work. Ask about family and financial problems. Young patients are likely to have been made sterile by the treatment. Total body irradiation and the use of alkylating agents are more likely than other treatments to cause permanent sterility. Women more often regain fertility than men. Ask tactfully whether the patient is aware of this and whether harvesting of oocytes or sperm was undertaken.
8. Ask how effective the treatment has been. Does the patient feel better or worse than before and what medium- and long-term prognosis has he or she been given?
9. Ask whether there have been specific transplant-associated problems. Ask specifically about the symptoms and signs of graft versus host disease (GVHD) and the other complications of allogenic transplantation (Table 8.24).
10. Ask about the patient's current medications including any regular injections (e.g. intravenous immunoglobulin (IVIG), bisphosphonates, rituximab), and check for side-effects and adherence.

Table 8.24 Complications of allogenic bone marrow transplant

EARLY COMPLICATIONS	LATE COMPLICATIONS
Induction-related: • Mucositis • Cystitis • Interstitial pneumonitis (usually CMV, PCP or RSV infection) • *Aspergillus, Candida, Nocardia* lung infection • Pulmonary haemorrhage • Non-cardiogenic pulmonary oedema • Idiopathic pneumonia syndrome (transplant-related lung injury) • Renal impairment Graft failure Infection Immunodeficiency Acute GVHD Veno-occlusive (sinusoidal obstructive) disease of the liver (hepatomegaly, ascites, jaundice)	Treatment-related: • Gonadal toxicity • Cataracts • Neurological Chronic GVHD including bronchiolitis obliterans Infection Relapse of treated condition Second malignancy Immunodeficiency

CMV = cytomegalovirus; GVHD = graft versus host disease; PCP = *Pneumocystis* pneumonia; RSV = respiratory syncytial virus

11. Ask about the impact of disease and hospital admissions on the patient at each point of their illness, and currently.
12. Ask about any regular screening relating to their condition and for age-appropriate cancer screening.

The examination

Examine for persisting or recurrent signs of the condition for which the bone marrow transplant was performed.

1. Examine for signs of chronic GVHD. These include skin changes similar to those of scleroderma, dry eyes and mouth (sicca syndrome), alopecia and bronchiolitis obliterans (signs of airflow obstruction).
2. Examine for hepatic enlargement and ascites (hepatic sinusoidal obstruction syndrome). Feel all the lymph node groups (e.g. enlarged as a result of a second malignancy, such as ALL or melanoma) and examine the eyes (e.g. secondary glioblastoma).
3. Look for signs of infection in the lungs and for herpes zoster.
4. Examine the hips (aseptic osteonecrosis).
5. Patients who have had radiotherapy may show evidence of hypothyroidism.
6. Look for any neurological signs.

Management

Detailed discussion about methods of transplantation will not be required.

1. Management after transplant begins with supportive treatment to prevent infection and bleeding before engraftment occurs. Platelet and blood transfusions may be required and the patient is usually kept isolated. Transfused products are irradiated to prevent GVHD from transfused lymphocytes. Most patients receive colony-stimulating factors to speed recovery. Platelet recovery is usually the slowest and tends to determine the time of discharge from hospital.
2. Patients who have had an allogenic transplant are at risk of GVHD. This risk is reduced if the HLA match is a highly compatible one (only one locus is mismatched).

Prophylaxis against GVHD with some combination of prednisone, methotrexate and cyclosporin is usual. The donor marrow may be treated to remove T cells to reduce the incidence of GVHD, but this increases the risk of graft rejection. The risk of GVHD is also increased by previous exposure to blood products and by previous pregnancy.

3. Acute GVHD can occur even when the major HLA antigens match. It occurs by definition in the first 3 months after transplant and is characterised by:
   - diarrhoea
   - skin rash
   - liver function test changes.

   Severe acute GVHD (generalised erythroderma or desquamation) reduces survival and requires aggressive treatment. It is usually treated with high doses of prednisone, antithymocyte globulin and monoclonal antibodies to T cells. Some centres use prophylactic GVHD treatment after transplant with methotrexate and tacrolimus or cyclosporin. Remember that the presence of some GVHD reduces the risk of tumour recurrence as a result of graft versus tumour activity.

4. Chronic GVHD develops after 3 months and affects up to half of transplant recipients. Patients develop an autoimmune-like illness with sicca syndrome, arthritis, cholestasis and bronchiolitis obliterans. It is treated with immunosuppression. It is rare for it to persist for more than 3 years.

5. Infection can be a problem at various times after transplant.
   a. Bacterial infection is most common during the early period before the neutrophil count reaches normal levels.
   b. Fungal infection can become a problem within a week of transplant, can be challenging to treat and clearance of infection becomes faster upon neutrophil recovery.
   c. *Pneumocystis jirovecii* infection and cytomegalovirus (CMV) infection can occur within a week of transplant but are uncommon after 3 months. Interstitial pneumonitis occurs in up to 10% of patients. This is usually the result of CMV infection and is treated with supporting measures and ganciclovir. CMV-negative recipients should receive only CMV-negative blood products, and CMV-positive patients should receive prophylactic ganciclovir.
   d. Antifungal prophylaxis with posaconazole or fluconazole, PJP prophylaxis with co-trimaxazole, and CMV prophylaxis with ganciclovir are usually indicated for allogenic bone marrow transplant,

6. Graft rejection is usually a result of the activity of functional host lymphocytes and is most common in patients who have not had their marrow ablated (e.g. those with aplastic anaemia).

7. Recurrence of leukaemia may be treated with infusion of more donor T cells, although this increases GVHD.

8. Hepatic sinusoidal obstruction syndrome occurs in up to 50% of patients. Most recover, but in severe cases treatment with tissue plasminogen activator may be indicated. The use of ursodeoxycholic acid may also diminish the incidence.

9. Overall, autologous bone marrow transplant is associated with similar but less severe complications. GVHD, however, does not occur. Transplant-related mortality is much less, at 1%–2%.

10. The prognosis varies with the indication for the treatment (Table 8.25). In general, malignant conditions have a better prognosis when treated with bone marrow transplant as a primary or secondary therapy than when it is used only after all else has failed. Patients with non-malignant conditions can often be very successfully treated with

Table 8.25 Survival of bone marrow adult transplant patients

CONDITION	5-YEAR SURVIVAL RATE (%)
Acute myeloid leukaemia (AML)	50
Acute lymphoblastic leukaemia (ALL)	50
Chronic myeloid leukaemia (CML), chronic phase	70
CML accelerated	40
CML blast crisis	15
Chronic lymphocytic leukaemia (CLL)	50
Hodgkin disease	50
Non-Hodgkin lymphoma	40
Aplastic anaemia	90
Severe combined immunodeficiency	90
Thalassaemia	90

bone marrow transplant. For example, aplastic anaemia patients can expect up to 90% disease-free survival. Opinions differ about the use of bone marrow transplant as initial treatment for these patients.

11. Remember, as with any complicated and life-threatening illness, to pay great attention to the patient's ability to cope and the availability of support at home; these are important matters that you must be able to discuss.

Possible lines of questioning

1. Was bone marrow transplant the first treatment used for *this* patient?
2. Have there been episodes of infection and neutrophilia since the transplant? How were these managed?
3. Has *this* patient planned to deal with symptoms of infection?
4. Have you found evidence of graft versus host disease?

Chapter 9

The rheumatological long case

It's better to be dead, or even perfectly well, than to
suffer from the wrong affliction.

Ogden Nash (1902–71)

Joint and mobility problems are common in long-case patients, even when this is not
the central abnormality. Elderly and obese patients often have osteoarthritis (OA), which
limits their ability to exercise and lose weight. A modified GALS (gait, arms, legs and
spine) assessment can be a quick way to identify the importance of these matters to the
patient (and to the long case itself).

Ask:

1. Have you been troubled by pain or stiffness in your back or muscles or joints? Where?
2. How are you affected by this? Can you walk up and down stairs? Can you get out
   of a chair easily? Can you dress and wash yourself?

Examine:

1. **Gait: g**et the patient to walk to the end of the room, turn around and come back.
   Note the length of stride, smoothness of walk and turning around, stance, heel strike
   and arm swing. Is walking painful? Hemiplegic, Parkinsonian, foot drop and other
   neurological gaits should be obvious.
2. **Arms, legs and spine:**
   a. From behind – look at the spine for scoliosis, muscle bulk of the shoulders, paraspinal
      muscles, gluteal muscles and calves, and the iliac crests for loss of symmetry.
   b. From the side – look for normal lordosis and thoracic kyphosis. Ask the patient
      to bend; look for normal separation of lumbar spinous processes.
   c. From in front – look for asymmetry or wasting of major muscle groups (shoulders,
      arms and quadriceps). Is there deformity of the knees, ankles or feet?
   When arthritis seems likely to be an important part of the case, take the time to test
   movement. Look for restricted, asymmetrical or painful movements.
1. **Spine** – rotation: say 'Turn your shoulders as far as you can to the right, and now
   to the left'; lateral flexion: 'Slide your hand down the side of the leg on the right

side, and now on the left'. Cervical spine – lateral flexion: 'Bend your right ear down towards your shoulder; now on the other side'; flexion and extension: 'Look up and back as far as you can; now put your chin on your chest'.

2. **Shoulders (acromioclavicular, glenohumeral, sternoclavicular joints)** – say 'Put your right hand on your back and reach up as far as you can as if to scratch your back; now the left'; 'Put your hands up behind your head and your elbows as far back as you can'.

3. **Elbows (extension)** – say 'With your elbows straight, put your arms down beside you'.

4. **Hands and wrists** – say 'Straighten out your arms and hands in front of you'. Look for fixed flexion deformity of the fingers and swelling and deformity of the hands and wrists or wasting of the small muscles of the hands. 'Turn your hands up the other way': look at the palms for swelling or muscle wasting. Is supination smooth and complete? Is there external rotation of the shoulder used to make up for limited supination? Test for grip strength: 'Squeeze my fingers as hard as you can'. Test finger joints: 'Touch the tip of each finger with your thumb'.

   If the hands seem abnormal, ask the patient to perform some functional testing: doing up buttons, undoing jar lids, etc.

5. **Legs and hips** – say 'Lie down on the bed for me'. Look at leg length and, if suspicious, measure true leg length from the anterior superior iliac spine to the medial malleolus and apparent length from the umbilicus to the medial malleolus. Test knee flexion: 'Bend your knee and pull your foot up towards your bottom'. Meanwhile, put your hand on the patella and feel for crepitus. Test for osteoarthritis of the hip by internally rotating the hip. Flex the knee to 90° and move the foot laterally. Pain and limitation of movement occur early with osteoarthritis.

6. **Feet** – look for arthritic changes especially at the metatarsophalangeal (MTP) joints, bunions, swelling, calluses, etc.

The examination will have to be varied for very immobile patients, but with practice it can be performed rapidly.

Possible lines of questioning

1. What was your assessment of *this* patient's general mobility and ability to cope with normal activities?
2. Did he or she have a normal gait?
3. Could he or she get up easily from a chair?
4. Did he or she need any walking aids? Were they adequate in your opinion?

Remember the patterns of joint involvement (Table 9.1).

Rheumatoid arthritis (RA)

This is the most common of the inflammatory arthritides and is a very common long case in which the diagnosis is usually straightforward and the patient has many physical signs. The peak incidence of the onset of rheumatoid arthritis is in the fourth decade of life and it is three times as common in women as in men. There may be a family history and there is an association with human leukocyte antigen (HLA)-DR4 (70%).

Table 9.1 Patterns of joint involvement

CONDITION	PATTERNS	CLUES
Rheumatoid arthritis (RA)	Symmetrical – wrists, MCPs, PIPs, MTPs with or without large joints	Never DIPs, CMC or temporomandibular joints
Axial spondyloarthropathy	Large joints – lower limb, spine, SI joints	Not hand small joints
Psoriatic	1. Like RA 2. Large joint lower limb 3. DIPs or PIPs or both 4. Arthritis mutilans	Psoriatic rash, nail changes Dactylitis Enthesitis
Gout	Asymmetrical – CMCs, DIPs, PIPs, big toe MTP	Tophi Rare in young women
Osteoarthritis (OA)	Asymmetrical – CMCs, DIPs, PIPs, big toe MTP (often first affected)	Swelling is bony, not boggy
SLE	Symmetrical – PIPs, MCPs, sometimes large joints	Rashes

MCP = metacarpophalangeal; PIP = proximal interphalangeal; MTP = metatarsophalangeal; DIP = distal interphalangeal; CMC = carpometacarpal; SI = sacroiliac; SLE = systemic lupus erythematosus.

If left untreated, the disease leads to progressive and irreversible joint damage and deformity (Fig. 9.1a). Life expectancy is reduced by 10 years.

The history

1. Ask when the diagnosis was made and whether diagnosis seems to have been delayed – the onset of RA in patients over the age of 60 is associated with a worse prognosis for those who are rheumatoid factor (RF) positive. Delay in diagnosis and treatment also leads to a worse outcome.
2. Ask about the presenting features – most patients present with vague generalised symptoms, such as fatigue, anorexia and non-specific musculoskeletal pains; a minority present with obvious oligoarticular arthritis; a few present with severe constitutional symptoms and acute arthritis. Morning stiffness that lasts for more than an hour and continues for more than 6 weeks is characteristic of inflammatory arthritis, but not of osteoarthritis.
3. Ask about the initial treatment.
4. Ask about the disease progression and which joints have been involved. The lumbar spine is never involved and the distal interphalangeal joints are only rarely affected. Find out how active the disease is currently: number of painful joints, duration of morning stiffness.
5. Enquire about the alterations in treatment over time and any complications encountered.
6. Ask about the non-articular features of the disease:
   a. skin – Raynaud's phenomenon, leg ulcers (Fig. 9.1b)
   b. eyes – dry eyes (and mouth; Sjögren's syndrome), scleritis, episcleritis or scleromalacia perforans, cataracts (caused by steroids); iritis does not occur
   c. sore throat, hoarseness or neck pain – suspect cricoarytenoid joint disease
   d. recurrent headaches at the base of the skull or arm – tingling from C1–2 subluxation (remember to tell the examiners you would like to see a lateral flexion cervical spine X-ray)

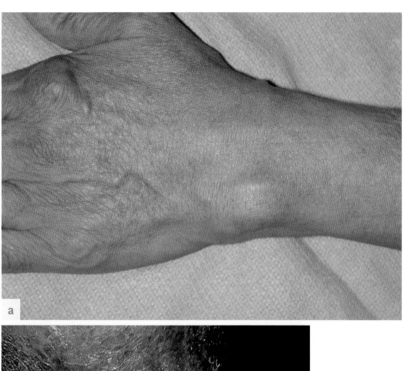

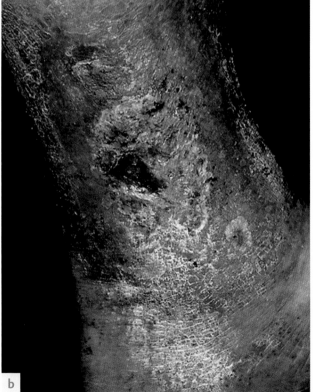

Figure 9.1 **Rheumatoid arthritis: (a) joint damage and deformity in the hand; (b) leg ulcer.**

(a) W R Frontera, J K Silver and T D Rizzo. *Essentials of physical medicine and rehabilitation,* 3rd edn. Fig. 41.1A. Saunders, Elsevier, 2015, with permission. (b) T P Habif. *Clinical dermatology,* 5th edn. Fig 3.66. Mosby, Elsevier, 2009, with permission.

   e. lungs – dyspnoea due to diffuse interstitial lung disease or pleural effusion; pain as a result of pleuritis
   f. heart – chest pain due to pericarditis, valve disease (from rheumatoid nodules), increased risk atherosclerosis and ischaemic heart disease (as with all chronic inflammatory diseases)
   g. renal – drug use, amyloid (all rare)
   h. nervous system – peripheral neuropathy, mononeuritis multiplex, cord compression (due to cervical spine involvement (C1–2 subluxation) or rheumatoid nodules), entrapment neuropathy (particularly carpal tunnel syndrome)
   i. blood – anaemic symptoms due to chronic disease, iron deficiency (from blood loss), folate deficiency (diet), Felty's syndrome (rheumatoid arthritis with leukopenia and splenomegaly, and non-healing leg ulcers)
   j. systemic – fever, weight loss, fatigue
   k. vasculitic – digital arteritis, ulcers, mononeuritis multiplex, pyoderma gangrenosum.
7. Ask about drug complications:
   a. aspirin (pain or nausea, gastric erosions or peptic ulcers causing bleeding, tinnitus)
   b. NSAIDs (ulceration, renal impairment, increased cardiac risk)
   c. methotrexate (MTX) is often used and has a number of side-effects that need to be monitored (hepatic and pulmonary toxicity, low white cell count and thrombocytopenia); the patient should know not to drink alcohol while taking MTX – an alternative drug (to MTX, not alcohol) is leflunomide (side-effects: diarrhoea, alopecia, liver toxicity)
   d. penicillamine (nephrotic syndrome, thrombocytopenia, rashes, mouth ulcers, alteration in taste and, rarely, systemic lupus erythematosus (SLE), polymyositis, myasthenia gravis, Goodpasture's syndrome or pulmonary infiltration)
   e. cyclosporin – monitor renal function and blood pressure
   f. hydroxychloroquine (nausea, pigmentation, bull's eye retinopathy – needs regular ophthalmological review)
   g. sulfasalazine (rash, nausea, haematological abnormalities, abnormal liver function tests, reversible oligospermia)
   h. anti-tumour necrosis factor (TNF) monoclonal antibody or other biological disease-modifying agent (increased risk of infections including reactivation of TB, positive ANA, lymphoma and demyelination)
   i. steroids.
8. Ask about the major current problem – such as decreasing hand function, paraesthesiae, severe pain, etc.
9. Find out about the current activity of the disease. This can be assessed historically by asking about the number of joints that have recently been involved with active synovitis, the severity and duration of early-morning stiffness (very important), functional ability, changes in weight and the degree of systemic ill health. A severe course is more likely if there is the early appearance of rheumatoid nodules, an insidious onset and constitutional symptoms.
10. Enquire about past medical history, especially regarding peptic ulceration, drug reactions or renal disease.
11. Enquire about social background – ability to cope at home, ability to climb steps, independence in daily activities, ability to perform fine-motor activities, the work environment, availability of support services. Smoking is a risk factor for rheumatoid arthritis, particularly in developing anti-CCP (cyclic citrullinated peptide) positive rheumatoid arthritis. The risk falls after smoking is stopped.

12. Ask about a family history (first-degree relatives) of rheumatoid arthritis, lupus, blood clots, diabetes (type 1), thyroid disease and miscarriages. Other types of autoimmune disease may be present in close relatives.

The examination

A thorough general examination (Table 9.2) is important. In addition to assessing for synovitis in *every* joint, look particularly at the following:

1. general appearance – steroid complications, weight; remember that the pain arises mostly from the joint capsule and that acutely inflamed joints are held in the flexed position to increase the volume of the capsule and reduce pain
2. the hands – including vasculitis and hand function; the wrist joints are almost always affected
3. the arms – the elbow and shoulder joints, rheumatoid nodules and axillary node enlargement
4. the face – check the eyes for Sjögren's syndrome, scleritis, episcleritis, scleromalacia perforans, cataracts, anaemia and signs of hyperviscosity in the fundi; enlarged parotid glands (Sjögren's syndrome); the mouth (dryness, dental caries, ulcers); listen for a hoarse voice and palpate the temporomandibular joints (crepitus); *note:* rheumatoid arthritis does not cause iritis
5. the neck – for signs of cervical spine involvement
6. the chest – the heart for pericarditis, conduction defects, and aortic and mitral regurgitation; the lungs for pleural effusion, fibrosis, nodules, infarction and Caplan's syndrome

Table 9.2 Rheumatoid arthritis

1. GENERAL INSPECTION
Cushingoid appearance
Weight

2. HANDS (EXAMINE ALL JOINTS)

3. ARMS
Entrapment neuropathy (e.g. carpal tunnel)
Subcutaneous nodules
Elbow joint
Shoulder joint
Axillary nodes

4. FACE
Eyes – dry eyes (Sjögren's), scleritis, episcleritis
Scleromalacia perforans
Cataract (steroids, chloroquine)
Fundi – hyperviscosity
Face – parotids (Sjögren's)
Mouth – dryness, ulcers, dental caries, temporomandibular joint (crepitus)

5. NECK
Cervical spine
Cervical nodes

6. CHEST
Heart – pericarditis, valve lesions
Lungs – effusion, fibrosis, infarction, infection, nodules (and Caplan's syndrome)
Tuberculosis (steroids)

7. ABDOMEN
Splenomegaly (e.g. Felty's syndrome)
Epigastric tenderness (drugs)
Inguinal nodes

8. HIPS

9. KNEES

10. LOWER LIMBS
Ulceration (vasculitis)
Calf swelling (ruptured synovial cyst)
Peripheral neuropathy
Mononeuritis multiplex
Cord compression

11. FEET

12. OTHER
Urine – protein, blood (drugs, vasculitis, infection, amyloidosis)
Rectal examination (blood)

7. the abdomen – for splenomegaly and epigastric tenderness
8. the hips and knees
9. the lower legs – for ulcers, calf swelling (ruptured Baker's cyst), neuropathy, mononeuritis multiplex and signs of cord compression
10. the feet
11. the peripheral nervous system – for peripheral neuropathy or mononeuritis multiplex (caused by vasculitis)
12. the skin – for cutaneous vasculitis (ischaemic ulcers on the legs or brown discoloured areas in the nail beds; *note:* exclude psoriasis); if there is erythema and heat over a single joint, consider gout
13. urine analysis – for protein and blood, and rectal examination for blood (if there is a history suggestive of NSAID complications).

Differential diagnosis

Consider the differential diagnosis of a deforming symmetrical chronic polyarthropathy:
1. rheumatoid arthritis
2. psoriatic arthropathy and other seronegative spondyloarthropathies
3. chronic tophaceous gout (rarely symmetrical)
4. primary generalised osteoarthritis
5. SLE (usually but not always non-deforming).
   Remember that the causes of arthritis plus nodules include:
1. rheumatoid arthritis (seropositive)
2. SLE – rare
3. rheumatic fever (Jaccoud's arthritis) – very rare
4. amyloid arthropathy (most usually in association with multiple myeloma).
Note: gouty tophi and xanthoma may sometimes be confused.

Investigations

To support the diagnosis (remembering that this is primarily a clinical diagnosis; see Table 9.3), investigations include:
1. **serological tests**
   a. rheumatoid factor – 70% of patients are seropositive; patients may at first be seronegative and seroconvert later. (*Note:* Most patients are RF positive if they have nodules or associated vasculitis; remember that more than 10% of well people over the age of 65 have RF and that it is commonly found in association with infections and other inflammatory conditions, in relatives of patients with rheumatoid arthritis and transiently after some vaccinations.)
   b. anti-citrullinated cyclic peptide – this is more specific (97%); it is associated with a more severe disease course and erosive disease
2. **X-ray films of involved joints** – changes to look for are:
   a. soft-tissue swelling
   b. symmetrical joint space narrowing (OA causes asymmetrical narrowing) (Figs 9.2 and 9.3) and erosions
   c. juxta-articular osteoporosis
   d. marginal joint erosions (Fig. 9.4).
   Investigations used to assess the activity of the disease include:
1. ESR or CRP – remember that the differential diagnosis of a raised ESR in rheumatoid arthritis includes:
   a. active disease
   b. amyloidosis

Table 9.3 Criteria for the diagnosis of rheumatoid arthritis (RA) in newly presenting cases (2010 ACR / EULAR RA criteria)

	SCORE
Target population (who should be tested?) – patients:	
1. who have at least one joint with definite clinical synovitis (swelling)	
2. with the synovitis not better explained by another disease	
CLASSIFICATION CRITERIA FOR RA	**SCORE**
(score-based algorithm: add score of categories A–D; a score of ≥ 6 / 10 is needed for classification of a patient as having definite RA)	
A. JOINT INVOLVEMENT	
1 large joint	0
2–10 large joints	1
1–3 small joints (with or without involvement of large joints)	2
4–10 small joints (with or without involvement of large joints)	3
> 10 joints (at least one small joint)	5
B. SEROLOGY (AT LEAST ONE TEST RESULT IS NEEDED FOR CLASSIFICATION)	
Negative RF *and* negative ACPA	0
Low-positive RF *or* low-positive ACPA	2
High-positive RF *or* high-positive ACPA	3
C. ACUTE-PHASE REACTANTS (AT LEAST ONE TEST RESULT IS NEEDED FOR CLASSIFICATION)	
Normal CRP *and* normal ESR	0
Abnormal CRP *or* abnormal ESR	1
D. DURATION OF SYMPTOMS	
< 6 weeks	0
≥ 6 weeks	1

ACPA = anti-citrullinated protein antibody; CRP = C-reactive protein; ESR = erythrocyte sedimentation rate; RF = rheumatoid factor.

© 2010 American College of Rheumatology and European League Against Rheumatism. Rheumatoid Arthritis Classification Criteria 2010. *Arthritis and Rheumatism* 2010; 62(9):2569–81.

   c. infection

   d. Sjögren's syndrome

2. haemoglobin measurement – the severity of normochromic anaemia usually correlates with activity

3. anti-CCP, and RF titres

4. the presence of progressive erosions on serial X-ray films.

Treatment

1. Remember that the aim of modern treatment is to induce complete remission of the disease by suppressing the inflammatory process. This means early diagnosis and introduction of disease-modifying antirheumatic drugs (DMARDs). The traditional DMARDs will control the disease effectively for many patients, but the newer biological

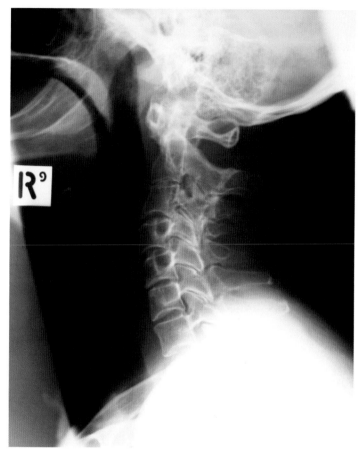

Figure 9.2 **Cervical spine X-ray of a patient with rheumatoid arthritis. Note the erosions and loss of joint space. Special views are needed to exclude erosion of the odontoid process.**

Figure reproduced courtesy of The Canberra Hospital.

therapies allow many more patients to have the disease controlled. The general principles of treatment include:

- education
- physiotherapy, including exercise and splinting of the joints to prevent deformity
- occupational therapy
- smoking cessation
- rest of inflamed joints
- drug treatment aimed at reducing pain and inflammation (with aspirin, other NSAIDs or COX-2 inhibitors) and at preventing progression of the disease. The risk of gastrointestinal toxicity of the traditional NSAIDs (i.e. peptic ulceration) is reduced by the use of the COX-2 inhibitors; however, all can cause dyspepsia and renal disease (e.g. acute interstitial nephritis) and worsen renal function in patients with diabetic or atherosclerotic kidney disease; all NSAIDs are associated with an increased risk of myocardial infarction. If there is aspirin allergy, sodium salicylate is an alternative.

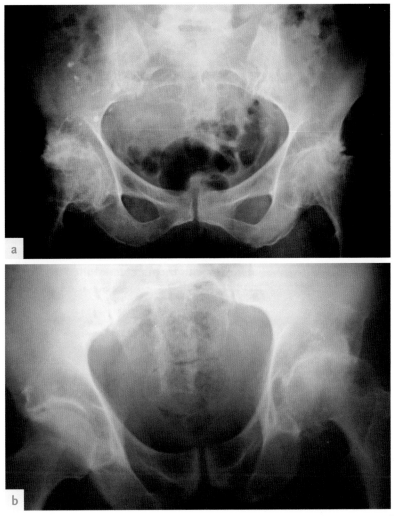

Figure 9.3 (a) X-ray of the pelvis of a patient with rheumatoid arthritis; note the severe destructive changes on both sides – very different from (b). (b) Osteoarthritis of the left hip; note the asymmetrical loss of joint space.

Figures reproduced courtesy of The Canberra Hospital.

2. The use of DMARDs is now recommended early on for patients with active progressive disease, especially if there is evidence of joint destruction (Table 9.4). These drugs include:
   - methotrexate (MTX)
   - sulfasalazine
   - hydroxychloroquine
   - cyclosporin
   - leflunomide
   - azathioprine
   - penicillamine
   - gold (oral or injected).

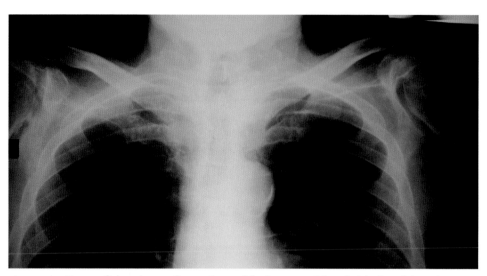

Figure 9.4 X-ray of the chest of a patient with rheumatoid arthritis involving the shoulder; note the erosions of the humeral heads with subluxation and erosions of the distal clavicles.

Figure reproduced courtesy of The Canberra Hospital.

Table 9.4 Risk factors for destructive disease
1. High-titre RF or positive anti-CCP
2. Constitutional symptoms
3. Insidious onset
4. Erosions early on X-ray
5. Rheumatoid nodules early
6. HLA-DR4

These medications have a slow onset of action (weeks for methotrexate to months for gold). There is evidence that they can lead to healing of bone erosions. Monitoring should include:
- full blood count
- urine testing for proteinuria
- specific tests for certain drugs, such as liver function tests for methotrexate, or ophthalmological examination and assessment of visual fields for hydroxychloroquine.
3. Methotrexate is the most commonly used of these drugs; it can be given orally or intramuscularly, usually 10–25 mg weekly, but starting with a low dose. It is usually better tolerated than the other DMARDs and is often the drug of first choice and given early in the course of the disease to decrease inflammation and sometimes the development of synovitis. MTX may sometimes cause an increase in the number of rheumatoid nodules. It can be given alone or in combination with hydroxychloroquine and sulfasalazine. Folic acid is given daily to decrease the risk of side-effects of MTX, especially mouth ulcers. Safety monitoring includes full blood count and liver function tests. Adverse reactions include rash, abnormal liver function tests (transaminases), leukopenia, thrombocytopenia and interstitial lung disease. It should not be given to patients with glucose-6-phosphate dehydrogenase deficiency.

4. Alternative agents in use include leflunomide (a pyrimidine antagonist that inhibits the proliferation of T cells).
5. The biological agents are generally second-line treatments because of their cost, but their use has increased greatly recently. Table 9.5 shows the current prescribing rules for these drugs, while Table 9.6 lists their side-effects and precautions for their use.

Table 9.5 Rules for use of biological agents for the treatment of rheumatoid arthritis

1. Failure of at least 6 months of treatment with a traditional DMARD
2. Treatment must include MTX and combinations of hydroxychloroquine, leflunomide or sulfasalazine

DMARD = disease-modifying antirheumatic drug; MTX = methotrexate.

Table 9.6 Side-effects and precautions for use of biological agents

1. Local reactions at injection sites (usually mild)
2. Infusion reactions – nausea, flushing, headache or palpitations (often well managed with antihistamines)
3. Delayed infusion reactions – fatigue, rash, arthralgia and myalgia (may require steroid use or cessation of treatment)
4. Increased risk of serious infections – patients should avoid undercooked eggs and meat (*Listeria* and *Salmonella* organisms)
5. Reactivation of TB (screen for TB before use – Mantoux, interferon gamma (IFN-γ), chest X-ray)
6. Contraindicated for patients with active hepatitis B or C
7. Contraindicated for patients receiving immunosuppression
8. Live vaccines are contraindicated
9. Possible increased incidence of non-melanoma skin cancers
10. Not recommended in pregnancy, though no evidence of problems

There are two main types of biological agents: the TNF (tumour necrosis factor) inhibitors and the non-TNF inhibitors.

THE TNF INHIBITORS

These drugs block the activation of TNF-α, which is an inflammatory cytokine found in the synovium of RA patients. Suppression of synovitis with these agents can almost completely prevent joint and bone destruction. All the TNF inhibitors have to be given by intravenous infusion or subcutaneous injection. The five drugs currently available (Table 9.7) are equally effective and can be used in combination with methotrexate. Failure to respond occurs in 30% of patients and for them it is worth trying another drug in the same class or a non-TNF inhibitor.

Table 9.7 TNF inhibitors for adults with RA

1. Infliximab: IV infusion initially 3 mg/kg at 0, 2 and 6 weeks and then 8-weekly (with MTX)
2. Adalimumab: SC injection 40 mg 2nd-weekly
3. Certolizumab pegol: SC injection of 400 mg at 0, 2 and 4 weeks, then every 4th week
4. Etanercept: SC injection 25 mg twice weekly or 50 mg weekly
5. Golimumab: SC injection 50 mg every 4th week (with MTX)

MTX = methotrexate; TNF = tumour necrosis factor.

THE NON-TNF INHIBITORS

These DMARDs inhibit proinflammatory cytokines other than TNF (see Table 9.8 for a list of currently available drugs).

Table 9.8 Non-TNF inhibitors and side-effects
1. Abatacept: a T cell co-stimulation inhibitor; monthly IV infusion or subcutaneous injection (hypersensitivity reactions, increased risk of serious infections)
2. Anakinra: an IL-1 receptor antagonist; daily SC injection (injection site reactions, neutropenia). Less effective than the other drugs in this class
3. Rituximab: antibody against CD20 B cell antigen; two 1000 mg IV infusions 2 weeks apart (infusion reactions, serious infection – URTI, UTI, sinusitis, progressive multifocal leukoencephalopathy)
4. Tocilizumab: IL-6 inhibitor; monthly IV infusion 8 mg/kg (URTI, neutropenia, increased lipids, abnormal LFTs)
5. Tofacitinib: Janus kinase inhibitor (increased risk of infections including herpes zoster, liver dysfunction)
IL = interleukin; LFT = liver function test; URTI = upper respiratory tract infection; UTI = urinary tract infection; TNF = tumour necrosis factor.

HINTS

Drugs in rheumatological disease
1. Methotrexate is useful for any form of bad joint disease.
2. Patients on biological agents may have serious infections without the usual signs.
3. Ankylosing spondylitis should be treated with NSAIDs first.
4. SLE should be treated with hydroxychloroquine.
5. Avoid big doses of steroids in scleroderma patients (see Table 9.9).
6. If a patient is unwell, consider stopping a disease-modifying agent but do not stop steroids.
7. Drugs are safe if monitored.

6. The main indications for steroid use are:
   • new or uncontrolled disease as a bridge until suppressive treatment with slow-acting DMARDs becomes effective
   • vasculitic complications of rheumatoid arthritis (where high doses are needed)
   • chronic low-dose treatment, which may be justifiable in the elderly
   • local steroid injections for acute involvement of a joint (these may give prolonged relief from pain and swelling, and improve function).
7. Surgery may be very effective treatment for severely diseased joints. Hip, shoulder and knee replacements are the most successful operations. Arthroplasty and relief of contractures can be of value, especially in the hands.

The prognosis of this chronic, but often intermittent, disease varies. Only a small minority of patients have no permanent joint problems 10 years after diagnosis, and half have a disability that interferes with work by this time. The greater the number of involved joints at the outset and the more abnormal the inflammatory markers, the worse is the prognosis. Life expectancy is reduced by up to 7 years as a result of the increased risk of gastrointestinal bleeding, the increased risk of infection and a threefold increased risk of atherosclerosis. The use of methotrexate has been shown to halve excess mortality, including that from cardiovascular disease.

At each visit, assess the patient for disease activity and function (Box 9.1).

Table 9.9 What drugs to use in rheumatoid arthritis and other autoimmune conditions

RHEUMATOID ARTHRITIS	ANKYLOSING SPONDYLITIS	SCLERODERMA
MTX with or without: hydroxychloroquine, sulfasalazine, leflunomide, prednisone	NSAIDs and exercise Try different NSAID	Treat Raynaud's MTX
No better after 6 months: add biological agent	No better at 3 months: add biological agent	If getting worse, ILD or cardiac involvement: cyclophosphamide, autologous stem cell transplant Keep steroid dose below 15 mg
Note: Always screen for TB and hepatitis B and C (serology) before using a biological agent.		
ILD = interstitial lung disease; MTX = methotrexate.		

Box 9.1 Routine assessment of patients with rheumatoid arthritis

1. Fatigue
2. Morning stiffness
3. Weight loss
4. Functional limitations
5. Acute-phase reactants (erythrocyte sedimentation rate, C-reactive protein)

PREGNANCY AND RHEUMATOID ARTHRITIS

The disease tends to abate during pregnancy but, in order to reduce the risk of fetal toxicity and assist conception, some drugs should be adjusted:

- Methotrexate should be stopped 3 months before conception.
- Leflunomide should be stopped until it is no longer detectable in the serum.
- Sulfasalazine can cause reversible oligospermia and men should stop this 3 months before attempted conception.
- Aspirin and NSAIDs can interfere with implantation; they can be used in the second trimester, but later in pregnancy can cause premature closure of the ductus arteriosus and interfere with labour.
- Steroids increase the risk of maternal diabetes and cleft palate in the baby.
- The safety of biological agents is uncertain.
- Methotrexate should not be used by breastfeeding mothers.
- NSAIDs and low-dose steroids are considered safe for breastfeeding mothers.

Possible lines of questioning

1. What is your impression of the activity of *this* patient's disease?
2. Has he or she a good understanding of the side-effects of these disease-modifying drugs?
3. How severely affected is *this* patient's mobility?
4. Would you recommend changes to drug or other treatment for *this* patient?
5. What is the history of steroid use for *this* patient?
6. Is there evidence of osteoporosis?

Osteoarthritis

This common problem will affect many long-case patients. It may not be the main medical problem, but it may be one that affects the patient's life severely. It affects 80% of people over 55 years of age, and 95% of people over 65. Osteoarthritis is associated with obesity and diabetes (Table 9.10) and may be one of the reasons a patient cannot exercise and lose weight. It should be possible from the history and examination to distinguish this from an inflammatory arthritis, although many patients may have both.

Osteoarthritis involves synovial joints. Weight-bearing joints (the hip and the knee) and the proximal interphalangeal (PIP) and distal interphalangeal (DIP) joints of the hands and the first MTP joint of the foot are most often affected (Fig. 9.5). There is usually loss of articular cartilage, meniscal damage, laxity of surrounding ligaments, formation of osteophytes and changes to subchondral bone.

Generalised nodal OA is particularly common in women and is characterised by the presence of Heberden's (DIP) and Bouchard's (PIP) nodes. These are posterolateral swellings on the sides of the finger extensor tendons. They gradually harden. There is often a period when the nodes are developing when the joints are painful, but this usually resolves and hand function remains preserved. The condition is genetic. A woman has a 1 in 3 chance of developing the condition if her mother has been affected. The characteristics of the condition are set out in Box 9.2.

Table 9.10 Risk factors for osteoarthritis
• Family history and genetics – especially knee and hip
• Developmental problems: hip dysplasia, slipped femoral epiphysis
• Repetitive loading: athletes, manual workers, squatting (knee arthritis in Indian and Asian populations)
• Biomechanical problems: Paget's disease, ligament rupture, meniscectomy
• Obesity (mechanical and possibly related to release of cytokines from adipose tissue)
• Trauma
• Hormonal: aromatase inhibitors, oestrogen deficiency

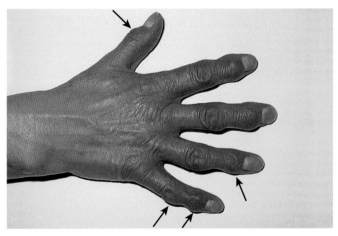

Figure 9.5 **Osteoarthritis of the hand.**

A Stevens, J S Lowe and I Scott. *Core pathology*, 3rd edn. Fig. 24.17. Elsevier Ltd, 2009, with permission.

Box 9.2 Generalised nodal osteoarthritis

- Interphalangeal joints affected
- Heberden's and Bouchard's nodes
- Joints enlarged, owing to osteophyte formation
- Onset in middle age
- Women more often affected
- Usually good eventual function of hands
- Increased risk of osteoarthritis of other joints, e.g. knees

---

Box 9.3 Examination findings – osteoarthritis of the hip

- Antalgic gait (to avoid pain: spends less time in stance phase)
- Gluteal and quadriceps wasting
- Restriction and pain on internal rotation of the hip when it is flexed; this is the earliest and most sensitive finding
- Later all movements are restricted and there may be fixed flexion and external rotation deformity.
- Tenderness of the anterior part of the groin lateral to the femoral pulse
- Ipsilateral leg shortening may occur when the femoral head has migrated and there is severe joint space loss

---

KNEE OA

Arthritis begins in the patella–femoral and medial–tibiofemoral compartments and spreads to involve the whole knee. Patients feel pain in the medal or anterior aspect of the knee and down into the tibia, especially when they walk up or down stairs, or get out of a chair or car. Bending to put on shoes can be difficult. Posterior knee pain suggests a complicating Baker's cyst.

HIP OA

The superior aspect of the joint is most often affected. It is quite often unilateral. Migration of the femoral head in a superolateral direction may occur and indicates a poor prognosis. Medial OA of the joint is less common, has a better prognosis, is usually bilateral and more often affects women.

Hip pain is usually felt deep in the anterior part of the groin. Radiation to the anterolateral thigh, the knee, shin or buttock is variable. Secondary trochanteric bursitis may occur and is suggested by lateral pain, worse when the patient lies on that side. The same activities that exacerbate knee pain affect the hip. The common examination findings are shown in Box 9.3.

OA OF THE SPINE

The cervical and lumbar areas of the spine are most involved (cervical and lumbar spondylosis). Pain is felt in the lower back or neck but can radiate to the arms, buttocks or legs if nerve root compression has occurred. Pain is better after rest and worse with movement. There may be reduced movement of the spine and loss of lumbar lordosis. The straight leg-raising test may be abnormal. Neurological signs may be present in the arms and legs.

Box 9.4 Causes of early-onset osteoarthritis

Localised
- Previous trauma

Poly or pauciarticular
- Juvenile arthritis
- Haemochromatosis
- Acromegaly
- Ochronosis
- Avascular necrosis
- Charcot's joint
- Spondylo-epiphyseal dysplasia

The history

Ask:
1. How long has the arthritis been a problem? (See Box 9.4.)
2. Has there been swelling or inflammation of the joints (suggesting an inflammatory arthritis rather than osteoarthritis)?
3. What joints have been involved? – the DIP, shoulders, hips, knees and proximal MCP joints are often affected.
4. Are the joints stiff in the morning? – patients with osteoarthritis do not have much morning stiffness.
5. Is there a family history?
6. Have there been injuries to the joints (e.g. from playing sport)?
7. Has the patient been able to lose weight?
8. What limitations are there with respect to mobility and exercise?
9. Are walking sticks or frames needed?
10. How does the patient manage around the house – ADLs, etc.?
11. Is he or she able to drive or work?
12. What treatment has been tried – drug treatment, joint injections, exercise and physiotherapy, alternative treatments, surgery, weight loss?
13. What drugs have been used?
14. Have there been side-effects, especially from NSAIDs?
15. Have these treatments helped?

The examination (Box 9.5)
1. Examine the joints that have been giving the patient problems.
2. Look for deformity, loss of range of movement, ligamentous laxity, scars from previous surgery, and joint pain on movement.
3. Test joint function (e.g. by getting the patient to walk, use their hands, etc.).
4. Look at the effectiveness of walking aids.

Management

NON-PHARMACOLOGICAL

Many treatments will probably have been tried, but consider:
1. exercise:
   a. stretching and mobility exercises can help maintain joint range of motion
   b. aquatic exercise may be possible for patients with severe restriction

---

Box 9.5 Examination findings – osteoarthritis of the knees

- Jerky, antalgic gait, favouring worse side
- Varus or sometimes valgus deformity
- Weakness and wasting of quadriceps
- Joint-line or periarticular tenderness
- Flexion and extension reduced
- Joint crepitus
- Bony swelling around the joint line

---

    c. an exercise bicycle so that exercise is not weight-bearing

    d. supervised or group exercise works better for reduction of pain than independent exercise at home

2. use of mobility aids:

    a. a stick used in the opposite hand

    b. knee braces and foot orthoses

3. loss of weight – this is the most important modifiable risk factor for osteoarthritis. A 10% loss of weight achieved by diet and exercise has been shown to reduce symptoms by 50%.

DRUG TREATMENT

1. **NSAIDs** are the usual first-line treatment. They are probably somewhat more effective than paracetamol, but at the expense of their well-known gastrointestinal and cardiovascular side-effects. Using a proton pump inhibitor with a NSAID reduces GI bleeding risk in older patients (≥ 60 years) or those with a history of peptic ulcer. There is no good information about the optimal duration of treatment.

2. **Paracetamol** (up to 4 g/day) has been a common choice for osteoarthritis because of concerns about NSAID side-effects. There is not much evidence, however, that it is more effective than placebo, especially for knee pain, and there have been concerns about acute liver failure with large doses (> 4 g daily).

3. **Topical NSAIDs** have been shown to be useful for knee and hand arthritis and seem safer than oral NSAIDs. Topical capsaicin can be a useful adjunct.

4. **Intra-articular injections of steroids** give 1–2 weeks of relief and improve mobility. They are useful for acute exacerbations. Frequent use can cause cartilage and joint damage and involve some risk of infection.

5. **Opioids** can be given topically or orally and are more effective than placebo for knee arthritis, but the benefits are modest. Their use is associated with more adverse events than is the case with NSAIDs. These include cardiovascular events, fractures and an increased mortality.

6. **Duloxetine** is a centrally acting serotonin reuptake inhibitor. It has been shown to be superior to placebo and can be used in combination with NSAIDs.

SURGERY

Joint replacement can be very helpful when other treatment has failed. Arthroscopic procedures have not been shown to be effective for knee arthritis beyond what medical treatment can achieve.

COMPLEMENTARY MEDICINES

1. The most commonly used of these drugs is glucosamine. It seems no more effective than placebo in controlled trials.

2. Fish oil and chondroitin have similarly failed to show advantages over placebo for knee pain.

Possible lines of questioning

1. How would you manage *this* obese patient with severe osteoarthritis of the knees?
2. What would you advise *this* woman with hip arthritis and a history of ischaemic heart disease about the use of NSAIDs? Is aspirin use a problem?
3. How would you assess *this* patient's surgical risk and likely postoperative course for knee replacement surgery?

Ankylosing spondylitis (spondyloarthritis, SPA)

Patients with this chronic condition are more commonly seen as short cases, but the problem may form part of a long-case patient's problems.

The classification of this group of diseases is in a state of flux. The term axial spondyloarthropathy now includes:

- ankylosing spondylitis
- reactive arthritis and sexually acquired reactive arthritis (SARA)
- psoriatic arthritis and spondylitis
- enteropathic arthritis and spondylitis
- juvenile-onset spondyloarthritis.

The axial skeleton, peripheral joints and extra-articular structures are affected (Fig. 9.6).

In some populations, 90% of patients are HLA-B27 positive. Between 1% and 6% of people with HLA-B27 have the disease.

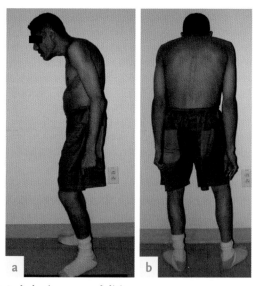

Figure 9.6 **(a and b) Ankylosing spondylitis.**

H N Herkowitz, S R Garfin, F J Eismont et al. *Rothman-Simeone the spine,* 6th edn. Fig. 35.1. Saunders, Elsevier, 2011, with permission.

Ankylosing spondylitis is diagnosed when sacroiliitis is present on X ray in a patient with other features of axial spondyloarthritis.

It affects men two to three times as often as women and rarely begins after the age of 45 – the median age of diagnosis is 23.

The history

The patient will be likely to know the diagnosis. Ask:

1. The age of diagnosis and symptoms leading up to the diagnosis:
   - Lower aching back pain with some hours of morning stiffness is common. Pain tends to occur over the lower back, buttocks and posterior thighs.
   - Nocturnal exacerbation is often a feature of ankylosing spondylitis.
   - There may be tenderness over bony processes including the spinous processes, ischial tuberosities, iliac crests, greater trochanters, costochondral junctions and heels.
   - Thirty per cent of patients develop hip and shoulder pain.
   - Asymmetrical peripheral joint involvement occurs in a similar proportion.
2. How was the diagnosis made – X-rays, MRI, or HLA assessment (see Table 9.11)?
3. What treatment has been used? Find out:
   - which drugs, if any, have been used
   - whether they have helped with symptoms
   - whether the patient knows if radiological and serological test results have improved
   - whether there have been problems with side-effects (see Table 9.6)
   - whether joint surgery has been required (e.g. hip replacement)
   - whether other manifestations of the disease required treatment (e.g. uveitis and topical steroids).
4. How has this debilitating disease affected the patient's ability to work, exercise and perform ADLs? What symptoms are present at the moment? How limited is the patient by these?
5. How is the treatment being monitored?
6. Have there been features of reactive arthritis – urethritis, conjunctivitis?
7. Has the patient any psoriasis?
8. Has there been a diagnosis of inflammatory bowel disease?

Table 9.11 Diagnosis of axial spondyloarthritis (SPA)
1. Age less than 45
2. ≥ 3 months of back pain
3. HLA-B27 plus two or more of:
• inflammatory back pain
• heel pain (enthesitis)
• uveitis
• dactylitis (diffuse swelling of digits – toes or fingers)
• inflammatory bowel disease
• family history of SPA or HLA-B27
• elevated CRP
• response to NSAIDs
4. Sacroiliitis on X-ray or MRI[a]
[a]MRI shows three or more corner inflammatory lesions in two slices or more.
CRP = C-reactive protein.

9. Has there been testing for HIV infection? Reactive arthritis and psoriatic arthritis exacerbations are associated with HIV infection.
10. Were the symptoms preceded by gastrointestinal or genitourinary infections? Reactive arthritis is often preceded by such infections.
11. The extra-articular manifestations include:
    - uveitis (40%)
    - fatigue and anaemia
    - prostatitis and sterile urethritis
    - aortic regurgitation (20%)
    - osteoporosis
    - symptoms of cauda equina syndrome (late)
    - upper lobe interstitial lung disease (late and rare).

Diagnosis

Persistent back pain in a young person that is worse at night should suggest the diagnosis. The presence of associated features and raised inflammatory markers makes the diagnosis more likely (Table 9.11). The most important differential diagnosis is malignancy.

Find out whether the patient knows the results of any of these investigations.

The examination

Examine the patient as set out for the short-case ankylosing spondylitis (p. 513).

Management

1. An exercise program is usually recommended to help the patient maintain flexibility.
2. Non-steroidal anti-inflammatories have been shown to relieve symptoms and slow radiographic progression.
3. For the many patients who progress despite this treatment, anti-TNF-α treatment with infliximab or etanercept has been very successful in improving symptoms and markers of disease activity. Even patients with severe deformity have obtained improvement. The doses used are similar to those used for rheumatoid arthritis.
4. Find out what drugs have been used, whether they helped symptoms, any side-effects, if joint surgery is being considered, and how the disease is affecting the patient's life (and family).

Possible lines of questioning

1. What precautions and advice would you give *this* patient before starting anti-TNF-α treatment?
2. What is your assessment of *this* patient's functional state?

Systemic lupus erythematosus

This multisystem disorder occurs usually in patients between 20 and 40 years of age.
- Women are more often affected than men (8 : 1) and there is an increased incidence in families (monozygotic twins have a 50% concordance).
- There are associations with HLA-DR2, with HLA-DR3, and with homozygous deficiencies of the early components of complement.

Table 9.12 American Rheumatism Association criteria for SLE

1. Malar rash – sparing the nasolabial folds
2. Discoid rash
3. Photosensitivity rash
4. Oral ulcers
5. Arthritis – non-erosive and affecting two or more peripheral joints
6. Serositis – pleurisy or pericarditis, with audible rub, effusion or ECG changes
7. Renal disorder – persistent proteinuria > 0.5 g / day or cellular casts
8. Neurological disorder – seizures or psychosis not related to drugs or metabolic abnormalities
9. Haematological disorder – haemolytic anaemia, leukopenia (< 4000 / µL), lymphopenia (< 2000 / µL), thrombocytopenia (< 100,000 / µL)
10. Immunological disorder – anti-DNA antibodies in abnormal titre, or anti-Smith (anti-Sm) antibody, or positive antiphospholipid antibodies
11. Antinuclear antibody disorder – abnormal ANA titre > 1 : 160

Note: Four or more manifestations of the 11 must be present serially or simultaneously.

ANA = antinuclear antibody; SLE = systemic lupus erythematosus.

- It presents diagnostic as well as long-term management problems. The diagnosis requires at least four of the 11 published criteria either currently or in the past (Table 9.12). Fewer than four criteria are often labelled 'possible lupus'. Non-specific positive autoimmune tests with some evidence of inflammation can be referred to as 'undifferentiated connective tissue disease'.

HINT

A weakly positive ANA test (see below) is very common and should not be used to make a diagnosis of lupus (but it often is, so be careful about accepting the label).

The history

1. Ask about the presenting symptoms (Table 9.13):
   a. general symptoms – malaise (nearly all patients), weight loss (60%), nausea and vomiting (50%), thrombosis of veins or arteries (15%)
   b. musculoskeletal symptoms (95%) – arthralgia, arthritis (typically symmetrical and non-erosive), myalgia and myositis
   c. dermatological symptoms (85%) – skin rash, alopecia, oral and nasal ulcers
   d. fever (77%)
   e. neuropsychiatric symptoms (60%) – delirium, dementia, convulsions, chorea, neuropathy, loss of vision (optic neuritis), stroke, headache, symptoms resembling multiple sclerosis, anxiety and depression
   f. renal tract symptoms (50%) – haematuria, oedema, chronic kidney disease (just about any type of glomerulonephritis)
   g. respiratory tract symptoms (45%) – pleurisy
   h. cardiovascular symptoms (40%) – pericarditis, myocarditis, valvular lesions, premature coronary artery disease (increased atherosclerosis)
   i. haematological symptoms (50%) – lymphadenopathy, anaemia
   j. gastrointestinal symptoms (30%) – nausea, diarrhoea, intestinal pseudo-obstruction, perforation

Table 9.13 Summary of systems review for SLE	
1. Apthous ulcers	6. Dry eyes and mouth
2. Serositis	7. Thrombosis
3. Raynaud's	8. Miscarriages
4. Alopecia	9. Nephritis
5. Photosensitivity rashes	
SLE = systemic lupus erythematosus.	

Table 9.14 Drugs inducing SLE
1. Procainamide (most patients are ANA positive within 1 year; 15%–20% develop SLE)
2. Hydralazine (most patients are ANA positive within 1 year; 5%–10% develop SLE)
3. Isoniazid[a]
4. Methyldopa[a]
5. Penicillamine[a]
6. Chlorpromazine[a]
7. Anticonvulsants[a] particularly phenytoin (not sodium valproate)
Note: There is an increased incidence of drug-induced lupus in slow acetylators who will develop a positive ANA and clinical manifestations sooner than rapid acetylators. Drug-induced lupus is more common in the elderly because of the more frequent use of drugs in this group. There is usually no renal or nervous system disease, no antibody to dsDNA and improvement may occur if the drug is withdrawn.
[a]Rarely cause overt SLE, but ANA is commonly positive.
ANA = antinuclear antibody; SLE = systemic lupus erythematosus.

    k. thrombophlebitis, recurrent abortions or fetal death in utero (suggests antiphospholipid syndrome)
    l. sicca symptoms (secondary to Sjögren's syndrome)
    m. difficulties with activities of daily living and ability to work as a result of the effect of this chronic and relapsing disease on the patient's life.

2. Ask about any drug history (e.g. procainamide, hydralazine – causes of an SLE-like syndrome) (Table 9.14). Remember, newer antiarrhythmic and antihypertensive drugs have made classical drug-induced lupus less common and typically the symptoms resolve rapidly with cessation of the drug; autoantibody levels (anti-histone) diminish slowly. Anti-TNF drugs can also cause a lupus-like syndrome with a positive ANA and anti-double-stranded DNA (anti-dsDNA); minocycline and hydralazine do this too, but with these drugs ANCA (antineutrophil cytoplasmic antibody) is positive as well.

3. Ask about any treatment given and any complications of treatment.

4. Ask about problems during pregnancy and use of contraception. Pregnancy is especially risky if the disease is active. Progesterone or low-dose oestrogen contraception is advisable.

5. Ask about protection from sunlight. This reduces the risk of photosensitivity rashes and flares of systemic disease.

6. Enquire about the family history.

7. Enquire about the patient's understanding of the implications of this chronic and incurable disease and its prognosis. Remember, though, that current treatment allows a 90% 10-year survival rate compared with 50% 30 years ago.

The examination (Table 9.15)

1. Inspect the patient for weight loss and Cushingoid appearance (because of steroid treatment) and assess the patient's general mental state.
2. Examine all the skin for a classical malar rash (Fig. 9.7), a discoid erythematous raised rash (Fig. 9.8) or a photosensitivity rash.

   Remember that discoid lupus erythematosus (DLE) occurs in 20% of SLE patients. This disfiguring skin disease leads to permanent hair loss with telangiectasia, scaling,

Table 9.15 Systemic lupus erythematosus (SLE)	
1. GENERAL INSPECTION Cushingoid Weight Mental state **2. HANDS** Vasculitis Rash Arthropathy (symmetric polyarthritis) **3. ARMS** Livedo reticularis Purpura Proximal myopathy (SLE, steroids) **4. HEAD** Alopecia, lupus hairs Eyes – scleritis, cytoid lesions, etc. Mouth – ulcers (painless), infection Rash (e.g. butterfly) – spares the nasolabial folds Cranial nerve lesions Cervical adenopathy	**5. CHEST** Cardiovascular system – endocarditis Respiratory system – pleural effusion, pleurisy, pulmonary fibrosis, collapse or infection **6. ABDOMEN** Hepatosplenomegaly **7. HIPS** Aseptic necrosis **8. LEGS** Feet – small joint synovitis Rash Proximal myopathy Cerebellar ataxia Neuropathy (uncommon) Mononeuritis multiplex **9. OTHER** Urine analysis (proteinuria) Blood pressure (hypertension) Temperature chart

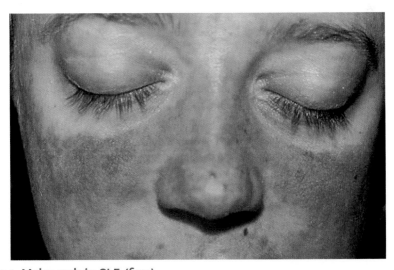

Figure 9.7 **Malar rash in SLE (face).**

B J Beck. Mental disorders due to a general medical condition. *Comprehensive clinical psychiatry.* Ch 21:257–81. On-line Archives of Rheumatology, 2008, with permission.

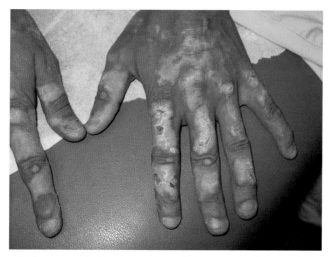

Figure 9.8 Discoid lupus rash. Note sparing of the proximal interphalangeal joints, a typical SLE feature.

M Dall'Era. *Kelley's textbook of rheumatology.* Saunders, Elsevier, 2013, with permission.

circular erythematous lesions and follicular plugging. There is often destruction of skin appendages. DLE can occur without other features of SLE.

3. Look at the hands for vasculitis, which can produce nail-fold infarcts and ischaemia or gangrene, and rash (e.g. photosensitivity, diffuse maculopapular rash).

4. Look for Raynaud's phenomenon and arthropathy (fusiform swelling of the PIP joints or synovitis, possibly in a rheumatoid arthritis distribution – 10% develop swan-neck deformity and ulnar deviation of the fingers). This non-erosive arthropathy is referred to as Jaccoud's arthritis.

5. Look at the forearms for livedo reticularis and purpura as a result of vasculitis or thrombocytopenia. Test for proximal myopathy caused by actual disease or secondary to steroid treatment.

6. Inspect the head. Look for alopecia. Lupus hairs are characteristic: they occur above the forehead and are short, broken hairs that grow back quickly after hair loss (except in patients with DLE).

7. Look at the eyes for keratoconjunctivitis sicca and for pale conjunctivae due to anaemia, and look at the fundi for cytoid lesions (hard exudates secondary to vasculitis) (Fig. 9.9).

8. Look in the mouth for ulcers and infection. Note any facial rash (butterfly photosensitivity rash (30%), discoid lupus or diffuse maculopapular rashes). Feel the cervical and axillary nodes.

9. Examine the chest. In the cardiovascular system, note signs of pericarditis or murmurs. (Libman–Sacks endocarditis is a very uncommon cause of clinical signs.)

10. In the respiratory system, note signs of pleural effusion, pleuritis, interstitial lung disease or atelectasis.

11. Examine the abdomen for splenomegaly (usually mild) and hepatomegaly. Feel for abdominal tenderness.

12. Examine the hips for signs of aseptic necrosis.

13. Examine for proximal weakness in the legs, cerebellar ataxia, hemiplegia and transverse myelitis. Assess mental status (cognitive changes, even psychosis).

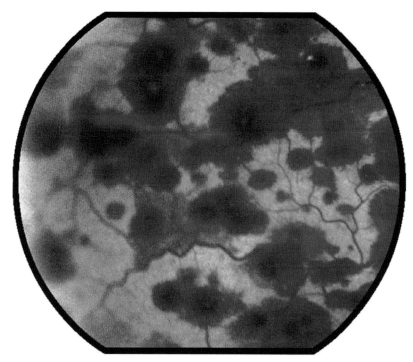

Figure 9.9 **Cytoid lesions in fundi. This patient also has a haemorrhagic fundus from SLE.**

L Yannuzzi. *The retinal atlas.* Ch 6. Elsevier 2010, with permission.

14. Also examine for neuropathy (mainly sensory) and mononeuritis multiplex, as well as thrombophlebitis and leg ulceration.
15. Look at the urine analysis for evidence of renal disease (haematuria and proteinuria).
16. Take the blood pressure (it may be elevated in renal disease). Also, look at the temperature chart for fever, indicating active disease or secondary infection.

Investigations

1. Diagnosis depends on a combination of the symptoms, signs and laboratory test results (see Tables 9.12 and 9.16). Almost all cases are ANA positive, which is a very sensitive but not specific test (if ANA is negative, check for Sjögren's syndrome A/B (SSA/SSB) antibodies). Very specific tests for SLE are anti-dsDNA (including titre, 100% specific) and anti-Smith (anti-Sm – positive virtually only in SLE).
2. Patients who do not fit the criteria may have another connective tissue disease. Mixed connective tissue disease (MCTD) is suggested by the overlapping clinical features of scleroderma, polymyositis and SLE and the presence of characteristic antibodies to nuclear ribonucleoprotein (nRNP), which is one of the extractable nuclear antigens. Anti-nRNP is present in high titre and produces a speckled pattern on fluorescent antibody testing in patients with MCTD. When these patients are followed for many years, they may start to resemble patients with progressive systemic sclerosis or SLE, or may continue with a relatively undifferentiated connective tissue disease.

HINTS

Features of mixed connective tissue disease include:
1. Overlapping features of SLE, polymyositis and systemic sclerosis
2. High titre of anti-U1-RNP antibodies
3. Pericardial effusion
4. Raynaud's, swollen hands, fatigue and arthritis
5. Pulmonary arterial hypertension (PAH) is main cause of death
6. Treat symptoms with steroids, antimalarials, NSAIDs and immunosuppression (cyclophosphamide for PAH)

Table 9.16 Antibodies associated with connective tissue and other autoimmune diseases

DISEASE	ANTIBODIES ASSOCIATED
Systemic lupus erythematosus	Anti-single-stranded DNA (anti-ssDNA) – not specific (useless!)
	Anti-dsDNA (70%) – high titres are specific
	Anti-Sm (30%) – specific for lupus
	Anti-RNP (30% in low titre) – high titre in MCTD
	Anti-Ro-SS-A (30%) – associated with primary Sjögren's syndrome, congenital heart block; can cause nephritis
	Anti-SS-B (15%) – associated with Sjögren's syndrome
	Antihistone (drug-induced SLE usually from hydralazine, or procainamide; 95%)
	Antiphospholipid (50%) – include anticardiolipin and lupus anticoagulant
	Antierythrocyte (60%) – occasionally causes anaemia
	Antilymphocyte (70%) – possible leukopenia
Systemic sclerosis	Anticentromere (lcSSc: 70%)
	Antinucleolar, anti-Scl-70 (dcSSc; ILD 30%)
	Anti-RNP, anti-SS-A (dcSSc, PAH, myositis)
	Antinuclear antigen (90%)
	Anti-PM-Scl (myositis)
	Anti-Th/To (lcSSc, PAH)
Sjögren's syndrome	Anti-SS-A (70%), anti-SS-B (60%)
MCTD	Anti-U1-RNP (100%)
Polymyositis and dermatomyositis	Anti-Jo-1 (polymyositis: 30%; dermatomyositis: 30%)
	Anti-Mi2 (10% dermatomyositis)
	Anti-SRP (aggressive disease)
Granulomatosis with polyangiitis (GPA)	Proteinase 3 ANCA (90% sensitivity and specificity)
Goodpasture's	Glomerular basement membrane (90% sensitivity and specificity)
Graves disease	TSH-receptor (sensitivity 80%, specificity 95%)
Idiopathic thrombocytopenic purpura (ITP)	GpIIb/IIIa (sensitivity 80%, specificity 90%)
Primary biliary cholangitis	Anti-mitochondrial (sensitivity 90%, specificity > 90%)

ANCA = antineutrophil cytoplasmic antibody; dcSSc = diffuse cutaneous systemic sclerosis; ILD = interstitial lung disease; lcSSc = limited cutaneous systemic sclerosis; MCTD = mixed connective tissue disease; PAH = pulmonary arterial hypertension; RNP = ribonucleoprotein; Sm = Smith; SRP = signal recognition protein; TSH = thyroid-stimulating hormone.

3. MRI scans and lumbar puncture (increased protein and mononuclear cells) may be indicated if central nervous system lupus is suspected. Central nervous system symptoms often correlate poorly with serological measures of the activity of the disease. Do not miss bacterial meningitis in SLE.

4. Haematological tests:
   a. Anaemia – normochromic, normocytic and related to the chronic inflammatory processes – is very common. Immune haemolytic anaemia is less common and the Coombs' test then gives a positive result.
   b. The ESR tends to be elevated but the CRP is often normal, except during episodes of serositis.
   c. Leukopenia (especially lymphopenia) occurs in over half the patients and may be caused by antibody directed against leukocytes.
   d. The lupus anticoagulant and anticardiolipin antibodies, or both, are found in about 10% of cases. Characteristically, there is a prolonged partial thromboplastin time with kaolin (PTTK), which is not corrected by the addition of normal plasma. It is associated with thrombosis rather than bleeding.
   e. Thrombocytopenia occurs in 15% of cases and is associated with anti-platelet antibodies.

5. Immunological tests:
   a. The characteristic abnormalities are the presence of autoantibodies (see Table 9.16). ANAs are present in 99% of cases and are usually detectable from the time of onset of symptoms. The antigens involved include ssDNA and dsDNA, SSA and SSB, and Sm antigen (an acidic nuclear protein). Many antibodies persist even when the disease is quiescent. Antibodies to dsDNA and Sm are the most specific for SLE and are therefore the most useful diagnostically. The latter, however, is not very sensitive.
   b. Complement abnormalities are usual during exacerbations of the disease, with a reduction in total haemolytic complement (CH50) and in the components of the classical pathway (C3 and C4). The combination of a low CH50 and normal C3 suggests an inherited deficiency of complement components and is strongly associated with SLE. The finding of high levels of anti-dsDNA and lower complement levels is usually associated with active disease and especially renal involvement.
   c. Positive RF occurs in 10% of cases at low titre. Skin biopsy in SLE can be helpful; positive immunofluorescence of the basement membrane in involved skin occurs in 95% of patients.

Treatment

Current work suggests that appropriate treatment to suppress exacerbations of SLE will prolong life. Many patients have mild disease without life-threatening complications. The prognosis of SLE is generally good. There is a 90% 10-year survival rate; the major causes of death are infections, renal failure, lymphoma and myocardial infarction.

1. Arthralgias, myalgia and fever respond to rest and NSAIDs.
2. Exposure to sunlight should be avoided and sunscreen used.
3. Hydroxychloroquine is very effective for skin and joint manifestations, reduces the risk of renal involvement and improves survival. Annual retinal and visual field examinations must be performed in patients on this drug because of the cumulative risk of retinal toxicity. Although it is a category D drug, it is often used in pregnancy, where its benefits outweigh the risks.
4. Raynaud's phenomenon may respond to calcium channel antagonists.
5. Steroids are indicated for central nervous system involvement, pericarditis, myocarditis, pleurisy, severe haemolytic anaemia and thrombocytopenia. Use of high initial doses

with gradual reduction once improvement occurs is the proper method of treatment.

6. Hypercoagulability (thrombotic episodes and antiphospholipid antibodies) should be treated with warfarin for life, with a target INR of 2.5–3.

7. Management of renal disease is difficult. Renal biopsy usually shows abnormalities, but often only mild changes. Virtually any type of glomerulonephritis may occur. Renal biopsy is indicated early on if there is any clinical or biochemical evidence of renal disease or if the urine sediment is abnormal. Four main groups of biopsy abnormalities can be identified:
   - mesangial proliferation
   - focal glomerulonephritis
   - diffuse proliferation
   - membranous proliferation.

   Mesangial proliferation has the best prognosis – disease is unlikely to progress. Diffuse proliferative glomerulonephritis has the worst prognosis and aggressive treatment (e.g. high-dose pulse steroids plus cyclophosphamide) is recommended. Membranous proliferation has a low rate of response to treatment. SLE is not a contraindication to dialysis or renal transplant in those patients who develop chronic kidney disease, but there is a higher than average risk of graft failure.

8. Calcium and vitamin D supplements should be offered to protect against osteoporosis. Bisphosphonates should be considered if long-term steroid treatment is likely.

9. Azathioprine is indicated as a steroid-sparing agent. Methotrexate can also be used, particularly if arthritis is prominent.

   Cyclophosphamide is a more toxic alternative. Intermittent pulses of cyclophosphamide may be helpful. These agents are particularly indicated in active glomerulonephritis.

10. Mycophenolate is now accepted in treatment guidelines as a less toxic alternative to cyclophosphamide in the treatment of renal lupus. A number of new biological agents are being tested in clinical trials. Autologous stem cell transplant is also an experimental treatment.

11. Anti-B cell treatment has been used for SLE. Rituximab and belimumab have shown modest efficacy. They are currently available under special access schemes. A few patients have a dramatic response to these drugs.

12. Exacerbations of lupus may occur in pregnancy and postpartum.
   - Hydroxychloroquine should be continued throughout pregnancy as there are better outcomes for mother and baby.
   - Spontaneous abortions are common in women with antiphospholipid antibodies. Treatment with anticoagulation (heparin plus low-dose aspirin – never prescribe warfarin) may be effective in reducing the risk of abortion.
   - Steroids may be used in pregnancy because, except for dexamethasone, these do not cross the placenta.
   - Women with the anti-Ro (SSA/SSB) antibody may have babies with permanent complete heart block and transient erythematous rashes.
   - Cervical dysplasia is common and women younger than 26 years should be offered human papilloma virus vaccine.

13. Improved survival has meant that cardiovascular complications are now the most common cause of death. This is probably due to the chronic inflammation associated with the disease. Aggressive control of cardiovascular risk factors and particularly avoidance of smoking is very important.

   The risk of lymphoma is also increased and screening may be indicated.

Systemic vasculitis

Patients with a systemic vasculitic illness will often be used for the long-case examination because of the complex nature of these illnesses and the frequent need for hospital admission. The fact that these illnesses tend to affect multiple body systems across numerous specialties is ideal for testing candidates' general approach to internal medicine. The majority of cases seen in the examination will have a vasculitis such as granulomatosis with polyangiitis (Wegener's granulomatosis), giant cell arteritis or polyarteritis nodosa. Occasionally, less common adult vasculitides, such as eosinophilic granulomatosis with polyangiitis (EGPA) (Churg–Strauss syndrome) or microscopic polyarteritis, will be encountered.

The long-case examination for the patient with systemic vasculitis requires the candidate to take a careful history and examine the patient in a thorough general manner, as well as to look for specific abnormalities in each disease. Candidates will be expected to have a good knowledge of the various investigative tools available to diagnose vasculitis. The course of treatment will invariably be discussed in this type of case, particularly the side-effects of long-term medications and likely prognosis.

The history

In most cases, the onset of a systemic vasculitic illness is subacute rather than acute. The patient has often seen several practitioners before a diagnosis is made. The history will be critical in determining the diagnosis if the patient has a systemic vasculitis and presents a diagnostic problem, or indeed if the diagnosis is clear and there are significant management problems.

1. First, ask about the systemic features that would suggest a vasculitic illness: fatigue, malaise, fever, myalgia and arthralgia will be very frequent in these patients. Ask about vasculitic skin rash, which would normally be in the form of palpable purpura. Ask about the pattern of joint involvement.
2. Next, ask about a history of renal disease, particularly hypertension or chronic kidney disease, and any gastrointestinal symptoms.

THE HISTORY TYPICAL OF IMPORTANT VASCULITIDES

1. **Granulomatosis with polyangiitis (GPA)** – the new name for Wegener's granulomatosis (small or medium-sized vessel inflammation causing a pulmonary–renal syndrome): the upper and lower respiratory tract are almost invariably involved and frequent symptoms include:
   - nasal congestion and sinusitis
   - rhinorrhoea

- bloody nasal discharge
- cough (which is initially a dry cough, but may evolve into haemoptysis)
- breathlessness.

2. **Giant cell arteritis:** patients are generally in the sixth–eighth decade of life. About 20% of patients with polymyalgia rheumatica develop giant cell arteritis. The usual specific symptoms are:
   - severe bitemporal headache
   - less commonly, visual disturbance (e.g. diplopia) or visual loss
   - jaw claudication (quite specific), scalp tenderness or occasionally tongue claudication. Other focal neurological symptoms can also occur.

3. **Polyarteritis nodosa** (medium-sized arteries): the specific symptoms depend on which arteries are involved – coronary arteries, mesenteric arteries or renal arteries. Suspect this possibility if there are multiple systems involved (e.g. foot drop – vasculitis of the vasa nervorum – with chest and abdominal pain). Skin changes include ulceration, palpable purpura and infarction. Severe hypertension may result from renal involvement. Ask about risk factors for hepatitis B (recently acquired in one-third of cases). The peak incidence is between 40 and 50 years and men are twice as often affected as women.

4. **Eosinophilic granulomatosis with polyangiitis (EGPA)** (small vessels causing a pulmonary–renal syndrome): this is the new name for Churg–Strauss vasculitis; patients almost invariably have asthma first, then a peripheral eosinophilia. Ask about a previous history of:
   - asthma
   - allergic rhinitis, nasal polyps
   - eczema
   - cough and breathlessness
   - peripheral nervous system disease, in the form of either symmetrical peripheral neuropathy or mononeuritis multiplex
   - serositis leading to pleural and pericardial effusions.

5. **Microscopic polyarteritis (polyangiitis)** (small vessels causing a pulmonary–renal syndrome): the major problem is usually with renal impairment and lung disease, which may not have any specific symptoms. Systemic symptoms of vasculitis are generally very prominent.

6. **Mixed essential cryoglobulinaemia** (small vessels are affected – due to rheumatoid factor bound to IgG): patients present with:
   - palpable purpura of the extremities
   - Raynaud's disease
   - arthritis
   - neuropathy.

   Hepatitis C is common.

The examination

1. The patient with systemic vasculitis usually looks unwell. Check for fever, sinus tachycardia, pallor and signs of recent weight loss.
2. Look for livedo reticularis (a net-like pattern – Fig. 9.10). The differential diagnosis includes cholesterol atheroembolism after a vascular procedure, antiphospholipid syndrome and vasculitis. Other mimics of vasculitis include atrial myxoma, bacterial endocarditis and thrombotic thrombocytopenic purpura (TTP).
3. Other physical signs will be more specific to the actual underlying illness:
   - **Granulomatosis with polyangiitis:** look for the classical collapse of the nasal septum (a saddle-shaped nose (Fig. 9.11), which also occurs in relapsing polychondritis).

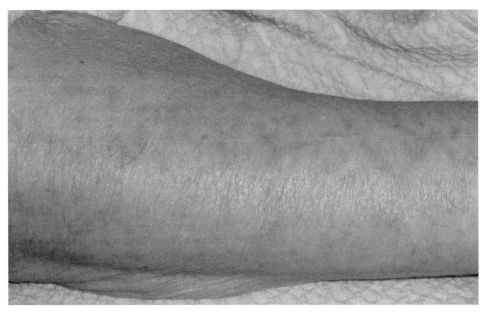

Figure 9.10 Livedo reticularis and erythematous macules of the forearms.

J Dion. Livedo reticularis and erythematous macules of the forearms indicating cutaneous microscopic polyangiitis. *American Journal of Medicine* 2010; 123(11), with permission.

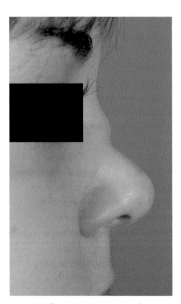

Figure 9.11 Saddle-shaped nose deformity in granulomatosis with polyangiitis (Wegener's granulomatosis).

H S Bennett. Restylane – a temporary alternative for saddle nose deformity in nasal Wegener's granulomatosis – how we do it. *British Journal of Oral and Maxillofacial Surgery* 2010; 49(4), with permission.

There may be evidence of tachypnoea and crackles throughout the lung field. Fluid overload may occur in the setting of worsening chronic kidney disease.

- **Giant cell arteritis:** tender and indurated temporal arteries will often be present. There may be abnormal eye signs if there is retinal involvement. Focal neurological signs should be sought.
- **Polyarteritis nodosa:** there may be evidence of painful skin nodules in rare cases, as well as palpable purpura and livedo reticularis. Look for mononeuritis multiplex.
- **EGPA:** look for signs of allergic disease, such as swollen nasal turbinates, nasal polyps and evidence of bronchospasm. Examine the peripheral nervous system carefully, looking for single nerve lesions or symmetrical peripheral neuropathy generally affecting the lower limbs.
- **Microscopic polyarteritis:** urinalysis is the key – look for any evidence of proteinuria or haematuria.
- **Mixed essential cryoglobulinaemia:** look for Raynaud's disease, palpable purpura and peripheral neuropathy. Assess for signs of liver disease (hepatitis C).

Investigations

Investigations will be critical in determining the diagnosis in systemic vasculitis.

1. In most cases a biopsy of affected tissue is the most reliable way of making the diagnosis; other investigations will raise the suspicion that vasculitis is the problem and direct the clinician to a suitable biopsy site.
2. It will often be necessary to exclude systemic infection, malignancy or generalised autoimmune disease.
3. In vasculitis, the ESR is invariably raised, often at levels of > 70 mm/h. There is frequently a normochromic normocytic anaemia and there may be neutrophilia. The platelet count may be elevated.
4. Renal function will often be impaired in granulomatosis with polyangiitis, polyarteritis nodosa and microscopic polyarteritis.
5. Abnormal liver function tests, particularly elevated transaminase levels, may be found in granulomatosis with polyangiitis and in polyarteritis nodosa. Liver function abnormalities are also reported in giant cell arteritis.
6. Urine abnormalities will often be found in the form of urinary casts and the presence of dysmorphic red blood cells in the urine, particularly in granulomatosis with polyangiitis, microscopic polyarteritis and polyarteritis nodosa.
7. The chest X-ray will often show a bilateral diffuse interstitial abnormality in granulomatosis with polyangiitis (see Fig. 16.31, p. 458) and a peripheral fluffy, patchy infiltrative pattern in EGPA.
8. **Granulomatosis with polyangiitis:** the critical investigation is the antineutrophil cytoplasmic antibody (c-ANCA). This will be present in a vast majority of cases of granulomatosis with polyangiitis. Further testing of this antibody will reveal the presence of anti-pr3 antibodies. The presence of a typical clinical syndrome with a positive c-ANCA and pr3 antibodies is virtually diagnostic of granulomatosis with polyangiitis. The need for a tissue biopsy may be avoided if these tests are positive. Occasionally, patients with upper airways disease only will not have a positive c-ANCA test.
9. **Giant cell arteritis:** diagnosis depends on a positive tissue sample. Treatment with steroids must not be delayed until a biopsy can be performed to make a definite diagnosis (the biopsy can be done within 2 weeks of starting steroids). Temporal artery biopsy should reveal the diagnosis as long as a generous biopsy is taken by the surgeon, but the artery on the other side may need to be sampled in some cases.

SITE	CLINICAL PROBLEM	PREVALENCE (%)
Table 9.17 Clinical findings in patients with polyarteritis nodosa		
Muscles and joints	Myalgia, arthritis	65
Kidneys	Hypertension, renal impairment	60
Gut	Nausea, vomiting, abdominal pain, bowel, liver or pancreatic infarcts	45
Peripheral nervous system	Mononeuritis multiplex, peripheral neuropathy	50
Central nervous system	Strokes and seizures	25
Skin	Purpura, infarcts, Raynaud's phenomenon	40
Heart	Cardiac failure, infarction, pericarditis	35
Genitourinary	Ovarian, testicular pain or infarction	20

10. **Polyarteritis nodosa:** tissue samples are often not available. Many organs may be involved (Table 9.17). If symptoms or signs point this way, a biopsy of nerve, muscle or testis may be diagnostic; renal biopsy is not helpful. CT or MRI angiography is often helpful in this illness, particularly of the mesenteric arteries, hepatic and renal arteries but possibly also of the coronary arteries (CT rather than MRI). Bead-like aneurysmal dilatation of the arteries is suggestive of polyarteritis.

11. **EGPA:** 50% of patients will have a positive perinuclear (p) ANCA test. The other important diagnostic tool is the tissue biopsy, which will reveal intense eosinophilia. Sural nerve biopsy will sometimes be required in the setting of neuropathy and this will show vasculitis.

12. **Microscopic polyarteritis:** this is characterised by a positive p-ANCA result. This antibody is directed against myeloperoxidase. Renal biopsy is usually necessary to establish the diagnosis.

13. p-ANCA is rare in other inflammatory diseases, but common in patients with vasculitis (c-ANCA is specific for granulomatosis with polyangiitis). ANCA titres do not correspond with the clinical severity of the patient's illness and they may be only markers of disease. Remember that p-ANCA tests may be positive, but myeloperoxidase (MPO) negative, in other conditions including inflammatory bowel disease, autoimmune hepatitis and primary sclerosing cholangitis, as well as in healthy individuals (5%).

Treatment

Systemic vasculitis will generally require aggressive immunosuppressive medication. Failure to suppress the vasculitis aggressively can result in permanent injury, progressive deterioration and death.

1. **Granulomatosis with polyangiitis (deadly if untreated):** high-dose corticosteroids and daily oral cyclophosphamide should be instituted. Trimethoprim-sulfamethoxazole is adjunctive therapy. Biological agents are being investigated for treatment of granulomatosis with polyangiitis. Rituximab shows the most promise, but should not be used at this stage unless other agents have failed.

2. **Giant cell arteritis:** high-dose oral corticosteroids are required, typically for 1–2 years.

3. **Polyarteritis nodosa:** the untreated 5-year survival rate is less than 20%. A combination of high-dose prednisone and cyclophosphamide will usually be very effective (90%

long-term remission). Treatment may often be discontinued after remission is obtained and the long-term prognosis is very good. Interferon alpha, or the antiviral drug vidarabine, may help to induce remission if there is associated hepatitis B infection.

4. **EGPA:** the eosinophilic vasculitis of the Churg–Strauss syndrome is generally very steroid responsive, but occasionally other cytotoxic agents need to be used. Steroids alone have been shown to increase the 5-year survival rate from 25% to 50%.

5. **Microscopic polyarteritis:** corticosteroids combined with immunosuppressive agents are usually required, with renal support in patients who develop chronic kidney disease.

6. The duration of treatment for all of these vasculitic illnesses needs to be individualised. Patients with giant cell arteritis can come off treatment after about 2 years, but some have disease for several years. Most of the other diseases will require maintenance therapy.

7. Patients often suffer the effects of long-term steroid therapy and immunosuppression, such as osteoporosis, hypertension, diabetes and accelerated vascular disease. Prevention should be aggressively pursued. Infection (e.g. *Pneumocystis* pneumonia) is common in this group and can be serious or fatal.

8. Patients on cyclophosphamide need careful monitoring of their blood count and careful counselling to ensure adequate fluid intake and avoid haemorrhagic cystitis. They also deserve an annual urinalysis for haematuria once therapy is ceased; haematuria may indicate the development of bladder cancer.

Possible line of questioning

How would you monitor *this* patient for problems with his or her drug treatment?

Antiphospholipid antibody syndrome

Antiphospholipid antibody syndrome is a disease that not infrequently requires patients to be admitted to hospital for its various complications. It may therefore crop up as a long case in the examination. The disease can be either primary or secondary. The secondary form is usually a complication of other autoimmune conditions and vasculitides, the most common of which are SLE and temporal arteritis. The main antibody in this disease is directed against the phospholipid–beta$_2$-glycoprotein 1 complex, on which it exerts a procoagulant effect. It has also been described in HIV infection.

The history

Patients with antiphospholipid antibody syndrome commonly suffer thrombosis (Table 9.18).

1. Ask about venous thromboses. The most common site is the deep lower limb or pelvic veins, but the axillary veins can be involved.

2. Ask about arterial thromboses. Stroke and myocardial infarction are the most common arterial complications.

3. Enquire about a history of recurrent first-trimester and later abortion. Antiphospholipid antibody syndrome is far more common in females and otherwise unexplained first-trimester abortions are characteristic of this disease. Other obstetric complications include intrauterine growth retardation and an increased tendency for hypertension in pregnancy.

Table 9.18 Clinical manifestations of the antiphospholipid antibody syndrome

1. Cardiac – myocardial infarction, valvular heart disease, pulmonary hypertension
2. Haematological – haemolytic anaemia, thrombocytopenia, migraine, epilepsy, transverse myelopathy
3. Renal – renal vein thrombosis
4. Endocrine – Addison's disease (adrenal vein thrombosis)
5. Neurological – cerebral ischaemia (stroke, multi-infarct dementia)
6. Gastrointestinal – bowel ischaemia
7. Obstetric – recurrent abortions, intrauterine growth retardation
8. Dermatological – livedo reticularis, ulcers

4. Ask about bleeding problems associated with thrombocytopenia, skin changes (especially livedo reticularis), central nervous system complications such as migraine and chorea, and eclampsia or pre-eclampsia with the HELLP syndrome: **H**aemolysis, **E**levated **L**iver enzymes, **L**ow **P**latelets.
5. Ask about features of the underlying disorder, such as SLE, which suggest the patient has a secondary form of antiphospholipid antibody syndrome.

The examination
Unless the patient has an active thrombosis, there are unlikely to be any abnormal physical signs. However, look especially for:
1. signs of any associated autoimmune diseases, particularly skin rashes and joint abnormalities in SLE, and dry eyes and mouth in Sjögren's syndrome
2. livedo reticularis rash on the lower limbs
3. heart murmurs from sterile valve vegetations.

Investigations (see also pp. 202–4)
1. The detection of IgG anticardiolipin antibodies is diagnostic for the antiphospholipid antibody syndrome if the antibodies are in high titre and found in the correct clinical context. IgM anticardiolipin antibodies may be detected, although these are less specific.
2. The lupus inhibitor is a related antibody (both are antibodies to phospholipid) that confers an even greater risk of thrombosis and pregnancy complications. The lupus inhibitor is also associated with a prolonged activated partial thromboplastin time (aPTT) not corrected in a mixing study.
3. Antibodies to beta$_2$-glycoprotein 1 (β_2-GP 1) in high titre may be present in the appropriate clinical setting.
4. In patients with suspected antiphospholipid antibody syndrome, it is worth checking the ANA and other autoimmune serology as indicated, as well as measuring the platelet count. The Venereal Disease Research Laboratory (VDRL) test may be falsely positive.

Treatment
1. Any patient with thrombotic complications of the antiphospholipid antibody syndrome should be considered for treatment with anticoagulants for life (consider whether the benefits exceed the risks for individual patients).
2. The patient with anticardiolipin antibodies but no clinical abnormalities presents a difficult clinical situation. There are no data to support routine anticoagulation in this situation, but clearly there is a risk of arterial thrombosis.

3. The patient who has had obstetric problems in the past but no history of thrombosis also presents a dilemma for clinicians. The literature supports the use of anticoagulation therapy only in those with anticardiolipin antibodies or lupus inhibitor in whom a thrombotic complication has previously occurred.

4. Women who have suffered recurrent abortion will require treatment during pregnancy. Low-molecular-weight heparin would normally be used throughout the pregnancy, with the addition of low-dose aspirin. There is no good evidence that corticosteroids improve survival of the fetus.

Systemic sclerosis (scleroderma)

Definitions

- Limited cutaneous systemic sclerosis (lcSSc) is characterised by skin changes of the distal extremities and the face (70%). These patients are usually anticentromere positive.
- CREST is a subset of lcSSc.
- Diffuse cutaneous systemic sclerosis (dcSSc) (30%) involves skin involvement proximal to the elbows and knees. There is chest, abdominal or internal organ involvement.

This is a progressive disease of multiple organs. Although rare, it crops up commonly in examinations. It is more common in women than in men (5:1). The 5-year survival for dcSSc patients at diagnosis is only 70%. Asian patients have a higher incidence of diffuse disease and of interstitial lung disease. There is a slightly increased risk of disease for people who have a first-degree relative affected.

The history

1. Ask about symptoms:
   a. dermatological symptoms – Raynaud's phenomenon (commonly the first symptom), tight skin, disability from sclerodactyly
   b. arthritis – arthropathy in a rheumatoid distribution, carpal tunnel symptoms
   c. gastrointestinal symptoms – dysphagia, heartburn (oesophagitis), diarrhoea (malabsorption)
   d. renal tract symptoms – hypertension, chronic kidney disease, scleroderma renal crisis
   e. respiratory symptoms – symptoms of interstitial lung disease, pleurisy, known diagnosis of pulmonary hypertension
   f. cardiac symptoms – symptoms of pericarditis, palpitations (arrhythmias), symptoms of cardiac failure (dilated cardiomyopathy)
   g. other symptoms – erectile dysfunction, hypothyroidism, history of non-melanoma skin cancer.
2. Consider the differential diagnosis (Table 9.19). Graft versus host disease can mimic scleroderma. Also ask about a history of exposure to polyvinyl chloride (PVC), L-tryptophan (eosinophilic myalgia syndrome) and drugs (e.g. bleomycin, pentazocine).

Table 9.19 Differential diagnosis of scleroderma

These rare conditions are not associated with Raynaud's phenomenon or antinuclear antibodies:

1. Eosinophilic fasciitis
2. Morphea
3. Scleroderma
4. Nephrogenic systemic fibrosis
5. Diabetic cheiroarthropathy

Nephrogenic systemic fibrosis can occur in dialysis patients exposed to gadolinium during an MRI. Also ask about drugs likely to aggravate Raynaud's phenomenon (e.g. beta-blockers); a possible association with silicone breast implants seems to have been negated. Don't miss diabetic-induced skin thickening.

3. Ask about treatment received (e.g. D-penicillamine) and any side-effects (see Table 9.21).
4. Enquire about degree of disability – function at home, ability to work, financial security. Scleroderma may be classified as limited or diffuse.

HINTS

- Limited cutaneous systemic sclerosis (face, hands and feet) is associated with a risk of pulmonary arterial hypertension.
- Diffuse cutaneous scleroderma is associated with a risk of interstitial lung disease, serositis and acute renal failure (scleroderma renal crisis).

In CREST (typically a more limited form of scleroderma, usually with oesophageal involvement, which causes dysphagia), sclerodactyly is usually limited to the distal extremities and/or face. The signs are:
Calcinosis (calcific deposits in subcutaneous tissue at the ends of the fingers) (Fig. 9.12)
Raynaud's phenomenon (resulting in loss of tissue pulp at the ends of the fingers)
(o)**E**sophageal involvement
Sclerodactyly (tightening of the skin on the fingers) (Fig. 9.13)
Telangiectasia.

Progressive pulmonary fibrosis (ILD) is more common in patients with diffuse disease who have topisomerase 1 antibodies. Pulmonary hypertension is six times more common in patients with limited disease; it tends to occur late in the course of the disease. Patients with rapidly progressing dyspnoea are more likely to have pulmonary hypertension than ILD. These lung conditions are the main causes of mortality for scleroderma patients.

Localised scleroderma is called *morphea*. It presents as single or multiple plaques of skin induration.

The examination (see Table 9.20)

1. Make a general inspection for weight loss (due to malabsorption or dysphagia).
2. Look at the hands. Look for the signs of limited scleroderma. These include sclerodactyly (tightening of the skin of the fingers – see Fig. 9.13) with extension up to the elbow, telangiectasia, finger tapering, pitting scars, signs of calcinosis (calcific deposits in subcutaneous tissue at the ends of the fingers – see Fig. 9.12) and the effects of Raynaud's phenomenon (loss of tissue pulp at the ends of the fingers). Nail-fold capillaroscopy is useful, but few have the skill. The presence of dilated tortuous vessels (giant loops) almost always indicates an underlying connective tissue disorder of some sort. Assess hand function.
3. Look at the arms for skin changes and assess proximal weakness (myositis).
4. Examine the head. Note any alopecia. Look at the face for 'salt-and-pepper' pigmentation, loss of wrinkling, 'bird-like' or 'mouse-like' facies (because of puckering of the mouth) and telangiectasia. Check for any difficulty in closing the eyes, dryness of the eyes (Sjögren's syndrome) and pale conjunctivae (anaemia). Check for any difficulty in opening the mouth wide and for dryness and puckering of the mouth.

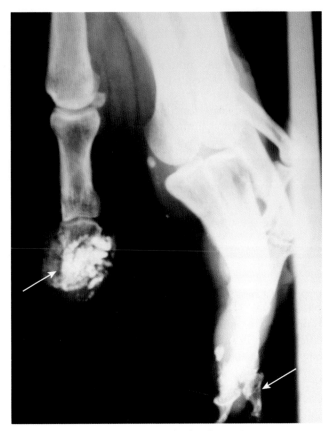

Figure 9.12 X-ray of the hands showing marked calcinosis (arrows).

Figure reproduced courtesy of The Canberra Hospital.

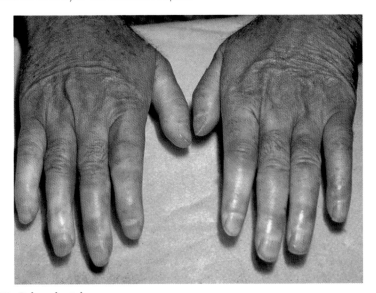

Figure 9.13 Sclerodactyly.

W D James, T Berger, D Elston. *Andrews' diseases of the skin: clinical dermatology*, 11th edn. Fig 8-25. Saunders, Elsevier, 2011, with permission.

Table 9.20 Systemic sclerosis

1. GENERAL APPEARANCE

'Bird-like' facies

Weight loss (malabsorption)

Anaemia (malabsorption, bleeding from a watermelon stomach)

2. HANDS

CREST – calcinosis, atrophy of distal tissue pulp (Raynaud's disease), (o)esophageal involvement, sclerodactyly, telangiectasia

Dilated capillary loops

Small joint arthropathy and tendon crepitus

Fixed flexion deformity

Hand function

3. ARMS

Oedema (early) or skin thickening and tightening

Pigmentation

Vitiligo

Hair loss

Proximal myopathy

4. HEAD

Alopecia

Eyes – loss of eyebrows, anaemia, dryness (Sjögren's syndrome), difficulty with closing

Mouth – dryness, puckered, difficulty with opening

Pigmentation

Telangiectasia

5. DYSPHAGIA

Ask patient about swallowing

6. CHEST

Tight skin ('Roman breast plate')

Heart – cor pulmonale from pulmonary hypertension, pericardial effusion, pericarditis, failure, arrhythmias, ischaemia

Lungs – fibrosis, reflux pneumonitis, chest infections, lung carcinoma, vasculitis

7. LEGS

Skin lesions

Vasculitis

Small joint arthropathy

Patellar crepitus

8. OTHER

Blood pressure (hypertension in renal involvement)

Urine analysis (proteinuria)

Temperature chart (infection)

Stool examination (steatorrhoea)

Cancer elsewhere (non-melanoma skin cancer)

5. Look at the chest for the 'Roman breast plate' effect as a result of skin tightening.
6. Examine the cardiovascular system for pericarditis, arrhythmias, cor pulmonale and cardiac failure (due to myocardial fibrosis).
7. Examine the respiratory system for interstitial lung disease, reflux pneumonitis, infection, lung carcinoma and vasculitis.
8. Look for jaundice and xanthelasma (primary biliary cholangitis occurs rarely with CREST). Scratch marks may be visible from pruritus.
9. Look at the legs for vasculitis and ulceration.
10. Take the blood pressure.
11. Check the urine analysis and temperature charts.

Investigations

1. The ESR may be raised. Anaemia may be present owing to chronic disease, iron deficiency (secondary to bleeding from oesophagitis), folate or vitamin B_{12} deficiency (secondary to malabsorption), or a microangiopathic haemolytic anaemia, which is usually associated with acute renal crises.
2. Hypergammaglobulinaemia (particularly IgG) is present in 50% of cases. Rheumatoid factor is present in 25% and ANA is found in most cases. Anti-Scl-70 is positive in a minority with diffuse scleroderma. Anticentromere antibody is particularly associated with CREST (up to 70%) (see Table 9.16).
3. Investigations for malabsorption and dysphagia may be necessary.

4. Assess visceral involvement with chest X-ray films, gastroscopy or oesophageal manometry, depending on the clinical presentation.
5. Regular screening for ILD and pulmonary hypertension should be routine:
   a. respiratory function tests, high-resolution CT of the chest for ILD
   b. echocardiography and, if pulmonary arterial hypertension is suspected, a right heart catheter and 6-minute walk test.

Treatment

This debilitating chronic disease will expose the patient to the need for recurrent investigations and adjustments to treatment. These matters need careful explanation from the outset. Prognosis is worse in men and those with renal or late-onset disease. Patients with skin and gut involvement, but without other organ disease, have the best prognosis.

1. Symptomatic treatment includes avoiding vasospasm (by avoiding smoking, beta-blockers and cold weather). Aggressive treatment of reflux with proton pump inhibitors is important to prevent the formation of oesophageal strictures. Nifedipine, phenoxy-benzamine, prazosin or methyldopa may help Raynaud's phenomenon. The prostacyclin analogue iloprost has shown promise for Raynaud's phenomenon in scleroderma. The endothelin antagonist bosentan is available in some places for the treatment of digital ischaemia. Morphea may respond to ultraviolet-A (UVA) light.
2. Artificial tears are useful for dry eyes and NSAIDs may help with joint symptoms.
3. Treat malabsorption (particularly bacterial overgrowth, with antibiotics).
4. D-penicillamine (an immunosuppressant drug that also interferes with collagen cross-linking) may be helpful for skin disease and may improve survival. It has been usual to start treatment with a low dose. Randomised studies have shown no advantage of higher doses. The drug has a number of severe side-effects (Table 9.21). Monthly full blood counts are usually recommended.
5. Cyclophosphamide is used if there is lung involvement and may improve other complications of the disease, especially if used early. Treatment is usually given for 9 months.
6. Pericarditis, inflammatory myopathy and early ILD may respond to steroids.
7. A number of drugs are approved for the treatment of pulmonary arterial hypertension (PAH) in scleroderma patients (Table 9.22).

Table 9.21 Side-effects of d-penicillamine

SEVERE	MORE MINOR
Glomerulonephritis and nephrotic syndrome	Alteration of taste
Myasthenia gravis	Skin rashes
Thrombocytopenia	Fever
Leukopenia	Nausea
Aplastic anaemia	Anorexia

Table 9.22 Drugs approved for the treatment of pulmonary arterial hypertension

1. Endothelin receptor antagonists: bosentan and ambrisentan
2. Phosphodiesterase inhibitors: sildenafil and tadalafil
3. Prostanoids: intravenous epoprostenol and inhaled iloprost

8. Aggressive treatment of hypertension to prevent chronic kidney disease is vital – ACE inhibitors are the drug class of choice. An ACE inhibitor is often given to patients even with abnormal renal function to prevent or treat hypertensive renal crises. Dialysis is not contraindicated. A sudden increase in blood pressure should prompt investigations for acute kidney injury and microangiopathic haemolytic anaemia, which occur in renal crises.

9. Many other drugs have been tried for patients with scleroderma, including angiotensin receptor blockers, selective serotonin reuptake inhibitors, serotonin antagonists, topical nitrates and platelet inhibitors. There are no controlled trials showing that treatment can reverse the course of the disease.

HINT

In systemic sclerosis, early diagnosis and treatment of interstitial lung disease and pulmonary arterial hypertension improve the prognosis; regular screening is most important.

Chapter 10

The endocrine long case

I would like to see the day when somebody would be
appointed surgeon somewhere who had no hands, for
the operative part is the least part of the work.

Harvey Cushing (1869–1939)

Osteoporosis (and osteomalacia)

Osteoporosis is increasingly encountered in the long-case examination. It would be
unusual not to see at least one patient with osteoporosis or at risk of the condition
during the exam day.

- Osteoporosis will commonly form part of another medical problem.
- The patient may be a postmenopausal woman, or even more often someone who is
  taking corticosteroids for an acute or chronic inflammatory illness or following organ
  transplant. The risk begins after use of 7.5 mg of prednisone or more for more than
  3 months.
- Osteoporotic fractures can affect 30% of postmenopausal women over their lifetime.
  Many older women have undergone bone densitometry screening and may be aware
  that they have asymptomatic osteoporosis.
- Patients who have had a hip fracture or who have evidence of an endocrine disorder,
  malabsorption, liver disease, Crohn's disease or bone marrow disease, or who are
  taking certain medications, should have the possibility of osteoporosis considered
  while they are being evaluated (Table 10.1).

The history

1. Ask about a history of fractures, particularly fractures of the wrist (the risk increases
   from age 55), hip (risk increases from age 70), humerus and ribs, and vertebral
   compression fractures (especially T12), which may have occurred with minimal stress
   (the risk increases from age 55). Acute back pain that subsides over weeks or months
   and then recurs may be caused by compression fractures.
2. If the patient has had a hip fracture, ask about any secondary complications, including
   pulmonary thromboembolism and nosocomial infections.

Table 10.1 Major secondary causes of osteoporosis

1. Drugs
   a. Steroids
   b. Chronic heparin therapy
   c. Thyroxine over-replacement
   d. Lithium
   e. Phenytoin
   f. Cyclosporin
   g. Aromatase inhibitors
2. Gastrointestinal diseases
   a. Malabsorption syndromes (e.g. coeliac disease, Crohn's disease, gastric bypass)
   b. Chronic cholestasis (e.g. primary biliary cholangitis)
3. Malnutrition
   a. Anorexia nervosa
   b. Scurvy
   c. Alcoholism
4. Bone marrow disorders
   a. Multiple myeloma
   b. Disseminated carcinoma
   c. Lymphoma
   d. Leukaemias
5. Connective tissue diseases
   a. Marfan's syndrome, Ehlers–Danlos syndrome
   b. Osteogenesis imperfecta
   c. Rheumatoid arthritis
6. Endocrine diseases
   a. Hyperthyroidism
   b. Hyperparathyroidism
   c. Cushing's syndrome
   d. Growth hormone deficiency
   e. Hyperprolactinaemia
   f. Hypogonadism
7. Other causes
   a. Systemic mastocytosis

3. Ask about symptoms of bone pain, which may be diffuse, and proximal muscle weakness. These features may occur with osteomalacia (characterised by defective bone mineralisation in adults).
4. Ask about:
   • risk factors for osteoporosis (see Table 10.1).
   • the menstrual history and age of onset of menopause
   • symptoms of thyroid excess or thyroid hormone replacement (thyroxine)
   • symptoms or a history of anaemia.
5. Ask about bone pain and proximal weakness (osteomalacia, usually due to vitamin D deficiency – then you must exclude malabsorption) (see Table 10.2).
6. Ask whether the patient has had a DEXA (dual X-ray absorptiometry) scan (see Investigations).

Table 10.2 Causes of osteomalacia

1. Unavailability of vitamin D:
  a. vitamin D malabsorption (e.g. coeliac disease, pancreatic insufficiency, cirrhosis)
  b. abnormal vitamin D metabolism (e.g. chronic kidney disease, pseudohypoparathyroidism)
  c. decreased vitamin D bioavailability (e.g. inadequate sunlight, nephrotic syndrome, peritoneal dialysis)

2. Phosphate unavailability caused by phosphate-binding antacids, hereditary hypophosphataemia, tumour-induced osteomalacia (e.g. fibrous dysplasia of bone) and Fanconi's syndrome type 1 or 2
3. Normal anion gap metabolic acidosis (e.g. distal renal tubular acidosis (type 1) with hypokalaemia and hypercalciuria, often caused by autoimmune disease such as Sjögren's syndrome or SLE)

Table 10.3 Sun exposure and maintenance of normal Vitamin D levels in moderately fair-skinned people requires
6–7 minutes of sun exposure to the arms, face and hands in the mid morning or afternoon in summer
9–13 minutes of exposure in winter in Northern Australia
11–15 minutes of exposure in winter in Central Australia (Brisbane or Perth)
16 (Sydney)–30 minutes (Hobart) of exposure of as much skin as practical in winter in the middle of the day

Table 10.4 Risk factors for falls and fractures[a]
• Previous minimal trauma fracture
• Female
• Age > 70
• Loss of 3 cm or more in height and back pain suggesting vertebral fractures
• History of falls
• Family history of hip fracture
• Steroid use (3 months of 7.5 mg prednisone or more)
• Premature menopause or hypogonadism
• Sedative or alcohol use
• Low weight or undernutrition
• Prolonged immobility, little physical activity
• Balance problems
• Smoking
• Vitamin D deficiency
[a]Remember that these are interconnected

7. Take a careful drug history. Medications that cause osteoporosis include steroids, alcohol, heparin, thyroxine over-replacement, anticonvulsants (by affecting vitamin D metabolism) and cyclosporin.

8. Enquire about a poor diet (a low-fat diet often limits calcium intake) or inadequate sunlight exposure if the patient is a nursing home resident, has dark skin, or has a history of renal disease or phenytoin use (all risk factors for osteomalacia) (Tables 10.2 and 10.3). Ask about the patient's exercise history, as physical activity throughout life preserves bone mass. Cigarette smoking reduces skeletal mass.

9. Determine any risk factors for falls (Table 10.4): a greater risk of falls increases the risk of fracture at any level of osteoporosis. Has the patient insight into his or her falls risk? Have exercises that might improve balance (e.g. Tai Chi) been recommended

and used? Has the house been assessed for risk: loose rugs, slippery surfaces, railings, etc.? Does the patient take sedative or antidepressant tablets or drink alcohol?
10. Does the patient wear hip protectors?
11. Determine the social effect of the disease (e.g. immobility, pain, fear of falling).
12. Have vitamin D levels been measured? Were they reduced?
13. Ask about sun exposure (see Table 10.3).

The examination

There are usually no signs of osteoporosis unless a recent fracture has occurred.
1. Examine for bone tenderness and proximal weakness (osteomalacia). Look for bowing of the legs (rickets).
2. Look for signs of thyroid disease and Cushing's syndrome.
3. Thoracic kyphosis is an important sign of vertebral fractures. The occiput to wall distance can be used to follow the condition.
4. Ask about previous falls. Examine for falls risk (e.g. use the get up and go test; see Ch 13, p. 373).
5. Assess weight and general nutritional status.

HINT

Vitamin D deficiency is increasingly commonly diagnosed in people of all ages. Consider this in all patients with reduced bone density and especially in those with bone pain or muscle weakness. Risk factors include lack of exposure to sunlight (nursing home residents), fear of sunburn, dark skin and modest dress.

Investigations

1. Ask for the DEXA scan results.
   Bone densitometry using dual-energy X-ray absorptiometry (DEXA) of the lumbar spine and/or proximal femur remains the test of choice for evaluation of bone mineral density (BMD; see Table 10.5). *Osteopenia* is used to refer to a bone mineral density between 1 and 2.5 standard deviations (SD) below peak bone mass; *osteoporosis* refers to a bone mineral density of more than 2.5 SD below peak bone mass. The measurement is often given as a T score. This is the number of SD by which the measured bone density falls below the average for a young normal person of the same sex. Thus, a T score of less than −2.5 defines osteoporosis.
2. Review the serum calcium and alkaline phosphatase results. In osteoporosis, serum calcium and alkaline phosphatase levels should be normal. Alkaline phosphatase is usually elevated

---

Table 10.5 Indications for bone mineral density (BMD) assay

- Fracture occurring after minimal trauma
- All women ≥ 65 years and men ≥ 70 years (but guidelines vary)
- Monitoring of known low BMD after at least 1 year
- Monitoring of bone loss after prolonged steroid use or as a result of hypogonadism
- Monitoring of bone loss in primary hyperparathyroidism, chronic liver disease, chronic kidney disease, Crohn's disease, known malabsorption and rheumatoid arthritis
- Measurement of BMD 12 months after change in treatment for known low BMD

Table 10.6 Tests in bone disease					
DISEASE	CALCIUM	PHOSPHATE	25-OH VITAMIN D	PARATHYROID HORMONE	ALKALINE PHOSPHATASE (BONE)
Osteoporosis	N	N	N	N	N
Osteomalacia or rickets due to malabsorption or dietary lack	Low–N	Low–N	Decreased	Increased–N	Increased
Osteomalacia with renal bone disease	Variable	Increased–N	Variable	Increased–N	Increased
Familial hypophosphataemic rickets	N	Decreased	N	N	Increased
Primary hyperpara-thyroidism	Increased	Decreased–N	N	Increased–high N	Increased
Paget's disease	N	N	N	N	Increased
N = normal.					

in all forms of osteomalacia. Check 25-OH vitamin D levels (not 1,25-OH vitamin D) if there are any risk factors for osteomalacia. If there is vitamin D deficiency, serum 25-OH vitamin D levels are usually low (e.g. vitamin D malabsorption, chronic liver disease, lack of exposure to sunlight – especially common in nursing home patients).

Assessment of calcium, parathyroid hormone (PTH) and vitamin D levels will usually distinguish the most important causes of osteomalacia and allow specific diagnostic tests to be appropriately directed (Table 10.6). A sustained elevation of alkaline phosphatase should lead to consideration of osteomalacia, as well as Paget's disease and metastatic malignancy to bone.

3. A FBC and ESR estimation should be ordered to look for evidence of myeloproliferative disease, and renal and liver function tests should be ordered to exclude renal or hepatic disease.

4. Thyroid-stimulating hormone should be measured to rule out thyrotoxicosis.

5. If osteoporosis is unexpectedly severe, then a serum protein electrophoresis (SPEP) (electrophoretogram) should be considered to rule out multiple myeloma. In men, a serum testosterone level is worthwhile.

A Z score < 2 SD below the age-related mean suggests a possible secondary cause for reduced bone density

6. Ask to review any skeletal X-rays.
   • In osteoporosis of the spine, there is characteristic loss of trabecular bone in the vertebral body, including accentuation of the vertebral endplates. The vertebral trabeculae become more prominent with the loss of horizontal trabeculae. Also look for collapse, anterior wedging and the codfish deformity (from expansion of the intervertebral disc; see Fig. 10.1).
   • In osteomalacia, X-rays may show some decrease in bone density with coarsening of trabeculae and blurring of the margins. A specific abnormality is Looser's zones (pseudo-fractures) in the long-bone shafts; these are ribbon-like zones of rarefaction. Other characteristic abnormalities may include a triangular (trefoil) pelvis and biconcave collapsed vertebrae. If there is secondary hyperparathyroidism present

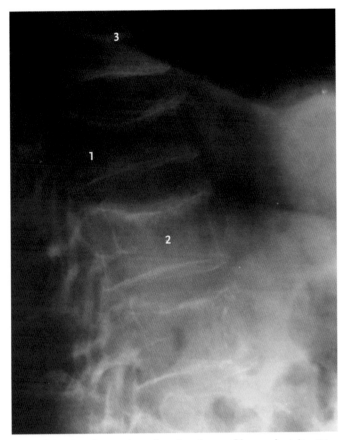

Figure 10.1 **X-ray of the lumbar spine showing loss of bone density (1), codfish deformity (2) and anterior wedging (3).**

Figure reproduced courtesy of The Canberra Hospital.

with osteomalacia, then bone cysts, erosion of the distal ends of the clavicles and subperiosteal resorption in the phalanges may be seen.

7. In difficult cases, an iliac crest bone biopsy with double tetracycline labelling can help to distinguish osteoporosis from osteomalacia.

8. Consider undertaking tests for secondary causes of osteoporosis if the clinical picture suggests this may be helpful.

Treatment

Established osteoporosis is currently not reversible with medical therapy. Early intervention can prevent progression of osteoporosis and is of value. Secondary causes of osteoporosis should be identified and corrected if present.

ANTIRESORPTIVE THERAPY

1. **Calcium:** because calcium absorption decreases with age, calcium therapy has a modest benefit in both early and late postmenopausal women. Consumption of 1200–1500 mg of calcium daily in adults over the age of 65 is advisable. Remember, though, the increased risk of cardiovascular events and renal calculi associated with calcium supplementation

2. **Vitamin D supplementation:** encourage sun exposure if that is possible. Moderate or severe vitamin D deficiency (serum 25-OH D < 25 nmol/L) should be treated with high-dose supplements of vitamin D of 3000–5000 IU/day for 6–12 weeks, and then 1000 IU/day from then on. Elderly women in nursing homes who have inadequate intake should receive supplementation of vitamin D 800 IU/day and calcium 1200 mg/day. This has been shown to reduce non-vertebral fracture risk.

3. **Generally recommend ceasing smoking, avoiding excess alcohol consumption:** institute fall prevention measures and prescribe regular weight-bearing exercise. Consider a hip protector.

4. **Weight-bearing exercise:** walking, dancing, tennis, etc. Resistance training exercise: lifting weights (not too heavy). These have been shown to increase bone mineral density and reduce the risk of falls.

5. **Bisphosphonates (risendronate and alendronate):** these drugs increase bone mineral density in postmenopausal women and have been shown to reduce the risk of fracture for postmenopausal women with osteoporosis by 50%. Patients unable to tolerate oral bisphosphonates because of upper GIT problems can be given the drug as an infusion once every 3 months or, with some of the newer agents, once a year. Intravenous treatment should be avoided in people with moderate or severe chronic kidney disease. The oral drugs can cause oesophageal ulceration that presents with odynophagia, usually within 1–2 months of commencing therapy. Osteonecrosis of the jaw is another serious but rare side-effect, which is more likely to occur with intravenous formulations in the presence of previous dental infections. A dental review may be indicated before treatment is begun. These drugs are now indicated for patients aged over 70 who have a BMD T score of −3 or less and for those who have had a fracture after minimal trauma.

   Alternative drugs for people who are unable to take bisphosphonates include:
   a. **denosumab** – a humanised monoclonal antibody that reduces osteoclastogenesis by binding RANKL (receptor activator of nuclear factor kappa-B ligand)
   b. **strontium ranelate** – its effectiveness for preventing hip fractures has not been established, but there is evidence for its use in protecting against vertebral and rib fractures. It should be taken at bedtime at least 2 hours after eating.

6. **Oestrogen:** hormone replacement therapy will prevent loss of cortical and trabecular bone in postmenopausal women. Therapy is probably more effective if started earlier in menopause as bone loss is most rapid then. Because oestrogen increases the risk of endometrial carcinoma, combination with progesterone is important unless a hysterectomy has been performed. A past history of endometrial cancer is a contraindication. There is an increased risk of breast cancer, as well as DVT and pulmonary embolism. Cardiovascular risk is also increased and hence its use in postmenopausal women has declined.

7. **Selective oestrogen receptor modulators:** raloxifene, closely related to tamoxifen, reduces the risk of spine fractures. It increases the risk of DVT, but lowers the risk of breast cancer (and is not associated with an increased risk of endometrial cancer). Tamoxifen is a mixed oestrogen receptor antagonist and agonist that prevents bone loss. It increases the risk of endometrial cancer.

8. **Calcitonin:** there have been inconsistent results with calcitonin and any effect is smaller than with other therapies. The drug can be given subcutaneously or intranasally. Administration can cause nausea, flushing and inflammation.

BONE FORMATION THERAPY

1. **Parathyroid hormone (PTH) peptide (teriparatide):** this drug is very effective for osteoporosis but very expensive. It is given subcutaneously for 18 months. After this,

antiresorptive treatment should be restarted. It is generally reserved for people who have a fracture while taking a bisphosphonate and have a T score of −3.0 or less.

2. **Men with osteoporosis:** men who have osteoporosis and androgen deficiency should be given androgen replacement unless there is a history of prostatic carcinoma. Bisphosphonates and teriparatide are efficacious; the role of raloxifene is not clear.

3. **Steroid-induced osteoporosis:** this is very important because, if prednisone is considered likely to be needed for a number of months or longer, then measures to prevent bone loss are important from the time steroids are begun, particularly in postmenopausal women or when high doses are needed. Co-administration of bisphosphonates is of value here. Calcium and 25-OH vitamin D in combination have also been shown to be effective. These are the only drugs that have been shown to reduce fracture risk for patients on steroids. Other general measures, such as cessation of smoking and a regular exercise regimen, are probably important and should be recommended to the patient.

4. **Surgical treatment of fractures:** this is often required. Frail elderly patients with other medical problems require careful assessment of anaesthetic risk.

Vertebral fractures may cause severe pain that requires potent analgesics. Bed rest should be as brief as possible. Injection of bone cement into the vertebral body (vertebroplasty) may relieve acute severe pain but seems to be of limited benefit in controlled studies and has fallen out of favour.

Possible lines of questioning

1. Is *this* patient's fracture risk adequately managed?
2. Does *this* patient with a renal transplant qualify for a DEXA scan?
3. Are other investigations warranted for *this* patient with vertebral fractures before she receives treatment for osteoporosis?
4. What is your assessment of this patient's risk of falls?

Hypercalcaemia

Hypercalcaemia is a common medical problem and therefore can appear in a long case. It is most likely to be a diagnostic problem. Most patients (90%) have hyperparathyroidism or malignancy (Table 10.7). The asymptomatic patient usually has hyperparathyroidism. A malignant condition that is advanced enough to cause hypercalcaemia is likely to have also caused other symptoms. The diagnosis is often made from a routine blood test and the patient may have no symptoms.

The history

If the patient tells you that he or she has high calcium levels:

1. Enquire about the non-specific symptomatic manifestations. These include tiredness, weakness and episodes of confusion. Enquire about anorexia and constipation, as well as nausea and vomiting; acute abdominal pain from acute pancreatitis may have occurred. Enquire about polyuria and polydipsia. Ask about a history of hypertension or a slow heart rate.

2. Enquire about a history of peptic ulcer or renal colic ('stones, moans, bones and abdominal groans') from primary hyperparathyroidism. Ask about joint pain from

Table 10.7 Causes of hypercalcaemia

WITH NORMAL OR ELEVATED PTH
1. Primary hyperparathyroidism (from a solitary adenoma, or rarely multiple endocrine neoplasia)
2. Tertiary hyperparathyroidism
3. Familial hypocalciuric hypercalcaemia

WITH LOW PTH
1. Malignancy (e.g. metastatic breast cancer, lung or renal cancer releasing humoral mediators, haematological malignancies)
2. Increased vitamin D (excess ingestion, granulomatous disease) (increased 25-OH vitamin D)
3. Increased bone turnover (e.g. hyperthyroidism, thiazide diuretics, vitamin A intoxication)
4. Other (e.g. lithium: increases parathyroid hormone)

CKD = chronic kidney disease; PTH = parathyroid hormone.

pseudogout (chondrocalcinosis in primary hyperparathyroidism). Enquire about a past history of hypertension (hyperparathyroidism).

3. Ask the patient whether he or she was known to have had a neck mass in the past or has had an operation to remove the parathyroid gland. In most cases a single adenomatous gland is found, but masses can be multiple. Surgical parathyroidectomy is the definitive treatment for primary hyperparathyroidism. Most neck masses will be coincidental thyroid nodules rather than a benign or malignant parathyroid tumour.

4. Ask whether the patient has had an eye examination and, if so, whether calcium was seen (band keratopathy). Also, ask whether X-rays of the bones have been taken. In hyperparathyroidism, X-rays of the hand may show subperiosteal reabsorption with a moth-eaten appearance on the radial sides of the phalanges and in the distal phalangeal tufts (osteitis fibrosa cystica), as well as in the distal clavicles.

5. Determine whether there is any past history of malignant disease, including diseases that metastasise to bone (e.g. carcinoma or myeloma) or haematological disease such as lymphoma (ectopic vitamin D production).

6. Ask about drugs, including thiazide diuretics and lithium, and ingestion of calcium or vitamin D.

7. Enquire about known chronic kidney disease, a cause of secondary hyperparathyroidism because of resistance to parathyroid hormone and growth of the size of the glands. These enlarged glands then produce partly non-suppressible parathyroid hormone and hypercalcaemia.

8. Ask about symptoms of thyrotoxicosis or phaeochromocytoma. Ask about recent immobilisation.

9. Check whether there is a family history of high serum calcium levels, such as familial hypocalciuric hypercalcaemia (autosomal dominant). Classically, a patient with this condition has had hypercalcaemia since a relatively young age, with only a slight elevation in the serum parathyroid hormone level at most, and with a personal or family history of unsuccessful neck exploration; it does not require any therapy. A family history of hypercalcaemia may also occur with the multiple endocrine neoplasia syndromes MEN1 and MEN2A. These are both autosomal dominant conditions. These patients may have symptoms related to the other features of their MEN syndrome (e.g. peptic ulceration from the Zollinger–Ellison syndrome – a result of a tumour causing excess gastrin secretion and therefore increased gastric acid production).

10. Many patients are asymptomatic and had hypercalcaemia detected on a routine set of biochemical tests. Hyperparathyroidism has been recognised much more commonly since automated biochemical analyses have become routine.

The examination

1. Look for any evidence of a neck scar from parathyroid surgery, as well as forearm scars from re-implantation of the parathyroid gland from the neck.
2. Evaluate the patient for evidence of malignancy, including lymphadenopathy or organomegaly.
3. Look for evidence of renal failure.
4. Carefully evaluate the respiratory system for any evidence of sarcoidosis, as well as tuberculosis or histoplasmosis.
5. Take the pulse for bradycardia, a result of a high serum calcium level. Measure the blood pressure for evidence of phaeochromocytoma.
6. Examine for signs of thyrotoxicosis.
7. Look for pigmentation from Addison's disease.
8. Examine for proximal weakness and signs of pseudogout in the joints.
9. Examine the cornea for band keratopathy (calcification horizontally across the centre of the cornea).

Investigations

1. Look at the total serum calcium level. Remember that apparently high calcium levels can be the result of haemoconcentration while the blood is being collected. Correct for hypoalbuminaemia: add 0.02 mmol/L to the serum calcium concentration for every 1 g/L by which the serum albumin level is less than 40 g/L. The calcium level at which symptoms occur varies, but most patients have symptoms when the corrected calcium level reaches 3 mmol/L. Higher levels are associated with tissue calcification and the risk of renal failure, especially if the phosphate level is normal or increased by renal impairment. Once the calcium level approaches 4 mmol/L, unconsciousness and cardiac arrest can occur.
2. Measure the parathyroid hormone level. If elevated, primary hyperparathyroidism is the most likely diagnosis (PTH can be inappropriately in the high normal range in 10%; phosphorus should be low). If the patient is taking lithium or thiazide, the test should be repeated after discontinuing drug treatment, because these drugs may influence both calcium and PTH secretion.
3. In a young otherwise asymptomatic person with a marginal elevation of parathyroid hormone, a 24-hour urine calcium examination should be requested to exclude familial hypocalciuric hypercalcaemia (FHH). Alternatively, collect a fasting morning spot urine and measure the urine calcium:creatinine clearance ratio (< 0.01 in FHH). This autosomal dominant condition is caused by faulty calcium sensing by the parathyroid glands and renal tubules.
4. If there is a low or undetectable parathyroid hormone level, consider the possibility of underlying malignancy or granulomatous disease.

      Measure PTH-related protein (PTHrP), and perform a bone scan and a serum protein EPG to look for malignancy.

      An increased level of 1,25-OH vitamin D supports the possibility of a granulomatous disorder, including:
   - sarcoidosis
   - tuberculosis
   - berylliosis

- leprosy
- lymphoma.

5. Ask to review the chest X-ray. Investigations to look for malignancy if suspected may then be required (e.g. protein electrophoresis, CT scan, etc.).

Treatment

There is evidence that asymptomatic patients with hyperparathyroidism who are not treated have increased bone loss compared with controls. Significant increases in fracture risk (especially of the wrist and spine) have been demonstrated.

1. If the diagnosis is hyperparathyroidism and the patient is symptomatic, has renal stones or has a reduced bone density, surgical parathyroidectomy is usually indicated. If the patient is asymptomatic, treatment is more controversial, but younger patients (< 50 years) with higher serum or 24-hour urine calcium levels will usually be offered surgery. Preoperative localisation is commonly performed using a combination of ultrasound and sestamibi scanning as this may enable a minimally invasive operation.
2. Note whether there has been hypocalcaemia after surgery. If there is no residual parathyroid tissue left, lifelong vitamin D therapy is necessary; alternatively, autotransplantation of parathyroid tissue into the forearm may be offered.
3. Primary hyperparathyroidism is associated with vitamin D deficiency. Treatment is controversial if the patient is unfit for surgery, but cautious vitamin D replacement is probably safe and desirable.
4. In patients with malignant hypercalcaemia the underlying tumour should be treated. Steroids are often effective in lowering the serum calcium level. With granulomatous disease, steroids are also effective in lowering the calcium level (but avoid if infection is the cause); chloroquine may be useful in patients who cannot tolerate steroids. Lithium treatment may need to be stopped. Hypercalcaemia does not necessarily mean lithium toxicity.
5. Familial hypocalciuric hypercalcaemia rarely causes symptoms and should not be treated with parathyroidectomy. Consider screening all first-degree relatives.
6. In an emergency, rehydration with intravenous saline and frusemide is indicated for hypercalcaemia. Parenteral calcitonin lowers calcium levels only transiently. The use of intravenous bisphosphonates is very effective.

Possible lines of questioning

1. How would you decide whether *this* patient's hypercalaemia is due to malignancy and what investigations would help?
2. How would you manage *this* patient with hypercalcaemia detected on a routine blood test?

Paget's disease of the bone (osteitis deformans)

This is usually a disease of the elderly, but it may occur in younger patients. In populations from western or southern Europe up to 10% of people over the age of 85 are affected. The condition is characterised by excessive resorption of bone and increased formation of new bone in an irregular 'mosaic' pattern. Bone turnover may be increased 20 times early on in the course of the disease. The aetiology is unknown, but it may be caused by a persistent paramyxovirus infection of osteoclasts. There are reports of familial occurrence (15% have a family history) and of autosomal dominant inheritance. Mutations of the *SQSTM1* gene are a cause. The condition is rare in Asian populations. It presents as a management problem.

The history

1. Ask about symptoms that led to the diagnosis:
   a. isolated elevation of alkaline phosphatase on routine blood testing
   b. an incidental finding on an X-ray (common)
   c. bone pain
   d. secondary osteoarthritis
   e. change in height or hat size
   f. progressive bone deformity or pathological fracture; gait abnormalities associated with change in length of a long bone
   g. neurological symptoms – hearing loss,[1] neurological gait disturbance (suggestive of basilar invagination with long tract signs, cerebellar involvement or spinal cord compression), cranial nerve symptoms, headache
   h. symptoms of congestive cardiac failure
   i. symptoms of renal colic (as there is an increased incidence of calcium nephrolithiasis in this disease, especially during the resorptive phase)
   j. gout, secondary to increased bone turnover
   k. sarcoma of bone (very rare – less than 1% of cases, occasionally multicentric)
   l. symptoms of hypercalcaemia – thirst, polyuria, nausea, coma (a rare occurrence even in immobilised patients, or alternatively caused by coexisting primary hyper-parathyroidism, which is common)
   m. pathological fractures, especially of the convex side of weight-bearing bones, which can be multiple.
2. Enquire about articular pain, which may be caused by secondary osteoarthritis in joints adjacent to sites of Pagetic involvement, and true bone pain. Secondary osteoarthritis is characterised by pain and stiffness, which improves with joint movement; alternatively, it may initially be exacerbated by weight-bearing and relieved by rest. True bone pain is more often constant or gnawing and is worse at night. A sudden exacerbation of bone pain may indicate a pathological fracture or the development of an osteosarcoma.
3. Ask about treatment, its effectiveness and side-effects.
4. Enquire about disability at home and work. Remember, though, that most patients are asymptomatic.

The examination (Table 10.8)

1. Inspect generally for short stature and obvious deformity (Fig. 10.2).
2. Look at the face. Measure the skull diameter (> 55 cm may be abnormal). Look for prominent skull veins, feel for bony warmth (actually caused by vasodilatation in the skin) and auscultate for systolic bruits. Examine the fundi for angioid streaks (Fig. 10.3), and for papilloedema or optic atrophy, which are rare. Also, assess visual acuity and visual fields.

---

[1]Deafness is usually conductive rather than sensorineural and is due to osteosclerosis of the temporal bone rather than compression of the auditory nerve.

Table 10.8 Paget's disease	
1. GENERAL INSPECTION Short stature Limb deformity Obvious osteosarcoma (bony swelling) **2. FACE** Skull diameter (measure) Auscultate skull (bruits) Fundi – angioid streaks, optic atrophy Hearing (ossicle or VIII nerve involvement) Other cranial nerves (foramina overgrowth or basilar invagination) **3. NECK** Short neck (basilar invagination) Jugular venous pressure – cardiac failure (high output)	**4. BACK** Deformity Tenderness Warmth Bruits **5. LEGS** Bowing femur, tibia Tenderness, warmth, swelling bones Hip examination (movements) Knee examination **6. GAIT** **7. NEUROLOGICAL ASSESSMENT OF LIMBS** (Spinal cord compression, basilar invagination) **8. OTHER** Urine (blood) Height (measure)

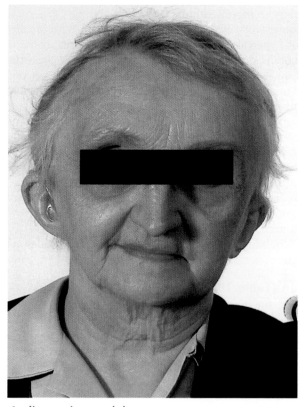

Figure 10.2 **Paget's disease in an adult.**

M C Hochberg, A J Silman, J S Smolen et al., *Rheumatology*, 5th edn. Fig 202.7. Elsevier, 2011, with permission.

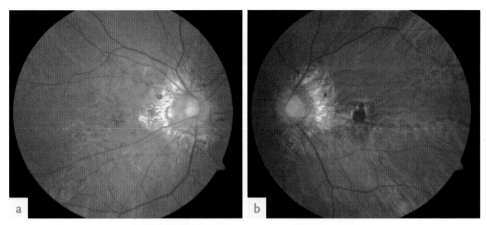

Figure 10.3 **Angioid streaks in fundus.**

S J Ryan. *Retina*, 5th edn. Fig 69.1 a and b. Elsevier, 2012, with permission.

3. Test to see whether hearing is decreased as a result of ossicle involvement or eighth nerve compression. Remember, *all* the other cranial nerves may rarely be affected owing to overgrowth of foramina or basilar invagination, so examine them carefully.
4. Look at the neck for basilar invagination. These patients have a short neck and low hairline, the head is held in extension and neck movements are decreased.
5. Assess the jugular venous pressure and examine the heart for signs of cardiac failure due to a hyperdynamic circulation.
6. Examine the back. Note any deformity, especially kyphosis. Tap for tenderness. Feel for warmth. Auscultate for systolic bruits over the vertebral bodies.
7. Look at the legs for anterior bowing of the tibia and lateral bowing of the femur. Feel for warmth. Note any changes of osteoarthritis in the hips and knees. There may be limitation of hip movements – especially abduction, which suggests protrusio acetabuli – and fixed flexion deformity of the knees. Be careful, as the bones may be tender.
8. Sarcomas (a feared, but rare, complication) should be looked for, particularly in the femur, humerus and skull; they usually present as tender, localised swellings. They can be multiple.
9. A full neurological examination is necessary for signs of spinal cord compression and basilar invagination, which may even cause quadriparesis. If the patient is mobile, do not forget to assess walking for any disability. Cerebellar signs may also rarely occur with basilar invagination.
10. Check the urine analysis (for blood, as renal stone incidence is increased) and measure the patient's height (for serial follow-up).

Investigations

These are indicated in symptomatic patients requiring treatment and in asymptomatic subjects to determine the extent of skeletal involvement. Paget's disease is occasionally confused with osteoblastic bone secondaries (e.g. from prostate, Hodgkin's disease) or fibrous dysplasia.

1. Testing for hypercalcaemia may be worthwhile for any patient who is immobilised.
2. The serum alkaline phosphatase level is an indicator of disease activity, as is the urinary hydroxyproline level. Other biochemical markers of bone turnover will also be increased (e.g. osteocalcin, urine or serum cross-links of collagen).

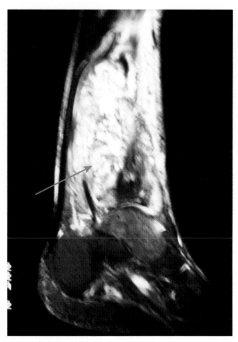

Figure 10.4 **MRI of the lower leg of a patient with Paget's disease. A large osteosarcoma of the tibia can be seen (arrow).**

Figure reproduced courtesy of The Canberra Hospital.

3. Radiologically, the bones most often involved are the pelvis, femur, skull and tibia (see Figs 10.4 and 10.5). Look for bony enlargement, increased density, an irregular widened cortex and cortical infractions (incomplete pseudofractures) on the convex side of the bowed long bones. The early lytic phase of the disease, presenting with a flame-shaped osteolytic wedge advancing along the bones, is often overlooked. Secondary arthritic changes may occur (e.g. in hips). Bone scanning is more sensitive than an X-ray in assessing the extent of disease. CT scanning or MRI may be useful in the investigation of an atypical lesion, especially if sarcoma is suspected.

Treatment

The indications for treatment are bone pain, progressive deformity or complications such as neural compression or high-output cardiac failure, and as a prelude to orthopaedic surgery. Treatment of patients with Pagetic involvement of weight-bearing bones may be indicated to attempt to prevent deformity and pathological fracture. Proof of benefit is not available, however.

1. Simple analgesics (paracetamol) or NSAIDs, including COX-2 inhibitors, should be used first to control pain. Orthopaedic procedures such as total hip replacement may be indicated.
2. A number of drugs are available that reduce bone resorption:
   a. An oral bisphosphonate (e.g. alendronate) is usually the first-line treatment for a defined period (usually 6 months). These drugs are effective at reducing hydroxy-proline excretion and often relieve symptoms, but may exacerbate bone pain initially. They also impair bone mineralisation and may cause osteomalacia. However, bone

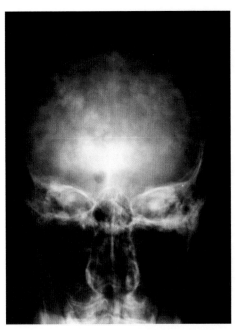

Figure 10.5 **Skull X-ray of a patient with Paget's disease. Note the bony enlargement of the cranium.**

Figure reproduced courtesy of The Canberra Hospital.

turnover is reduced and new bone is usually more normal in structure. The bisphosphonates should be given in combination with calcium supplements and vitamin D. Ulcerating oesophagitis causing dysphagia is an important side-effect. The bisphosphonates are not generally indicated for asymptomatic patients. Intravenous infusions of the potent bisphosphonate pamidronate may produce prolonged suppression of Pagetic activity and may normalise bone turnover in patients with mild disease without adverse effects on bone mineralisation or bone formation.

b. Calcitonin of salmon or human origin, given subcutaneously, often improves bone pain and may be useful in the treatment of neurological complications. Although side-effects (nausea, flushing and diarrhoea) are common and may limit treatment in up to 20% of patients, it is still second-line therapy. Resistance to salmon calcitonin after 1–2 years may indicate the development of neutralising antibodies. Serum alkaline phosphatase levels and urinary hydroxyproline levels are useful guides to the effect of treatment: a 50% reduction in either test value indicates a good response to treatment.

c. Mithramycin, given intravenously, can be very effective. It is reserved for occasions when rapid remission is required (e.g. spinal cord compression). There may be significant increases in bone lysis and predisposition to fractures with this drug, as well as bone marrow depression.

3. Surgery, including osteotomy for mis-shapen femurs, may be useful. It is important for the patient to avoid immobilisation in the postoperative period because of the risk of hypercalcaemia.

4. The appearance of osteosarcoma (see Fig. 10.4) is associated with a poor prognosis. Preoperative chemotherapy followed by amputation – the current treatment for spontaneously occurring tumours – is being evaluated.

Possible lines of questioning

1. Do you think *this* patient has any evidence of neurological complications of Paget's disease?
2. What would be your strategy for drug treatment for *this* patient and what would you tell him or her about the likely success and complications of the treatment?

Acromegaly

Although an uncommon condition (three to four new cases per million people a year), acromegaly is a chronic illness and common as a long or a short case. It can be a component of multiple endocrine neoplasia type 1 (MEN1).

The history

The patient will probably know the diagnosis, although if the condition has been suspected only recently then investigations may still be under way. The patient may be in hospital for these tests because of a complication of the condition or, perhaps more likely, may have been brought in for the clinical examinations.

1. Find out when the diagnosis was made and how long ago; in retrospect, the patient may have had symptoms for years. The average time taken to make the diagnosis is more than 10 years.
2. Ask why the diagnosis was suspected. The onset of abnormalities is usually very gradual. The common features of the condition are listed in Table 10.9. Ask what changes the patient has been aware of and whether these have improved with treatment. Bony and acral changes are irreversible and early diagnosis is worthwhile.
3. Ask about the associations and complications of the condition. The mortality rate for untreated acromegaly is about twice that of the age-matched population, mostly as a result of an increased risk of cardiovascular disease. There is also an increase in the incidence of colonic polyps and carcinoma of the colon.

Table 10.9 Symptoms and signs in acromegaly	
Acral enlargement[a]	Macroglossia
Cardiac failure	Muscle weakness
Carpal tunnel syndrome	Osteoarthritis
Diabetes mellitus	Paraesthesiae
Enlarged jaw and facial features[a] (see Fig. 10.6)	Peripheral neuropathy
Erectile dysfunction and hypogonadism	Skin tags and colon polyps
Galactorrhoea	Soft-tissue enlargement[a]
Goitre	Sweating[a]
Headache[a]	Symptoms of sleep apnoea
Hypertension	Visual disturbance (field defect)
Hypopituitarism	
[a]In > 50% of patients.	

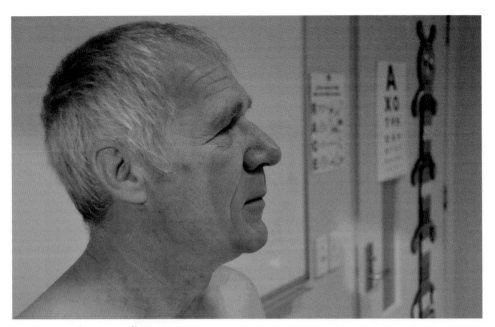

Figure 10.6 **Acromegalic appearance.**

4. There is now a recognised association with obstructive sleep apnoea and questions should be asked about snoring, daytime sleepiness and other relevant symptoms. The reason for the association is the enlargement of the tongue and swelling of the upper airway.
5. Ask if the patient knows what investigations have been performed (see Investigations below).
6. Ask about current and past treatment and how helpful this has been. Pituitary surgery and radiotherapy have a number of complications.
7. As with any chronic illness, the effect of acromegaly on the patient's life may be severe. Ask about occupation and ability to work.

The examination
See pages 481–4 and Fig. 10.6.

Investigations
1. The preferred test is measurement of insulin-like growth factor I (IGF-I). Unlike growth hormone (GH), which is affected by exercise and diet, the level of IGF-I does not fluctuate and the absolute level reliably reflects the average GH level. The result must be interpreted according to the patient's age – levels are highest at puberty and decline with age. There is also physiological elevation of the level in pregnancy.

   The diagnosis is usually confirmed with a glucose tolerance test, where GH suppression (normal to < 0.3 µg/L) is measured in response to a glucose load. Failure of suppression is characteristic of acromegaly, but the test is non-specific and may be abnormal in renal impairment, thyrotoxicosis and diabetes.
2. In 25% of acromegalic patients, the prolactin level is elevated and this can be associated with galactorrhoea. Other pituitary hormone levels may be low because of interference with normal pituitary function by the large mass of the tumour. Baseline pituitary

> **Box 10.1 Basal tests of pituitary function**
>
> - 9 a.m. cortisol
> - Testosterone or oestradiol
> - Luteinising hormone
> - Follicle-stimulating hormone
> - Prolactin
> - Thyroid-stimulating hormone and free thyroxine

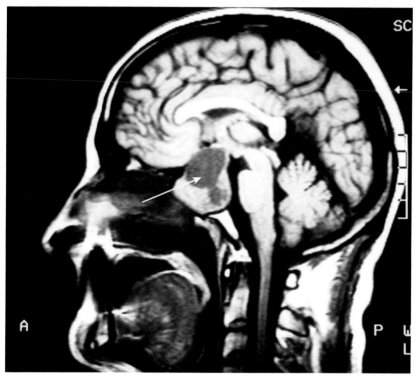

Figure 10.7 MRI of the brain showing a large pituitary tumour (arrow).

Figure reproduced courtesy of The Canberra Hospital.

function should be assessed, with measurements of prolactin, cortisol, thyroid-stimulating hormone (TSH), thyroxine (T_4), follicle-stimulating hormone (FSH) and luteinising hormone (LH) (Box 10.1).

3. Imaging is performed once an elevated IGF-I is confirmed. MRI scanning is the modality of choice as it provides excellent anatomical definition of the tumour (Fig. 10.7); 70% of tumours are macroadenomas (> 1 cm). If the tumour is close to the optic chiasm then visual field assessment should be performed.

Treatment

The aim of treatment is to prevent excess GH production without interfering with normal pituitary function.

Early diagnosis makes treatment easier and more effective, and IGF-I testing makes the diagnosis easier.

Acromegaly is cured when the IGF-I level is normal and GH is suppressed to less than 1.2 mIU/L after an oral glucose load. However, symptomatic relief can be obtained without complete cure.

Investigate for complications:

- HbA_{1c}
- sleep study
- echocardiogram
- colonoscopy.

Medical treatment with long-acting somatostatin analogues is increasingly useful, both before surgery and afterwards if removal is incomplete. Overall, surgery remains the treatment of first choice.

SURGERY

1. Trans-sphenoidal pituitary surgery is effective and remains first-line treatment. Selective resection of the benign adenoma and preservation of pituitary function is possible in 50%–80% of surgically treated cases. If cure is defined as a return of IGF-I to the normal range, then surgical cure is less often obtained. Nevertheless, symptoms are almost always greatly relieved by surgical debulking of the tumour.
2. The perioperative mortality rate should be less than 1%.
3. Uncommon complications include cerebrospinal fluid rhinorrhoea, diabetes insipidus and stroke. Hypopituitarism follows eventually in about 10% of patients.

MEDICAL TREATMENT – PATIENTS NOT CURED BY SURGERY

1. Long-acting somatostatin analogues, such as octreotide LAR and lanreotide autogel, are available. These drugs mimic the inhibition of GH release by somatostatin. They have the advantage that they are sufficiently long-acting to be effective when given by subcutaneous or intramuscular injection. The usual dose of octreotide LAR is 20 mg by intramuscular injection 4-weekly, but this can be increased or decreased depending on the GH and IGF-I levels. Lanreotide autogel is given as a starting dose of 60 mg by SC injection 4-weekly. Unlike somatostatin, these drugs do not significantly inhibit insulin secretion. Unless surgery or radiotherapy has cured the disease, treatment must be continued indefinitely. Symptoms such as headache, arthralgia and sweating improve after a few weeks. Biochemical remission occurs in up to 70% of patients. The drugs sometimes cause a 50%–70% reduction in the size of the tumour, which can make surgery easier. Side-effects of treatment are usually relatively mild and include discomfort at the injection site, diarrhoea, anorexia, abdominal bloating and cholelithiasis.

   Long-acting depot injections are now available but expensive. For this reason, they are usually reserved for patients in whom other treatment has not been completely successful or is contraindicated.
2. Cabergoline is also available for treating acromegaly. It causes a paradoxical suppression of GH release in acromegalics but, at tolerated doses, remission is not usually obtained. Side-effects include nausea, anorexia and hypotension. The drug is most often used as adjunctive treatment after radiotherapy or surgery.

RADIOTHERAPY

Radiotherapy is usually considered as a second-line treatment where surgery has not been completely effective.

1. Conventional radiotherapy delivers about 5000 cGy to the pituitary over 5 weeks. It works only slowly. GH levels take a year to fall by 25%. Even after 10 years, few

patients achieve normal IGF-I levels. Hypopituitarism is common after radiotherapy, but other side-effects are rare.

2. Newer, more promising techniques use computerised MRI to deliver larger doses accurately to the gland ('stereotactic radiosurgery').

SCREEN FOR COMPLICATIONS

1. Cardiovascular: echocardiography 5- to 10-yearly (heart failure, valve disease).
2. Gastrointestinal: colonoscopy for polyps – at diagnosis and as required for surveillance.
3. Thyroid: thyroid examination and thyroid function tests (TFTs) regularly.
4. Metabolic: check blood pressure, check lipids annually, fasting blood sugar level (BSL) annually.
5. Musculoskeletal: ask about symptoms, carpal tunnel, arthropathy.

Possible lines of questioning

1. What screening would you recommend to *this* acromegalic patient for complications of the disease?
2. How would you explain to *this* patient the benefits of surgery compared with non-surgical treatment of his acromegaly?

Types 1 and 2 diabetes mellitus

This is a common subject for the long case since patients with diabetes are always available. A large proportion of long-case patients have type 2 diabetes, often as part of the 'metabolic syndrome'. Diabetes usually presents a management rather than a diagnostic problem. The examiners like this disease because it tests very practical management skills.

> **HINT**
>
> Candidates are often tempted to unleash a set piece *diabetes long-case formula* on the examiners. Don't do it. Tailor the presentation to the actual patient you have seen.

Juvenile diabetes (immune-mediated diabetes) is called type 1 and maturity-onset diabetes (non-immune-mediated diabetes) is called type 2. Most type 1 diabetes (type 1A) is associated with autoimmune destruction of islet cells, but a small proportion of these diabetics do not have these abnormalities (type 1B). Table 10.10 lists the antibodies known to be associated with type 1 diabetes. The cause of type 1B diabetes in these patients is not known, but it is more common in Asian populations. Type 2 diabetes is increasingly found in obese adolescents and children. More than 90% of diabetics have type 2 disease.

- Don't forget the criteria for diagnosis of diabetes mellitus – a fasting (overnight) blood sugar level of 7.0 mmol/L or higher on at least two separate occasions or, in the absence of fasting hyperglycaemia, a 2-hour postprandial glucose level of 11.1 mmol/L or higher.

Table 10.10 Type 1 diabetes – associated antibodies

1. Insulin autoantibody (IAA)
2. Insulinoma-associated protein 2 antibody (IA-2)
3. Zinc transporter 8 antibody (ZnT8)
4. Glutamic acid decarboxylase antibody (GADA)

Table 10.11 Causes of glucose intolerance

1. Diabetes mellitus
2. Counter-regulatory hormone excess (rare):
   - Acromegaly
   - Cushing's syndrome
   - Phaeochromocytoma
   - Glucagonoma (associated with necrolytic erythema)
3. Pregnancy
4. Drugs:
   - Steroids or oral contraceptives
   - Streptozotocin
   - Calcineurin inhibitors (tacrolimus and cyclosporin)
   - Thiazide diuretics (temporary and mild, secondary to hypokalaemia)
   - Olanzapine
   - Phenytoin, diazoxide (insulin secretion inhibited)
5. Pancreatic disease:
   - Chronic pancreatitis or carcinoma
   - Haemochromatosis (decreased insulin production with or without increased insulin resistance)
6. Chronic liver disease (insulin resistance)
7. Syndromes:
   - Lipoatrophic diabetes (generalised lipoatrophy, hepatomegaly, hirsutism, hyperpigmentation, hyperlipidaemia)
   - Type A syndrome (usually young women with acanthosis nigricans and polycystic ovary disease)
   - Type B syndrome (acanthosis nigricans (see Fig. 10.8) and autoimmune disease)
8. Inherited:
   - Monogenic diabetes (maturity onset diabetes of the young (MODY) – *HNF1A* and glucokinase mutations)
   - Diabetes insipidus; diabetes mellitus, optic atrophy and deafness (DMOAD)

- Fasting blood glucose levels between 6.1 and 7.0 mmol/L are considered to represent impaired fasting glucose levels. In a patient with symptoms of diabetes, a random BSL of > 11.1 mmol/L is diagnostic.
- There is evidence that complications of diabetes may occur in some populations when the fasting glucose level is over 6.1 mmol/L.
- An HbA_{1c} level of > 48 mmol/mol (> 6.5%) is consistent with a diagnosis of diabetes and often used in place of a formal glucose tolerance test to make the diagnosis, except in pregnancy (see p. 307).

The history

1. Ask about the age at which diabetes was diagnosed and its manner of presentation – thirst, polyuria and polydipsia, weight loss, infection, ketoacidosis, asymptomatic glycosuria. Remember the rare causes of glucose intolerance (Table 10.11).

Table 10.12 Dietary recommendations for type 1 and type 2 diabetes
• Protein 10%–20% kJ/day
• Saturated fat < 10% kJ/day
• Polyunsaturated fat 10% kJ/day
• Carbohydrate (50%–55%) and monounsaturated fats for the rest
• Artificial sweeteners as required
• Fibre 30 g/day
• Minimise cholesterol intake (< 300 mg/day)

2. Ask about the treatment initiated at diagnosis and major changes that have occurred over time (insulin is required for survival in type 1 diabetes, which usually has an onset below age 30 years; in type 2 diabetes, control typically becomes more difficult with time).

3. Ask about the diet prescribed (Table 10.12). People with diabetes are educated regarding the requirements of a healthy diet. In addition, most type 1 diabetes patients are taught carbohydrate counting. This allows them to work out the carbohydrate content of their meals. They then base their rapid-acting insulin dose on their carbohydrate intake, for example 1 unit for every 10 g of carbohydrate.

   What has happened to the patient's weight since the diagnosis was made?

4. Ask whether oral hypoglycaemic drugs have been used or are being taken.

5. Ask about insulin treatment – how much and when taken. The usual dose is 0.5 units/kg/day, with 40% of the dose comprising a long-acting insulin. Also ask where the insulin is injected and by whom, and find out the type of insulin syringe used (e.g. a pen injector).

6. Ask about the progress of the disease:
   a. assessment of control adequacy – does the patient use a home blood glucose monitoring meter? If the patient is blind, is the glucometer a talking version? Which glucose reagent strip is used and which meter? (Remember that different meters require different reagent strips.) Enquire how often the test is done, the usual results, at what time of day the test is performed (pre- or postprandial or both) and whether the dose is adjusted at other times (e.g. gastrointestinal upset). Ask about recent glycosylated haemoglobin (HbA$_{1c}$) results. Ask about symptoms of poor control:
      i. hyperglycaemia – polyuria, thirst, weight loss, intermittent blurring of vision, hospital admissions with ketoacidosis (type 1 diabetes only)
      ii. hypoglycaemia and hypoglycaemia awareness – ask the patient to describe the symptoms and how they are managed; ask specifically about morning headaches, morning lethargy and night sweats (symptoms suggestive of nocturnal hypoglycaemia), weight gain and seizures; ask about the time of day in relation to food, alcohol, exercise and insulin injection
   b. involvement of other systems:
      i. vascular system – ischaemic heart disease, intermittent claudication, cerebrovascular disease
      ii. nervous system – peripheral neuropathy, autonomic neuropathy (causing erectile dysfunction, fainting, nocturnal diarrhoea), amyotrophy
      iii. eyes – regular visits to an ophthalmologist or retinal photography at the diabetes clinic and treatment received (ask especially about laser treatment)

    iv. renal system – dysuria, nocturia, oedema, hypertension; is the patient taking an ACE inhibitor or AR blocker for renal protection; has there been proteinuria?

    v. skin – boils, vaginitis and balanitis, *Candida*, necrobiosis lipoidica.

7. Ask about drug history – steroids, thiazides, oral contraceptives, beta-blockers.
8. Ask about associated other diseases – history of pancreatitis, Cushing's syndrome, acromegaly.
9. Enquire about social background – type of work, living conditions (living alone or with family), coping with giving insulin (associated blindness, etc.), eating habits, financial situation, driving (type of licence held – testing of BSL before driving).
10. Ask about variations in weight and a regular exercise program. Have diet and exercise led to a fall in weight since the diabetes was diagnosed?
11. Ask about cardiovascular risk factors, including family history, serum cholesterol level, smoking and hypertension, and drug and non-drug attempts at control of these factors (except family history).
12. Enquire about family history of diabetes and obstetric history (e.g. big babies, stillbirths), and other risk factors for type 2 diabetes (Table 10.13).
13. Ask whether the patient has an 'action plan' for hypoglycaemic symptoms and what this involves (Table 10.14).

The examination

Detailed examination is essential; look specifically for causes and complications of the disease (Figs 10.8 and 10.9). In particular, don't forget to look at the retina. Inspect the

---

Table 10.13 Risk factors for type 2 diabetes

- Family history (first-degree relatives)
- Age over 45
- Overweight (BMI > 27 kg/m^2)
- Race (Australian Aboriginals – at risk with BMI > 22 kg/m^2; Māori, Pacific Islander)
- Previous abnormal fasting glucose (6.1–7.0 mmol/L)
- Gestational diabetes
- Hypertension
- Polycystic ovaries

Table 10.14 Particular considerations for type 1 diabetes

1. Insulin is always required
2. Absolute lack of insulin makes BSLs unstable
3. BSL testing at least four times a day is optimal
4. Much higher risk of severe hypoglycaemia (10-fold at least)
5. Much higher risk of life-threatening ketoacidosis
6. Severe disruption to normal life – > 1000 BSL tests a year
7. Complicated and constant adjustments of insulin doses
8. Vascular and renal complications occur later, but still at a young age for most patients
9. Vascular complications common once proteinuria occurs
10. Lifelong aggressive cardiovascular risk factor control essential
11. Associated autoimmune abnormalities are common – if clinically indicated, test for thyroid and coeliac disease

BSL = blood sugar level.

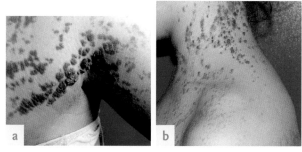

Figure 10.8 **Acanthosis nigricans. (a) View of the axillar region. (b) View of the neck and anterior chest wall.**

I Tonguc, S Cenc, D Iscen, K Yildiz. Acanthosis nigricans and an alternative for its surgical therapy. *Journal of Plastic, Reconstructive and Aesthetic Surgery* 2008; 62(1):148–50, with permission.

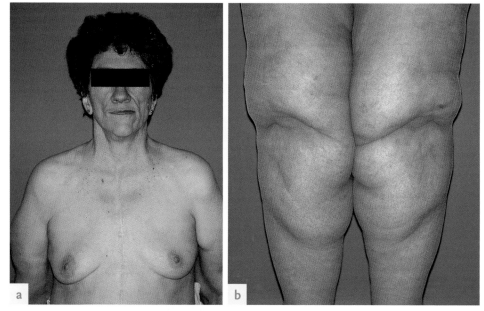

Figure 10.9 **Partial lipodystrophy, acquired. (a) Face. (b) Hypertrophy of subcutaneous fat on the lower half of the body.**

W D James, T Berger, D Elston. *Andrews' diseases of the skin: clinical dermatology*, 11th edn. Fig 23-9. Saunders, Elsevier, 2011, with permission.

feet and assess for peripheral neuropathy. Test the urine. If the patient is obese, assess BMI and waist circumference.

Management

The general aim is to regulate diet, exercise and insulin so as to allow the patient to lead a normal life while avoiding short- and long-term complications.

In adults with type 1 diabetes, multiple injection regimens are preferred because the improved control prevents or retards the progression of complications.

THE NEWLY DIAGNOSED PATIENT WITH DIABETES

The major management decision here is whether insulin is required. In some cases this will be obvious (e.g. for the type 1 patient with ketoacidosis), but for many elderly obese diabetics the position is not so clear. If insulin is not indicated at presentation, attempt to gain control first by weight loss and diet, followed by oral hypoglycaemic agents.

1. **Weight loss:** weight loss to achieve ideal body weight increases insulin sensitivity. Abdominal obesity (waist:hip ratio > 0.9 for women and > 0.8 for men) increases the risk of metabolic complications. Realise that there is some disagreement about the ideal diet, but achieving ideal weight (whatever that is) is essential.

> **HINT**
>
> Helping patients to lose weight can be difficult and frustrating (see Ch 13). It is best to be realistic with the examiners and say that numerous strategies to help the patient lose weight have been unsuccessful (if true) and that significant weight loss may not be possible (then talk about bariatric surgery if this is a reasonable option).

Usually weight loss fails. If the patient expresses some willingness to keep trying, suggest a realistic strategy and target weight. Examples include:
a. getting the patient to join a walking group
b. hydrotherapy for patients with joint pain
c. use of a pedometer or exercise mobile app. as a way of promoting exercise.

2. **Diet:** the recommended diet (see Table 10.12) should be tailored to the patient's requirements and activities. For example, kilojoule recommendations for a 20-year-old man undertaking normal activities are 175 kJ/kg of body weight and for a 75-year-old man they are 140 kJ/kg. Distribution of carbohydrate should be worked out on an individual basis. Fat intake should be kept to ≤ 30% of kilojoules for patients who are not overweight and considerably less for obese patients. The distribution of kilojoules is more important for insulin-requiring patients, who should usually have about 20% for breakfast, 35% for lunch, 30% for dinner and 15% for supper. Patients who use short-acting insulin before each meal may be able to vary the insulin dose to suit the meal. The diet should include high-fibre foods and monounsaturated fats. Polyunsaturated fats can raise triglyceride levels, but monounsaturates tend to reduce them. Patients with nephropathy may be advised to restrict protein intake, usually to about 10% of kilojoule intake.

3. **Oral hypoglycaemic agents:** the use of oral hypoglycaemic agents is first-line treatment for type 2 patients where diet has not been successful. Table 10.15 shows the National Health and Medical Research Council (NHMRC) treatment chart for type 2 diabetes.
a. Metformin is the only available biguanide and is regarded as the agent of choice in the obese patient with type 2 diabetes. It is contraindicated for patients with an eGFR < 30 mL/min/1.73 m^2. Side-effects of biguanides include:
i. diarrhoea, anorexia, nausea and occasionally vomiting
ii. vitamin B_{12} malabsorption
iii. lactic acidosis (the risk is increased in the elderly and in patients with cardiovascular, liver and kidney disease); the drug is contraindicated in heart failure

Table 10.15 Treatment chart for type 2 diabetes
1. Diet modification, weight loss, exercise ↓
2. Metformin or sulfonylurea if intolerant of metformin ↓
3. **Add one of:** sulfonylurea +/− metformin, thiazolidinedione, acarbose, SGLT-2 inhibitor, GLP-1 agonist ↓
4. **Add or substitute:** thiazolidinedione, acarbose or GLP-1 agonist / DPP-IV inhibitor or insulin
DPP-IV = dipeptidyl peptidase IV; GLP-1 = glycogen-like peptide 1; SGLT-2 = sodium–glucose linked transporter 2.

    iv. interaction with radiocontrast materials; the drug should be stopped on the day of a procedure requiring contrast and for 48 hours afterwards

    v. metformin rarely causes hypoglycaemia and there is a synergistic effect when it is used in combination with sulfonylureas.

  b. The sulfonylureas used now are second-generation drugs (e.g. gliclazide, used for obese patients; glipizide, used for thin patients; and glibenclamide). The mechanism of action of sulfonylureas is to increase insulin secretion. Side-effects of current sulfonylureas are rare apart from the following:

    i. Prolonged hypoglycaemia – this is greatest with glibenclamide, which is therefore not recommended for those over the age of 60; gliclazide and glipizide are as effective and are safer.

    ii. They are usually added to metformin therapy rather than used instead of it.

    The effectiveness of the sulfonylureas is variable and rates of secondary failure vary between agents. Primary failure occurs in 40% of cases and secondary failure in 3%–30%; only 20%–30% of patients continue with satisfactory control. Substitution of one drug for another may be worth trying (Table 10.16).

    Eventually secondary failure of sulfonylureas occurs owing to progressive decline in beta cell numbers.

  c. Thiazolidinediones (TZDs) are used as third-line treatment oral hypoglycaemic drugs. They are used less than they had been previously because of problems with weight gain and exacerbation of heart failure (see Table 10.16). They reduce insulin resistance, blood sugar levels and triglycerides. Pioglitazone and rosiglitazone are available in Australia: their use is restricted to patients whose HbA_{1c} is over 7% during the preceding 3 months and who are on maximum tolerated doses of metformin and a sulfonylurea. Patients on insulin must also be on metformin and have a raised HbA_{1c}. Liver function tests must be performed every 2 months for the first year and the drug stopped if the alanine aminotransferase (ALT) level rises above 2.5 times normal. The drugs are associated with small rises in HDL and LDL cholesterol and with peripheral oedema. Some are associated with an increased risk of ischaemic heart disease. They are contraindicated for patients with class III or IV heart failure.

  d. Acarbose inhibits intestinal alpha-glucosidase, slowing polysaccharide degradation and absorption. It is a useful agent taken before meals with other treatment. Side-effects include flatulence, diarrhoea and abdominal pain, but there is no major toxicity.

  e. The gliptins (DPP-IV inhibitors) sitaglitin, vidagliptin, saxagliptin and linagliptin increase the levels of incretin peptides (e.g. glucagon-like peptide) by inhibiting

Table 10.16 Oral hypoglycaemic agents

DRUG	FEATURES	EXPECTED FALL IN HbA$_{1c}$ (%)	PROBLEMS	CKD CRCL (mL / min)
Metformin	No weight gain	1–2	Lactic acidosis, gastrointestinal, contraindicated in severe CKD	Stop when < 60
Sulfonylureas	Work quickly	1–2	Weight gain, hypoglycaemic risk	Stop when < 30
Thiazolidinediones	Little risk of hyopoglycaemia, help lipids	0.5–1.5	Weight gain and fluid retention, ischaemic heart disease, increased fractures, macular oedema, osteoporosis, bladder cancer (pioglitazone)	No change needed
Gliptins	No weight gain, not much hypoglycaemia	0.5–1.2	Headache	Adjust dose (except linagliptin)
Exenatide	Weight loss	0.8–1.5	Nausea, pancreatitis	Stop when < 30
Acarbose	No weight gain	0.5–0.8	Flatulence, faecal incontinence	
SGLT-2 inhibitors	Weight loss, lower systolic BP, fewer cardiovascular deaths	0.25–0.5	Nausea, hypoglycaemia risk with insulin, candida	Stop when < 60 (dapagliflozin); < 45 (empagliflozin)

CKD = chronic kidney disease; CRCL = creatinine clearance.

their degrading enzyme. Insulin release is increased and glucagon suppressed. They can be used only in combination with metformin or a sulfonylurea except for linagliptin, which can be used with both. They are weight neutral and can be used in elderly patients, but chronic kidney disease is a relative contraindication. They have to be injected.

f. GLP-1 analogues: exenatide is a glucagon analogue resistant to DPP-IV degradation. It has to be given by injection twice a day. It can be especially useful for overweight patients.

g. SGLT-2 inhibitors: these drugs slow gastric emptying and reduce glucagon secretion. They tend to cause weight loss. They have to be injected and should be stopped if the creatinine clearance falls below about 60 mL/min. A number of these drugs, including recently dapagliflozin, have been shown to improve cardiovascular outcomes quite dramatically in diabetic patients.

INSULIN THERAPY

1. Insulin requirements initially are generally between 0.4 and 1.0 U/kg/day. An anorectic agent should be considered when requirements exceed 1.5 U/kg/day. Insulin therapy is often begun on an outpatient basis and, under these circumstances, small doses

Table 10.17 Available insulins	
NAME	**TYPE**
HUMAN INSULINS **Short-acting** Actrapid Humulin R	 Neutral Neutral
Intermediate- and long-acting Humulin NPH Protaphane	 Protamine suspension Protamine suspension
Biphasic mixtures: Humulin 30/70 Mixtard 30/70 Mixtard 50/50	 Protamine suspension + neutral Protamine suspension + neutral Protamine suspension + neutral
INSULIN ANALOGUES **Rapid-acting** Humalog Aprida NovoRapid	 Lispro Glulisine Aspart
Biphasic analogue insulins: Novomix 30 Humalog mix 25 Humalog mix 50	 Aspart + aspart protamine Lispro + lispro suspension Lispro + lispro suspension
Long-acting Lantus Levemer	 Glargine Detemir

(e.g. 0.25 U/kg/day) sufficient to prevent ketosis are used with a view to avoiding hypoglycaemia.

Modern insulins are either recombinant human insulin or analogue insulin (Table 10.17). Analogue insulins have been genetically altered to maintain their monomeric form when injected subcutaneously. This better mimics physiological insulin release.

Possible insulin regimens include:

- Type 1 diabetes: a basic bolus regimen, using a once-daily long-acting insulin analogue and short-acting insulin analogue at mealtimes (see Table 10.17), or a continuous subcutaneous insulin infusion (CSII) using an insulin pump. Extra insulin is given at mealtimes after calculation of the insulin:carbohydrate ratio and measurement of the blood sugar. Extra rapid-acting insulin is given if necessary.
- Type 2 diabetes: basal insulin is used in combination with metformin.

The administration of intraperitoneal insulin via the dialysate can be useful in the management of patients on continuous ambulatory peritoneal dialysis (CAPD), and continuous intraperitoneal infusion has been attempted in some centres.

Human insulin has replaced the highly purified (monocomponent) insulins. Many patients reported altered symptoms of hypoglycaemia and a more rapid onset of symptoms after changing to human insulin. Aim for euglycaemia: ideally the glucose level should be between 3.5 and 7.0 mmol/L throughout the day and night.

2. Insulin resistance is defined as a requirement of more than 200 units per day. Causes of insulin resistance are:
   a. obesity (decreased receptor number)
   b. insulin antibodies (uncommon, and an indication for a more purified insulin)
   c. circulating antagonist hormones – growth hormone (e.g. in puberty), cortisol, thyroxine, glucagon
   d. association with acanthosis nigricans (e.g. receptor abnormalities, lipodystrophies). Remember, injecting into a lipoatrophied site may cause poor control because of unpredictable absorption.

3. Insulin allergy has been uncommon since the widespread introduction of human insulins, but they can cause immediate local reactions (e.g. pruritus, local pain) or delayed reactions (e.g. swelling). Urticaria and anaphylaxis can also occur. Treatment in mild cases is with antihistamines and local steroids, but desensitisation is important in severe cases. Insulin allergy is more common in patients who stop and start insulin therapy.

4. Fasting hyperglycaemia is a major management problem. The 'Somogyi effect' refers to rebound morning hyperglycaemia following nocturnal hypoglycaemia, which is thought to be caused by the release of counter-regulatory hormones. This is now, however, a matter of considerable debate. The treatment is to reduce the evening insulin dose. The 'dawn' phenomenon is early-morning hyperglycaemia in the *absence* of nocturnal hypoglycaemia; the treatment is to increase the insulin coverage without inducing hypoglycaemia.

5. Causes of hypoglycaemia in a previously stable diabetic on insulin therapy are:
   a. decreased food intake, increased exercise or weight loss
   b. injection errors
   c. diabetic renal disease
   d. rare causes – high level of insulin antibodies, malabsorption, hypothyroidism, autoimmune adrenal insufficiency, panhypopituitarism or an insulinoma.

6. Glycated haemoglobin (HbA_{1c}) gives an indication of control over the preceding 3 months.

   Newly diagnosed patients should aim for tight blood sugar control (HbA_{1c} <50 mmol/mol – 6.8%), and those with advanced disease and who already have cardiovascular complications for less tight control (e.g. < 60 mmol/mol). Spurious readings may occur in kidney failure, iron deficiency, haemoglobinopathies and pregnancy.

DIABETES EDUCATION

Because diabetes is a lifelong disease, detailed education by the team looking after the patient is important. Regular follow-up is essential (Table 10.18).

1. Blood glucose level (BGL) monitoring with a glucose meter is essential for all patients who can manage it – initially, testing several times a day before and 2 hours after

Table 10.18 What to do if BSL targets not met after drug adjustment
1. Make sure the patient understands the point of treatment.
2. Look again at diet, weight and exercise program.
3. Ask about adherence; begin by asking about side-effects and then ask whether the patient has been able to take the medication.
4. Exclude infection and use of new medications that would interfere with sugars, e.g. steroids.
BSL = blood sugar level.

meals, and before bed, may be necessary; later, in stable diabetes, twice-daily testing may be enough.

2. Exercise promotes glucose utilisation; in the well-controlled diabetic it is important to reduce the dose of regular insulin before exercise or supplement with glucose. (*Note:* Exercise in the poorly controlled diabetic may precipitate ketoacidosis because of increased release of counter-regulatory hormones.)

MANAGEMENT OF CHRONIC COMPLICATIONS

Complications are probably a result of damage caused by glycosylated proteins. Convincing evidence that tight control prevents or reverses complications is now available. Following the Diabetes Control and Complications Trial and the more recent United Kingdom Prognosis in Diabetes Study (UKPDS), clinicians now agree that rigorous control of blood sugar levels and aggressive control of blood pressure (< 140/90)[2] and other cardiovascular risk factors is essential. These measures are probably more effective in the early stages of the disease.

1. The blood pressure can be managed with any antihypertensive drug, but the use of an ACE inhibitor (ACEI) or an angiotensin II receptor blocker (ARB) – but not both – is strongly indicated when proteinuria has been detected, and is often used routinely.

2. Lipid control with the statins is being assessed in a number of trials. The high cardiovascular risk of these patients suggests that aggressive lipid-lowering with one of these drugs will be of value. Remember to control other risk factors, such as smoking (for retinopathy and vascular disease) and alcohol intake (for neuropathy and hypertriglyceridaemia). Aspirin prophylaxis is controversial, but prophylaxis should be recommended for patients with macrovascular complications.

3. Ideally, all patients should be assessed every 2 years by an ophthalmologist. Less sophisticated fundoscopy may miss early diabetic retinopathy (see Table 16.43, p. 490). Retinal cameras can now be used at the clinic to take clear retinal photographs, which can be repeated often and 'read' by an ophthalmologist. Retinopathy almost always precedes diabetic nephropathy.

4. Diabetic nephropathy is a common cause of chronic kidney disease and results from arteriolar disease or glomerulosclerosis (classic Kimmelstiel–Wilson lesion or, more commonly, diffuse intercapillary glomerulosclerosis). The evolution of diabetic nephropathy has been well studied and can be divided into the following stages:
   a. glomerular hyperfiltration
   b. microalbuminuria
   c. dipstick proteinuria
   d. proteinuria in the nephrotic range
   e. end-stage kidney disease.

5. Microalbuminuria is defined as a urinary albumin excretion of 20–200 µg/min (measured using sensitive immunoassays) on more than two occasions in the absence of urinary tract infection and intercurrent illness. The albumin:creatinine ratio may be a more sensitive way of assessing the presence of significant proteinuria. Regular screening for microalbuminuria is now considered an important component of good diabetes management. The microalbuminuria stage is probably reversible with a combination of ACEI or ARB therapy, strict metabolic control and possibly dietary protein restriction.

---

[2] The ACCORD study.

6. Once proteinuria develops, progression to end-stage kidney disease is common over a period of about 5–10 years. The rate of progression may be modified by:
   a. control of hypertension – ACEIs are the agents of choice, but it is important to be aware of the risk of hyperkalaemia as a result of hyporeninaemic hypoaldosteronism and deteriorating kidney function in patients with renovascular disease
   b. treatment of urinary tract infections
   c. dietary protein restriction
   d. possibly improving glucose control.
   ACE inhibition is indicated as soon as proteinuria is detected. ARBs are an alternative for those intolerant of ACEIs. ACEI and ARB combination treatment may reduce proteinuria further, but has little additive effect on blood pressure and is associated with an increased risk of acute kidney failure. There is an increased incidence of papillary necrosis with urinary tract infection.

7. The best form of management for end-stage chronic kidney disease in a diabetic is peritoneal dialysis and early kidney transplantation. Remember that diabetics with chronic kidney failure almost invariably also have retinopathy, which may be worsened by haemodialysis.

8. For type 1 diabetics with severe systemic complications or end-stage kidney disease, whole-organ pancreas (with or without kidney) transplantation is a promising therapeutic option. A number of successful kidney/pancreas transplants have been performed. Patients are generally euglycaemic without hypoglycaemic treatment. This is the treatment of choice for diabetics with kidney failure.

9. Be aware of continuous glucose monitoring systems and whether the patient is using the technology. Remember, it measures the interstitial fluid glucose (with a several-minute time lag in terms of blood sugar level). These devices improve glycaemic control in type I diabetes.

10. Is an insulin pump being used? Short-acting insulin is given and if discontinued there is a risk of diabetic ketoacidosis so education in important. Use with continuous glucose monitoring reduces the risk of hypoglycaemia.

THE PREGNANT PATIENT WITH DIABETES

Remember that blood sugar levels are normally lower in pregnancy. A woman with no diabetic history should be screened for gestational diabetes in the 24th–28th week. A 75 g glucose load is given and the blood sugar is measured 1 and 2 hours later. Abnormal results (gestational diabetes) are: fasting > 5.1, 1 hour > 10.0, 2 hours > 8.5 mmol/L.

1. High-risk women (previous gestational diabetes, BMI > 35, maternal age > 40) should be tested at 12–16 weeks.

2. Insulin requirements vary during pregnancy owing to the effects of human placental lactogen (HPL). In the first trimester, insulin requirements usually remain unchanged or may decrease, but in the second trimester some increase in insulin requirements occurs owing to rising HPL levels. By the third trimester, insulin requirements are usually at least 50% higher than before pregnancy, but after delivery there is a dramatic decrease in insulin requirements.
   In general, insulin is used alone for pregnant women with pre-existing diabetes, and diet, metformin or insulin for gestational diabetics.

3. Blood glucose control should be improved as much as possible before conception in a diabetic woman wanting to undertake pregnancy. HbA_{1c} should be normalised, as strict metabolic control at the time of conception has been shown to prevent the

otherwise increased incidence of congenital malformations in the offspring of diabetic mothers. The complications of poor control seen in the infant are:

a. congenital malformations such as spina bifida (incidence about 6%, double the normal rate)

b. macrosomia

c. intrauterine fetal death in the later stages of pregnancy

d. hypoglycaemia after delivery

e. complications related to immaturity (e.g. respiratory distress syndrome, hypocalcaemia, jaundice).

4. Use of home blood glucose monitoring, with testing of both pre- and postprandial glucose levels, is essential. Strict glucose control must be maintained during labour and delivery. Paediatric services and a neonatal intensive care unit should be available. Remember that statins, ACE inhibitors and ARBs *must* be ceased in pregnancy.

Possible lines of questioning

1. What strategies can you suggest to help *this* patient lose weight?

2. How would you manage *this* patient whose blood sugars have not improved despite a recent increase in treatment?

3. How would you explain to *this* patient the advantages and disadvantages of beginning insulin treatment?

4. Has *this* patient a good understanding of her risk of hypoglycaemia and a plan to deal with it?

Chapter 11

The renal long case

When the patient dies the kidneys may go to the pathologist, but while he lives the urine is ours.

Thomas Addis (1881–1949)

Chronic kidney disease (chronic renal failure)

Chronic kidney disease (CKD) by itself is not a particularly common main problem for the long case. However, it is a difficult and important topic and kidney disease is often present in that very common long case: the obese diabetic with hypertension and vascular disease. Renal transplant patients are commonly seen in the exam.

Keep in mind the current CKD classification and the causes of and risk factors for progression of CKD (Tables 11.1–11.3). The patient will usually know that he or she has renal disease. Methodical questioning to establish the diagnosis, cause, management and complications is necessary.

Fast facts on the eGFR

- The estimated glomerular filtration rate (eGFR) is a useful tool for communicating to patients. It conveys the level of renal function. One can simplify it as a percentage of global kidney function. The normal range is 80–120 mL/min (thus the average is 100 mL/min). This means that if the eGFR is 30 mL/min patients can be told they have 30% of normal renal function.
- CKD patients often know their eGFRs.
  - The measurement tends to underestimate normal or near-normal renal function.
  - The serum creatinine should be stable for a number of days for an accurate eGFR reading, so eGFR is *not* helpful for assessing acute kidney injury.
    - In elderly people there is controversy about its interpretation. An eGFR of more than 45 mL/m^2 in an old person without proteinuria is not associated with an adverse renal prognosis.
    - For black populations the laboratory reading should be multiplied by 1.2.
    - The measurement of eGFR is not accurate in pregnancy.

Table 11.1 Stages of chronic kidney disease

STAGE	DESCRIPTION	eGFR (mL/min)
1	Kidney damage but normal GFR	> 90
2	Kidney damage and mild GFR reduction	60–89
3	Moderate reduction in GFR	30–59
4	Severe reduction in GFR	15–29
5	Kidney failure	< 15

eGFR = estimated glomerular filtration rate.

Table 11.2 Causes of chronic kidney disease

1. Diabetes mellitus – 33%
2. Glomerulonephritis – 24%
3. Hypertension – 14%
4. Polycystic kidneys – 7%
5. Reflux nephropathy
6. Analgesic nephropathy
7. Uncertain

Table 11.3 Risk factors for progression of chronic kidney disease

1. Low birth weight (fewer than normal nephrons to start with)
2. Hypertension
3. Acute kidney injury
4. Proteinuria
5. Smoking
6. Hyperuricaemia
7. An increase in glomerular pressure (pregnancy, obesity, diabetes)

- In people with low muscle mass the number may be an over-estimate of renal function.
- The eGFR helps to determine when preparation for dialysis should begin (but gives no information about the cause of the renal dysfunction). For example, the Initiating Dialysis Early and Late (IDEAL) study suggested that dialysis should commence when the eGFR is 7–10 mL/min.
- Arteriovenous fistulas for haemodialysis are not usually ready to use for at least 3 months after the surgery. Nephrologists prepare for vascular access surgery when the eGFR is about 15–20 mL/min.
- A pre-emptive renal transplant is sometimes performed when the eGFR is about 15 mL/min.
- It is important to note that eGFR falls with ageing. The rate of fall is slower for females (≈ 0.7 mL/min/year) than for males (≈ 1 mL/min/year). The falls start at

approximately the age of 35. Hence, when assessing an 85-year-old man, you could expect that his eGFR should be about 50 mL/min. If he has had a nephrectomy, he should have about 25 mL/min eGFR.

- If there is discrepancy between the calculated and expected eGFR, the nephrologist or astute candidate will suspect the presence of causes of reduction of eGFR other than ageing.
- The eGFR is not accurate in patients with limb amputation because of their loss of muscle mass.

The history
QUESTIONS REGARDING SYMPTOMS, DIAGNOSIS AND AETIOLOGY

1. Early symptoms of renal failure include:
   - nocturia
   - lethargy
   - loss of appetite
   - fluid retention
   - pruritus.
     Severe CKD (GFR < 15–20 mL/min/1.73 m^2) can cause:
   - pericarditis
   - serositis
   - encephalopathy
   - gastrointestinal bleeding
   - uraemic neuropathy.
     Patients are sometimes diagnosed following an episode of haematuria or loin pain. A first episode of overt renal failure may have been precipitated by a further insult, such as:
   - use of drugs such as NSAIDs, trimethoprim or, less commonly now, aminoglycoside administration
   - use of radiocontrast injections
   - infection
   - use of angiostensin-converting enzyme inhibitors (ACEIs) or angiotensin II receptor blockers (ARBs) (if there is bilateral renal artery stenosis)
   - dehydration
   - anaemia.
     Many patients are asymptomatic and have a family history. Sometimes haematuria or proteinuria has been detected during a routine or insurance medical examination or during pregnancy.
2. **Glomerulonephritis** (Table 11.4). Determine whether there is a history of:
   - proteinuria
   - haematuria
   - oliguria
   - oedema
   - sore throat
   - sepsis
   - rash
   - haemoptysis
   - renal biopsy.
     Run through the various causes listed below with the patient or ask 'Have you been told what the cause of your kidney trouble is?' This question may save a lot of time and trouble.

HINTS

Ask yourself after you have taken the history: 'What is the cause of this patient's CKD?' Consider:

1. **Glomerulonephritis:** has the patient had a kidney biopsy? Was there any specific change in therapy following the biopsy? For example, in IgA nephropathy, if there are significant chronic changes and reduced kidney function, data suggest there is little point in starting high-dose steroids. On the other hand, if there are no severe chronic changes (eGFR >80 mL/min and proteinuria <0.5 g/day) a 6-month trial of prednisolone (≈ 1 mg/kg/day) may be indicated to attempt to induce a remission, if supportive therapy with ACEIs or ARBS hasn't helped.

2. **IgA nephropathy** is associated with intermittent macroscopic haematuria, synpharyngitic haematuria (typically following soon after a mild upper respiratory tract infection) or persistent microscopic haematuria. Even so, it is important to consider other causes of haematuria (e.g. bladder transitional cell carcinomas, kidney stones).

3. **Diabetic nephropathy:** this is now the most common cause of CKD in Australia. These patients don't usually undergo a renal biopsy. However, it may be indicated in patients with diabetes where non-diabetic renal disease is suspected, for example those without micro- and macrovascular complications of diabetes, or where the duration of diabetes is short.

4. **Hypertensive nephropathy:** this is an unusual diagnosis. However, most patients with CKD are hypertensive and improving blood pressure (BP) control is often a mainstay of therapy aimed at slowing the rate of progression of CKD of any cause. Because of its place in therapy, detailed knowledge of the patient's blood pressure and its management is crucial. Trials have suggested that angioplasty for atheromatous renal artery stenosis is no more effective than medical therapy; similarly, despite early enthusiasm, renal artery sympathectomy (denervation) has not proven to be effective in most patients with resistant hypertension.

5. **Analgesic nephropathy:** this is now a truly rare condition but patients very occasionally turn up at exams.

6. Don't forget to ask about a **family history** of kidney disease. Clearly, it is important not to miss polycystic kidney disease (see below). However, diabetes, hypertension, reflux nephropathy and various forms of glomerulonephritis (GN) can also have an inherited basis. This can be important even when discussing the possibility of living related donors for kidney transplantation, for example.

7. **Interstitial nephritis:** acute interstitial nephritis can be a result of drug allergy, an immune reaction or an infection (Table 11.5). It is an important cause of chronic interstitial nephritis and CKD.

8. **Unknown cause:** this group of patients usually present with chronic changes in their kidneys or small shrunken kidneys that cannot be safely biopsied. Serological tests for causes of kidney diseases are negative.

Ascertain treatment details (e.g. antihypertensives, immunosuppressives, antiplatelet therapy, dialysis).

1. **Diabetic nephropathy:** ask about other complications and therapy. An ACEI or ARB (but not both) is preferred for all cases with diabetic nephropathy. The creatinine should be monitored after treatment is begun. An increase in serum creatinine of less than 30% is acceptable and may indeed indicate a degree of renal protection – reduced glomerular pressure increases the creatinine but protects the kidneys in the long run. A rise in creatinine of more than 30% usually means the drug should be stopped.

Table 11.4 Classification of glomerulonephritis (GN)

PRIMARY

Diffuse

1. Minimal change – most common cause of nephrotic syndrome in children
2. Membranous GN (Box 11.2)
3. Proliferative
   - Post-streptococcal (and after other infections)
   - Mesangiocapillary
   - Crescentic
   - Mesangioproliferative

Focal

1. IgA nephropathy (Box 11.1)
2. Focal segmental glomerulosclerosis (FSGS) – most common cause of nephrotic syndrome (Box 11.3)

GLOMERULONEPHRITIS AS PART OF A SYSTEMIC DISEASE

1. Systemic lupus erythematosus (SLE)
2. Granulomatosis with polyangiitis (GPA)
3. Polyarteritis nodosa (PAN)
4. Goodpasture's syndrome
5. Henoch–Schönlein purpura
6. Infective endocarditis
7. Cryoglobulinaemia ± hepatitis C
8. Myeloma
9. Diabetes mellitus
10. Haemolytic uraemic syndrome (HUS)

Box 11.1 IgA nephropathy – associations

- HIV infection
- Chronic liver disease
- Inflammatory bowel disease
- Coeliac disease

Box 11.2 Causes of membranoproliferative glomerulonephritis

a. Hepatitis C
b. Autoimmune diseases
c. Indolent infections (malaria, syphilis)
d. Essential cryoglobulinaemia
e. Malignancies
f. Drugs – penicillamine, NSAIDs, anti-TNF drugs
g. Mercury or gold poisoning

NSAID = non-steroidal anti-inflammatory drug; TNF = tumour necrosis factor.

Box 11.3 Causes of focal segmental glomerulosclerosis

- Primary
- Familial
- HIV infection
- Morbid obesity
- Heroin use
- Reflux nephropathy

Table 11.5 Causes of acute interstitial nephritis
ALLERGIES Proton pump inhibitors, penicillin, NSAIDs, gadolinium contrast material
IMMUNE Transplant rejection, autoimmune nephritis
INFECTIONS TB, bacterial pyelonephritis, leptospirosis
TOXINS Mushrooms, myeloma light chains

HINT

Distinguish the nephrotic syndrome (Table 11.6) from the nephritic syndrome (Table 11.7) and the types of glomerulonephritis (GN) (see Table 11.4).

Nephrotic – protein leakage across the glomeruli:
- severe proteinuria (urine protein > 3.5 g / 24 hours)
- hypoalbuminaemia
- oedema.

Nephritic – inflammation or injury within the glomeruli allowing protein, red blood cells and white blood cells into the renal tubule; there is:
- reduced glomerular filtration
- proteinuria
- haematuria, pyuria
- hypertension
- reduced renal function.

Patients with very low eGFRs (< 20 mL / min) should have the drug stopped, but if there is no improvement in eGFR it can usually be restarted.

2. **Polycystic kidney disease (PKD):** ask about family history (the condition is usually autosomal dominant – called ADPKD), how the disease was diagnosed, haematuria, polyuria, loin pain, hypertension, headache, subarachnoid haemorrhages and visual disturbance (intracranial aneurysm).

   Also ask about deafness and a history of persistent haematuria (hereditary nephritis – Alport's syndrome).

3. **Reflux nephropathy:** ask about childhood renal infections, cystoscopy, operations, treatment (e.g. regular antibiotics) and enuresis.

4. **Hypertensive nephropathy:** ask about how the disease was diagnosed, duration and control of hypertension, treatment and compliance with medication, angiography and family history.

5. **Connective tissue disease:** think especially of systemic lupus erythematosus and scleroderma.

6. Find out whether the patient is aware of the **long-term prognosis**. If he or she is not yet on dialysis, has this been discussed? Is the patient likely to be eligible for dialysis or the transplant list?

7. Ask when the **underlying condition** was **diagnosed** and how it is being **treated**. The progression to end-stage kidney disease may be rapid or very prolonged.

HINT

Autosomal dominant polycystic kidney disease
The extrarenal manifestations of ADPKD include:
- liver cysts/hepatomegaly
- pancreatic cysts
- splenic cysts
- thyroid cysts
- seminal vesicle cysts
- intracranial cerebral aneurysms
- hypertension
- diverticular disease
- hernias.

Table 11.6 The nephrotic syndrome

CLINICAL FEATURES
1. Proteinuria (> 3.5 g/24 h)
2. Hypoalbuminaemia (serum albumin < 30 g/L)
3. Oedema
4. Hyperlipidaemia (increased LDL and cholesterol levels)

CAUSES
1. Primary (80%)
Idiopathic membranous glomerulonephropathy is the most common cause in adults over 40 years of age. Other primary causes include focal glomerular sclerosis, membranoproliferative glomerulonephritis and minimal change nephropathy

2. Secondary
Systemic disease – diabetes mellitus (the most common by far), SLE, Hodgkin's disease (minimal change), solid tumours (membranous), amyloid, multiple myeloma
Infection – hepatitis B (membranous), HIV (IgA nephropathy, collapsing focal sclerosis), infective endocarditis
Drugs – D-penicillamine, probenecid, non-steroidal anti-inflammatory drugs, heroin

Note: Renal vein thrombosis is a complication and rarely a cause of the nephrotic syndrome.

Table 11.7 Causes of nephritic syndrome

ABNORMALITY	CAUSE OF NEPHRITIC SYNDROME (%)	COMPLEMENT (C) FINDINGS
IgA nephropathy	25	Normal
Lupus (SLE)	20	Low C3 and C4
Pauci-immune crescentic GN	20	Normal
Membranoproliferative GN	10	Low C3 or C4 or both
Thrombotic microangiopathy	5	Low C3 sometimes
Postinfectious GN	5	Low C3
Anti-glomerular basement membrane disease (Goodpasture's)	3	Normal
C3 glomerulonephropathy	< 1	Low C3
GN = glomerulonephritis.		

Table 11.8 Principles of management of chronic kidney disease
1. Fluid intake and diet
2. Anaemia
3. Acidosis
4. Phosphate / calcium / bones
5. Cardiovascular risk reduction
6. Consider vascular access
7. Consider when to start dialysis
8. Consider suitability for transplant compared with conservative treatment

Table 11.9 Foods high in potassium
FRUIT
Bananas, figs, avocados, rhubarb (really a vegetable)
VEGETABLES
Spinach, parsnips, tomatoes (really a fruit), sprouts, potatoes; boiled vegetables contain less potassium
SNACKS
Chocolate, nuts, toffee
DRINKS
Wine, beer, cider (spirits contain less potassium, though more alcohol)
SALT SUBSTITUTES
These are usually potassium chloride

QUESTIONS REGARDING MANAGEMENT (TABLE 11.8)

1. **Conservative management:**
   a. Ask about:
      - follow-up
      - medications
      - diet
      - salt and water allowance
      - investigations performed (particularly renal biopsy)
      - whether erythropoietin has been given subcutaneously in an attempt to elevate the haemoglobin.
   b. Has the patient been advised to restrict protein intake? There is controversy about the value of protein restriction in delaying end-stage renal failure. Patients with nephrotic syndrome should be much less restricted. The concern about protein restriction is that it leads to more rapid loss of muscle mass without much delay in end-stage renal failure.
   c. Has potassium restriction been recommended? Potassium accumulates in patients with severe CKD and intake is often restricted to 70 mmol / day (Table 11.9). Has the patient been told about food that should be avoided because of its potassium content?
   d. What effect have the disease and the dietary and other restrictions had on the patient's quality of life and his or her family?
   e. Some kidney disease can be treated and this can at least slow the progression to end-stage chronic kidney disease. Ask about specific treatment including:
      - rituximab for induction and relapse and azathioprine for maintenance for antineutrophil cytoplasmic antibody (ANCA)-associated vasculitis

Table 11.10 Principles of treatment of hypertension in CKD patients

1. Multiple drugs are often required
2. ACEI or ARB first
3. A rise in creatinine is to be expected
4. A loop diuretic may help by reversing volume expansion
5. Dihydropyridine calcium antagonists may delay disease progression in hypertensive patients, compared with thiazide diuretics
6. Aldosterone antagonists can be used in patients with reasonable residual renal function, but the serum potassium must be monitored
7. In difficult cases a loop and thiazide diuretic can be used together and may help reduce the potassium level

ACEI = angiostensin-converting enzyme inhibitor; ARB = angiotensin II receptor (AR) blocker; CKD = chronic kidney disease.

Table 11.11 Dialysis

PERITONEAL DIALYSIS (CAPD OR APD)	
Advantages	Simple, reliable and safe (from a cardiovascular point of view). Removes large fluid volumes. Allows greater freedom of diet and fluid intake. Preferable for diabetics. Performed daily rather than a few days a week, can be done at home. Better if unstable cardiovascular system. APD exchanges done at night.
Disadvantages	Peritonitis, exit-site infections (around catheter). Protein loss (7–10 g / day usually; 30–40 g / day with peritonitis). Basal atelectasis. Abdominal hernias, obesity and previous surgery are contraindications. Does not control uraemia in hypercatabolic patients. Hyperglycaemia. Catheter displacement. 'Peritoneal membrane failure'. Perforation of bladder and bowel (rare). Hydrothorax (rare). May develop hernias.
HAEMODIALYSIS	
Advantages	Takes approximately 18 hours per week (4–5 hours three times / week, plus set-up time). No protein loss. Large volumes can be ultrafiltrated.
Disadvantages	Circulatory access problems (thrombosis, infection of vascular access). Heparin may increase bleeding. Increased cardiovascular instability. Anaemia. Osteodystrophy. Dialysis dementia (aluminium). Patient less involved in treatment. Dietary compliance still needed. Fluid overload and high potassium levels can still be significant problems, especially after the longer interval between dialysis sessions each week.

Note: Mortality from dialysis is caused by myocardial infarction (60%) or sepsis (20%) in most cases. Acquired cystic disease in native kidneys may occur; < 5% are malignant. Arthropathy and carpal tunnel syndrome may occur in long-term dialysis patients owing to amyloid (beta$_2$-microglobulin) deposition.

APD = automated peritoneal dialysis; CAPD = chronic ambulatory peritoneal dialysis.

- treatment for thrombotic microangiopathy with ADAMTS13 for thrombotic thrombocytopenic purpura and eculizumab for haemolytic uraemic syndrome
- polycystic kidney patient and treatment with tolvaptan
- immunosuppression for other vasculitic kidney disease such as systemic lupus erythematosus (SLE)
- treatment of hypertension (Table 11.10)
- advice about smoking cessation and avoidance of nephrotoxins.

There is no evidence that good glycaemic control helps established diabetic nephropathy.

2. **Dialysis** (Table 11.11)**:** ask about haemodialysis or peritoneal dialysis, including where performed, how often, how many hours per week, relief of symptoms with

treatment and subsequent complications. Also ask about shunts, other operations (e.g. renal tract operations, parathyroidectomy) and medications taken.

3. **Transplant work-up and management:** ask when and how many, whether from living relative or cadaver, postoperative course, improvement, symptoms since transplantation, medications, follow-up and long-term complications (e.g. neoplasia, steroid complications).

4. **Bladder management for reflux or neurogenic bladder.**

5. **Social arrangements and activities of daily living.** Ask about:
   a. employment
   b. the family's ability to cope
   c. travel
   d. sexual function
   e. the financial situation.

QUESTIONS REGARDING COMPLICATIONS

1. **Conservatively treated patients:** ask about symptoms of:
   - anaemia
   - bone disease
   - secondary gout or pseudogout
   - pericarditis
   - hypertension
   - cardiac failure
   - fluid overload
   - peripheral neuropathy
   - pruritus
   - peptic ulcers
   - impaired cognitive function
   - poor nutrition.

   Have the doses of renally excreted drugs given for other conditions been reduced? Remember that, although most drugs that require a loading dose are begun at their usual dose (and then continued at a reduced maintenance dose), digoxin, which has an altered volume distribution, must have its loading dose reduced.

   These patients will also need treatment for anaemia, potassium control and dietary restriction to minimise symptoms of uraemia.

2. **Dialysis patients:** ask about:
   a. Haemodialysis (HD) (see Table 11.11):
      i. How long has the patient been on dialysis?
         - The longer the duration of dialysis, the more likely it is the patient will develop complications from the dialysis.
         - Patients will typically have more problems with arteriovenous fistulae and are more likely to dialyse via a catheter, for example.
         - A long duration on dialysis for patients on the transplant waiting list means they have no living donors, or they may be highly sensitised and can't easily be matched for transplant.
      ii. Where does he or she dialyse?
         - In a satellite unit or at home?
         - Typically, home patients are more likely and able to increase the frequency and duration of their dialysis treatment.
         - Satellite dialysis is easy for many patients but transport to and from the dialysis unit may be difficult. The times allocated may not be convenient for patients, especially if they work.

iii. What is the current dialysis prescription?
- This includes the ideal (euvolaemic/ideal) dry weight, the frequency of dialysis (typically 3 days/week, the duration of each session (usually 4.5–5 hours), the typical fluid removal required at each dialysis session (the more fluid removal required, the greater the fluid intake and the lower the urine output must be).
- Ask about the patient's pre-dialysis and post-dialysis BP and if he or she modifies or omits antihypertensives on dialysis days (usually to avoid post-dialysis hypotension).
- Most patients don't know the dialysate being used and may or may not know about the blood flow rate or pump rate (usually ≥ 300 mL/min).
- Are water-soluble vitamins given after dialysis?
- Is the patient on an anticoagulant other than typical heparin or enoxaparin given at each dialysis session? The heparin is usually ceased an hour before the dialysis session finishes to reduce the risk of bleeding.
- Ask about problems with dialysis access (e.g. cannulation difficulties) or why the patient is using a chronic haemodialysis catheter rather than an AV fistula.
- Ask whether there have been changes in any of the above that may explain the patient's symptoms or problems.

iv. What is the patient's dialysis access history?
- Is there an arteriovenous fistula in a native vein, or a graft with interposed artificial blood vessel (typically fashioned from polytetrafluoroethylene (PTFE)), or is a chronic dialysis catheter used? These catheters are usually tunnelled to reduce infection risk and are situated in the internal jugular vein.
- The subclavian vein is not the usual site because its use more commonly leads to central vein stenosis.
- Ask the patient how many different access sites there have been. The scars on the forearms, upper arms, thighs and from catheters on the upper chest wall should all be explained.
- Patients with catheters are more likely to have slower blood flow.

v. Ask the patient about any symptoms that occur on or after dialysis.
- These may include nausea, vomiting, hypotension, cramps or collapse.
- Hypotensive patients are not uncommonly given a saline bolus to help their low BP, but this may impair their ability to achieve their assigned ideal dry weight.

b. Peritoneal dialysis (PD) (see Table 11.11): there are two main types of peritoneal dialysis – continuous ambulatory peritoneal dialysis (CAPD) and automated peritoneal dialysis (APD).

i. CAPD is typically a manual process involving daytime drain and fill cycles of PD fluid. Typically, the fill volume is 2 litres and 4 cycles/day are commonly used. This gives the patient weekly volumes of 56 litres.

ii. APD involves a bedside machine to carry out the draining and filling of the abdominal cavity while the patient sleeps. This has the advantage of giving free time during the day.

Commonly, patients now do a mixture of both techniques, especially if they have stayed on PD for many years. They have an APD cycler at night and may also do some daytime exchanges in order to improve fluid and electrolyte control (or dialysis adequacy).

Ask:

i. How long has the patient been on PD?

ii. Have there been infections of the exit site or episodes of peritonitis? These increase the risk of failure of the technique and may eventually lead to the need for removal of the catheter and a change to haemodialysis.

      iii. Does the patient still pass urine?
- This means there is still residual renal function.
- Anuric patients are more likely to have problems with inadequate dialysis and problems with adequate fluid removal on dialysis.

  c. **Medications:** obtaining an accurate list of medications helps in identifying problems that are being treated. Some medications are used commonly for dialysis patients:
    i. erythropoietin-stimulating agents (ESAs) – these may be given parenterally on dialysis by the dialysis staff if a patient is on HD
    ii. parenteral iron is commonly used in the HD units and intermittently in PD patients
    iii. phosphate binders (calcium-containing and non-calcium-containing binders)
    iv. vitamin D analogues (1,25-OH vitamin D)
    v. other vitamins
    vi. antihypertensives
    vii. also possibly sodium bicarbonate for acidosis.

  d. **Nutrition:** inadequate dialysis can lead to weight loss and malnutrition.
    i. Dietary advice is commonly required to help manage hyperkalaemia, phosphate control and fluid control (water intake).
    ii. As many patients commonly have diabetes, these patients also need advice for glucose control.
    iii. Sodium restriction and water restriction help BP control.
    iv. Hyperlipidaemia and osteoporosis problems can be managed (at least partly) with reduction of dietary intake of saturated fats and increase in calcium intake.

  e. **Other questions** to ask should include:
    i. Is the dialysis patient on the transplant list? If the transplant is planned in the short term, there may be less need for permanent haemodialysis vascular access.
    ii. Does the patient have an advance care directive ('living will')?
    iii. Has the patient been immunosuppressed previously (e.g. for treatment of previous glomerulonephritis or a previous transplant)? This may increase the risk of malignancies or infections.

3. **Transplant patients:** for patients with recent transplants, ask about:
- graft pain or swelling (failure of graft function, rejection)
- infection
- urine leaks
- steroid and immunosuppression side-effects.
  For those with long-term renal grafts, ask about:
- serum creatinine levels
- proteinuria
- recurrent glomerulonephritis (dense deposit disease)
- avascular necrosis
- skin cancer
- reflux nephropathy.
  Find out about adherence to drugs and whether the patient knows about rejection episodes and treatment (e.g. with pulsed-dose steroids or muromonab-CD3).

The examination (Table 11.12)

A complete physical examination is always essential. Look particularly for the following.
1. General appearance – mental state, hyperventilation, Kussmaul's breathing, hiccupping, the state of hydration and tachypnoea from fluid overload. Ask the patient to show you any old scars from access sites, transplant or other surgery.

Table 11.12 Chronic kidney disease (renal failure)

1. GENERAL INSPECTION

Mental state

Hyperventilation (acidosis), hiccups

Tachypnoea (fluid overload)

Cushingoid (steroids)

Scars

Sallow complexion

Hydration, JVP

Scaly skin (vitamin deficiency)

Fever

2. HANDS

Nails – Terry's nails, brown lines

Bruising

Asterixis

Neuropathy

3. ARMS

Bruising

Blood pressure (lying and standing)

Vascular shunts (feel for buzz, auscultate for bruit)

Pigmentation

Scratch marks

Urea frost (whole crystal deposits – terminal uraemia)

Myopathy

4. FACE

Eyes – anaemia, jaundice, band keratopathy

Mouth – dryness, fetor

Rash (vasculitis, etc.)

Facial hair – cyclosporin

Saddle nose (GPA)

5. CHEST

Heart – pericarditis, failure

Lungs – infection

6. ABDOMEN

Scars – dialysis, operations

Kidneys – transplant kidney, renal mass, polycystic kidneys

Tenckhoff catheter, exit-site infection

Bladder

Liver

Lymph nodes

Ascites

Bruits

Rectal (prostatomegaly, bleeding)

7. LEGS

Oedema – nephrotic syndrome, cardiac failure, etc.

Bruising

Pigmentation

Scratch marks

Gout

Neuropathy

Vascular access

8. BACK

Tenderness

Oedema

Spina bifida scar

9. URINE ANALYSIS

Specific gravity, pH

Glucose – diabetes

Blood – 'nephritis', infection, stone, etc.

Protein – 'nephritis', etc.

10. URINE SEDIMENT

Red cells

Casts

11. OTHER

Blood pressure – lying and standing

Fundoscopy – hypertensive and diabetic changes, etc.

GPA = granulomatosis with polyangiitis; JVP = jugular venous pressure.

2. Hands – nails for white transverse opaque bands or lines in hypoalbuminaemia; a brown arc near the ends of the nails (Terry's nails – Fig. 11.1) in CKD, palmar crease pallor. Look for the dry, scaly skin that results from vitamin deficiency vasculitis.

3. Arms – vascular shunts at the wrist, scars from old vascular access sites, asterixis and peripheral neuropathy, bruising, pigmentation, scratch marks, subcutaneous calcification, myopathy, fistulae and skin cancers, especially squamous cell carcinomas. Blood pressure lying and standing (do not take the blood pressure from an arm with a shunt in situ).

4. Face – eyes for jaundice, anaemia and band keratopathy (caused by hypercalcaemia); mouth (dry, fetor); rash (e.g. SLE); and a Cushingoid appearance.

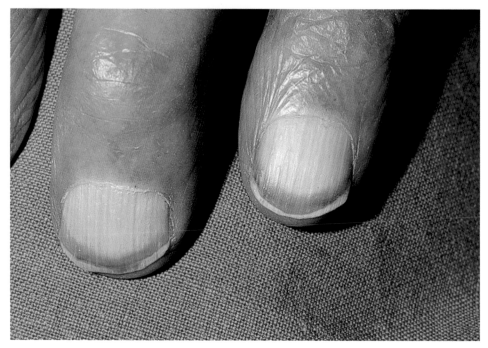

Figure 11.1 **Terry's nails in chronic kidney disease. There is proximal pallor with distal brownish colour.**

G M White, N H Cox (eds). *Diseases of the skin: a color atlas and text*, 2nd edn. St Louis, Mosby, Elsevier, 2006, with permission.

5. Chest – pericardial rub, cardiac failure, lung infection, pleural effusion and venous hum (shunt). Presence of central venous catheter for access to dialysis or scars from previous catheters.
6. Abdomen – palpable kidney or polycystic kidneys, scars (due to dialysis or transplants), renal artery bruit (a systolic bruit, or occasionally a systolic–diastolic bruit in the upper abdomen, suggests possible renal artery stenosis or even bruits over a transplanted kidney with an atrioventricular fistula from a kidney biopsy), bladder enlargement, rectal examination (for prostatomegaly, urethral mass and signs of blood loss), nodes (lymphoma, cytomegalovirus or other infections if the patient is immunosuppressed), ascites (dialysis or other causes), and femoral bruits and pulses.
7. Urine – for blood, protein, specific gravity, pH, glucose, urine microscopy and examination of the urinary sediment for casts.
8. Legs – oedema, bruising, pigmentation, scratch marks, peripheral neuropathy, vascular access and myopathy.
9. Back – bone tenderness and sacral oedema.
10. Fundoscopy.

Investigations

1. Determine renal function:
   a. glomerular filtration rate (GFR) – creatinine clearance (creatinine clearance levels of <10 mL/min are considered indications for dialysis) and plasma creatinine/urea level; the eGFR is routinely calculated by laboratories and the patient may know these results

b. tubular function – plasma electrolyte levels, urine specific gravity and pH, glycosuria, serum potassium, serum phosphate and uric acid, aminoaciduria, serum calcium and plasma albumin levels

c. urine analysis and urinary protein excretion (protein-to-creatinine ratio)

d. others if necessary – CT scan for renal artery stenosis or urinary tract obstruction (think about the risks of the contrast).

2. Determine renal structure:

a. ultrasound – renal size and symmetry, signs of obstruction; small kidneys (suggest chronic disease) and the presence or absence of ureteric jets – indicating patent ureters

b. CT scan – if contrast is to be used; hydration with IV saline does offer some renal protection; now, even the use of normal saline loading before and after the use of contrast material is of uncertain benefit

c. cystoscopy and retrograde pyelography

d. other – renal artery Doppler study, CT renal angiography.

3. Consider investigations aimed at assessing the widespread effects of CKD – blood count; serum ferritin and iron saturation level; midstream urine examination; calcium, phosphate and alkaline phosphatase levels; parathyroid hormone level; nerve conduction studies; arterial Doppler studies.

4. Decide whether there are features that favour chronic over acute kidney disease: nocturia, polyuria, longstanding hypertension, renal osteodystrophy, peripheral neuropathy, anaemia, hyperphosphataemia and hyperuricaemia. The differentiation of acute and chronic renal failure is also aided by determining kidney size. Kidneys are usually small in chronic kidney disease, but the exceptions to this rule include:

- diabetic nephropathy (early)
- polycystic kidneys
- obstructive uropathy
- acute renal vein thrombosis
- amyloidosis
- rarely other infiltrative diseases (e.g. lymphoma), which can all produce CKD but maintain normal kidney size.

   In general, however, kidneys enlarge or maintain normal size in acute kidney disease and are small in CKD.

5. Look for anaemia and the presence of burr cells in the peripheral blood film, which are usually indicative of CKD but may also occur in acute renal failure (e.g. in SLE), thrombotic thrombocytopenic purpura and the haemolytic uraemic syndrome.

6. Always ask about previous urine analyses, such as insurance examinations, in which proteinuria may have been detected and followed up, thus giving a clue about chronic glomerulonephritis.

7. Consider investigations aimed towards the likely underlying disease process – measurement of antinuclear antibody, hepatitis B surface antigen, hepatitis C, HIV, complement, immune complexes, serum and urine immunoelectrophoresis as well as urinary kappa and lamda light chains, micturating cystogram, urine cytology and renal biopsy.

Treatment

This most chronic disease (Table 11.13) has profound effects on the patient and his or her relatives. The association between the patient and the renal physician and nursing staff becomes a very intense one, often lasting many years. It is important to ask detailed questions about the way the patient copes with the condition, whether work and travel are possible, and what the patient feels about the long-term prospects. Also, ask whether a dialysis patient has considered accepting a kidney from a live donor.

Table 11.13 Complications and treatment of chronic kidney disease

ANAEMIA

Causes include erythropoietin deficiency, poor nutrition (especially folate deficiency), blood loss, reduced iron absorption, haemolysis, bone marrow depression, chronic disease and aluminium toxicity.

Treatment should include prophylactic folate supplements for dialysis patients. Erythropoietin is very effective for the chronic anaemia of renal failure and can normalise the haematocrit. Erythropoietin-stimulating agents (ESAs) are commonly used in conjunction with intravenous iron supplements given IV late in dialysis (as oral iron is poorly absorbed in end-stage renal disease). The serum ferritin should be maintained at > 100 but less than 600, and transferrin saturation at > 20%. The target haemoglobin should be between 100 and 120 µg/L.

BONE DISEASE

Maintenance of normal calcium and phosphate levels is the key to preventing the problem.

Treatment with phosphate binders (e.g. calcium carbonate, sevelamer, lanthanum or sucroferric (to bind phosphate in the gut), vitamin D analogues and low calcium concentration in dialysis fluids is necessary. Aluminium is no longer used as a phosphate binder.

1. Osteomalacia – diagnosis by:
   a. X-ray films (decreased density, Looser's zones)
   b. low calcium, phosphate and vitamin D levels
   c. high serum alkaline phosphatase level
2. Tertiary hyperparathyroidism – diagnosis by:
   a. X-ray film (microcysts on radial side of the middle phalanx, erosion of the clavicular ends, 'rugger jersey' spine (see Fig. 11.2), telescoped terminal phalanges, metastatic calcification of vessels)[a]
   b. high phosphate and very high parathyroid hormone (PTH) levels, and a high calcium level
3. Osteoporosis
4. Osteosclerosis
5. Aluminium-induced bone disease
6. Adynamic bone disease (reduced bone formation) is the most common type of bone disease in dialysis patients owing to over-suppression by phosphate binders; *note:* PTH is low

PERIPHERAL NEUROPATHY

This is now uncommon in patients receiving adequate dialysis. It is more often a result of diabetes than of CKD itself. Combined pancreatic islet and renal transplant may help.

HYPERTENSION

This needs careful monitoring and control of salt and fluid balance as well as judicious use of antihypertensive drugs (an ACEI or ARB slows disease progression).

INFECTION

These patients are at risk of infection because of the kidney disease itself, the immunosuppressive drugs given to treat glomerulonephritis and their need for frequent intravenous vascular access.

ACIDOSIS

This is often treated with dialysis and carefully monitored. Sodium bicarbonate often helps.

HYPERKALAEMIA

This should be treated with a low-potassium diet and ion-exchange resins if necessary. Dialysis is very effective.

[a]This is now a rare occurrence. Increased PTH that does not respond to medical treatment is managed with parathyroidectomy.
ACEI = angiostensin-converting enzyme inhibitor; ARB = angiotensin II receptor (AR) blocker.

It is also always important to consider whether conservative therapy (no dialysis or transplantation) has a role in this patient – considering the patient's condition and wishes after being fully informed (see below).

1. Treat reversible causes of deterioration. These include:
   • hypertension
   • urinary tract infection
   • urinary tract obstruction

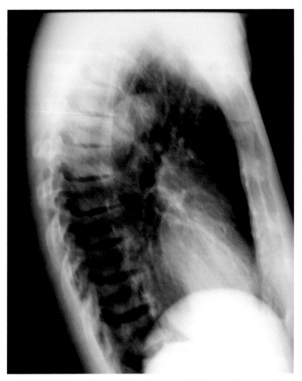

Figure 11.2 **Spine X-ray of a patient with chronic kidney disease showing alternating dense and radiolucent bands – 'rugger jersey spine'.**

Figure reproduced courtesy of The Canberra Hospital.

- dehydration
- cardiac failure
- drug use (e.g. radiocontrast, NSAIDs, aminoglycosides, cyclosporin)
- hypercalcaemia
- hyperuricaemia with urate obstruction
- hypothyroidism or rarely hypoadrenalism.

2. Monitor and control the blood pressure very carefully. Treat lipids.
3. Carefully attend to salt and water balance and acidosis.
4. Normalise the calcium and phosphate levels with diet, phosphate binders or calcitriol. Non-calcium-based phosphate binders (e.g. sevelamer) improve mortality compared with calcium-based ones. Treatment of secondary hyperparathyroidism with the drug cinacalcet has not been shown to improve mortality or risk of vascular events in dialysis patients.
5. Restrict dietary protein. However, although this may delay slightly the need for dialysis, it leads to wasting and protein malnutrition. It is no longer universally recommended.
6. Assess and treat sexual dysfunction.
7. Dialyse when indicated (see below).
8. Consider transplantation.

The absolute indications for dialysis (see Table 11.11) are:
1. uraemic symptoms despite conservative management (eGFR about 7 mL/min)
2. volume overload despite salt and water restriction and diuretic use
3. hyperkalaemia unresponsive to conservative measures

4. progressive deterioration of renal function (dialyse before symptoms develop)
5. acute renal failure (dialyse early).

Note: Dialysis may be started earlier to avoid these complications, but there is no evidence that mortality is improved by this strategy.

DIALYSIS

It is very important to consider that patients may not be suitable for dialysis or may have unrealistic expectations of the benefits of dialysis. Patient education about dialysis options and non-dialysis management is necessary in a timely manner for all patients with worsening CKD.

Not all end-stage CKD patients should be dialysed. Consider:
1. age and co-morbidities
2. conservative treatment
3. type of dialysis
4. suitability for later transplant
5. lack of benefit in starting before symptoms have occurred.

Patient's wishes

Find out their wishes and assess how well informed they are if possible. Patients with a number of co-morbidities who are over 75 have a poor survival (80% 3-year mortality) whether dialysed or not. Seventy per cent of nursing home patients started on dialysis have died within 12 months. Peritoneal dialysis gives patients a slight survival advantage over haemodialysis, but only for the first year.

Remember the common complications of dialysis:
1. sudden cardiac death
2. vascular disease
3. extravascular calcification – accelerated aortic stenosis, calciphylaxis
4. amyloidosis (β_2-microglobulin).

A number of dialysis trials are been undertaken including high-dose versus low-dose dialysis, high flux versus low flux, increased frequency of haemodialysis, and haemodiafiltration versus haemodialysis. These strategies haven't shown evidence of survival benefit.

ANTICOAGULATION

Atrial fibrillation is common in CKD and dialysis patients. Their risk of stroke is high and warfarin reduces this risk by 14%, but the price is an increased risk (of 44%) of significant bleeding. The decision to recommend anticoagulation is a complicated one and depends on an individual analysis of the bleeding and stroke risk. The role of the newer anticoagulants (NOACs) is uncertain in patients with CKD stages 4–5; apixaban has been approved in the United States for dialysis patients.

Possible lines of questioning

1. Is *this* patient a candidate for a renal transplant?
2. At what point do you think *this* patient will require dialysis? Would you recommend peritoneal or haemodialysis? Why?
3. How adherent do you think *this* patient is with his or her treatment recommendations?
4. How would you investigate *this* patient with newly diagnosed chronic kidney disease to establish the aetiology? Do you think there are any reversible factors?

Renal transplantation

Renal transplantation is now a widely accepted, commonly performed treatment for end-stage chronic kidney disease. Unfortunately, patients continue to have a number of problems that may bring them into hospital and make them available for examinations. Cadaveric transplantation is generally more common than the use of matched family donors. Specific contraindications to renal transplantation include:

- recent malignancy
- an untreatable focus of infection
- old age, severe frailty or chronic disease, e.g. cardiac failure, severe peripheral vascular disease
- untreated ischaemic heart disease.

The prognosis continues to improve and the newer immunosuppressives have made a substantial difference to survival rates. The 1-year graft survival rate is now more than 95% and 15-year graft survival is 50% in experienced centres. The selection of patients for transplant is difficult, but the pool of available donor kidneys has enlarged over recent years because:

- ABO-incompatible transplants are much more common and have outcomes similar to ABO-compatible transplants. The recipient must be pre-treated to remove anti-A or anti-B antibodies that could cause a hyperacute rejection.
- Paired kidney exchange (PKE) has increased the potential for receiving a compatible kidney if one's current potential donors (e.g. family members) are incompatible. Donors give a kidney to another donor–recipient pair and receive a compatible kidney in return.
- Kidneys can now be used that previously were thought to be marginal – e.g. donation after cardiac death (DCD) kidneys.
- Attempts have been made to increase cadaveric donation rates by public information programs, donor coordinators in public hospitals, etc.
- There are also new trials of therapies for highly sensitised individuals, who would otherwise wait many years or never have an offer of a kidney transplant.

The history

1. Ask the patient about the cause of the original renal failure. Find out how long the transplant has been in situ and whether this is the patient's first transplant. Ask whether the kidney came from a relative or was a cadaveric graft.
2. The patient should be well informed about previous rejection episodes and how these have been managed. Find out whether this is the reason for the current admission. Clinically, rejection may be marked by fever, swelling and tenderness over the graft. The patient should be aware of all these signs. There is also often a reduction in urine volume. A rise in creatinine level is usual. Ask about recent graft biopsies, which may have been necessary to assess rejection, recurrence of disease or drug toxicity.
3. Find out what immunosuppressive drugs the patient is taking and in what doses. He or she should know whether changes in doses have been required recently because of problems with any of the drugs. Ask about the history of steroid use.
4. The patient may know whether he or she and the donor were CMV positive.
5. Ask about specific complications of immunosuppression.
   a. Calcineurin inhibitors (tacrolimus or cyclosporin) can result in significant side-effects. The drugs can be associated with:
      - renal impairment
      - hair disorders – hirsutism with cyclosporin, alopecia with tacrolimus

- tremor
- gout (with cyclosporin)
- abnormal liver function tests (especially bilirubin)
- hypertension
- hyperkalaemia
- hypomagnesaemia
- gingival hypertrophy and rarely
- haematological malignancy.

b. Mycophenalate is associated with an increased risk of infections and leukopenia, as well as upper and lower gastrointestinal symptoms.

c. The mTOR inhibitors sirolimus and everolimus are associated with:
- proteinuria
- hyperlipidaemia
- leucopenia
- pneumonitis
- tendon rupture
- slow wound healing (see below).

d. Ask about ischaemic heart disease and peripheral vascular disease, infections and malignancy, as the incidence of these conditions remains higher than in the general population.

The examination

1. Look particularly at the skin for squamous and basal cell carcinomas.
2. Note any signs of Cushing's syndrome and hirsutism (e.g. from cyclosporin).
3. Examine the abdomen carefully, noting the position and site of the allograft and whether it has any tenderness or bruits. Don't forget to look for scars from previous transplants, too! Were these non-functioning organs removed or not?
4. Look for old vascular access sites for haemodialysis and decide whether there will be problems finding sites for access for further dialysis if this is required.
5. Examine the lungs for signs of infection and the mouth for *Candida*. Inspect the gums. Note gouty tophi. Look at the temperature chart.

Investigations

1. It is important to obtain the serum creatinine level and, if possible, establish whether the serum creatinine level has been rising or falling since the time of transplantation. A slightly elevated creatinine level is considered acceptable in patients treated with calcineurin inhibitors (CNIs) as these drugs interfere with renal function. Patients usually know their creatinine and eGFR results. If they don't, there may be some doubt about their adherence with treatment and understanding of their disease.
2. The electrolyte levels and liver function test results are important. Cyclosporin can cause hepatotoxicity and renal impairment, as can cytomegalovirus infection of the liver. A white cell count should be obtained to look for leukocytosis (infection or steroids) and leukopenia (e.g. excessive doses of mycophenolate, mTOR inhibitors, azathioprine, valganciclovir or trimethoprim-sulphamethoxazole combination).

   These drugs' doses are usually adjusted according to the neutrophil count. The haemoglobin is usually normal in patients with a successful transplant and good function.
3. The results of blood cultures should be sought if there has been any suggestion of recent infection. Urinary tract infection must also be considered and early urine microscopy is helpful.
4. Consider viral infections with PCR testing for, for example, cytomegalovirus (CMV) and BK virus – these can alter the white cell count and renal function.

Table 11.14 **Contraindications to renal transplant**
ABSOLUTE
Malignant disease (2 years of remission after treatment before transplant considered)
Severe ischaemic heart disease
Active vasculitis or anti-basement membrane disease
Occlusive aortoiliac disease
Continuing sepsis
RELATIVE
Older than 75 years
High risk of recurrence in transplant
Ureteric or bladder disease (may need ileal conduit inserted before transplant)
Other co-morbidities

5. Exclude prerenal and postrenal disease. A renal scan and ultrasound with measurement by Doppler is useful for estimating renal artery blood flow.

Management

1. The majority of patients receiving chronic dialysis are candidates for renal transplantation; the contraindications are listed in Table 11.14. Generally, transplantation improves patients' quality of life and is less expensive than dialysis over time.
2. Most patients are given three immunosuppressive drugs for kidney transplants. The most common combination is prednisolone, tacrolimus and mycophenolate mofetil. Cyclosporin and azathioprine are much less common first-choice agents as they have been shown to be less effective. Monoclonal antibodies are commonly used for induction therapy at the time of surgery.

   mTOR inhibitors are also commonly used and patients may be changed to these agents especially if calcineurin inhibitors (e.g. tacrolimus and cyclosporin) have caused renal transplant toxicity. They may be specifically indicated to reduce skin and other malignancies. However, their use is associated with poor wound healing, leukopenia, hyperlipidaemia and proteinuria. Hence these agents should be stopped before surgery and restarted after healing is complete. Often the patients have to be changed back to a CNI temporarily over this period.

   Immunosuppressants include:
   a. **Mycophenalate mofetil** can be used with allopurinol, and can cause leukopenia as well as upper gastrointestinal symptoms (nausea, weight loss) or more commonly diarrhoea; typical doses are 500–1000 mg twice daily (CellCept) or 360–720 mg twice daily.
   b. **Tacrolimus** is a CNI. Trough levels should be monitored (5–10 ng/mL). It can cause renal dysfunction, alopecia and hypertension but (unlike cyclosporin) not gout, hirsutism or gum changes.
   c. **Sirolimus** and **everolimus** are mTOR inhibitors, given daily orally. Their adverse effects include a reduced white cell count (use with caution in combination with mycophenalate), increased lipids and proteinuria. Monitor trough levels. They delay wound healing and should be replaced before surgery with tacrolimus and restarted when wound healing has been achieved (typically 1–3 months later).
   d. **Azathioprine** has largely been replaced by mycophenalate (resulting in less acute rejection), but some patients with older transplants may still be taking azathioprine.
   e. **Prednisone** is given in maintenance doses of approximately 7.5–10 mg daily after about 6 months and usually 5 mg/day by 12 months post-transplant surgery.

3. **Prophylactic anti-infective medications** include:
   a. Most if not all new transplant patients are treated with oral valganciclovir for CMV prophylaxis for the first 6 months post-surgery.
   b. Prophylaxis for *Pneumocystis jirovecii* (PJP) with trimethoprim-sulfamethoxazole – it has been recommended that this agent be continued forever, owing to the risk of late *Pneumocystis* infections. Atovaquone may be a suitable alternative, in cases of toxicity to trimethoprim-sulfamethoxazole.
   c. The influenza vaccine is recommended in all suitable patients.
   d. Opportunistic infections typically occur a month or more post-transplant. *Toxoplasma*, *Nocardia* and *Aspergillus* are now less common with current immunosuppressive protocols; viral infections (especially CMV) dominate. Infection must be aggressively diagnosed (e.g. by blood cultures and lung biopsy) and treated. When infections are life-threatening, immunosuppressive treatment, apart from prednisone, should be suspended. CMV prophylaxis with ganciclovir (for CMV-negative patients with a CMV-positive donor) and PCP prophylaxis with co-trimoxazole may be indicated.
4. **Acute rejection episodes:** these are still treated with pulsed high-dose steroids and usually an increase in the general level of immunosuppression (Table 11.15).

Table 11.15 Causes of renal allograft rejection

HINT: consider surgical problems, thrombophilia or SLE.

TIME FRAME	CAUSE	POSSIBLE REASONS
Very early (hours to days)	Renal artery or vein thrombosis	Surgical problems Thrombophilia or SLE
	Ureteric leak	Small bladder
	Delayed graft function	Long graft ischaemia time, older donor, elevated tacrolimus level
	Hyperacute rejection	HLA mismatch Previous transplant Pre-formed anti-HLA antibodies
Early (weeks)	Acute rejection, non-adherence to treatment or inadequate immunosuppression	HLA mismatch Previous transplant Pre-formed anti-HLA antibodies
Months	Renal artery stenosis, BK virus infection and nephropathy	Use of ureteric stent, intense immunosuppression, disease of donor kidney, damage to graft during harvesting
Years	Chronic allograft injury (usually mediated by antibodies)	Insufficient immunosuppression, non-adherence Previous acute rejections
At any time	Cyclosporin or tacrolimus toxicity	High doses, serum levels not monitored Concurrent use of P450 cytochrome-inhibiting drugs
	Infection	
	Recurrence of original kidney disease, e.g. minimum change GN (early) IgA nephropathy or membranous GN (later)	Recurrence in a previous transplant

GN = glomerulonephritis; HLA = human leukocyte antigen; SLE = systemic lupus erythematosus.

5. **Chronic rejection:** the differential diagnosis is:
   a. chronic allograft nephropathy
   b. recurrent glomerulonephritis (e.g. focal segmental glomerulosclerosis (FSGS) or membranous GN)
   c. de novo glomerulonephritis
   d. chronic antibody-mediated rejection – an increasingly recognised problem – which may be treated by plasmapheresis, immunoglobulin infusions or even different immunosuppressives such as rituximab.
6. A gradually rising creatinine level may be a sign of calcineurin toxicity (which, if caused by interstitial fibrosis, is not reversible) or of chronic rejection. This is a difficult clinical problem, but graft biopsy can be used to decide whether the calcineurins should be stopped or immunosuppression changed.
7. Some diabetic patients with end-stage CKD will have undergone kidney/pancreas transplants. They may have additional problems with pancreatic drainage (bladder or to gut) and leakage.

Possible lines of questioning

1. Did *this* patient have complications during renal transplant surgery? How were they managed?
2. Has *this* transplant patient had rejection episodes? How were they diagnosed and treated?
3. What changes to immunosuppressive treatment have been required during the period since *this* patient's transplant?
4. What complications of immunosuppressive treatment have occurred?

Chapter 12

The neurological long case

The brain is a wonderful organ. It starts working the
moment you get up in the morning and does not stop
until you get into the office.

Robert Frost (1874–1963)

Multiple sclerosis

This is a common chronic disease. Patients suffering from multiple sclerosis (MS) are readily available for the clinical examinations. They are mostly very well informed about, and interested in, their disease. MS usually begins in early adult life and is more common in women than in men (2:1). The disease is much more common among people who lived as children in regions far from the equator. Exposure to Epstein–Barr virus (EBV) infection at an older age increases risk and the condition is rare in seronegative individuals. Numerous alleles associated with risk have been identified, but *HLA-DRB1* has the strongest association.

The most common pattern of disease is called *relapsing–remitting multiple sclerosis* (RRMS). In untreated patients the rate of relapse is 0.65 attacks a year, though this is highly variable between patients. Episodes of fever or fatigue associated with a temporary worsening of symptoms are not considered to be relapses and are called *pseudorelapses*. In most cases, complete or almost complete resolution of symptoms occurs in this phase of the disease. After 10 years, up to 50% of patients begin to develop a progressive accumulation of disability – *secondary progressive MS* (SPMS). However, with the advent of newer pharmacological agents and more aggressive, earlier treatment, it is anticipated that long-term progression will be improved. Other types are *primary progressive* (10%), where disability slowly develops over time and there are no relapses or flares, and *progressive relapsing* (5%), where disability slowly develops over time and there are also relapses or flares without recovery.

Table 12.1 **Sites of demyelinating lesions on MRI scanning**	
1. Corpus callosum	4. Optic nerve
2. Juxtacortical white matter	5. Periventricular white matter.
3. Spinal cord	6. Pons, cerebellar peduncles and cerebellum

The history

The disease usually begins with an episode of acute neurological disturbance, which is called a *clinically isolated syndrome (CIS)*. However, the clinical diagnosis requires at least two neurological events separated in time and place within the CNS. MS is primarily a clinical diagnosis, but the use of MRI scanning has led to the McDonald criteria for diagnosis. These allow for the diagnosis after a single neurological episode if the MRI shows a separate area typical of MS (see Table 12.1).

1. Ask about the presenting symptoms (listed here in approximate order of importance):
   a. episodes of spastic paraparesis, hemiparesis or tetraparesis (may present as gradually progressive disease in late-onset MS)
   b. episodes of limb paraesthesiae (due to posterior column, medial lemniscus or internal capsule involvement)
   c. episodes of visual disturbance – loss of acuity, pain on eye movement, loss of central visual field (optic neuritis), diplopia
   d. episodes of ataxia, dysarthria and tremor – Charcot's triad (due to cerebellar or posterior column involvement)
   e. band sensations around trunk or limbs
   f. urinary urgency, incontinence of faeces
   g. less common symptoms, such as:
      • vertigo, symptoms of cranial nerve disorders (e.g. tic douloureux)
      • erectile dysfunction
      • depression
      • euphoria
      • dementia
      • seizures
      • bulbar dysfunction (pseudobulbar palsy).

2. Ask about factors that worsen symptoms, such as:
   a. heat (hot baths, etc.) – this is referred to as Uhthoff's phenomenon
   b. infection
   c. fever
   d. pregnancy
   e. exercise.
   Disease activity tends to be less during pregnancy; relapse is common postpartum.
3. Ask about family history: MS is seven times more common in immediate relatives (sibling risk is 5%).
4. Ask about social disability – sexual function, ability to work, financial problems.
5. Ask about place of birth: MS is more common in subjects who spent their childhood in temperate latitudes rather than in tropical regions. Smoking is also a risk factor.
6. Find out what treatments have been tried and with what success and any side-effects. Various unproven treatments are often tried by patients with this incurable disease. Ask whether any of these have been used.

> **HINT**
>
> Unlike patients with cerebrovascular disease, MS patients do not develop cortical symptoms such as neglect and aphasia. However, cognitive dysfunction is frequently overlooked as a source of disability, especially in SPMS.

The examination

1. The signs can be very variable. Focus on the reported symptoms and look for signs related to them. Look particularly for signs of spastic paraparesis and posterior column sensory loss, as well as cerebellar signs. You must objectively quantify the main neurological deficit and any effect on function.
2. Examine the cranial nerves. Look carefully for loss of visual acuity, optic atrophy or swelling. Check colour saturation and look for a relative afferent pupil defect (RAPD), especially if acuity is reduced. Internuclear ophthalmoplegia is an important sign and is almost diagnostic in a young adult. It can also occur in patients with SLE or Sjögren's syndrome, who may have disease confined to the CNS, or with brain stem tumours or infarcts. Internuclear ophthalmoplegia is weakness of adduction in one eye as a result of damage to the ipsilateral medial longitudinal fasciculus; there is nystagmus in the abducting eye. In MS, internuclear ophthalmoplegia is often bilateral. Other cranial nerves may rarely be affected by lesions within the brain stem (III, IV, V, VI, VII, pseudobulbar palsy).
3. Test for Lhermitte's sign (an electric-shock-like sensation in the limbs or trunk following neck flexion). This can also be caused by other disorders of the cervical spine, such as subacute combined degeneration of the cord, cervical spondylosis, cervical cord tumour, foramen magnum tumours, nitrous oxide abuse and mantle irradiation.
4. Rarely, signs suggesting neuromyelitis optica (NMO, or Devic's disease) are present (unilateral or bilateral optic neuritis and transverse myelitis occurring within a few weeks of one another). Patients are typically children or young adults. Patients may experience the sudden onset of visual loss and pain on eye movements, associated with weakness, numbness and sometimes paresis of the arms or legs, along with sensory disturbances and loss of bladder and bowel control. Unlike MS there is no

cerebellar or cognitive impairment and the brain MRI is usually normal, though brain stem lesions can also be seen in some patients. The presence of specific aquaporin-4 antibodies in up to 70% of patients helps distinguish the condition from MS. NMO is pathologically very different to MS, and requires different treatment.

Investigations

The differential diagnosis of multiple CNS lesions includes:

- SLE
- Sjögren's syndrome
- Behçet's disease
- small vessel ischaemia
- acute disseminated encephalomyelitis
- meningovascular syphilis
- paraneoplastic effects of carcinoma
- sarcoidosis
- multiple emboli from any source.

It is important to distinguish MS affecting predominantly the spinal cord from other diseases – especially subacute combined degeneration of the cord (more common in the older population) and spinal cord compression presenting with root pain and persistent levels of sensory loss.

MS is essentially a clinical diagnosis, but the following tests may be helpful.

1. MRI is the imaging modality of choice (Fig. 12.1). Table 12.1 lists the typical sites of changes. Typical changes are present in the great majority of patients with MS. Gadolinium contrast studies show leakage into the brain from blood vessels for up to some months after the formation of a new lesion. T2-weighted images will show persisting changes that are probably due to a combination of oedema, gliosis and inflammation. The extent of these abnormalities – the burden of disease – correlates to some extent with the clinical severity, though brain stem and spinal cord lesions cause particular disability. The presence of numerous gadolinium-enhancing lesions indicates a worse prognosis. CT scan may reveal low-density, sometimes contrast-enhancing, plaques in white matter (subcortical or periventricular, but only in 10%–50% of cases). CT scanning is no longer in routine use for diagnosis of MS.

2. Visual-evoked responses are delayed in 80% of established cases and indicate previous optic neuritis (important if there is only one other clinically detectable lesion present). Auditory-evoked responses and somatosensory-evoked responses may be abnormal, but are not usually diagnostic.

3. Cerebrospinal fluid in chronic MS contains oligoclonal immunoglobulin G (IgG) bands (70%) and an altered IgG:albumin ratio. Myelin basic protein may be elevated in acute demyelination. There are usually < 50 white cells per millilitre in the cerebrospinal fluid, but acute severe demyelination may result in a cell count > 100/mL.

4. Antimyelin antibodies are of uncertain value.

A definite diagnosis is not possible without the presence of two or more CNS episodes, usually separated in time and place; the first may be a clinical abnormality and the second detected by MRI or visual-evoked responses (Macdonald's criteria – Table 12.2). These include objective CNS changes, usually involving long-tract signs and symptoms: pyramidal, cerebellar, optic nerve, posterior columns and medial longitudinal fasciculus. Gradual progression of symptoms may be used to make the diagnosis if typical cerebrospinal fluid (CSF) abnormalities are present. The MRI should show four distinct areas of abnormality at least 3 mm in diameter. There should be no other explanation for the symptoms (see above).

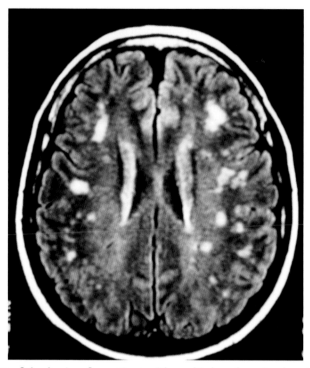

Figure 12.1 **MRI of the brain of a patient with multiple sclerosis showing numerous plaques (white patches).**

Figure reproduced courtesy of The Canberra Hospital.

Treatment

There are two aspects to treatment of these patients:

1. supportive and symptomatic treatment
2. immunomodulation / immunosuppression.

In addition, there are many support groups and organisations for patients with MS. These often give sensible advice to these distressed people and should be recommended to patients. It is most important, however, that the diagnosis is secure before patients are labelled with this condition with its numerous long-term implications.

1. The course of the disease:
    a. **relapsing–remitting MS:** relapses with or without complete recovery, but stable between episodes; offer early disease-modifying therapy
    b. **secondary progressive MS:** about half of the patients with relapsing–remitting MS develop secondary progressive MS within 10 years; they experience gradual progression of their symptoms without distinct episodes
    c. **primary progressive MS:** these patients have increasing symptoms without distinct episodes from the start and there are no disease-modifying therapies as yet
    d. **progressive relapsing MS:** in these patients there is gradual worsening, with episodes of deterioration occurring later in the course of the illness.
2. General support is essential. During exacerbations, bed rest with meticulous nursing is vital. Treatment of bladder dysfunction, severe spasticity (e.g. with baclofen), urgency (e.g. with amitriptyline), tic douloureux and facial spasm (e.g. with carbamazepine

Table 12.2 Macdonald's criteria for the diagnosis of multiple sclerosis

The diagnosis of multiple sclerosis requires establishing disease disseminated in both space and time.

DISSEMINATION IN SPACE
Dissemination in space requires ≥ 1 T2 bright lesions in two or more of the following locations:
- periventricular
- juxtacortical
- infratentorial
- spinal cord

If a patient has a brain stem / spinal cord syndrome, the symptomatic lesion(s) are excluded from the criteria, not contributing to the lesion count.

DISSEMINATION IN TIME
Dissemination in time can be established in one of two ways:
- a new lesion when compared with a previous scan (irrespective of timing)
- T2 bright lesion and / or gadolinium enhancing
- presence of asymptomatic enhancing lesion and a non-enhancing T2 bright lesion on any one scan.

PRIMARY PROGRESSIVE MULTIPLE SCLEROSIS (PPMS)
In addition to the above criteria, the diagnosis of primary progressive multiple sclerosis has also been revised. The diagnosis now requires:
- ≥ 1 year of disease progression (this can be determined either prospectively or retrospectively)
- plus two of the following three criteria:
  - brain dissemination in space (≥ 1 T2 bright lesions in ≥ 1 of juxtacortical, periventricular, infratentorial areas)
  - spinal cord dissemination in space (≥ 2 T2 bright lesions)
  - positive CSF (oligoclonal bands and / or elevated IgG index).

Dr Bruno Di Muzio and A. Prof Frank Gaillard. McDonald diagnostic criteria for multiple sclerosis. Radiopaedia. org (http://radiopaedia.org/articles/mcdonald-diagnostic-criteria-for-multiple-sclerosis), with permission.

and physiotherapy) is important. Intention tremor can be treated with propranolol or clonazepam.

3. Drug treatment: (Table 12.3) immunomodulators and immunosuppressants:
   a. Interferon (IFN) β1a and interferon β1b have been shown to reduce the frequency of exacerbations by about one-third when used at an early stage of disease, and to reduce the accumulation of CNS white matter lesions. They are more effective for the relapsing forms of the disease (see below). There is evidence that these drugs improve survival. Remember the risk of hepatotoxicity and leukopenia; monitor blood tests.
   b. Glatiramer acetate (subcutaneous) takes up to a year to provide benefit; the drug can induce non-cardiac chest pain or shortness of breath. It is of similar efficacy to interferon. Bradycardia can be a problem.
   c. Natalizumab (monoclonal antibody to alpha$_4$-integrin) is more effective than these agents, especially for RRMS, but its use is restricted to patients with very aggressive disease because 1 in 600 patients treated develop progressive multifocal leukoencephalopathy (PML) owing to brain infection with the John Cunningham agent. A *negative* JC virus (JCV) antibody test means a very low risk (1 in 10,000) of developing PML. A JCV-*positive* patient who has had previous treatment with immunosuppressing drugs and more than 2 years of natalizumab treatment has a 1 in 90 chance of developing PML.
   d. Ocrelizumab is an anti-CD20 monoclonal antibody infusion for RRMS. It can reactivate hepatitis B so you must screen for HBsAg and anti-HBc prior to prescribing.

Table 12.3 Disease-modifying drugs available for the treatment of MS

DRUGS	DOSE	MAJOR SIDE-EFFECTS	MINOR SIDE-EFFECTS	PREGNANCY CATEGORY	MONITORING REQUIRED
INJECTABLE					
IFN-β	SC 3 times a week or 2nd-daily	Hepatotoxicity, cytopenia	Injection site reactions, flu-like symptoms, depression	D	LFTs and FBC 1, 3 months then annually
Glatiramer acetate	SC daily	Hepatotoxicity, cytopenia	Injection site reactions (lipoatrophy)	B1	LFTs and FBC at start and annually
ORAL					
Teriflunomide	Daily	Hepatotoxicity, cytopenia, infections	Nausea, diarrhoea, loss of hair	X	LFT and FBC monthly for 6 months then 6–9-weekly; monitor for skin malignancy
Fingolimod	Daily	Hepatotoxicity, macular oedema, lymphoedema, bradycardia, herpes zoster and simplex infections	Back pain, headache	D	6 h cardiac monitoring – first dose
Dimethyl fumarate	Twice a day	Lymphopenia, proteinuria, PML	Flushing, GIT symptoms	B1	Urine protein, FBC at start and annually
IV					
Natalizumab	Monthly	PML, hepatotoxicity	Headache, infusion reactions	C	MRI brain at start and 6-monthly, LFTs, FBC at start
Ocrelizumab	Induction – two doses, 2 weeks apart, then maintenance 6-monthly	Infusion reactions, infection, malignancy – most notably breast	Infusion reactions, URTI	C	FBC, Neurologist follow-up

FBC = full blood count; FN-β = interferon beta; GIT = gastrointestinal tract; ITP = idiopathic thrombocytopenic purpura; LFT = liver function test; PML = progressive multifocal leukoencephalopathy: SC = subcutaneous; TFT = thyroid function test.

e. Fingolimod is an oral agent. It works via the sphingosine-1-phosphate receptor to prevent lymphocyte tracking through lymph nodes. It causes reversible lymphopenia. It has been shown to be more effective than interferon, with relapse rates of 25% at 2 years. Side-effects include macular oedema and increased infection risk. It should not be given to people without varicella immunisation or known previous exposure and immunity. Patients should also be screened for herpes simplex, hepatitis serology and TB exposure. The ECG should be monitored for 6 hours for QT prolongation and arrhythmias with first dosing. PML has been described in a handful of patients.

f. Teriflunomide is the active metabolite of leflunomide. It is probably less effective than the other oral drugs but has predictable if unpleasant side-effects. Hair loss and gut upset are common; haematological and liver abnormalities are rare. It is important to monitor for skin malignancy.

g. Dimethyl fumarate has had good trial results. It is generally well tolerated. Severe lymphopenia can occur but is rare; flushing and gut upset are common but often improve with time.

h. Alemtuzumab is a monoclonal antibody against CD52, with high potency and limited need for regular dosing. However, B-cell-mediated autoimmunity is a problem in the early phase post-dose; autoimmune thyroid disease, anti-glomerular basement membrane (GBM) glomerulonephritis and idiopathic thrombocytopenic purpura (ITP) have all been described.

i. Prior to monoclonal therapies, patients may have been treated with methotrexate, azathioprine, cyclophosphamide or mitoxantrone. Mitoxantrone was particularly used in the past in patients with rapidly progressive disease, but cardiac toxicity and subsequent malignancy limited its use. Occasionally, autologous stem cell transplant has been used.

RELAPSES

Pseudorelapses are an exacerbation or recurrence of previously improved symptoms and are related to an intercurrent infection. Treatment of the infection is indicated.

1. Acute 'true' relapses are treated with methylprednisolone – 500–1000 mg/day for three doses if they are severe (impair mobility, vision, etc.). Plasmapheresis and intravenous gamma globulin may help relapses when steroids fail. Treatment of relapses may hasten recovery, but does not improve the long-term outlook or reduce the risk of further relapses.

2. At 15 years after the first episode, 80% of patients have significant symptoms that prevent them from working and require help with normal activities. If the initial episode is limited to a single abnormality and the MRI is normal, only 10% will go on to develop a second episode over the following 10 years. If the MRI is abnormal, up to 80% will experience further episodes.

3. Consider symptomatic management: there are a range of medications which can address spasticity, walking, bladder dysfunction and fatigue. Make sure you have a plan and can at least provide an overview of the available treatments every general physician should know.

4. As with all chronic and debilitating diseases, a discussion about the patient's expectations and prognosis and plans for the future is important.

Possible lines of questioning

1. Please summarise the course of *this* patient's symptoms of multiple sclerosis.
2. What treatments have been tried?
3. What do you think future possibilities for treatment for *this* patient are?
4. How would you explain the possible side-effects that future treatment would involve?
5. What would you advise *this* woman patient about the implications of pregnancy?
6. What is the impact on function and quality of life in this patient with MS? How would you address the issues?

Myasthenia gravis

This chronic autoimmune disease presents both diagnostic and management problems. Peak incidence in women is in the third decade of life, but in men it is in the seventh decade. Overall it is more common in women than in men (2:1). Exacerbations and remissions (incomplete) are common.

The history

1. Ask about symptoms at presentation:
   a. ocular – diplopia (90%), drooping eyelids
   b. bulbar – choking (weakness of pharyngeal muscles), dysarthria, difficulty (especially fatigue) when chewing or swallowing
   c. neck – dropped head
   d. limb girdle – proximal muscle weakness; there is fatigue on exertion and prompt partial recovery on resting.
2. Ask about a history of difficult anaesthesia (owing to prolonged weakness after muscle relaxation) and past episodes of pneumonia (as a result of bulbar and respiratory weakness).
3. Determine how the diagnosis was made, including whether electrodiagnostic studies were done and whether the patient had blood tests for acetylcholine receptor antibodies.
4. Ask about a history of thymectomy (i.e. previous treatment for myasthenia).
5. Enquire about other treatment – including drug dose and when the last dose was taken, intravenous immunoglobulin, plasma exchange or immunosuppressive therapy.
6. Ask about drug use, which may interfere with neuromuscular transmission (see below).
7. Ask about other organ-specific autoimmune disease associations (e.g. SLE, RA).
8. Enquire about the social history.

The examination

1. Examine for muscle fatigue, particularly the elevators of the eyelids and the oculomotor muscles (tested by sustained upward gaze), bulbar muscles (tested by counting or reading aloud) and the proximal limb girdles (tested by holding the arms above the head).
2. Look for the peek sign (orbicularis oculi weakness – ask the patient to close his or her eyes and keep them closed; within 30 seconds in myasthenia they will begin to separate and you will see the lower sclera).
3. Asking the patient to smile may produce a snarling expression. Speech on prolonged speaking may sound dysarthric or nasal because of weakness of the palate.
4. Weakness of neck flexion may be prominent.
5. Flap one arm for 10–30 seconds and then test shoulder strength together.
6. Look for a thymectomy scar.
7. Reflexes are preserved, there is no sensory loss and muscle atrophy is usually minimal.

Investigations

The **ice pack test** can be performed at the bedside if there is ptosis: fill a surgical glove with ice and place it on the closed eyelid for 2 minutes – if ptosis improves this is suggestive, but not diagnostic, of myasthenia.

Laboratory tests for myasthenia gravis (Fig. 12.2) include the following.

1. **Acetylcholine receptor antibodies (AChR-Ab)** – these occur in 80%–90% of cases, with false-positive results being rare (but the frequency of positive tests is lower in

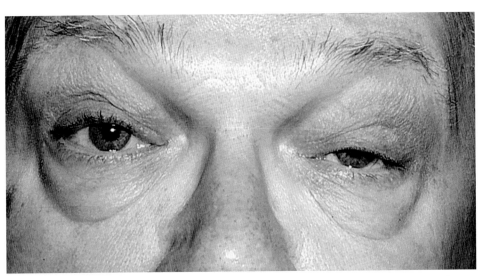

Figure 12.2 **Myasthenia (face). The patient has bilateral asymmetrical ptosis and needs to use the frontalis muscle to elevate the eyelids.**

S R Hamilton. *Albert and Jakobiec's principles and practice of ophthalmology*, 3rd edn. Elsevier, 2008, with permission.

pure ocular and inactive myasthenia gravis). The titre is not directly related to disease severity. Muscle-specific kinase antibodies (MuSK) are present in half of those AChR-Ab negative. Occasionally only antibodies to low-density lipoprotein receptor-related protein 4 (LRP4) are positive (1%); seronegative disease can occur (6%).

2. **Electromyogram (EMG)** – in myasthenia gravis, repetitive stimulation at low frequencies causes an asymptotic reduction (there is progressively less reduction with each shock) in muscle action potential amplitudes if that particular muscle is affected. Needle examination of affected muscles shows motor unit potential variation and, sometimes, fibrillation potentials and myopathic change. Single-fibre EMG shows increased jitter and blocking.

3. **Thymoma investigations** – chest X-ray, thoracic CT scan or MRI.

4. **Associated conditions** – hyperthyroidism and autoimmune diseases (check thyroid function tests, rheumatoid factor and antinuclear antibodies).

5. **Respiratory function tests** – these patients may have severe respiratory impairment.

Differential diagnosis

The differential diagnosis of proximal muscle weakness is important. The ocular muscle dystrophies also need to be considered. The Lambert–Eaton syndrome is occasionally confused with myasthenia gravis. This syndrome results from presynaptic failure of release of acetylcholine, caused by small cell carcinoma of the lung (in 50% of cases) or autoimmune disease. In the Lambert–Eaton syndrome:

• there is proximal muscle weakness and pain, and power may increase on repeated effort; reflexes are reduced or absent

• the ocular and bulbar muscles are usually spared

• the EMG is helpful (high-frequency stimulation causes an increment, whereas low-frequency stimulation causes a decrement and muscle action potential amplitudes are low).

Symptoms may be reduced by 3,4-diaminopyridine (DAP: safe and effective) or guanidine; steroids and plasma-exchange therapy can also be effective. Some patients with small cell carcinoma of the lung have a neurological remission if the tumour is completely removed. Treatment with D-penicillamine may cause a mild reversible form of myasthenia.

Treatment

The prognosis of myasthenia gravis is good: 50% of patients have a remission, although 5%–10% die from respiratory failure.

SYMPTOMATIC

1. Anticholinesterases are the mainstay of treatment in mild cases. Pyridostigmine is the usual one prescribed. Potassium supplements and potassium-sparing diuretics (e.g. spironolactone) may give additional improvement, but are rarely used these days.
2. It is important to avoid drugs that interfere with neuromuscular transmission, including streptomycin, gentamicin,[1] quinidine and procainamide. Immunise to prevent respiratory infections because of potential respiratory compromise (avoid live-attenuated flu or varicella-zoster vaccines if using immunosuppressive treatment).
3. Sudden worsening of the patient's symptoms so as to be life-threatening (because of respiratory failure) is called a myasthenic crisis. It is often precipitated by infection, which must be treated aggressively with antibiotics (though some, especially aminoglycosides, worsen myasthenia) and intensive respiratory support. Mechanical ventilation and a course of plasmapheresis may be required.
4. Sometimes the problem may be excessive anticholinesterase treatment (cholinergic crisis). Temporary suspension of drug treatment and monitoring of muscle strength may be all that is required for these episodes.

DISEASE-SUPPRESSING

1. Steroids are indicated for generalised severe disease when anticholinesterases are inadequate. They are then needed in the long term. They may aggravate disease initially (in the first week to 10 days), so all patients should be observed closely when treatment is commenced.
2. Failed steroid treatment in patients with severe disease is an indication for immunosuppressive drug therapy (e.g. azathioprine, cyclosporin, mycophenolate). Azathioprine has been shown to be effective as a steroid-sparing agent and to reduce relapses and prolong remissions, but it should not be used as initial management or on its own.
3. Thymectomy is advisable early on for many patients with generalised myasthenia gravis if they are AChR antibody positive. The exceptions are elderly patients or those with an easily inducible remission. Thymomas occur in 10% of cases (and, of these, 25% are malignant) and thymic hyperplasia occurs in 65%. Of such patients, after resection 70% show improvement and 25% of those who improve undergo remission. Causes of failed response to thymectomy include incomplete removal, ectopic tissue and fulminant disease.
4. Intravenous immune globulin (IVIG) can reverse a severe, life-threatening episode or refractory disease. Rituximab has been tried in desperate cases. This chimeric antibody attaches to the CD20 membrane site of B lymphocytes and attracts T-killer cells and antibodies that destroy the lymphocytes making the pathological antibodies.

---

[1] The restriction of use of antibiotics is controversial and many neurologists advise that there is little risk that can't be managed and that patients should receive the antibiotic indicated for their infection.

5. Plasmapheresis is useful in acute situations such as in myasthenic crisis, preparation for surgery or in the peripartum period. Very ill patients may need repeated treatments. Removal of the antibody from the blood in this way usually leads to rapid improvement.

Possible lines of questioning

1. Is there a possible differential diagnosis for *this* patient's muscle weakness and fatigue?
2. How would you investigate it?
3. Is screening for malignancy indicated for *this* patient?

Guillain–Barré syndrome

Acute inflammatory demyelinating polyneuropathy (AIDP) is not infrequent in the examination, as patients may be in hospital for an extended period and present management difficulties. It is the most common acute polyneuropathy and can affect both sexes and all ages.

The history

1. Ask about the presenting symptoms of ascending motor weakness, their time course and whether they are decreasing or increasing. The patient may report difficulty in breathing. Other symptoms include paraesthesiae or sensory loss (sensory neuropathy is usually minimal) and symptoms of cranial nerve palsies, particularly bulbar lesions (all cranial nerves except I, II and VIII can be affected). Back pain is a common complaint and may be intractable initially.
2. Ask about a preceding respiratory or gastrointestinal infection (which occurs in up to 50% of cases 1–3 weeks beforehand – *Campylobacter*, mycoplasma, EBV and influenza). Also enquire about other precipitating events, such as surgical operation, vaccination, intercurrent malignant disease (e.g. Hodgkin disease), SLE and HIV infection.
3. Find out how severe the disease has been at its worst. Some patients find themselves in ICU for many months with a prolonged and tortuous recovery. This may have significant impacts on how well they will recover both physically and psychologically.
4. Ask about previous episodes of disease (a relapsing course and the presence of sensory symptoms and proximal weakness suggest chronic inflammatory demyelinating polyneuropathy – CIDP).
5. Ask about evidence of autonomic neuropathy, such as postural hypotension, labile blood pressure, difficult-to-control arrhythmias and, rarely, sphincter dysfunction (see Table 16.42, p. 490).
6. Ask about neuropathic pain.
7. Enquire about the social history, recurrent falls, family support, etc.

The examination

1. Predominantly, distal muscle weakness without atrophy is present, although 25% have more proximal than distal weakness. The upper limbs may be more affected than the lower limbs. Tendon reflexes are reduced or absent concomitant with the degree of weakness. Muscle tenderness is common (one-third of cases).

2. Signs of autonomic neuropathy (severe postural changes in blood pressure and cardiac arrhythmias) must be looked for.
3. Sensory loss is usually minimal, but if present it affects the posterior columns (vibration and proprioception) more than the spinothalamic tracts.
4. Always measure forced expiratory time.
5. Examine for ophthalmoplegia, as its presence suggests the uncommon Miller Fisher variant (ophthalmoplegia, ataxia and areflexia).
6. Look for pressure sores and signs of deep venous thrombosis in bed-bound patients.

Investigations

Guillain–Barré syndrome is a clinical diagnosis. Helpful tests include the following:
1. **immune stimulus** – identify the immune stimulus by the Monospot test, cold agglutinins, tests for cytomegalovirus, HIV or *Campylobacter*
2. **cerebrospinal fluid examination** – look for a raised protein level and the relative lack of white blood cells in 90% of cases; 10% have 10–50 mononuclear cells/mL
3. **respiratory function tests (FEV$_1$, FVC)** – assess the progressive involvement of respiratory muscles; the patient can progress rapidly (even over hours) to respiratory failure requiring intubation and should be admitted to hospital, even if only mildly affected
4. **nerve conduction and electromyogram studies** – many nerves may have to be studied to find abnormalities because this disease is patchy, but abnormalities include slowed motor conduction, conduction blocks, increased distal motor latencies, reduced sensory action potentials and increased F wave latencies. EMG evidence of denervation takes 10 days to 3 weeks to appear and may indicate axonal involvement with a worse prognosis
5. **antiganglioside antibodies** – anti-GM1 and anti-GD3 (not sensitive) and anti-GQ1b antibodies are found in 90% of the Miller Fisher variant cases.

Differential diagnosis

Infections such as glandular fever, acute viral hepatitis, *Mycoplasma* pneumonia, *Campylobacter jejuni* and HIV can cause Guillain–Barré syndrome. Post-influenza vaccine disease is rare. The differential diagnosis of acute ascending motor paralysis includes diphtheria, polio, polyarteritis nodosa, acute intermittent porphyria, tick or snake bites and rhabdomyolysis, arsenic poisoning and botulism. Critical illness myopathy or polyneuropathy might be considered in some patients. Remember that diphtheria, botulism and myasthenia gravis usually begin with bulbar symptoms.

The differential diagnosis of autonomic neuropathy includes diabetes mellitus, alcoholism, acute intermittent porphyria and amyloidosis.
1. Chronic inflammatory demyelinating polyradiculopathy may begin in a similar way to Guillain–Barré but progress or relapse more than 2 months after it begins. Other patients with CIDP have more slowly developing motor and, to a lesser extent, sensory changes in proximal and distal muscles. Sensory changes including pain are more common in CIDP.
2. Diabetes and connective tissue disease are important differential diagnoses.

Treatment

Prognosis is good – most patients make a complete recovery over time (up to a year), but 2% die (usually of respiratory complications, pulmonary emboli or cardiac arrhythmias) and 10% have a major residual deficit. If the deficit does not diminish within 3 weeks or the patient has autonomic neuropathy, a poorer prognosis is more likely.
1. Physiotherapy is used to prevent contractures. Respiratory support in an ICU is essential if the vital capacity is less than 1 litre.

2. Immunosuppression, intravenous gammaglobulin and plasma exchange have all been shown to be effective treatment.
3. Plasmapheresis or intravenous gamma globulin shortens the time to recovery from respiratory paralysis and hastens the return of mobility. They are equally effective and combined treatment offers no additional benefit. Treatment should be begun as soon as possible. Rapid improvement is much more likely if treatment is begun within 2 weeks of the first symptoms. Relapses may occur and are more common after intravenous gamma globulin than after plasmapheresis.

Possible lines of questioning

1. Discuss the differential diagnosis of *this* patient's weakness.
2. How would you investigate *this* patient?
3. How do you see *this* patient progressing in the short, medium and long term?

Syncope, seizures and 'funny turns'

Patients presenting with a 'funny turn' can pose a difficult diagnostic problem as there are many possible explanations. The problem may be neurological, cardiac, endocrinological or psychiatric. A careful history and physical examination should enable the candidate to produce a sensible differential diagnosis and management plan. Treatment is usually fairly straightforward once the diagnosis is made.

The history

1. Presyncope refers to a sense of impending loss of consciousness, manifest as faintness or light-headedness, and is often associated with sweating, nausea, anxiety and visual dimming. These can be considered haemodynamic causes of dizziness (Box 12.1).
   a. Causes of this condition can include cardiac arrhythmias, postural hypotension, cough syncope and micturition syncope.

Box 12.1 Haemodynamic dizziness

1. Cardiac
   • Aortic stenosis, hypertrophic cardiomyopathy
   • Arrhythmia – bradycardia or tachycardia
2. Autonomic
   • Vasovagal
   • Autonomic neuropathy, e.g. diabetes mellitus
   • Multisystem atrophy, e.g. associated with Parkinson's disease
3. Drugs
   • Antihypertensives including vasodilators for prostatism
   • Antipsychotics
4. Hypovolaemia
   • Haemorrhage
   • Dehydration
   • Addisonian crisis
5. Cerebrovascular
   • Vertebrobasilar insufficiency (very rare)

b. Vasovagal syncope or presyncope can often be diagnosed clinically if the history is typical: an episode begins with clamminess, sweating and nausea and often occurs in a crowded room or after something upsetting has happened.

2. Epilepsy needs to be considered in the differential diagnosis. The diagnosis depends greatly on the characteristics of the seizures (Tables 12.4 and 12.5):

a. Focal epilepsy is usually accompanied by an aura or a warning (e.g. flashing lights, twitching of the face or a limb, unilateral tingling or numbness, buzzing noises or humming).

b. Generalised epilepsy may be associated with myoclonic jerks (juvenile myoclonic epilepsy), but frequently occurs with sudden loss of consciousness without warning.

c. Eyewitness accounts are crucial in making a diagnosis. Eyewitnesses are likely to find a seizure more frightening than a syncopal episode. Idiopathic generalised epilepsy is frequently symmetrical with tonic (stiffening) and then clonic (brief jerking movements) phases, whereas partial seizures with secondary generalisation may be associated with asymmetric posturing initially.

d. Eyewitnesses may have had the presence of mind to film the episode on their phones and review of these pictures can be very helpful.

e. If epilepsy has been diagnosed or is suspected, ask the patient how this has been discussed and what restrictions have been placed on his or her activities. How has the diagnosis affected him or her at home, at work and emotionally?

f. Remember that seizure activity may accompany cerebral hypoxia of any cause (e.g. Stokes–Adams attacks). A long period of drowsiness often follows a major seizure.

Table 12.4 Classification of epileptic seizures[a]

1. **Partial seizures** – the abnormal electrical discharge may remain localised or spread to other parts of the cortex:

a. Simple partial seizures do not affect consciousness. Examples may include isolated 'auras' of smells or *déjà vu* (a feeling that new events or people are familiar), or *jamais vu* (a feeling that known events or people are unfamiliar), or pure motor or sensory seizures.

b. Complex partial seizures involve altered consciousness when the seizure spreads to involve one or both temporal lobes. Patients may stare and not respond, and may posture, turn their head or perform automatic motor tasks.

c. Secondarily generalised seizures cause convulsions and occur when a partial seizure spreads to involve both hemispheres diffusely. These convulsions involve impaired awareness followed by generalised muscle contractions (tonic movements) and then rhythmical contraction and relaxation of muscles (clonic movements). They may be hard to distinguish from primary generalised seizures, but sometimes focal features such as asymmetric posturing or the report of a preceding aura help to make the diagnosis.

d. Jacksonian seizures are simple motor seizures characterised by rhythmical contraction of a group of muscles (typically of the fingers) that spread to the arm and then the ipsilateral side of the face.

e. Partial seizures may be preceded by an aura, particularly if the seizure activity begins in the temporal lobe. Patients may describe a feeling of *déjà vu*, of dread, or of abdominal pain that spreads to the chest. This aura is a form of partial seizure, of which the patient is aware.

2. **Generalised seizures** – involve both hemispheres from the start:

a. Primary generalised tonic and clonic seizures (GTCS) are convulsions that may occur with no warning. Tongue biting and incontinence are common, and a feeling of confusion and tiredness is common afterwards.

b. Absence seizures are generalised seizures that cause momentary loss of consciousness. They mostly happen in children. Up to 200 episodes a day may occur.

c. Myoclonic seizures are very brief jerky movements that occur without warning, often when the patient is tired or in the morning. They are associated with juvenile myoclonic epilepsy (JME).

[a]Remember that epilepsy is the condition of having seizures and a seizure is the event itself.

Table 12.5 Syncope vs seizure

SYNCOPE	SEIZURE
Onset precipitated by emotion, standing, micturition, showering	May occur during sleep or when patient lying down
Often a prodrome of lightheadedness, pallor, nausea, clamminess, fading vision and hearing	May begin with familiar aura (actually a focal seizure)
	Temporal lobe seizures may begin with anxiety and feeling of *déjà vu* or *jamais vu*
Twitching or brief tonic and clonic movements	Clear tonic and then clonic phase
No coordinated movements	May have focal lifting of arm, head turning and spread of jerking ('Jacksonian march' of focal-onset seizures)
Only briefly disoriented, not sleepy	Prolonged state of drowsiness and sometimes confusion afterwards (post-ictal symptoms)

3. Vertigo is the illusion of movement of the self or the environment. The sensation is often rotational. Often nausea, vomiting, imbalance and anxiety are associated.
   a. Causes of this condition include vestibular neuritis or labyrinthitis, benign paroxysmal positional vertigo (BPPV), Ménière's disease, stroke and MS. Cerebellar stroke characteristically causes severe associated nausea and vomiting, and is of sudden onset.
   b. Ask whether the vertigo is related to the position of the head (e.g. especially occurs when the patient turns over in bed or looks up or down). This symptom suggests benign paroxysmal positional vertigo. If vertigo is persistent or occurs at rest, the diagnosis *is not BPPV*.
4. Unsteadiness of gait may be secondary to a number of disorders of the peripheral or central nervous system. Cerebellar, sensory, extrapyramidal and myopathic diseases can all present in this way. Causes may include a range of pathologies from drug side-effects and stroke to neoplasms and degenerative disease.
5. Hypoglycaemia is an important, albeit rare, cause of 'funny turns' and must always be considered in the differential diagnosis. It is associated with hunger, sweating, tremor and tachycardia (owing to catecholamine release), as well as neurological dysfunction. Causes of hypoglycaemia include: too much insulin or oral hypoglycaemic agent and not enough food; reactive or postprandial, usually among patients with gastric surgery; or fasting (especially among patients with hypopituitarism, adrenal insufficiency, cirrhosis, alcoholism or rarely an insulinoma).
6. There are a number of cardiac causes of 'funny turns' or syncope (see Table 12.5):
   a. A dizzy feeling related to standing up and without any component of true vertigo suggests postural hypotension. This can be a complication of antihypertensive treatment, especially with vasodilating drugs, and occasionally occurs in patients with single-chamber ventricular pacemakers (pacemaker syndrome).
   b. Orthostatic hypotension is common in the elderly and in patients with autonomic neuropathy (e.g. secondary to diabetes mellitus).
   c. Episodes of complete heart block may complicate ischaemic heart disease or be caused by degenerative disease of the conducting system. These patients describe syncope occurring without warning. Unless they have been injured by the fall, they feel normal again immediately.
   d. Ventricular and supraventricular tachyarrhythmias may cause dizziness or syncope, possibly associated with palpitations. Ventricular arrhythmias are more likely in

patients with known structural heart disease (e.g. previous infarction). Remember that antiarrhythmic drugs can cause bradycardia and are associated in some cases with dangerous proarrhythmic effects.

e. Patients with severe aortic stenosis may present with exertional syncope, which may be associated with ischaemic-like chest pain.

7. Other conditions that need to be considered include episodes of hyperventilation or panic attacks. Patients who sigh often because of anxiety are rarely aware of any abnormality of their breathing. Their dizziness is often accompanied by a sensation of swaying.

Transient global amnesia sometimes presents as a 'funny turn' involving temporary disorientation and loss of memory without other focal neurology. Its hallmark is the sudden onset of repetitive questioning of family and friends about what is happening.

8. Psychogenic non-epileptic seizures (PNES – no longer called pseudoseizures or hysterical seizures) need to be distinguished from epilepsy as a cause of apparent syncope. They do not respond to anticonvulsant treatment. Unlike the seizures of epilepsy, they feature:
   * forced eye closure
   * prolonged episodes (> 5 minutes)
   * occurrence particularly when there is an audience (often the crowded waiting room)
   * unusual motor events – opisthotonus (back arching), pelvic thrusting, side-to-side movements, changes in the plane of movement (nodding then shaking of the head)
   * a normal EEG during the event.

   The patient may have been given this diagnosis. Investigations may have included prolonged video and EEG recording. This diagnosis is an important one as intubation and aggressive benzodiazepine therapy are associated with substantial morbidity.

9. Ask for a list of all the drugs the patient has been taking (Tables 12.6 and 12.7). Enquire about medications that increase the risk of vascular episodes, including oral contraceptives and some peripheral vasodilator drugs that can lower blood pressure. Also, ask specifically about sedatives, hypoglycaemic agents, anticonvulsants and drugs affecting cardiac conduction. Try to find out whether adherence has been a problem. Have anticonvulsant blood levels been monitored?

Table 12.6 Choice of anticonvulsant

Remember, treatment is generally not indicated for a first seizure without a CNS lesion. Although there is evidence to suggest a preference for certain first-line agents for certain seizure disorders, the effect sizes are quite small, so if other factors such as dosing frequency, side effects and interactions become issues, you could consider commencing with another agent.

	FIRST LINE	SECOND LINE	THIRD LINE
Focal or secondary generalised tonic–clonic seizures (GTCS)	Lamotrigine	Carbamazepine, sodium valproate	Gabapentin, phenytoin, pregabalin
GTCS	Sodium valproate	Lamotrigine, topiramate	Carbamazepine, phenytoin, phenobarbital, primidone
Absence	Ethosuximide	Sodium valproate	Clonazepam, lamotrigine, phenobarbital
Myoclonic	Sodium valproate	Clonazepam	Lamotrigine

Table 12.7 **Principles of drug treatment for epilepsy**

- Begin with a single first-line drug
- Begin with low dose and increase as required or until side-effects become a problem
- Keep regimen simple to improve adherence
- Failure of first-line drug – begin second line and gradually withdraw first
- Failure of second-line drug – add baseline drug at maximum tolerated dose (beware of drug interactions
- Failure – begin alternative second-line drug
- Failure – consider adherence problems and alternative diagnosis
- Use a minimum number of drugs

10. Both undiagnosed and diagnosed syncopal episodes can have legal and other implications. Ask how the condition has affected the patient's life and work:
    - Has driving or the operating of machinery been forbidden?
    - If so, for how long?
    - When might these be allowed again?
    - How does he or she manage work, shopping, getting to appointments?
    - Has this led to mood changes?
    - How does the family cope?

THE EXAMINATION

A complete examination of the neurological and cardiovascular systems is essential, but must be guided by the symptoms.

1. Check all the pulses. Decide whether atrial fibrillation is present. Test the blood pressure lying and standing for postural hypotension. Listen for murmurs (e.g. as a result of aortic stenosis, infective endocarditis, rheumatic heart disease or a prosthetic valve). Examine for peripheral vascular disease. Note the presence of an electronic pacemaker.
2. The fundi should be carefully examined for evidence of emboli, hypertensive changes, diabetic changes and ischaemic retinopathy. Test the visual fields (e.g. for homonymous hemianopia in stroke).
3. If indicated, perform the Hallpike test for benign paroxysmal positional vertigo. If vertigo is a symptom, examine eye movements carefully for nystagmus and skew deviation. Perform a head impulse test for vestibular hypofunction. Examine for limb and gait ataxia and sensation in the head and limbs.
4. Palpate over the temporal areas for the tenderness of giant cell arteritis.

Investigations

1. An ECG should be recorded (for evidence of ischaemic heart disease, arrhythmia or heart block). Look for a long or short QT interval. Patients in sinus rhythm, but with bifascicular or trifascicular block, may be having episodes of complete heart block. Intermittent episodes that may be a result of cardiac arrhythmias (brady- or tachycardias) can be investigated with Holter monitor recordings. When episodes are infrequent but severe, an implanted cardiac 'loop' recorder can be used. These small subcutaneous devices will record loops of ECG. They can be programmed to record heart rate above or below a certain number and will store the ECG from the preceding few minutes if activated by the patient with a magnet.

   Suspected epilepsy is investigated with an MRI scan and EEG. A first seizure must be investigated to exclude cerebral tumours, vascular malformations and strokes.

2. Normal results from these tests *do not exclude epilepsy* and a slightly abnormal EEG does not make the diagnosis of epilepsy in someone with atypical symptoms. Video and EEG monitoring can be required to make the diagnosis and can be used where patients have not responded to two antiepileptic drugs to help clarify the diagnosis and to exclude pseudoseizures.

In patients with a suspected transient ischaemic attack (TIA – transient focal neurological symptoms are essential to this diagnosis), it is worthwhile ordering an FBC, ESR (elevated in temporal arteritis and in connective tissue disease), fasting plasma glucose (for evidence of diabetes or hypoglycaemia), cholesterol (for hyper-cholesterolaemia), cortisol (if hypotensive) and urinalysis (for evidence of renovascular disease).

3. Possible TIAs and strokes require investigation with at least a CT scan of the brain and often an MRI as well (see p. 352). Urgent carotid Doppler scans are indicated for symptoms that could be attributed to brain supplied by the anterior circulation.

Management

Treatment will depend on the final diagnosis and can include:

1. withdrawal of drugs
2. canalith-repositioning manoeuvres – can be very helpful for people with benign paroxysmal positional vertigo
3. pacemaker or defibrillator insertion – it is usually unwise to implant these devices without an established diagnosis
4. use of anticonvulsants (Table 12.8)
5. for patients with vasovagal syncope – reassurance and explanation and advice about recognising the triggers and symptoms that may precede an episode may be all that is required.

A diagnosis of epilepsy will have serious consequences for the patient and his or her work, ability to drive, play sport, etc. Much explanation and discussion will be required about the condition and what treatment involves as far as effectiveness and side-effects are concerned. Find out from the patient whether these matters have been discussed.

Table 12.8 Commonly used anticonvulsants and their side-effects

In general, any of these can be used to treat partial epilepsies but some (carbamazepine, gabapentin, phenytoin and pregabalin) can make generalised epilepsy worse. The newer drugs are not especially more effective than older ones, but may have fewer side-effects. Combinations of drugs are used when one fails.

DRUG	COMMON PROBLEMS	SERIOUS PROBLEMS
Carbamazepine	Dizziness, sedation, hyponatraemia	Aplastic anaemia, Stevens–Johnson syndrome, rash
Gabapentin	Sedation, oedema, weight gain	Drowsiness, dizziness, ataxia
Lamotrigine	Acne, insomnia, headache and dizziness, diplopia	Stevens–Johnson syndrome, rash, hepatic failure
Phenobarbital	Sedation, ataxia, nausea	Stevens–Johnson syndrome, rash, hepatic failure
Phenytoin	Sedation, oedema, weight gain	Stevens–Johnson syndrome, rash, blood dyscrasia, hepatic failure, lupus-like syndrome, cardiac conduction abnormalities, gingival hyperplasia
Valproic acid	Hirsutism, weight gain, tremor	Hepatic failure, pancreatitis, thrombocytopenia

Transient ischaemic attack and stroke

Patients with a history of stroke or transient ischaemic episodes are common in the long-case exam. Cerebrovascular disease may sometimes be the main problem. Note that the correct terminology is a 'stroke' and not 'cerebrovascular accident'.

The history

The patient who has had a stroke or TIA is likely to know the diagnosis, but there may still be a differential diagnosis. It may be possible from the history to establish whether cerebrovascular disease and, in particular, TIAs explain the symptoms convincingly. Misdiagnosis of TIA is also common, so confirmation of the symptoms is essential.

TIAs occur suddenly; there is focal neurological loss that is maximal at onset and does not spread or intensify. By definition, the symptoms must resolve within 24 hours, although after an hour imaging changes are usually present on MRI. If so, it is termed a stroke. As such, true TIAs usually last from minutes to an hour. Specific enquiry should be made about unilateral weakness or clumsiness, difficulty in understanding or expressing spoken language, altered sensation unilaterally, and partial or complete loss of vision in one eye or bilateral blindness. Ten per cent of TIA patients have a completed stroke within 90 days, and 40% of strokes are preceded by TIAs.

HINT

Remember the criteria for recommending admission to hospital after a TIA (a score of 3 or more is an indication for admission):

1. Age > 60 = 1 point
2. BP > 140/90 mmHg = 1 point
3. Focal weakness during episode = 2 points
4. Speech impaired, no weakness = 1 point
5. > 60 min of symptoms = 2 points
6. 10–59 min of symptoms = 1 point
7. Diabetic patient = 1 point

Slurred speech is less helpful as a symptom in a possible TIA and faintness, confusion, simultaneous bilateral weakness and spinning sensations are not localising symptoms. If these are the main symptoms, it suggests that the diagnosis is not a TIA.

1. Ask whether the neurological deficits have lasted for longer than 24 hours. This is consistent with the syndrome of a completed stroke.

2. The absence of focal symptoms in a patient with severe headache and vomiting suggests subarachnoid haemorrhage. Vomiting and focal symptoms may occur with intracerebral haemorrhage, but headache is present in less than 50% of these patients.
3. In ischaemic stroke, the symptoms typically begin abruptly, often during sleep, and are not usually associated with headache or vomiting.
4. Enquire about risk factors for cerebrovascular disease (in particular hypertension (the most important), smoking, diabetes, family history and hyperlipidaemia).
5. Neck pain or previous neck manipulation may indicate arterial dissection.
6. Symptoms of connective tissue disease or thrombotic episodes may be relevant.
7. Vasculitis can be an occasional cause of stroke.
8. What residual deficit has the patient suffered?
9. How has this affected the patient's work, sport, his or her ability to look after him or herself, mood and thoughts about the future?
10. What investigations is the patient aware of?
11. Was thrombolysis attempted?
12. What treatment is being given now – antiplatelet drugs, anticoagulants, antihypertensives, cholesterol-lowering drugs?

HINT

Haemorrhagic stroke (17% of strokes) cannot be differentiated from ischaemic stroke clinically, although coma, seizures, vomiting, headache, meningism and a raised diastolic blood pressure are suggestive of haemorrhage.

The examination

1. Perform an appropriate neurological examination to establish the deficit and its effect on function (e.g. walking, writing, etc.). Be guided by the history.
2. Carotid bruits should be listened for, but their absence does not exclude tight carotid stenosis. Unfortunately, even if a bruit is present, this does not necessarily indicate tight common or internal carotid artery stenosis, because external carotid artery stenosis can also cause a bruit.
3. Examine the rest of the cardiovascular system for evidence of hypertension, atrial fibrillation, heart failure or a mechanical valve.

Investigations

1. A CT or MRI ± MRA scan of the head (Figs 12.3 and 12.4) should be performed for all patients with a TIA or stroke, as 5% of apparent TIAs are caused by structural lesions. A CT scan is also worth performing in patients with established stroke to exclude haemorrhage, as this alters management. CT perfusion imaging can be used to guide thrombolysis or endovascular clot retrieval. It would be useful to know what the patient received as it will give you an indication of the perceived severity of the stroke at the time relative to the patient's baseline function.

HINT

A non-contrast CT scan will easily exclude a haemorrhagic stroke. It may appear normal early (days) after an acute ischaemic stroke.

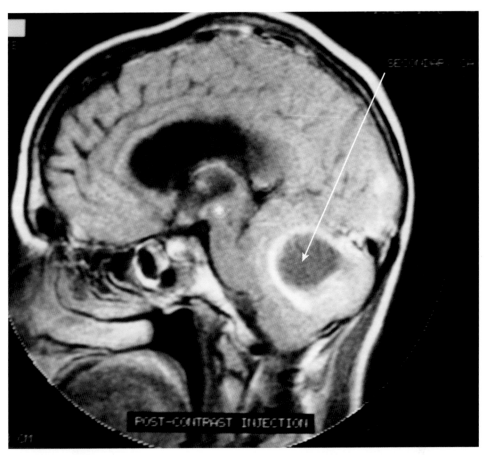

Figure 12.3 MRI of the brain showing a metastatic cerebellar tumour (arrow).

Figure reproduced courtesy of The Canberra Hospital.

2. A carotid ultrasound should be performed in patients who have carotid territory TIAs / stroke. Suggestive features of a carotid artery TIA / stroke include monocular visual loss, unilateral sensory disturbances or weakness, or aphasia. Vertebrobasilar TIAs, on the other hand, may cause bilateral visual loss, weakness or sensory disturbance, and crossed sensory and motor loss. If > 70% stenosis of the origin of the internal carotid artery on the symptomatic side is found, carotid angiography should be considered with a view to endarterectomy or angioplasty, which is of value in otherwise-fit patients.

3. A transoesophageal echocardiogram (TOE) and if indicated a bubble study should be considered. Order a TOE in any stroke patient with abnormalities on examination of the heart or with abnormalities on the ECG (or chest X-ray). It is also recommended when no other cause has been found for the episode as it may reveal a patent foramen ovale (PFO), a known cause of paradoxical embolism, in up to 30% of people. Catheter-based PFO closure is superior to medical therapy.

4. Patients with atrial fibrillation should have their thyroid function checked and an echocardiogram performed to look at left ventricular size – a predictor of risk of embolic events. Rarely, an intracardiac mass (usually a left atrial myxoma) is discovered. It is a rare cause of stroke and is often associated with systemic symptoms. Resection is usually possible.

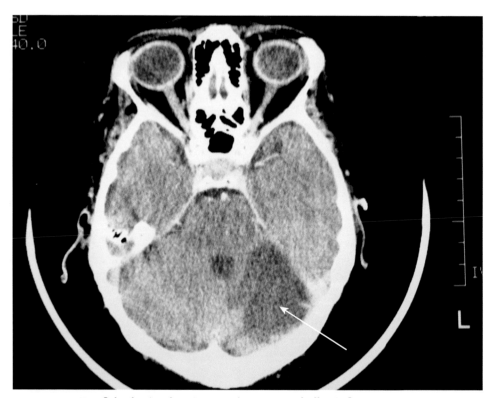

Figure 12.4 **CT of the brain showing a subacute cerebellar infarct (arrow).**

Figure reproduced courtesy of The Canberra Hospital.

5. In relatively young patients with a TIA/stroke (< 50 years of age), careful attention to the possibility of connective tissue disease is worthwhile. Check for antinuclear antibody, anticardiolipin antibody (because of antiphospholipid antibody syndrome) and for thrombophilia.

HINT

Causes of ischaemic stroke:
1. Embolus from the heart – 20%
2. Large artery disease – 20%
3. Subcortical (lacunar) – 25%
4. Cryptogenic – 30%
5. Vasculitis, genetic, venous sinus thrombosis – 5%

Treatment

This will depend on the diagnosis in the particular case. If a TIA is likely, you should plan to discuss vascular risk factor treatments, antiplatelet therapy and the role of carotid endarterectomy. The diagnosis is never TIA if neurology persists, even if improving.

1. Acute stroke can be treated with thrombolysis with recombinant tissue plasminogen activator (rtPA) up to 4.5 hours after the onset of symptoms, though the benefit is

larger the earlier the drug is given after symptom onset. If onset of symptoms (e.g. on waking up) is unclear then thrombolysis should not be given. It is best practice for this to be administered by someone experienced in the management of stroke. Clot retrieval is increasingly available for these patients. It can be performed after thrombolytic treatment. It can be dramatically effective and the window for successful treatment is extending. A CT scan must be performed to exclude haemorrhagic stroke.

2. There is a direct relationship between high blood pressure, smoking and cholesterol level and an increased risk of ischaemic stroke as well as coronary artery disease. Therefore, management of risk factors by conservative means or with drugs is essential.

3. The blood pressure is often elevated after an acute ischaemic stroke – do *not* lower unless malignant hypertension or thrombolysis is planned.

4. Antiplatelet therapy reduces the risk of stroke in patients prone to TIAs. Low-dose aspirin (between 75 and 100 mg per day) is a reasonable regimen to use. Clopidogrel is an adenosine diphosphate (ADP) inhibitor and a slightly more effective alternative to aspirin. It is generally used for people intolerant of aspirin, or sometimes for those who have recurrent events while taking aspirin. Recurrence of symptoms when patients are already taking aspirin is an indication for the combination of aspirin and dipyridamole or a change to clopidogrel. Aspirin and clopidogrel in combination have not been shown to be more effective than aspirin alone, mainly because of an increased risk of serious bleeding. At least 2 years of treatment is necessary after a TIA, but most would recommend the lifelong use of antiplatelet agents.

   In those with atrial fibrillation (AF) not caused by rheumatic heart disease, aspirin reduces the risk of a recurrent event by one-fifth and direct oral anticoagulant (DOACs) reduce it by one-half, similar in efficacy to warfarin. Most cardiologists and neurologists would now recommend a DOAC to any patient in AF who has had a definite or even a possible embolic event and in patients with an elevated (i.e. one point or more) CHA_2DS_2-VASc score (see p. 95). The risk of major haemorrhage with apixaban use is the lowest of all the DOACs, and the risk with DOACs as a group is less than with warfarin. If there are contraindications to DOACs (due to renal dysfunction or medication interaction), it would probably be appropriate to use warfarin rather than an empirical low-dose DOAC. In those who have rheumatic heart disease, mechanical prosthetic heart valves or other cardiac sources of emboli, long-term anticoagulation with warfarin is strongly recommended.

5. If the patient is taking warfarin, find out about problems managing the dose and INR tests. Does the patient know what recent INR results have been? How often is it tested?

6. Carotid endarterectomy or angioplasty and stenting is worth considering in patients with a TIA / small stroke in the carotid territory within the preceding 6 months who have documented severe (> 70%) stenosis of the origin of the internal carotid artery on the symptomatic side. It is most beneficial if performed early after TIA, though after stroke it can be delayed if there is a risk of haemorrhage. These patients have a 25% risk of having a completed stroke in the following 2 years. Surgery in such cases is definitely superior to medical therapy. A decision to operate should be based on the availability of surgical expertise and the complication (stroke) rate of a particular surgical unit.

Admission to an acute stroke unit improves outcome and 1-year mortality. These units provide expertise in care of the patient's airway, assessment of swallowing, use of feeding tubes and prevention of pressure sores and they provide access to rehabilitation units. They can also provide occupational therapists to make home visits and appropriate equipment to ensure a patient has the best chance of returning home. These are important issues to assess in discussion of a stroke patient's treatment.

Possible lines of questioning

1. What would you tell *this* patient about his or her risk of stroke over the next few years?
2. Would you recommend closure of *this* patient's patent foramen ovale?
3. Has *this* patient had the best possible rehabilitation and care?
4. What anticoagulant or antiplatelet regimen should this patient be on?

Chapter 13

Other important long cases

Humanity has but three great enemies: fever, famine
and war; and of these by far the greatest, by far the
most terrible, is fever.

Harvey Cushing (1869–1939)

Pyrexia of unknown origin

Although not a common long case, pyrexia of unknown origin (PUO) presents both
diagnostic and management problems. The term 'pyrexia of unknown origin' previously
was used for patients with a fever > 38.3°C for more than 3 weeks for whom no diagnosis
has been made during a week of intensive study. The criteria have been relaxed slightly
to include fever of unknown cause after 3 days of intensive investigations in hospital,
or after 3 outpatient visits or a week of outpatient investigations. The common causes
of PUO are listed in Table 13.1.

The history
1. Ask about the chronological development of symptoms.
    a. Gastrointestinal tract symptoms should be sought. Consider:
       - Crohn's disease
       - metastatic cancer in the abdomen
       - subphrenic abscess
       - diverticular abscess
       - cholangitis
       - appendiceal abscess
       - liver abscess
       - Whipple's disease.
       Note any preceding acute infections (e.g. diarrhoeal illness, boils).
    b. Chest pain may suggest pericarditis, multiple pulmonary emboli or, rarely,
       intraluminal dissection of the aorta.
    c. Joint pain may suggest:
       - rheumatoid arthritis (RA)
       - systemic lupus erythematosus (SLE)

Table 13.1 Important causes of pyrexia of unknown origin

1. NEOPLASMS
   a. Lymphoma, leukaemia
   b. Solid tumours
   c. Primary – renal, lung, atrial myxoma, colon, pancreas, liver
   d. Secondary – metastatic disease (including melanoma, sarcoma)

2. INFECTIONS
   a. Bacterial – tuberculosis, atypical mycobacteria, abscess (e.g. pelvic, abdominal, dental), brucellosis, endocarditis, pericarditis, osteomyelitis, cholangitis, pyelonephritis, leptospirosis
   b. Viral, rickettsial and chlamydial – hepatitis, human immunodeficiency virus (HIV), cytomegalovirus (CMV), Q fever, psittacosis
   c. Parasitic – malaria, amoebiasis, trichinosis, toxoplasmosis

3. CONNECTIVE TISSUE DISEASES
   a. Rheumatoid arthritis, systemic lupus erythematosus, rheumatic fever, adult Still's disease
   b. Vasculitis – polyarteritis nodosa, temporal arteritis, Wegener's granulomatosis

4. MISCELLANEOUS
   a. Drug fever, e.g. NSAIDs, antibiotics, phenytoin, quinidine
   b. Inflammatory bowel disease, Whipple's disease
   c. Granulomatous disease – granulomatous hepatitis, sarcoidosis (uncommon)
   d. Multiple pulmonary emboli, intraluminal aortic dissection
   e. Thyroiditis
   f. Haematomas – retroperitoneal space (consider especially if on anticoagulants)
   g. Haemolysis
   h. Habitual hyperthermia (usually young women with low-grade fever, but no organic disease)
   i. Thermoregulatory disorders (rare – abnormal temperature-regulating mechanism)
   j. Cyclic neutropenia
   k. Factitious fever

- vasculitis
- atrial myxoma
- endocarditis.
   d. Dysuria or rectal pain may indicate prostatic abscess or urinary tract infection.
   e. Headache and joint or muscle pain may indicate giant cell arteritis.
   f. Night sweats may indicate:
   - lymphoma
   - tuberculosis (TB)
   - brucellosis
   - endocarditis
   - an abscess.
2. Ask about place of residence and overseas travel (e.g. malaria, amoebiasis, fungal infections).
3. Ask about contact with domestic or wild animals or birds and consider:
   - psittacosis
   - brucellosis
   - Q fever
   - histoplasmosis
   - leptospirosis
   - toxoplasmosis.

4. Ask about close contact with persons who have TB.
5. Enquire about occupation and hobbies:
   * veterinary surgeon
   * farmer (fungal infection, raw milk ingestion, hypersensitivity pneumonitis)
   * intravenous drug use (contaminants, e.g. quinine).
6. Ask whether you may enquire about sexual practices:
   * risk of HIV infection
   * sexually transmitted disease
   * pelvic inflammatory disease.
7. Ask about evidence of immunocompromised host (e.g. cytomegalovirus (CMV), *Pneumocystis jirovecii*).
8. Find out about medication used:
   * drug fever (antibiotic allergy, e.g. sulfonylureas, penicillin)
   * arsenicals
   * iodides
   * thiouracils
   * antihistamines
   * NSAIDs
   * antihypertensives (methyldopa, hydralazine)
   * antiarrhythmics (procainamide, quinidine).
9. Ask about anticoagulant use (accumulation of old blood in a closed space, e.g. retroperitoneal, perisplenic).
10. Ask about iatrogenic infection including:
    * catheter
    * arteriovenous fistula
    * prosthetic heart valve.
11. Ask about factitious fever (Table 13.2) from injection of contaminated material or tampering with thermometer readings – suspect the former diagnosis if there is an excessively high temperature, or the latter in the absence of tachycardia, chills or sweats; this is more common in medical or paramedical personnel.

The examination
1. Look at the temperature chart, if available, to see whether the fever pattern is characteristic. The temperature tends to fall to normal each day in pyogenic infections, TB and lymphoma, whereas in malaria the temperature can return to normal for days before rising again.

Table 13.2 Features suggesting factitious fever
1. Patient looks well
2. Temperature >41°C
3. Absence of diurnal temperature variation
4. No sweating as temperature comes down
5. Temperature normal when taken under supervision
6. History of self-harm, previous self-injection sites
7. Normal CRP or ESR
8. Infection with multiple commensal organisms
9. Photographic record of infection site

CRP = C-reactive protein; ESR = erythrocyte sedimentation rate.

2. Inspect the patient: note whether he or she appears ill or not, whether there is cachexia (suggesting a chronic disease process) and any skin rash, e.g.:
   - erythema multiforme
   - erythema nodosum
   - adult Still's disease (salmon-pink macular rash).
3. Pick up the hands and look for stigmata of infective endocarditis or any vasculitic changes, and for finger clubbing.
4. Inspect the arms for injection sites (intravenous drug abuse).
5. Palpate for epitrochlear and axillary lymphadenopathy (e.g. lymphoma, solid tumour spread, focal infections).
6. Examine the eyes for iritis or conjunctivitis (e.g. connective tissue disease, sarcoidosis) or jaundice (e.g. cholangitis, liver abscess). Look in the fundi for choroidal tubercles (miliary TB), Roth's spots (infective endocarditis), retinal haemorrhages or infiltrates (e.g. leukaemia). Note any facial rash (e.g. SLE). Feel the temporal arteries (temporal arteritis).
7. Examine the mouth for ulcers and gum disease and the teeth and tonsils for infection. Feel the parotids for parotitis and the sinuses for sinusitis.
8. Palpate the cervical lymph nodes.
9. Examine for thyroid enlargement and tenderness (subacute thyroiditis).
10. Examine the chest. Palpate for bony tenderness over the sternum and shoulders.
11. Examine the respiratory system (e.g. for signs of TB, abscess, empyema, carcinoma) and the heart for murmurs (e.g. infective endocarditis, atrial myxoma) or prosthetic heart sounds or rubs (e.g. pericarditis).
12. Examine the abdomen.
    a. Inspect for skin rash (e.g. the rose-coloured spots of typhoid, an uncommon long case).
    b. Palpate for:
       i. tenderness (e.g. abscess)
       ii. hepatomegaly (e.g. granulomatous hepatitis, hepatoma, cirrhosis, metastatic deposits)
       iii. splenomegaly (e.g. haemopoietic malignancy, infective endocarditis, malaria)
       iv. renal enlargement (e.g. obstruction, renal cell carcinoma).
13. Feel the testes for enlargement (e.g. seminoma, TB). Feel for inguinal adenopathy. Always ask for the results of the rectal examination (e.g. prostatic abscess, rectal cancer, Crohn's disease) and pelvic examination (pelvic pus). Look at the penis and scrotum for a discharge or rash.
14. Examine the nervous system for signs of:
    a. meningism (chronic meningitis)
    b. focal neurological signs (e.g. brain abscess, mononeuritis multiplex in polyarteritis nodosa).
15. Check the results of the urine analysis.

Investigations

1. Determine how many blood cultures have been obtained and the results.
   a. Ask to review the:
      i. blood count and smear (e.g. for neutropenia, eosinophilia, atypical lymphocytes)
      ii. liver function tests
      iii. electrolytes and creatinine.
   b. Look at the chest X-ray.
   c. Rule out urinary tract disease if suspected.

2. Selected serological tests may be helpful depending on the clinical setting (e.g. fungal, HIV, Q fever). An autoimmune screen – antinuclear antibody (ANA), erythrocyte sedimentation rate (ESR), C-reactive protein (CRP), an electrophoretogram (EPG) and complement levels – should be assessed if a connective tissue disease is suspected. However, remember that malignancy and infection can also cause an increase in acute-phase reactants and a low-titre ANA. Check the purified protein derivative (PPD) for TB exposure.

3. If abdominal disease is suspected or other tests have not provided a clue, obtain a CT scan.

4. Biopsy of involved tissue (e.g. bone marrow, liver, lymph node, skin, muscle) may lead to a definitive diagnosis. The clinical setting determines what should be biopsied.

5. Exploratory laparotomy when all other tests are negative and in the absence of any evidence of abdominal disease is usually unproductive.

Treatment

Therapy directed at the underlying disease should be the goal of assessment. Therapeutic trials in the absence of a diagnosis (e.g. antibiotics, antituberculosis therapy, NSAIDs, steroids) may result in resistant bacterial infection or drug toxicity and may make accurate diagnosis difficult. If the patient is thought to have a fever caused by a drug – a *drug fever* – it may be worth stopping the drug or using an alternative one. A possible drug fever makes trialling a change of drug worthwhile.

Possible lines of questioning

1. When would you decide to start *this* patient on antibiotics?
2. Can you give us a detailed account of *this* patient's occupational exposure to possible infection?

HIV / AIDS

Patients with human immunodeficiency virus (HIV) infection or the acquired immunodeficiency syndrome (AIDS) have become increasingly available for long-case examinations. This is now often a chronic disease and patients are getting older and likely to have problems such as ischaemic heart disease. Remember that the diagnosis of AIDS can be made when someone infected with HIV has a CD4$^+$ cell count of < 200 cells/μL or an HIV-associated disease. These patients present numerous diagnostic and management problems. The candidate will be expected to display a logical approach to the case and, of course, show a sympathetic attitude to the patient with this chronic disease. There needs to be a strong emphasis in the discussion on the psychological and social effects of the illness. Public health implications may also have to be addressed. Candidates should have an approach to pretest counselling for patients being tested for HIV.

The history

1. Ask about the presenting symptoms. As usual for long cases, the candidate must find out what symptoms or complications are currently affecting the patient. These must be assessed in the context of possible longstanding disease affecting many systems of the body.

2. Enquire when the virus was acquired. This is especially important in helping predict the likely level of immunosuppression. Not all patients are prepared to discuss this. Insistent questioning by candidates is not a good idea. There have been complaints from long-case patients that this has been handled insensitively.

   a. Find out about symptoms of a possible seroconversion illness in the past (Table 13.3). Approximately 50% of people have a seroconversion illness. It occurs 3–6 weeks after infection and often resembles glandular fever. Remember that, without treatment, the development of AIDS takes roughly 7–10 years from the time of seroconversion. The occurrence of a seroconversion illness does not seem to be associated with a worse prognosis.

   b. Note from the history any of the conditions likely to occur during the period of mild-to-moderate immunosuppression that precedes the development of AIDS and those related to severe immunosuppression that define the development of AIDS (see Table 13.4).

3. Ask about the mode of acquisition of infection. Co-morbidity differs between subgroups, so specific questions about risk factors are essential. For example, co-infections with syphilis or papilloma viruses and Kaposi's sarcoma is often found in the homosexual male subgroup, whereas hepatitis B and C infection, endocarditis, heroin nephropathy and other disorders related to drug abuse may complicate the disease in the intravenous-drug-using group. Many haemophilia A patients acquired HIV from pooled blood products.

4. Ask about sexual contacts. Contact tracing must be mentioned and the possibility of infection of sexual partners without their knowledge addressed. Ask the patient whether family and friends are aware of the diagnosis. Their attitude to this chronic illness may affect the patient's ability to cope.

Table 13.3 Features of the seroconversion illness

A seroconversion illness occurs in more than 50% of cases. There is usually some combination of the following symptoms:

- fever
- lymphadenopathy
- maculopapular rash
- arthralgia
- myalgia
- pharyngitis
- nausea
- vomiting
- diarrhoea
- headache
- meningism
- weight loss
- oral candidiasis.

Table 13.4 HIV-related conditions with severe immunosuppression

- *Pneumocystis jirovecii* pneumonia
- Kaposi's sarcoma
- Non-Hodgkin lymphoma
- Disseminated *Mycobacterium avium* complex infection
- Cytomegalovirus infection
- Cerebral toxoplasmosis
- Oesophageal candidiasis
- AIDS dementia complex

Note: This is a representative rather than an exhaustive list.

5. Ask about general constitutional symptoms. Symptoms of fever, lethargy and weight loss may indicate the AIDS-related complex or suggest an underlying opportunistic infection or malignancy.

6. Enquire about specific symptoms:

   a. respiratory – cough, dyspnoea, sputum; these may result from *P. jirovecii* pneumonia, lymphoid interstitial pneumonitis, TB, bacterial pneumonia or fungal pneumonia

   b. gastrointestinal – diarrhoea or weight loss as a result of cryptosporidiosis, microsporidiosis, mycobacterial infection or CMV colitis; odynophagia as a result of oesophageal candidiasis, herpes simplex virus (HSV) or CMV ulceration; vomiting and abdominal pain due to biliary tract disease; drug side-effects (e.g. didanosine-induced pancreatitis) – diarrhoea is usual when patients are treated with protease inhibitors

   c. neurological – meningism caused by cryptococcal meningitis; focal neurological symptoms or seizures as a result of space-occupying lesions, toxoplasmosis or non-Hodgkin lymphoma; cognitive decline as a result of HIV dementia or multifocal leukoencephalopathy; peripheral nervous system disease due to peripheral neuropathy, CMV radiculopathy or myopathy; manifestations of neurosyphilis

   d. renal – nephrotic syndrome from HIV-associated nephropathy; renal failure due to sepsis or drug side-effects

   e. ocular – deteriorating vision, which usually suggests advanced CMV retinitis

   f. dermatological – rashes may be caused by drug reactions, viral infection (e.g. herpes zoster virus (HZV) or HSV) or fungal infection; itch may be caused by scabies or drug reaction; nodules can be caused by Kaposi's sarcoma (Fig. 13.1) or bacillary angiomatosis; seborrhoeic dermatitis and psoriasis occur commonly

   g. mouth – ulcers (aphthous or viral) (Figs 13.2 and 13.3), gingivitis, periodontal disease, hairy leukoplakia or candidiasis

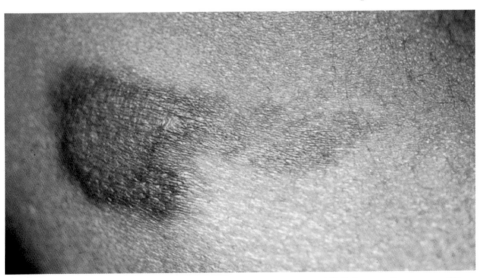

Figure 13.1 **Kaposi's sarcoma on the leg. The lesion is reddish-brown because of its vascular nature and accompanying haemosiderin deposition.**

J P Piccini, K R Nilsson. *The Osler medical handbook*, 2nd edn. Plate 19. © 2006 The Johns Hopkins University.

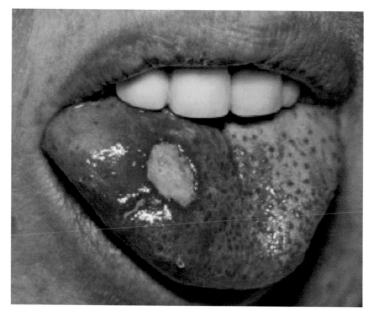

Figure 13.2 **Viral mouth ulcer. Immunocompromised patient with tongue ulcer and fissures secondary to herpes simplex virus.**

W D James, T Berger, D Elston. *Andrews' diseases of the skin: clinical dermatology*, 11th edn. Fig. 19-12. Saunders, Elsevier, 2011, with permission.

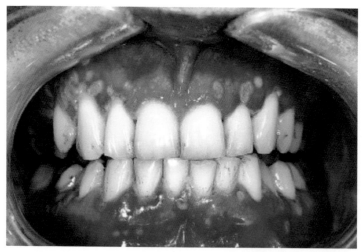

Figure 13.3 **Recurrent intraoral herpes simplex in an adult with numerous, widely scattered vesicles and ulcers in association with pain, tenderness and fever.**

D W Flint, B H Haughey, V J Lund et al. *Cummings otolaryngology: head and neck surgery*, 5th edn. Fig 91-32. Mosby, Elsevier, 2010, with permission.

h. cardiac – dyspnoea, chest pain or palpitations due to myocarditis or pericarditis, angina

i. haematological – anaemia (bone marrow suppression or infiltration, treatment with zidovudine); thrombocytopenia and neutropenia are less common.

7. Ask about previous treatment. Find out about antiretroviral drug and antibiotic treatment and about any adverse effects of these. Enquire about specific side-effects (Table 13.5). If the disease has recently been diagnosed, ask what treatment options have been discussed with the patient.

8. Ask about immunisation. Vaccination with live organisms is contraindicated if the CD4 count is < 200/μL and immune response to other vaccines is very poor.

Table 13.5 Side-effects of selected antiretroviral drugs

DRUG	SIDE-EFFECTS
A. NUCLEOSIDE REVERSE TRANSCRIPTASE INHIBITORS	
Zidovudine (AZT)	Headache, nausea, myopathy, bone marrow suppression; used in pregnant HIV-positive patients
Didanosine (ddI)	Diarrhoea, pancreatitis, peripheral neuropathy
Zalcitabine (ddC)	Mouth and oesophageal ulcers, pancreatitis, peripheral neuropathy
Lamivudine (3TC)	Side-effects uncommon
Stavudine (d4T)	Peripheral neuropathy, pancreatitis; do not use in pregnant women (fatal lactic acidosis)
Abacavir	Hypersensitivity syndrome (3%) – linked to HLA-B5701
B. NON-NUCLEOSIDE REVERSE TRANSCRIPTASE INHIBITORS	
Nevirapine	Rash, hepatitis (can be fatal)
Efavirenz	Dizziness, cognitive disturbance, insomnia, vivid dreams, fatigue, rash; teratogenic
Delavirdine	Rash
C. PROTEASE INHIBITORS – INTERACTIONS OCCUR WITH: SILDENAFIL, MIDOZALAM, ATORVASTATIN, RIFAMPICIN	
Indinavir	Nausea, diarrhoea, lipodystrophy, insulin resistance, hepatitis, renal calculi, hair and nail changes
Saquinavir	Diarrhoea, lipodystrophy, insulin resistance, hepatitis
Nelfinavir	Diarrhoea, lipodystrophy, insulin resistance, hepatitis
Amprenavir	Diarrhoea, nausea, perioral paraesthesia, lipodystrophy, insulin resistance
Ritonavir	Nausea, diarrhoea, taste disturbance, perioral paraesthesia, lipodystrophy, insulin resistance
D. ENTRY/FUSION INHIBITORS	
Enfuvirtide	Increased risk of pneumonia, local reaction at injection site
E. INTEGRASE INHIBITORS	
Raltegravir	Increased cholesterol, myopathy
HAART (highly active antiretroviral therapy) – this is combination treatment often with nucleoside reverse transcriptase inhibitors and protease inhibitors	Increased risk of hepatocellular injury and cholestasis with combination treatment

Table 13.6 Vaccination recommendations for HIV patients
• Pneumococcal
• Annual influenza
• Hepatitis A
• Chickenpox if seronegative
• Measles, mumps, rubella if measles serology is negative
• Human papilloma virus for those aged less than 40 years
• Meningococcus for those younger than 25 years

Vaccination is recommended once treatment has begun and the CD4 count has risen (Table 13.6).

9. Ask about previous investigations. The patient may be able to give much helpful information on previous investigations, including viral load results, T cell CD4$^+$ counts, MRI scans, CT scans, lumbar punctures, bone marrow biopsies and endoscopy.

10. Enquire about social, drug and alcohol history. The examiners will expect quite detailed knowledge of the patient's social, economic and family circumstances.

11. Ask about risk factors and treatment for cardiovascular disease:
    a. known ischaemic heart disease – angioplasty, coronary artery bypass graft (CABG)
    b. smoking – awareness of risk
    c. cholesterol level – statin treatment
    d. family history of ischaemic heart disease
    e. diabetes
    f. hypertension – treatment.

The examination

Note especially:

1. temperature
2. nutritional state (wasting is common in advanced disease); there may be fat loss on the face and fat gain over the limbs (retroviral drug effect)
3. skin (e.g. rashes – herpes zoster seborrhoeic dermatitis, exacerbation of psoriasis (Fig 13.4), molluscum contagiosum – pigmentation and the lesions of Kaposi's sarcoma)
4. mouth (e.g. hairy leukoplakia, Kaposi's sarcoma lesions, candida, periodontal disease, HSV mouth ulcers)
5. eyes – acuity, visual fields and fundoscopy (e.g. CMV retinal lesions)
6. cognition, gait and coordination (e.g. AIDS dementia)
7. chest – cough, sputum, crackles (e.g. opportunistic chest infection)
8. heart – cardiac failure, pericardial disease (e.g. AIDS cardiomyopathy)
9. abdomen – rectal examination, perianal disease (especially warts and HSV)
10. haematological system – lymph nodes and spleen.

Investigations

The patient is likely to have had many tests.

1. The standard screening test for HIV is an enzyme-linked immunosorbent assay (ELISA) or enzyme immunoassay (EIA) test. It tests against antigens of both HIV1 and HIV2 (the latter rare in Australia) and becomes positive in 3–7 weeks after infection so is usually negative in primary HIV infection. It has a sensitivity of more than 99%. Its specificity in low-risk populations is only about 90%. False positives can occur related to recent vaccinations, other viral infections and autoimmune diseases. The earliest detectable test

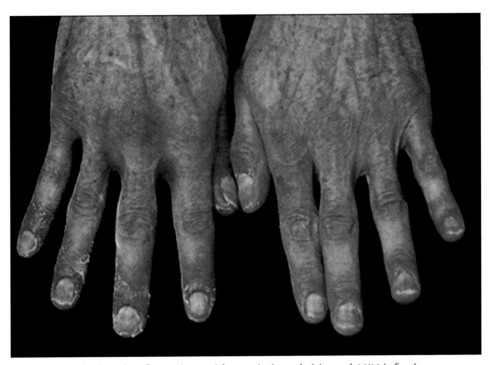

Figure 13.4 The hands of a patient with psoriatic arthritis and HIV infection.

M C Hochberg, A J Silman, J S Smolen et al. *Rheumatology*, 5th edn. Fig 107.1. Mosby, Elsevier, 2010, with permission.

is an HIV PCR DNA (within a few days of inoculation). The Western blot test is more specific and a negative Western blot means a positive EIA test is a false positive.

2. Other tests are used to assess the severity of the illness and immunocompromise, and to look for associated conditions (e.g. syphilis) and complications. The currently relevant tests will depend on the clinical presentation; however, certain tests are essential for all patients, either as a baseline or for monitoring (Table 13.7).

BASELINE

1. Immune function needs to be established at this point with a full blood count, $CD4^+$ level (levels < 200 cells/μL are associated with opportunistic infections) and HIV plasma serum viral load.

2. A delayed-type hypersensitivity skin test will help define cellular immune function: the lower the $CD4^+$ (T-helper cell) level (Table 13.8) and the higher the HIV viral load, the more advanced is the infection. $CD4^+$ levels may fall progressively to undetectable levels. Aggressive treatment of infections may allow continued survival of patients despite these low $CD4^+$ levels. Antiviral treatment may slow $CD4^+$ depletion or stabilise it for many years. About 5% of infected patients do not develop a reduction in $CD4^+$ counts even after more than 10 years without treatment. These patients are called 'non-progressors'.

3. It should also be established whether the patient has concurrent sexually transmitted disease (syphilis serology, hepatitis B serology) or TB (tuberculin test), and whether he or she is at risk of activation of latent infection (CMV, toxoplasma serology).

4. Renal and liver function should be checked prior to commencing antiviral drugs.

Table 13.7 Routine initial investigations for HIV patients

ALL PATIENTS

1. CD4⁺ count
2. Viral load
3. Hepatitis B surface antigen and core antibody
4. Hepatitis C antibody
5. Hepatitis A antibody (IgG)
6. Chest X-ray, which may reveal cardiac or pulmonary complications especially in acutely ill patients (Figs 13.5–13.7)
7. Cytomegalovirus antibody (IgG)
8. Serological tests for syphilis
9. Toxoplasma antibody
10. Liver function tests, eGFR

PATIENTS WITH CD4⁺ COUNT < 200 CELLS / μL

1. Hepatitis C RNA
2. Cryptococcal antigen
3. Stool examination for cysts, ova and parasites

PATIENTS WITH CD4⁺ COUNT < 100 CELLS / μL

1. Cytomegalovirus PCR
2. Mycobacterial blood cultures
3. Fundoscopy (pupils dilated)
4. ECG

eGFR = estimated glomerular filtration rate; IgG = immunoglobulin G; PCR = polymerase chain reaction.

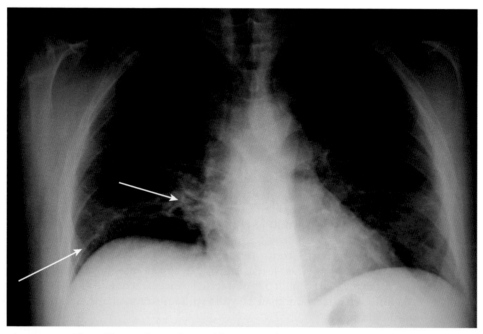

Figure 13.5 Chest X-ray of a patient with HIV and pneumocystis pneumonia. Note the perihilar and basilar reticular airspace opacities (arrows).

Figure reproduced courtesy of The Canberra Hospital.

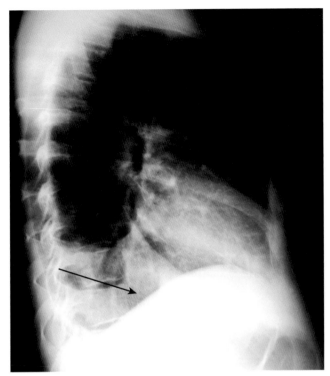

Figure 13.6 Lateral chest X-ray of a patient with HIV showing left lower lobe consolidation (arrow).

Figure reproduced courtesy of The Canberra Hospital.

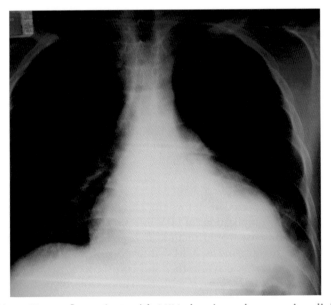

Figure 13.7 Chest X-ray of a patient with HIV showing a large pericardial effusion.

Figure reproduced courtesy of The Canberra Hospital.

Table 13.8 CD4⁺ level and common clinical features

CD4⁺ COUNT > 500 CELLS / µL
1. Primary infection
2. Generalised lymphadenopathy
3. Vaginal candidiasis

CD4⁺ COUNT 200–500 CELLS / µL
1. Herpes zoster
2. Oral candidiasis
3. Hairy leukoplakia (caused by Epstein–Barr virus)
4. Kaposi's sarcoma (caused by human herpes virus 8)
5. Pulmonary TB
6. Lymphoid interstitial pneumonitis
7. HIV-associated idiopathic thrombocytopenia

CD4⁺ COUNT < 200 CELLS / µL
1. *Pneumocystis* pneumonia
2. *Microsporidium* and *Cryptosporidium* infection
3. Oesophageal candidiasis
4. Peripheral neuropathy
5. Wasting
6. Miliary or extrapulmonary TB
7. Herpes simplex

CD4⁺ COUNT < 100 CELLS / µL
1. Cryptococcal meningitis
2. Cerebral toxoplasmosis
3. CNS lymphoma
4. Dementia
5. Non-Hodgkin lymphoma
6. Multifocal leukoencephalopathy

CD4⁺ COUNT < 50 CELLS / µL
1. Disseminated *Mycobacterium avium*
2. Disseminated cytomegalovirus infection – retinitis, gastrointestinal disease

MONITORING

The key investigations for monitoring progress are the HIV plasma viral load and the CD4⁺ T cell count (see Table 13.8). Serial full blood counts and biochemistry will help assess any complications of disease or therapy.

Treatment

1. Candidates will be expected to know the clinical features and general treatment options for common complications of HIV infection, especially opportunistic infection and malignancy. This list would include *P. jirovecii* (*carinii*) pneumonia, Kaposi's sarcoma, cerebral toxoplasmosis, CMV infection, *Mycobacterium avium* complex (MAC) infection, diarrhoeal syndromes and cryptococcal meningitis.
2. Primary prophylaxis for *P. jirovecii* with co-trimoxazole or pentamidine (if CD4⁺ count < 200 cells / µL) and MAC with azithromycin (if CD4⁺ count < 50 cells / µL) is an important consideration. If the CD4⁺ count is > 200 cells / µL for 3 months, prophylaxis can be ceased.

3. Herpes simplex prophylaxis with aciclovir and *Candida* prophylaxis with fluconazole or ketoconazole are appropriate for prevention after one episode has occurred.

4. Multiple antiretroviral agents are now available for the treatment of HIV (see Table 13.5). ART (active antiretroviral therapy) in combination has dramatically improved quality of life and life expectancy in HIV disease.

5. The optimal time to commence therapy must be considered. It is clear that symptomatic patients, or those with an increasing viral load (> 20,000 copies/mL) or a falling CD4$^+$ count (< 350 cells/μL), are definite indications, but most clinicians prefer to commence treatment in nearly all cases regardless of CD4$^+$ count. Pregnant infected women should be treated. Drugs should be used only in combination to prevent emergence of resistance and most regimens contain three or more drugs. Treatment is not curative and must be continued indefinitely.

6. Standard treatment begins with two NRTs (nucleoside reverse transcriptase inhibitors) (Table 13.9) and an NNRTI (non-nucleoside reverse transcriptase inhibitor), or protease inhibitor or integrase inhibitor together with abacavir or tenofovir.

7. Ongoing patient monitoring is routine. After starting ART, assess adherence and any side-effects within 2 weeks. Check a blood count, electrolytes and creatinine, liver function tests, glucose and lipids, and a urinalysis (depending on the agents used) every 3–6 months once stable. Check CD4 counts every 3 months. Assess HIV RNA 2 weeks after starting, then every 8 weeks until undetectable, then 3-monthly. After 2 years, if the viral load is undetectable, less frequent testing is usual.

8. Resistance testing is indicated for the treatment of the naive patient. Virological failure (> 200 copies/mL) results from lack of adherence or drug resistance, and resistance testing is also indicated.

9. ART reduces the risk of vertical transmission and probably also the risk of seroconversion following occupational exposure (e.g. needlestick injury), if given promptly.

10. In pregnancy, the aim of therapy is to make the patient's viral load undetectable. If the HIV RNA is more than 1000 copies, recommend caesarean section. Do not use dolutegravir.

11. Patients co-infected with hepatitis B virus (HBV) should have antiviral treatment that is also effective for that (e.g. lamivudine, emtricitabine). Surveillance for the development of hepatic carcinoma is also indicated for these patients.

12. Patients whose disease is well controlled by antiviral agents are more likely to die of cardiovascular disease than infection. This is partly as a result of their drug treatment (e.g. with protease inhibitors). Aggressive control of cardiovascular risk factors is indicated (Table 13.10). Hyperlipidaemia should be treated with pravastatin (which has less interaction with antiviral drugs).

Table 13.9 Commonly prescribed antiretrovirals

- Nucleoside reverse transcriptase inhibitors (NRTIs) – abacavir, emtricitabine, lamivudine, tenofovir
- Non-nucleoside reverse transcriptase inhibitor (NNRTI) – rilpivirine
- Protease inhibitors – atazanavir, darunavir
- Integrase inhibitors – raltegravir, dolutegravir

Table 13.10 Longer term management considerations for HIV patients

1. Smoking	4. Malignancy surveillance
2. Lipids	5. Vaccinations
3. Weight and exercise	6. Sexual health screening

Falls and the risk of falls

Elderly patients and patients on large numbers of medications are at risk of falling and injuring themselves. Many long-case patients are in these categories. If one of the examiners is a geriatrician then questions on this topic are very likely (from the other examiner). In some cases it may be one of the main problems that needs to be discussed.

The history

1. Ask:
   a. Have there been any falls? How many?
   b. Has the patient had any injuries, fractures?
   c. Has hospital admission or surgery been required?
   d. What were the circumstances – tripping, loss of balance, postural, nocturnal, going to toilet?
   e. Was the patient syncopal?
   f. Has the patient a pacemaker? Has it been tested recently?
   g. Has treatment been recommended or changed?
   h. Have changes been made to the house or have walking aids been recommended?
2. What medications is the patient taking? Ask particularly about:
   a. antihypertensive drugs
   b. sedatives, e.g. sleeping tablets
   c. alpha-blockers (often for prostatism)
   d. anti-Parkinsonian drugs
   e. anticholinergics
   f. opioid analgesics
   g. alcohol.
3. Is there a problem with mobility? Ask about:
   a. stroke or cerebellar disease
   b. muscle weakness
   c. arthritis
   d. spinal disease
   e. inappropriate footwear.
4. What insight has the patient into the problem?
   a. Is there adherence to suggestions about use of sticks, walking frames, etc.?
   b. Does the patient undertake risky activities: climbing ladders, clearing gutters, etc.?
5. Is there a problem with visual acuity?
6. Has there been a history of vertigo?
7. Has there been a diagnosis of osteoporosis (increased risk of fracture caused by a fall)?
8. Is there a history of vitamin D deficiency?

9. Has the patient lost confidence as a result of falls and is this affecting his or her ability to leave the house, drive, shop, etc.? Is the rest of the family affected?

The examination

1. Look for walking aids: sticks, walkers, orthotics, footwear.
2. Is the patient obese, frail?
3. Does the patient seem confused or disorientated?
4. Take the pulse.
5. Measure the blood pressure, both lying and standing if possible. Is there a postural drop? Is the patient symptomatic when standing?
6. Ask your patient to stand up unassisted (arms folded) to look for a proximal myopathy. Always perform a Romberg's test before walking your patient; ask your bulldog to supervise and assist the patient while you observe from a distance. Look for unsteadiness. Try heel-to-toe walking.
7. Perform the *get up and go* (GUG) test. Measure the time it takes the patient (wearing his or her regular shoes and with any aids) to get up from a chair, walk 3 metres, turn around and walk back, then sit. A normal person, up to the age of 79, can complete this in 10 seconds or less. Someone who takes longer may be at increased risk of further falls.
8. If the patient looks Parkinsonian, test comprehensively (p. 575).
9. Test vision – loss of acuity is associated with a higher risk of falls.
10. With the patient back in bed, perform cerebellar testing and look for peripheral neuropathy. Assess muscle strength.

Investigations

1. If there are focal neurological or cerebellar signs, CT or MRI scanning may be useful – focal lesion, normal pressure hydrocephalus.
2. Examine full blood count and electrolytes – anaemia, hyponatraemia.
3. If syncope is suspected, an ECG and Holter monitor or loop recorder may be useful – to look for conduction system disease.

Management

Assess for intrinsic factors (neuropathy, poor eyesight, urge incontinence, medications and others) and extrinsic risk factors (house set-up) contributing to the falls risk, and highlight these in your discussions along with addressing any harm minimisation strategies.

1. Review medications that may be causing problems:
   a. Can antihypertensives be stopped or changed?
   b. Are anti-Parkinsonian drugs optimal?
   c. Should sedatives and psychotropic medications be stopped?
   d. Are alternative analgesics possible?
2. Correct electrolytes or haemoglobin.
3. Recommend more appropriate footwear, prostheses and walking aids.
4. Gait exercise and balance training have been shown to improve outcomes.
5. Treatment of vitamin-D-deficient patients with supplements reduces the risk of falls by 14%, probably by improving muscle strength and gait.
6. Consider rehabilitation and physiotherapy.
7. Suggest new spectacles if needed.
8. Assess the house (hazards in the home account for up to 50% of falls): removal of loose rugs and installation of ramps, bars, etc.; removal of uneven floors and use of non-slipping surfaces on steps.
9. Does possible syncope need further investigation or treatment?
10. Is the patient's response to the episodes appropriate and how might this be improved?

The obese patient

The world of the FRACP long case is a place where there are even more obese patients than there are in the real world. These people often have a number of medical problems related to their weight. Even when obesity is a minor part of the long case, candidates need to have a plausible approach to the problem.

If obesity is defined as a BMI (body mass/height squared) of 30 or more, about a third of adults are obese.

The history

1. Ask general questions about the weight:
   a. the timing of weight gain and variations in weight over time
   b. a family history of obesity
   c. medications that may have contributed (Box 13.1)
   d. exercise – what, how often and for how long each time
   e. eating patterns (keep this general or time will disappear)
   f. insight into the problem and willingness to address it
   g. previous attempts to lose weight
   h. mood and symptoms of depression
   i. diabetes during pregnancy.
2. Ask about problems associated with obesity and their effect on ability to exercise and on normal activities:
   a. arthritis
   b. diabetes and its complications and treatment
   c. cardiovascular disease and risk factors (hyperlipidaemia, smoking, hypertension)
   d. sleep apnoea
   e. fatty liver
   f. other mobility problems, e.g. balance, bathing
   g. shopping for fresh food; ability to cook
   h. social life and work.

The examination

1. Examine for central obesity.
2. Calculate BMI.

Box 13.1 Medications associated with weight gain

1. Steroids
2. Hypoglycaemics – insulin, sulphonylureas, thiazolidinediones
3. Antipsychotics (atypical) – clozapine, risperidone
4. Anticonvulsants – carbamazepine, valproate
5. Tricyclic antidepressants

---

3. Measure waist circumference at the level of the iliac crest (> 88 cm for women or > 105 cm for men is associated with increased risk of diabetes, hyperlipidaemia, hypertension and heart disease independent of BMI).
4. Take the blood pressure (use a big cuff).
5. Look for signs of hypothyroidism or Cushing's.
6. Examine for complications of diabetes.

Management

1. Suggest management strategies – much depends on a patient's insight and motivation.
   a. **Keep a food diary:** can help patients appreciate their food intake accurately.
   b. **Exercise program:** should be tailored to limitations, e.g. arthritis (water aerobics).
      i. Ways of encouraging exercise include: pedometer, fitness watch, gymnasium program, exercise class.
      ii. Remember that exercise alone has modest effects on weight loss but can help maintain it.
   c. Reduce food intake – reduction of food intake by 2000–4000 kilojoules a day will cause 400–500 g of weight loss a week. A very low calorie diet may be considered for a patient requiring rapid weight loss (e.g. prior to surgery).
   d. Dietary advice and behavioural therapy may help.
   e. Remember that no particular weight loss diet has been shown to be better than any other, but enthusiasm for a particular diet may be valuable.
   f. Can any medications be changed?
   g. As with any other long-case situation where a change in behaviour is needed, your plan should include providing education to ensure understanding of the risks involved, involving family members and the patient's GP, setting goals and reviewing progress regularly, acknowledging difficulties and providing support while applying a non-judgmental approach.
2. **Drug treatment:**
   a. has generally been disappointing
   b. fat absorption (lipase) inhibitors have a modest benefit – 8 kg in a year in a placebo-controlled study; oily, loose stools are a problem
   c. sympathomimetic appetite suppressants tend to work only when being taken continuously and have side-effects including hypertension and arrhythmias.
3. **Surgery:** is the only treatment shown to improve prognosis. Type II diabetes mellitus may resolve. The operations are performed laparoscopically. The procedures may work partly by reducing gastric ghrelin release, which increases satiety as well as restricting intake capacity. Gastric banding has largely been replaced with gastric sleeve surgery where part of the stomach is removed. Roux-en-Y gastric bypass surgery is rarely performed now, but patients who have had the procedure may present to exams. Table 13.11 sets out the effectiveness and common complications of the operations.
   a. Surgery is usually reserved for those with BMI > 40 or > 35 but with complications of obesity.
   b. It must have acceptable surgical and anaesthetic risk.
   c. The patient must be enthusiastic and understand that long-term results still depend on changes to diet and exercise.
   d. Roux-en-Y gastric bypass can be dramatically effective and has been shown to reduce complications of obesity; however, the late complications of gastric bypass, which can include anastomotic stricture, bowel obstruction, marginal ulcer, hernia and malabsorption with vitamin deficiency, have made the operation unusual.

Table 13.11 Results and complications of bariatric surgery		
OPERATION	**EXPECTED WEIGHT LOSS (% OF EXCESS, LOWER LIMIT)**	**COMPLICATIONS**
Gastric banding	45	Band slippage, stricture or obstruction
Sleeve gastrectomy	55	Iron and vitamin B_{12} deficiency
Roux-en-Y	60	Stomal ulcer, dumping syndrome, hypoglycaemia, iron, vitamin B_{12} and vitamin D deficiency

HINT

A common manageable weight reduction goal to suggest is 10% of current body weight over 6 months at a rate of 0.5–1 kg a week.

Possible lines of questioning

1. What do you think of *this* patient's insight into his or her problem with obesity?
2. What strategies can you suggest for *this* patient to help him or her lose weight?
3. Is *this* patient a good candidate for bariatric surgery?

The preoperative assessment

Examiners who are running out of questions will often resort to 'How would you advise the surgeon and anaesthetist about *this* patient before elective surgery?' They can then sit back and expect the candidate to fill in the remaining time nicely (so don't be caught out).

The history
Ask about the following:
1. The operation:
   - What operation is being planned?
   - Is it an emergency?
   - Can it be performed under local anaesthetic (low risk)?
2. Co-morbidities (most will have been covered during the general history taking):
   a. Heart:
      - Is there a history of ischaemic heart disease?
      - Has the patient had recent angina or infarction?
      - Has there been treatment, e.g. recent coronary stenting?
      - What is the patient's exercise tolerance?
      - Have any tests of exercise capacity or for myocardial ischaemia been performed (e.g. exercise test, coronary angiogram, stress echo)?
      - Is there a history of heart failure (work out the NYHA class)?
   b. Lungs:
      - Has there been a diagnosis of COPD or asthma? Is the patient a smoker?
      - Have steroids been required?
      - What is the current exercise ability?
      - Has sleep apnoea been diagnosed?

c. Glands:
  - Is the patient diabetic, on insulin?
  - Is there a history of thyroid disease? Have thyroid function tests been performed recently?
  - Is there a history of Addison's disease?
d. Kidneys:
  - Is there a history of chronic kidney disease?
  - Does the patient know their eGFR?
e. Blood:
  - Is there a history of anaemia?
  - Have there been previous DVTs or pulmonary emboli?
  - Has the patient had thrombocytopenia?
f. Liver:
  - Is there a history of liver failure?
  - Is the patient hepatitis B or C (or HIV) positive?

3. Drugs:
  a. anticoagulants
  b. antiplatelets
  c. beta-blockers
  d. steroids
  e. insulin
  f. oral hypoglycaemics
  g. angiotensin-converting enzyme inhibitors (ACEIs)
  h. anticonvulsants
  i. analgesics.

Management

The history should help with a calculation of the risk of surgery and suggest measures to reduce this risk.

1. Heart:
  a. Consider the cardiac risk score (Table 13.12).
  b. Remember that perioperative stress testing is not indicated unless (1) patients have a poor exercise tolerance – < 4 METs (metabolic equivalent of tasks) – pharmacological testing may be needed, or (2) many risk factors.

Table 13.12 Revised cardiac risk index	
1 point for each of: • history of ischaemic heart disease • compensated heart failure • diabetes needing insulin • chronic kidney disease (creatinine > 170 µmol / L) • previous stroke • high-risk surgery (intrathoracic, intra-abdominal, abdominal or pelvic vascular)	
NO. OF POINTS	**RISK (OF CARDIAC DEATH, INFARCTION OR CARDIAC ARREST) (%)**
0	0.4
1	1.0
2	2.4
3 or more	5.4

c. In general, cardiac revascularisation is not indicated in preparation for non-cardiac surgery unless it was already needed. Beta-blocker treatment should not be started routinely except for high-risk surgery and for patients with more than one cardiac risk factor.

d. Beta-blockers, if needed, should be commenced some weeks before surgery at a low dose and adjusted upwards as tolerated. Patients already taking beta-blockers should continue them in the perioperative period.

e. Only emergency surgery should be undertaken within 3–6 months of a myocardial infarction.

f. Antiplatelet treatment:
   i. Aspirin should be continued throughout the operative period if possible for all patients with known ischaemic heart disease (exceptions include spinal and cerebral surgery).
   ii. Dual antiplatelet treatment should continue for at least 6 months (3 months for urgent surgery with modern drug-eluting stent) from the time of a drug-eluting stent insertion or acute coronary event and surgery delayed if possible. Heparin does not provide protection against stent thrombosis and is not useful as bridging treatment for these patients.
   iii. The second antiplatelet drug can be stopped 1 month after a bare-metal stent insertion for stable angina.

g. Anticoagulation:
   i. Warfarin can be stopped for 3–4 days before surgery and a NOAC 1–2 days before for a patient anticoagulated for atrial fibrillation who is at low risk of embolic events; otherwise bridging treatment with enoxaparin or unfractionated heparin is needed.
   ii. Patients with mechanical heart valves need bridging treatment.

2. Lungs:
   a. Mull over the risk factors for pulmonary complications of surgery (usually prolonged postoperative intubation) (Table 13.13).
   b. Remember that routine spirometry does not help predict problems and it should be reserved for patients with unexplained breathlessness.
   c. Smoking cessation at least 2 months before surgery reduces complications, but it is not so clear that a shorter period of cessation helps.
   d. Deep-breathing exercises and incentive spirometry before and after surgery do reduce pulmonary complications.

Table 13.13 Risk factors for perioperative pulmonary complications	
PATIENT	**SURGERY**
MAJOR Age Chronic obstructive pulmonary disease Co-morbidities, immobility Smoking Hypoalbuminaemia Chronic kidney disease	**MAJOR** Intrathoracic or abdominal surgery Surgery lasting more than 3 hours Emergency surgery General versus local or spinal anaesthesia
MINOR Obesity Sleep apnoea	

3. Glands:
   a. Diabetic patients usually stop oral hypoglycaemics up to 12 hours before surgery and may require short-acting insulin and frequent blood sugar level measurements. Type 1 diabetic patients must continue to receive insulin (because of risk of ketoacidosis).
   b. Patients with thyroid disease should be euthyroid if possible before surgery.
   c. Patient with adrenal insufficiency should be kept well hydrated and receive extra doses of hydrocortisone: 25 mg on the day of minor surgery and up to 100–150 mg for major surgery.
4. Kidneys:
   a. ACEIs are often withheld for a few days.
   b. Severe chronic kidney disease patients may end up on dialysis temporarily or permanently after major surgery (especially cardiac surgery); this must be discussed with them before surgery.
   c. Extra attention needs to be paid to fluid balance and the use of renally excreted or nephrotoxic drugs.
5. Liver:
   a. Liver function may worsen in chronic liver disease patients owing to hepatic ischaemia during surgery.
   b. Anaesthetic and other drugs have an increased half-life and may accumulate.
   c. Coagulation may be abnormal.
   d. The higher the Child–Pugh score the greater is the surgical risk (e.g. Child–Pugh B = 30% risk of death for general surgery).

When perioperative risk is only a fragment of the long case, candidates must learn to assemble information about risk factors from the patient efficiently and make sensible suggestions to the examiners about risk and its amelioration.

Possible lines of questioning

1. What would you advise the surgeon about *this* patient's antiplatelet treatment and his or her planned cholecystectomy?
2. What should be done about *this* patient who has a mechanical mitral valve and his or her warfarin treatment in the perioperative period?

Carcinoma of the breast

This common malignancy may be a current active problem or a previously treated disease that continues to affect the woman's health. It might occasionally be the long-case patient's main problem.

The history

1. Ask when and how the diagnosis was made: by breast self-examination or routine screening.
2. Ask about risk factors for carcinoma of the breast:
   a. previous breast cancer
   b. nulliparity
   c. first pregnancy at over the age of 30
   d. early menarche and late menopause

Box 13.2 Breast cancer staging

Stage I – 100% 5-year survival
- Tumour < 2 cm
- No involved nodes

Stage II – 86% 5-year survival
- Tumour < 2 cm but 1–3 involved nodes, or
- Tumour 2–5 cm and 0–3 involved nodes, or
- Tumour > 5 cm but no involved nodes

Stage III – 57% 5-year survival
- Tumour > 5 cm and 1–3 nodes
- Four or more nodes, or
- Tumour extending to the chest wall or skin

Stage IV
- Distant metastases

---

   e. postmenopausal obesity
   f. older age
   g. alcohol consumption
   h. family history
   i. previous ovarian cancer
   j. previous mantle irradiation.
3. Find out whether *BRACA1/BRACA2* gene testing has been performed. Up to 10% of women with breast cancer have this mutation or the *p53* mutation. Ninety per cent of familial breast cancer is associated with these genes.
4. Does the patient know whether the tumour was oestrogen or progesterone receptor positive? Also ask about the expression of human epidermal growth factor 2 (HER2) receptor status.
5. Try to find out whether the stage of the disease and prognosis (Box 13.2) have been discussed with the patient.
6. Ask about treatment.

The examination
1. Examine the breasts, axillary nodes and skeleton.
2. Be guided by the history to look for evidence of radiotherapy – skin erythema, tattoo marks – and of lymphoedema and the presence of secondaries.

Treatment
1. **Surgery:** lumpectomy is performed for ductal carcinoma in situ. Invasive carcinoma is treated with mastectomy and sentinel lymph node biopsy or lumpectomy, lymph node evaluation and breast irradiation. Breast-conserving surgery is not usually recommended for:
   - tumours > 5 cm
   - women with small breasts
   - women with involvement of the nipple or areola
   - multifocal tumours

- women who have had previous chest irradiation
- women with SLE or scleroderma.

Sentinel node biopsy has replaced axillary node dissection. If the node is negative, the risk of other node involvement is only about 5% and axillary dissection with its associated lymphoedema can be avoided.

2. **Radiotherapy:** this is not now indicated for most women after surgery, but is used if:
- the margins are not clear
- the tumour is larger than 5 cm
- there are four or more involved lymph nodes
- the tumour is inflammatory breast cancer.

This treatment improves local control and may improve survival. If three nodes are involved then adjuvant radiotherapy is more controversial.

Adjuvant treatment is meant to help prognosis by removing microscopic residual disease. Appropriate adjuvant is guided by:
- size of tumour
- progesterone receptor status
- oestrogen receptor status
- over-expression of *HER2/neu*
- hormone receptor negativity
- lymph node involvement
- patient's age and general health.

3. **Adjuvant endocrine treatment:** endocrine therapy can reduce the risk of recurrence by 50% and is indicated for oestrogen- or progesterone-positive cancers. Tamoxifen blocks the action of oestrogen on receptors and is used for premenopausal women, usually for 5 years. Oophorectomy can be performed for women unable to take tamoxifen. Tamoxifen is generally well tolerated, though there are several side-effects (Box 13.3).

Aromatase inhibitors are used for postmenopausal women who are receptor positive. Their side-effects are different from those of tamoxifen (Box 13.4).

4. **Adjuvant chemotherapy:** women younger than 50 years with involved lymph nodes should be offered conventional chemotherapy for 3–6 months. Typical regimens include two or three drugs from among:
- cyclophosphamide
- anthracyclines

Box 13.3 Side-effects of tamoxifen

- Risk of thromboembolism
- Risk of endometrial cancer
- Hot flushes
- Cataracts

Box 13.4 Side-effects of aromatase inhibitors

- Loss of bone mineral density
- Increased risk of fractures
- Musculoskeletal arthralgia syndrome – symmetrical pain and joint stiffness reversible on cessation of treatment

> **Box 13.5 Side-effects of breast cancer chemotherapeutic agents**
>
> - Nausea
> - Vomiting
> - Alopecia
> - Cardiotoxicity (anthracyclines, 5-fluorouracil)
> - Myelodysplasia
> - Leukaemia
>
> **Taxenes**
> - Peripheral neuropathy
> - Oedema
> - Bone marrow suppression
> - Amenorrhoea

- methotrexate
- 5-fluorouracil (5-FU)
- a taxene – paclitaxel or docetaxel.

Side-effects are common (Box 13.5).

Patients with triple-negative tumours (oestrogen, progesterone and HER2 negative) or with *HER2/neu* over-expression have an adverse prognosis and benefit from chemotherapy, particularly trastuzumab, a monoclonal antibody directed against the HER2 receptor. This is given for a year and can be used in combination with conventional chemotherapy. Recurrence rates are reduced by up to 50%.

Patients with previous anthracycline use, hypertension and who are over 50 years of age are at risk of developing heart failure with this drug. This is usually reversible. Three-monthly cardiac echoes are usually indicated.

5. Treated patients are followed clinically every 6 months for 5 years and then yearly. Monthly breast self-examination and annual mammography are recommended. At the moment, MRI is not indicated as a follow-up investigation.
6. Ask the patient about side-effects that might be a result of her particular treatment, and particularly about:
   a. weight gain
   b. osteoporosis
   c. cognitive dysfunction
   d. sexual problems, vaginal atrophy, dyspareunia
   e. depression and loss of self-confidence and self-esteem; concerns about surgical scars and breast appearance
   f. vasomotor symptoms
   g. early menopause
   h. whether she needs continuing contraception (which should not be with oral contraceptives)
   i. lymphoedema
   j. skin damage from radiation.

   Ask what treatment has been used to help manage side-effects.
   a. Topical oestrogens are thought safe and can help with vaginal atrophy.
   b. Vitamin D, calcium and exercise are used in osteoporosis.
   c. Antidepressants are often used for vasomotor symptoms, but CYP2D6 enzyme inhibitors (e.g. paroxetine, fluoxetine) should be avoided when patients are taking tamoxifen, which is activated by this enzyme.

7. Ask whether she has been involved in support groups, or has had help with breast prostheses, or breast reconstruction.

8. Finally, ask about the effect this terrible disease has had on the woman and her family, whether she can work and what she knows about her prognosis.

Metastatic breast cancer is generally an incurable disease with a median survival of 2 years. If secondaries are present at the time of diagnosis then surgical or radiation treatment is not used unless there are local symptoms that can be palliated. Surgical resection of secondaries does not improve survival. When a secondary is a recurrence of tumour, biopsy is necessary in most cases as the secondary may have different hormone receptors.

Hormone-receptor-positive tumours are treated with endocrine therapy, starting with tamoxifen in premenopausal women and aromatase inhibitors in postmenopausal women. Ovarian ablation can be used for premenopausal women. If the tumour has over-expression of *HER2/neu*, trastuzumab and chemotherapy are used. Triple receptor-negative tumours are treated with sequential single-agent chemotherapy. Combination chemotherapy is more toxic and does not improve survival. Metastatic bone disease can be treated with bisphosphonates. Dental monitoring is required because of the risk of osteonecrosis of the jaw. Painful bony secondaries are treated with local radiotherapy.

Possible lines of questioning

1. How do you feel *this* woman has coped with her Illness?
2. How would you manage *this* woman's painful bony metastases?
3. What would you tell *this* woman about the problems that might occur when she begins treatment with tamoxifen?

Chapter 14

Think like a physician, think like an examiner – an approach with long-case examples

I should have liked to be asked to say what I knew.
They always tried to ask what I did not know. When I
would have willingly displayed my knowledge, they
sought to expose my ignorance. This sort of treatment
had only one result: I did not do well in examinations.
Winston Churchill (1874–1965)

The cases set out below are examples of typical and realistic long-case patients. We have framed the case outlines from an examination perspective, including typical points likely to be raised in the discussion and clinical traps that candidates may fall into. Think about how you would cope with them and what sorts of questions you might predict.

Only the most important parts of the history are summarised, as might be obtained by the examiners (not how you would present the case).

CASE 1

Mr AH is a 76-year-old retired stockbroker. He is an outpatient.

Problem list provided to the examiners (reviewed after blinded clinical evaluation by the examiners):
1. Type 2 diabetes.
2. Asthma.
3. Hypertension.
4. Muscle cramps secondary to statin use.
5. Carcinoma of the prostate.
6. Carcinoma of the colon.
7. Social aspects.
8. Knee replacements.

Mr AH was due to have CT scans of his chest abdomen and pelvis as follow-up of his two malignancies and felt anxious about the results of these tests.

Carcinoma of the prostate was diagnosed in 2011 after a screening prostate-specific antigen (PSA) test. Management was radical prostatectomy and external radiotherapy.

He had a period of urinary incontinence, which has now resolved.

There was minor radiation proctitis.

Carcinoma of the colon was diagnosed in 2014 after a positive screening faecal occult blood test – anterior resection but no colostomy.

Several adjacent lymph nodes were involved.

His postoperative course was complicated by a period of bowel obstruction and he required parenteral feeding for 10 days.

He had a course of chemotherapy including, he thought, 5-fluorouracil (5FU) and a platinum-based drug. The main complications were nausea and painless peripheral neuropathy. The neuropathy has improved slightly.

Follow-up colonoscopies and CT scans have been normal so far.

There have been no bowel symptoms apart from some mild diarrhoea.

Type 2 diabetes was diagnosed in 2011. It has only ever been treated with diet. He has lost no weight since the diagnosis and is currently 100 kg (BMI 30). His HbA$_{1C}$ recently was 6.1. He has had no identified complications of diabetes. He checks his blood sugar level every few days.

He has had a recent episode of cough, wheeze and fever.

He reports recurrent childhood asthma, but no problems with missing school and no admissions to hospital.

His chest symptoms occur almost every winter and are debilitating; he produces large volumes of discoloured sputum.

He has been given five courses of antibiotics this year.

He thinks one set of sputum cultures has been performed, but doesn't know the result.

There have been no chest investigations for years.

Last year he had a nasal polyp removed.

Has frequent problems with a blocked nose and symptoms of sinusitis, which usually precede his chest symptoms; sometimes he uses intranasal steroids.

He has often been treated with a course of prednisone for 10 days by his local doctor for these illnesses.

He uses regular seretide, 2 puffs mane and salbutamol as required.

He has been treated for hypertension for 6 years with candesartan / hydrochlorothiazide.

He has been told he has a heart murmur, which needs review in a few years.

He associated the use of two different statins with muscle pains in the legs and has stopped them; he is unsure of his untreated cholesterol level.

He is moderately active; he plays golf using a cart and walks 3 km on 5 days a week. He is mostly limited by joint problems – two previous knee replacements and chronic back pain and two previous laminectomies – but also by dyspnoea and wheeze.

His wife, who is affected by dementia, has been admitted in the last few weeks to a nursing home that is half an hour's drive away. He drives to visit her 6 days a week. He lives with his 48-year-old son, who works but is mildly mentally retarded. He has three other children whom he sees often.

He smoked until 25 years ago and has a 25-packet-year history of smoking. He drinks four or five glasses of wine a day.

When asked what troubled him most, he described his worry about his forthcoming screening tests and the limitations caused by his frequent respiratory symptoms.

Examination

1. Obesity.
2. Abdominal and back and knee scars.
3. BP 135 / 70 mmHg; pulse 75 / minute and regular.
4. There were occasional expiratory wheezes; his cough was dry.
5. He had signs of mild aortic regurgitation and stenosis.
6. Peripheral neuropathy in stocking distribution – his hands were unaffected. Reflexes were absent distally and proprioception and vibration sense was reduced.

Discussion

First examiner

1. Diagnosis of respiratory symptoms: asthma versus COPD. Possibility of bronchiectasis. What investigations are indicated, e.g. CXR, HRCT of the chest, sputum culture (possibility of unusual organisms, e.g. atypical mycobacteria, *Pseudomonas*)? Investigation of sinusitis because this seemed to precipitate attacks. IgE for bronchopulmonary aspergillosis. Lifelong problem of recurrent infections – consider immunodeficiency and investigate. Consider aspirin sensitivity; however, he takes regular aspirin without difficulty.
2. Management of respiratory problems: once-daily seretide – is this appropriate? Is intermittent steroid treatment appropriate? Management of sinusitis, e.g. regular inhaled nasal steroids. Should he have antibiotics or steroids at home for use at onset of symptoms? Would postural drainage, a flutter valve or physiotherapy be helpful for his productive cough?

3. Is candidate happy with the current management of follow-up of the two malignancies? What to do if PSA is up again? Is it worth checking the CEA?
4. Strategy for treating lipids in view of his intolerance to statins.
5. Management of possible peripheral neuropathy.

Second examiner

1. How is he managing at home? Does he have problems with depression? Does he drink too much? What would you say to him about this?
2. Management of valvular disease. Which is the more significant lesion?

COMMENTS

This man appeared well and might have been included in the exam because of his two malignancies, but the more significant unresolved problem was his recurrent productive cough. Relevant issues relating to the pharmacological management could include review of sputum cultures for sensitivity guided therapy, use of a spacer, use of N-acetylcysteine (NAC) or hypertonic saline in the case of underlying bronchiectasis, spacer technique and vaccination. Non-pharmacological measures include pulmonary exercise rehabilitation, house dust mite eradication (if allergic), and assessment of overlapping disordered sleep breathing. Discussions regarding goals of care may be highly relevant. This is an excellent topic for discussion and it is likely the examiners would be keen to pursue this problem. You would also want to talk about diabetes management and cancer surveillance.

CASE 2

Mr RD is a 66-year-old retired public servant.

Problem list provided to examiners

1. Antibody deficiency.
2. Chronic wound on right thigh, previous necrotising fasciitis.
3. Type 2 diabetes.
4. Ischaemic heart disease.
5. Hypertension.
6. Hypercholesterolaemia.
7. Obstructive sleep apnoea.
8. Gastro-oesophageal reflux.
9. Hypothyroidism.
10. Opioid dependence.
11. Subacute bowel obstruction.
12. Inflammatory bowel disease, proctocolectomy in 2003.

His gut problems began in 2001 with bloody diarrhoea and a diagnosis of inflammatory bowel disease.

Biopsies were more suggestive of Crohn's colitis and he was treated for a few years with steroids and azathioprine. He was intolerant of sulfasalazine.

Biological agents were not available at that time and poor control of his symptoms led to a proctocolectomy and the need for an ileostomy drainage bag.

He had further surgery with relocation of his stoma in 2011 because of a parastomal infection.

There were recurrent admissions to hospital with subacute bowel obstruction. Opioid dependency developed at this stage.

In 2014 he had further surgery to relieve adhesions, which was largely successful.

His stoma works continuously and he empties it three times a day.

He does not know how much of the small bowel was resected.

His appetite has been poor since the wound problems and he has lost 20 kg. He takes Ensure supplements.

Two years ago he had surgical removal of two skin lesions on his right thigh. The wound broke down and numerous further operations were performed. The wound was complicated by necrotising fasciitis. Various organisms, including *E. coli* spp., were cultured. He has a photographic record of the wound, which he was keen to show. An immunoglobulin deficiency was diagnosed after investigations for failure of his wound to heal. He has intermittent human IV immunoglobin infusions.

He had two myocardial infarctions in 2002 and then a stent to the right coronary artery in 2003. He describes recurrent episodes of what he called 'unstable angina' requiring admission to hospital and narcotic analgesics in 2015, but an angiogram showed his stent was patent and there was no obstructive disease. His chest pain was atypical and not associated with ECG changes.

There was a history of hyperlipidaemia and hypertension, currently treated with atorvastatin 10 mg, and he is not currently on antihypertensives. He has not smoked for 18 years.

He takes clopidogrel rather than aspirin because of gastrointestinal side-effects associated with aspirin.

Type 2 diabetes was diagnosed in 2004. He measures his blood sugar level 'randomly'; results are between 4.5 and 9 mmol / L and he does not know his HbA_{1C}.

He has regular eye checks and has no nerve problems.

Metformin was associated with diarrhoea and he takes glimepiride. This dose has been reduced because of episodes of hypoglycaemia. He believes his renal function is normal.

He has had a diagnosis of obstructive sleep apnoea; this appears to be mild and is not being treated.

He lives at home with his wife, who is well. His son died 3 years ago from complications of type 1 diabetes. He has no particular financial worries. He drives and is moderately physically active. He uses morphine on a daily basis for thigh pain.

Examination

1. He appeared well nourished.
2. Blood pressure 130 / 80 mmHg, pulse 65 / minute and regular. No signs of heart failure.
3. The thigh wound was almost healed, except for a small area at the lower margin.

4. The stoma appeared satisfactory and the abdominal examination was otherwise normal.
5. There was no peripheral neuropathy.

Discussion

First examiner

1. History and management of IBD, including malabsorption and nutrition.
2. Ischaemic heart disease.
3. Candidates could be asked to speculate on the original cause of the thigh wound. Remember pyoderma gangrenosum and necrobiosis diabeticorum. Discussion about the slow healing should consider his antibody deficiencies as well as his Crohn's disease. The recurrent infection with bowel organisms and curious photographic record of the wound might make you think about a factitious cause.
4. While discussing the management of his IBD, also consider investigation of possible malabsorption, e.g. vitamin B_{12} deficiency, and tests for this, e.g. blood count, serum albumin, folate and B_{12} levels, vitamin D.

Second examiner

1. Possible ischaemic heart disease would lead to a standard spiel about risk factor control. But don't take the patient's assertion that he had experienced recent acute coronary syndromes at face value. Make sure you ask about the characteristics of the symptoms. Think: is the diagnosis incompatible with the angiography findings? What about the influence of the opioid dependence on the symptoms?
2. You may be keen to wheel out your usual diabetes presentation, but you may not be allowed to by the examiners.

There may be time for a brief discussion of the opioid problem. Be prepared to discuss issues relating to a behaviour change in a thorough but succinct manner. This allows more time to spend discussing other issues that you may be more expert in. Your response should be personalised and directly relevant to your patient (what has worked before, who are their support network, what is their understanding of the implications, etc.), and should include engaging other healthcare professionals, having a plan for follow-up and emphasis on establishing a good therapeutic relationship. Simply referring the patient will likely be graded as unsatisfactory by the examiners.

COMMENTS

This complicated patient could provide good candidates with an opportunity to look beyond what they were told to achieve a high mark. Never blindly believe the history – look for evidence to support your diagnoses, and always consider a different diagnosis in every long case (and in clinical practice).

CASE 3

Mrs AB is a 37-year-old outpatient and former hospital nurse. She has been unable to work for some years because of her illness.

In 2012, 2 weeks after the birth of her third child, she developed joint pains and swelling of the hands and feet. She had not had any rashes.

Investigations at the time led to a diagnosis of systemic lupus erythematosus (SLE).

She was treated with prednisone doses varying from 10 to 30 mg.

Steroid-sparing agents such as azathioprine and mycophenalate were tried, but led to side-effects; however, she is not sure what these were. Methotrexate caused febrile neutropenia. Diclofenac and hydroxychloroquine were not very effective.

In 2013 she had an episode of pleuritic chest pain, was diagnosed with pericarditis and was admitted to hospital and treated with prednisone, starting with 40 mg. Her symptoms resolved over a few days.

In 2014 she had sudden loss of vision in one eye and retinal vein thrombosis was found. She was then diagnosed with antiphospholipid syndrome and began treatment with warfarin.

In 2014–15 she had recurrent *Nocardia* infections – skin, muscles (calf) and brain. There was no neurological deficit, but she had severe headache. This was treated successfully with co-trimoxazole.

In 2015 she developed left-sided paraesthesiae and vertigo. A transient ischaemic attack (TIA) was diagnosed. A CT of the brain and carotid Dopplers were normal. Aspirin was added to her treatment.

In 2016 a pruritic rash developed on her legs and the co-trimoxazole was stopped.

Her steroid use was associated with a number of problems: weight gain from 65 to 95 kg; her BMI is now 35; she developed gestational diabetes needing insulin, but is now taking metformin. She is unsure of her current blood sugar level (BSL); she checks it every 4 days or so. She has not had a hypoglycaemic episode; she doesn't know her glycated haemoglobin (HbA_{1c}).

She smokes 15 cigarettes a day and her husband also smokes.

She looks after her three children at home; once a week she rides a bike with them, but her joints become very sore afterwards.

Joint symptoms and muscle weakness limit household work (e.g. putting out washing). Her husband works 6×12-hour days. She gets some support from her family at home.

She has an intrauterine device (IUD) for contraception and per vaginam (PV) bleeding has improved with a progesterone device.

There have been no other rashes.

She has no kidney disease as far as she knows. There has not been a problem with hypertension.

Her last INR was 1.4. She has monthly tests.

Her eyes are reviewed regularly.

She is keen to work again as a nurse or clerk, but has been told by her doctors that this is not possible.

She sees her main problem as her inability to work and exercise.

Examination

On the day of the exam the important examination findings were:

1. She was Cushingoid.
2. There was swelling without deformity involving the hands and wrists.

3. She had a healing rash on the legs (probably co-trimoxazole associated).
4. Her BP was 130/90 mmHg.
5. There was mild proximal muscle weakness – she could stand with effort from a chair without using her arms.
6. The left fundus was pale with 6/12 vision.

Discussion

First examiner

1. SLE:
   a. serology and diagnosis and role of follow-up blood tests
   b. management of joint symptoms: drugs, exercise, physiotherapy
   c. steroids and doses, any action plan needed
   d. future complications of SLE, especially kidneys
   e. *Nocardia* prophylaxis.
2. Diabetes:
   a. routine discussion: how diagnosed, family history
   b. vascular risk
   c. renal risk
   d. role of ACE inhibitors (ACEIs)
   e. BSL measurements
   f. weight loss
   g. smoking cessation strategies
   h. patient's understanding of prognosis.
3. Warfarin – INR monitoring and use of aspirin for antiphospholipid syndrome.

Second examiner

1. Contraception issues; aspects relating to management during possible pregnancy.
2. Prognosis and psychological state, patient's view of her main problem.

COMMENTS

1. Management problems of SLE and its treatment.
2. Complicated history needs to be presented succinctly and logically – probably best given chronologically.
3. Some common management areas for discussion (e.g. diabetes). This needs to be done smoothly – should be straightforward so a high standard would be expected.
4. Indication for and management of anticoagulation and management of initial or recurrent pericarditis are very likely areas for discussion depending on time available. Much detail about patient's management and understanding of warfarin will be expected. You would need to know where and how often INR readings are taken, how result is communicated to patient and who makes dose adjustments. What happened after the last reading of 1.4?
5. Management of stroke/TIA could be asked about, and use of warfarin and aspirin.
6. Plenty of scope for discussion of effect of illness on family, income, work, self-esteem and so on.
7. Need to be able to show how you would discuss the prognosis with the patient; this usually requires you to elicit an understanding of the factors limiting prognosis and their management rather than estimating the life expectancy.

CASE 4

Mr BC is a 68-year-old accountant in full-time work. He has come in for the exam from home. He has a younger wife and his youngest child is only 5 years old.

He has had a recent admission to hospital with a chest infection and was diagnosed with chronic obstructive pulmonary disease (COPD).

In 2001 he was diagnosed with chronic kidney disease (CKD). He had a biopsy but the diagnosis was unclear, at least to him. He was treated with haemodialysis for 18 months. He still has a functioning fistula in the left arm.

In 2002 he had a cadaveric transplant. Immunosuppression was with prednisone and azathioprine.

In 2003 he developed gout and was treated with colchicine and allopurinol. There has been no recurrence.

Azathioprine led to bone marrow suppression, admission to hospital and a requirement for blood transfusion. Azathioprine was stopped and cyclosporin started.

His current creatinine is 250 μmol/L. He doesn't know his eGFR (estimated glomerular filtration rate), but says his creatinine has been stable for many years, but had increased to 270 μmol/L during his recent admission.

His cyclosporin dose was reduced last year and mycophenolate was added to his treatment.

He is not worried about his current renal function.

In 2012 he had left and then right hip replacements. He thinks the left was because of avascular necrosis and the right was because of osteoarthritis. He is not aware of having had any bone density assessments.

His recent admission was with dyspnoea and productive cough – antibiotics and steroids were used to treat this, but have now been stopped.

COPD was diagnosed, but his spirometry measurements were not abnormal as far as he knows. He smoked until 5 years ago – 25 packet-years altogether.

His cough is still productive. He can walk 200 m on the flat; he plays golf with a cart.

He is being treated with Symbicort II (budesonide-formoterol), 2 puffs twice daily and salbutamol, 2 puffs PRN.

Obstructive sleep apnoea (OSA) was diagnosed in 2012. He snores and has mild daytime sleepiness, but never when driving. His sleep study was positive. He has been unable to tolerate a mask.

He has been overweight for many years and is currently 140 kg for 2 m of height. He has been unable to lose weight despite insight into his problem.

He has a long history of hypertension, which has been difficult to control since he developed kidney disease. His current treatment for this includes: diltiazem 180 mg daily, candesartan 16 mg daily, prazosin 5 mg BD and hydralazine 50 mg BD.

He had angioedema with an ACEI, and his angiotensin II receptor blocker (ARB) was initiated in hospital.

In 2015 he had symptomatic atrial fibrillation requiring two cardioversions. He takes amiodarone 200 mg twice daily for this and has had no symptomatic recurrences. He is anticoagulated with warfarin. His INR target is 2–3 and he is having weekly blood tests. His INR was 5.4 during admission when on antibiotics. He has had no bleeding problems.

He has peripheral oedema, which is worse with diltiazem. He has never used support stockings, but takes frusemide 80 mg daily. An episode of cellulitis in the legs occurred 2 years ago and required treatment with IV antibiotics.

He still works and supports his family (sedentary job, good employer), but he is not sure for how much longer he will be able to continue. He feels his breathlessness is his worst problem.

Examination

The examination revealed:

1. Obesity.
2. BP 120 / 80 mmHg, pulse 80 regular.
3. Not dyspnoeic at rest, loose cough.
4. Not clubbed.
5. Widespread polyphonic wheezes and coarse inspiratory crackles.
6. Reduced chest expansion.
7. Soft systolic ejection murmur, apex beat not palpable.
8. Peripheral oedema moderately severe and venous staining.
9. Transplant palpable in abdomen, left arm fistulae working.

Test results available to examiners:

1. Chest X-ray (CXR) increased lung markings, thickened bronchial walls, over-inflated chest.
2. ECG left bundle branch block, sinus rhythm.
3. Spirometry FEV_1 / FVC 71% little reversibility.
4. Echo severe left ventricular dyssynchrony, dilated left atrium, systolic function preserved.

Discussion

First examiner

1. a. What does patient see as his main problem? Does COPD explain all the symptoms and signs?
   b. What are the other possibilities, e.g. bronchiectasis, pneumocystis, bronchopulmonary aspergillosis?
   c. How to investigate and manage?
2. a. Current renal function satisfactory or a problem?
   b. What measures to investigate and treat, e.g. BP, chronic rejection, cyclosporin?
   c. Surveillance of current antirejection treatment, e.g. full blood count, skin, blood levels, indications for kidney biopsy?
3. AF management, amiodarone toxicity and surveillance, warfarin management.
4. Peripheral oedema significance and management – calcium antagonists, venous problems, right heart failure – any signs of this?

Second examiner

1. Obstructive sleep apnoea management – what else to do?
2. Chronic illness, work, money, etc. Patient insight into his prognosis?
3. Obesity – what approach? (if time)

COMMENTS

A long case with a number of active problems:

1. Recent lung disease perhaps not explained by COPD.
2. Renal function possibly deteriorating despite patient's claim of stable creatinine.
3. Opportunity to discuss management of surveillance of antirejection Rx.
4. Management of AF, and warfarin and amiodarone.
5. Approach to peripheral oedema not always or even usually heart failure, but possibility of right heart failure and pulmonary hypertension.
6. OSA and obesity.

The examiners would be keen for a differential diagnosis of his dyspnoea and lung disease, and pharmacological and non-pharmacological treatment. You would want to talk about transplant surveillance and management. There would be time for both.

CASE 5

Mr WP is a 60-year-old wheat farmer who is currently in hospital 100 km away from his home and farm.

In 2013 he discovered a painless testicular mass. There were no sweats or fevers. He underwent a single orchidectomy. He was unable to remember a preceding biopsy. Lymphoma was diagnosed.

He was treated with eight cycles of R-CHOP treatment delayed by drug side-effects (fever, oedema), but completed in 8 months and followed by maintenance rituximab.

In 2016 he relapsed. He developed back pain and left leg weakness. There were no bowel or bladder symptoms. He was admitted to hospital for 5 months and was unable to walk. There was numbness of the left leg and a necrotic ulcer developed on the heel. There was little improvement in power while he was in hospital.

He then had an episode of diplopia and ptosis without associated headache.

An MRI of the brain was performed. He was unsure of the result. During the same admission he had an episode of chest pain and dyspnoea. A CT pulmonary angiogram (CTPA) showed pulmonary embolism.

He was treated with intravenous and intrathecal methotrexate and anticoagulated with warfarin. An episode of pleuritic chest pain was diagnosed as pericarditis. He is not sure how this was treated.

He is currently awaiting autologous bone marrow transplant, having had stem cell harvesting.

He has lost 15 kg during this illness.

In the past he had a stroke in 2012. This was treated with clopidogrel.

A transoesophageal echo showed a patent foramen ovale (PFO). He had a long history of hypertension and hyperlipidaemia. He was never a smoker.

His main worries about his health are about his prospects of recovery and return to his family and the farm, which is currently being managed with difficulty by his son.

Examination

1. Left foot drop with S1 and L5 loss of sensation.
2. Absent reflexes in the left leg.
3. Moderate weakness of knee extension and flexion, mild weakness at hip.
4. Right leg normal power and reflexes.
5. Absent right testis.
6. Eye movements normal.

Investigations available to the examiners

1. Histology – large B cell lymphoma.
2. MRI brain-thickening of right 3rd nerve within the prepontine cistern.
3. MRI of foot showed osteomyelitis.
4. CTPA showed a pulmonary embolus in the lateral segment of the right middle lobe.
5. MRI of lumbar spine showed retroperitoneal lymphadenopathy on the left side of the pelvis and involvement from L4 to the sacral nerves extending to the cauda equina nerve roots.

Discussion

First examiner

1. Management of lymphoma and bone marrow transplant:
   a. a common transplant problem, immunosuppression surveillance
   b. lymphoma staging – presentation with non-lymph-node involvement and no B symptoms – implications for prognosis
   c. common side-effects of R-CHOP and rituximab
   Appropriate tests (as above) and their interpretation.
2. Management of osteomyelitis.
3. Management of leg weakness – including rehabilitation.
4. Loss of independence and prognosis.

Second examiner

1. Anticoagulation – management of TIA and PFO, use of clopidogrel versus aspirin.
2. Ability to work, run farm, etc. How has he coped with 5 months in hospital, far from his family?

COMMENTS

A complicated case involving:

1. diagnosis of lymphoma – discussion about staging, etc.
2. complications of treatment, first of drugs and then theoretically about complications of bone marrow transplant
3. disease recurrence with a variety of neurological problems and problems of immobility – necrotic ulcer, psychological
4. significant examination findings
5. need for anticoagulation; opportunity to discuss warfarin management

6. investigation of possible cerebral ischaemic episode, significance of PFO
7. patient's concerns about his prognosis: loss of income, separation from family, long period in hospital – all possible areas for discussion.

The examiners have plenty to choose from and are likely to want to discuss some problems in detail and to ensure the candidate has thought about the others by asking a few questions on each.

CASE 6

Mrs AP is a 72-year-old retired nurse who has come in for the exams.

She has a long history of hypertension, which has recently been difficult to control. A CT of the renal arteries showed 'thickening'.

She smoked for 18 years until 10 years ago. She has had lower back pain for 10 years, which was not relieved by a laminectomy. Spinal canal stenosis was diagnosed 4 years ago.

She has had a gain in weight over the last 5 years from 88 to 107 kg. Her BMI is 40.

A thyroidectomy was performed in 2013 following a biopsy that showed atypical cells. The tumour, however, was benign.

She is breathless on mild exertion, but not at rest.

She had a right hip replacement in 2005.

In 2015 she had a left hip replacement. She became very dyspnoeic 5 weeks later, with investigations for a DVT. There were multiple pulmonary emboli, but no DVT was found. She was treated with enoxaparin and then warfarin for 10 months.

Currently she can walk 30 metres on the flat. She is limited by dyspnoea and knee pain.

She has been diagnosed with asthma and an allergy to cats and dogs. She has three cats at home.

She suffered from childhood chest infections and sinusitis but no ear infections. She coughs up little phlegm and has never had an admission to hospital with asthma, or required steroid treatment.

In 2004 hypogammaglobulinaemia was diagnosed. She was given vaccinations for influenza, whooping cough, pneumonia (possibly pneumococcus and *Haemophilus influenzae*) and hepatitis.

She now receives monthly gammaglobulin injections. These were given IM for 5 years, then IV. She feels she is much improved and requires only one or two courses of antibiotics per year now.

She is currently taking atenolol 50 mg a day for hypertension and detected ventricular bigeminy (asymptomatic). She had had problems with previously prescribed ACEIs and ARBs, but can't remember what they were.

She is unable to drive and goes out only with a frame. Her husband does the shopping and housework.

Her main concern about her health was her back pain. She was not especially worried about her immobility or her weight.

Examination

1. Obese.
2. BP 150/80 mmHg.
3. Able to walk with great difficulty, but not apparently concerned.
4. Chest clear.
5. Forced expiratory time (FET) normal – 5 s.

Discussion

First examiner

1. History of childhood infections and asthma: Was this typical of hypogammaglobulinaemia? Did she have time off school? Admissions to hospital? Inability to play sport, etc.?
2. Dyspnoea – current causes: obesity, asthma, PE, or something else? How to investigate?
3. Back pain – has this been nocturnal? Is its current treatment satisfactory? This is her main worry.
4. Obesity – is she serious about weight loss? What is her attitude to illness? Is there some secondary gain?
5. Asthma – she has pets at home to which she is said to be allergic. How severe is it? Is current treatment satisfactory?
6. Immobility – what might be done?

Second examiner

1. What risks would further surgery involve? How would you advise her anaesthetist?
2. Hypertension – is it well controlled? Is there a need to investigate and consider renal artery angioplasty? Discuss use of a beta-blocker.
3. Does she have a GP coordinating her case? Does she have an advance care directive?

COMMENTS

1. Problem of a patient enthusiastic about her illnesses.
2. Sometimes difficult to get to the point during history-taking, but of course a problem for examiners as well. A more efficient approach when obtaining the history here would be to start with the current management of each condition, including medications, follow-up and complications, before returning to try and tease out the detailed chronological sequence.
3. Any illness that begins in childhood requires questions about its effect on education – time off school, playing of sport, socialising with other children and effect on final level of education.
4. Discussion about treatment of problems that seem severe, e.g. immobility, but do not really seem to worry the patient.
5. Some more straightforward medical problems, e.g. hypertension, possible renal artery stenosis, use of beta-blockers for an asthmatic.

This case has an interesting mix of significant medical but also of social, and perhaps psychiatric, problems. A good candidate needs a sensible and realistic approach to these probably insoluble aspects of the case.

CASE 7

Mrs CE is a 73-year-old outpatient with chronic renal failure and on haemodialysis.

The aetiology of her CKD was suspected to be analgesic nephropathy; she used large doses of aspirin and paracetamol for headaches for 25 years and stopped 30 years ago.

She has now been dialysing for 2 years. She has 5 hours three times a week. Her right arm fistula works well. She has had recurrent renal 'stones'.

She doesn't know her dry weight and is unsure about fluid, salt or dietary restrictions. She remembers having had some parathyroid problems while on tablets in 2014. Her calcium levels were too low and the tablets were stopped.

In 2012 her renal failure was precipitated after an episode of pancreatitis requiring ICU admission. She remembers severe abdominal pain, but little else of this illness. The pancreatitis has meant she is not suitable for peritoneal dialysis.

She passes no urine.

In 2009 she swallowed a fish bone and developed peritonitis and required emergency surgery.

In the past she drank 6–8 whiskies a day (more when friends visited) for 10 years. She is now a non-drinker.

She thinks her liver is normal now. There have been no problems with it or with exocrine pancreatic function.

Hypertension was diagnosed after this illness and is being treated with metoprolol 50 mg daily.

There is some exertional dyspnoea but no orthopnoea. Her back limits her more than shortness of breath. This has been present since she was assaulted by her first husband over many years.

She needs a knee replacement. She has had both her hips and the left knee replaced. Three lots of back surgery have been performed following her injuries. A new left knee replacement has been recommended after she fell on her knee a few months ago.

She has no history of ischaemic heart disease. She does not know whether her cholesterol level is elevated. She smoked for 20 years until 10 years ago.

There is a history of gout many years ago.

Her medications include:

- analgesics for her back (she is not sure what these are at the moment)
- Aranesp monthly (she doesn't know her current haemoglobin).

She first married at 16, and had a very difficult life with first husband.

She cannot drive. Her husband brings her to dialysis 40 minutes from home and does all the housework, shopping and cooking. He is very different from her first husband, whom she divorced 29 years ago. She remarried 5 years ago. She has two children, one of whom lives locally.

Gallstones have been found and an endoscopic retrograde cholangiopancreatography (ERCP) recommended. Gallstones were not found at the time of her pancreatitis.

She is very happy in her second marriage. Her main concern about her health is her immobility and constant back pain.

Examination

1. BMI 24.
2. Working fistula.
3. Blood pressure 120/80 mmHg, pulse 70/min. Grade 1/6 systolic ejection murmur.
4. Scars over cervical and lumbar spine.
5. Abdominal examination normal.
6. Peripheral pulses normal.
7. Reflexes normal.
8. Power limited by knee pain.

Discussion

First examiner

1. Discussion about details of illness that led to dialysis and analgesic nephropathy (now a rare condition).
2. Dialysis problems: diet, calcium levels, drugs, cardiovascular protection.
3. Patient's understanding of her illness.
4. Back pain management (one of her main concerns).
5. Is she a candidate for a transplant? Screening for transitional cell carcinoma.

Second examiner

1. Fitness for knee surgery.
2. Significance of murmur.

COMMENTS

1. This case involves the usual discussion about CKD and dialysis: cause of renal failure, choice of type of dialysis, patient's understanding of illness – dry weight, diet, haemoglobin, etc.
2. Analgesic nephropathy is now a rare cause of CKD, but candidates need to know something about it – including the risk of transitional cell carcinoma.
3. This woman had a very difficult life for many years with her first husband and now copes with her chronic illness cheerfully – some details about her domestic problems and their effect on her current state of mind are important.
4. Common further questions would involve asking about your management of her back pain and discussion of her suitability for knee surgery and transplant. These may not have clear-cut answers, but a sensible approach would be expected.

Long-case videos

A selection of examples of long cases is available from Student Consult (studentconsult. inkling.com).

In these videos, typical long cases are discussed by the authors and then presented by a candidate. The candidate's performance is discussed and assessed.

First case

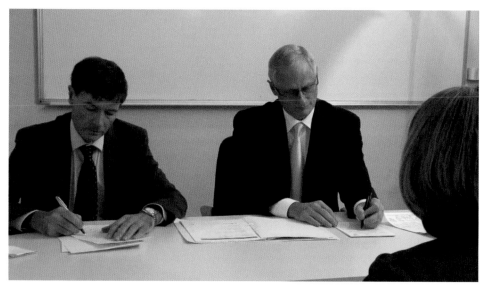

Examiners listen attentively to long case 1 presentation.

A woman with:
1. Cushing's disease – pituitary tumour – two operations and radiotherapy
2. obesity and fatty apron resection
3. adrenal tumour resection
4. persisting increased adrenocorticotrophic hormone (ACTH) excretion
5. type 2 diabetes – peripheral neuropathy
6. stroke with right hemiparesis
7. depression
8. thyroidectomy
9. acoustic neuroma.
    The patient's main concerns are about her mobility and depression.

Examiners' problem list
1. Mobility.
2. Depression.
3. Management of Cushing's.
4. Replacement pituitary treatment, management of surgery or acute illness.
5. Diabetic control and complications.
6. Cytomegalovirus (CMV) retinitis.
7. Osteoporosis.

Second case

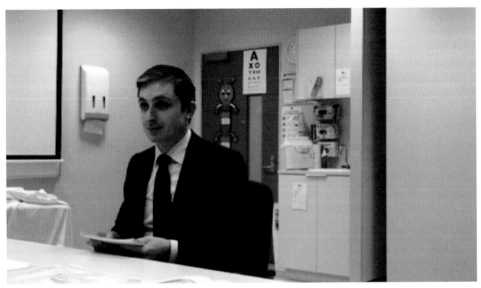

Candidate finishes presenting long case 2.

A 50-year-old woman with:
1. dermatomyositis and interstitial lung disease
2. cyclophosphamide, azathioprine and steroid use
3. chronic hepatitis B
4. osteoporosis
5. type 2 diabetes
6. unwillingness to continue some medications
7. proximal muscle weakness
8. stiffness in joints.

The patient's main concerns were about her morning stiffness and medications.

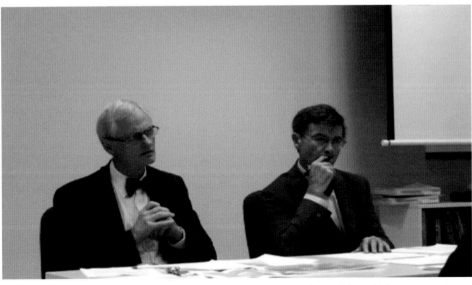

Professor Talley asks penetrating (but fair) questions of candidate in long case 2.

Examiners' problem list

1. Joint stiffness – differential diagnosis and management.
2. Prognosis of dermatomyositis, possibility of underlying malignancy and association with interstitial lung disease (ILD).
3. ILD.
4. Osteoporosis.
5. Medications.
6. Hepatitis B and its implications.

Third case

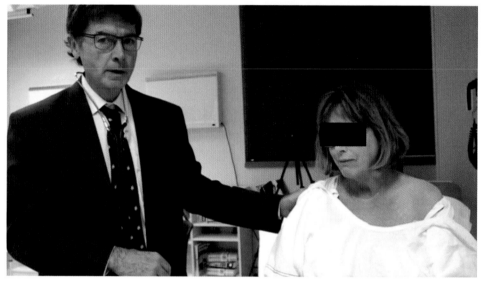

Dr O'Connor independently evaluating the patient prior to commencement of the long case.

A 58-year-old woman with:

1. a long history of SLE leading to renal failure and a renal transplant. Her SLE has been quiescent since her transplant.
2. She has had psychotic episodes on steroids.
3. Recently, after a period of confusion, she has been diagnosed with encephalitis. This has responded to immunoglobulin treatment.

She is limited by pain in her ankle of uncertain cause. She sees this as her main problem. She is keen to return to work.

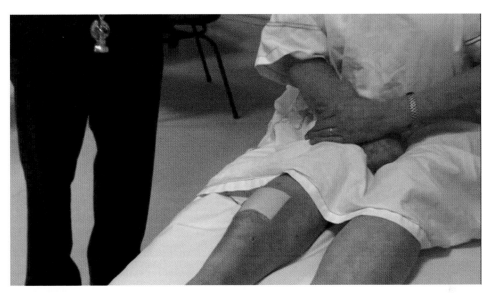

Long case 3.

Examiner's problem list
1. Ankle pain.
2. Persisting cognitive problems.
3. Management of transplant.
4. SLE not an active problem.
5. Social support.

Chapter 15

The short case

You see, but you do not observe.

Sir Arthur Conan Doyle (1859–1930)

The short case is a test of the candidate's ability to examine a patient smoothly, confidently and accurately. There is rarely the opportunity to go back and repeat the examination. It takes a long time to get used to being watched critically while examining. This is why it is important to practise short cases of every conceivable type so that the physical examination is performed automatically in the correct way. While proceeding, the candidate should be consciously synthesising the results, not trying to remember what to do next.

The stem

Written introductions (or *stems*) were introduced for the short cases in 2008. These have a standardised format, including the patient's name and age, followed by a brief description of the patient's symptoms, if there are any, and then a request to perform a particular examination. The stem is chosen by the examiners after they have assessed the patient. The written stem is given to the candidate or displayed on the door 1 or 2 minutes before the start of the case and is repeated verbally to the candidate when he or she enters the room. The idea is to give the candidate time to decide what to do.

If the patient has no symptoms, the stem may state this. If the case is an obvious 'spot diagnosis', the stem may give the diagnosis and ask for an appropriate examination to assess the severity, activity or functional effect of the condition on the patient – for example: 'Mrs Jones is a 60-year-old woman who has a long history of rheumatoid arthritis. Please make an assessment of the activity of the disease.'

If the stem contains specific instructions, these must be followed. For example, if the candidate is asked to examine a patient's gait, it is vital to get the patient to walk first. This may appear obvious, but many candidates have failed because they have not followed the examiners' instructions. If the stem says 'examine the lower cranial nerves', do not start with the eyes. The stem means that the problem will be somewhere between nerves VII and XII, so start with VII. In the short-case examination of a patient with bronchiectasis, the stem may be: 'This man has a cough. Please examine him.' The patient would have an obviously loose cough, typical of bronchiectasis. Candidates who ask the patient to cough would be off to a great start, but those who do not ask him to cough may risk a much poorer score. In reality, there is plenty of time, but you certainly do not want to run out of time before getting to the problem the examiners have raised.

The stem is never a trick. The examiner will become quite anxious if candidates begin to perform the wrong examination (e.g. a neurological examination of the hands when the problem is rheumatoid arthritis).

Timing

The time allowed for each short case is 15 minutes. Having a sense of time even early on in your exam preparation is always helpful. This means that time should be available for both examination and discussion. Patients are not really included just as quick 'spot diagnosis' cases alone, but if you do 'spot the diagnosis' it will be a golden opportunity to demonstrate systematically the associated signs in full. The examiners will expect a higher standard of examination when the diagnosis is fairly obvious.

Marking

With the previous marking system, a candidate could fail all the short cases and still pass the examination. This changed in 2014 so that everyone must pass at least one short case. The new marking system is more complicated in that passing no longer depends on achieving a certain mark and passing one short case but rather is calculated from a grid. The aim is that candidates should not pass unless one short case is passed. The most common short cases are cardiovascular and neurological problems. We suggest that candidates aim to examine each short case proficiently within 8 minutes.

Hand washing

Remember that infectious diseases physicians are everywhere. Ask to wash or wipe your hands before going into the short-case room (and do it). The examiners do not usually want you to wash them in the examination room because of the delay involved, but look around for somewhere to wash as you go out.

HINT

Wash your hands before and after examining. Some candidates keep a small bottle of hand gel in their bags so that they can be seen to wash their hands and are not delayed by having to search the room.

Starting off

It is a good idea, when introduced to the patient, to step over and politely acknowledge him or her. You do want to quickly establish rapport, as in any clinical encounter.

Shaking hands is no longer recommended, in view of the COVID19 pandemic, and don't forget hand hygiene. Always position the patient properly (e.g. at 45° for the cardiovascular examination or flat for the abdominal examination) and make sure that he or she is appropriately undressed for the relevant examination.

It is always worthwhile taking a moment to stand back and look at the whole patient. This may prevent you from missing an obvious spot diagnosis, such as myxoedema, a thymectomy scar in a patient with muscle weakness (myasthenia), muscle fasciculations in motor neurone disease, a psoriatic rash in a patient with arthropathy or a Cushingoid appearance in a hypertension examination. Practice really does help improve ability to see clinical associations. A candidate will almost always fail the case if a major sign is missed. The examiners decide what signs they feel are most important and, in practice, finding the majority of the agreed signs will result in a pass.

Approach to the patient

Do not ask the patient any questions about the diagnosis, but it is essential to say, 'Let me know if this is uncomfortable or if I hurt you', and, when examining the abdomen directly, to ask, 'Are you tender anywhere?' This is a test of bedside manner (and may give you a clue). Always try to make the patient comfortable and avoid totally exposing the patient or exposing parts that are not being examined. Look at the patient's face intermittently, particularly during the abdominal and hand examination, for signs that he or she is uncomfortable. It is distressing for the examiners to see from the patient's face that he or she is in pain and that the candidate is unaware of this or is ignoring it.

Blood pressure

The examiners do ask the candidate to take the patient's blood pressure as part of the cardiovascular examination. In the past the measurement was often provided when the candidate asked, 'Do you want me to take the blood pressure?' or said, 'I would now normally take the blood pressure'. This is not as simple as it sounds and many candidates can have considerable difficulty with this. In examinations, some candidates have looked shocked when told to go ahead and do what they had just offered to do; others struggled with an unfamiliar sphygmomanometer, while others looked as though they did not really know how to measure blood pressure.

> **HINT**
>
> Practise taking the blood pressure accurately under exam-type conditions, and be prepared to do so in your case. It may be worth bringing your own portable sphygmomanometer.

Candidates often worry about the need to look for radiofemoral delay when they are asked to do a cardiovascular case. This is not necessary unless the introduction mentioned hypertension (or you find hypertension when taking the blood pressure).

Performance

Remember that you are, in fact, demonstrating the signs (particularly in the case of a neurological short case) to the examiners. It is important to perform each manoeuvre accurately and deliberately. Be seen to be smooth and confident, as if you have done the examination a thousand times before. Perform a thorough examination on patients you see during your routine clinical care – remember, practising for the clinical examination will make you a much better physician! Also, try to be confident of each sign before moving on to another area (e.g. on finding an abdominal mass, concentrate on excluding the various possibilities and coming to a firm conclusion), and do not worry too much about the time it takes. Practice will facilitate formation of conclusions accurately and quickly.

Very occasionally, the examiners will pull a candidate away in the middle of an examination. This is why it is important to synthesise the data as you go. Do not get flustered by this – it usually means that enough of the examination has been completed for you to have discovered the important signs. Examiners do not ask for the interpretation of a particular sign in isolation (e.g. the collapsing carotid pulse in aortic regurgitation or the double apex beat in hypertrophic cardiomyopathy).

There may not be time to complete a complicated examination, particularly in a neurology case. A good candidate will tailor the examination so that nothing really important is left out by the end of the time available.

Usually there is no interruption until the examination is almost finished. We suggest that candidates keep on examining until told to stop, and then give a short list of the other steps they would like to have completed and why (e.g. urine analysis, rectal examination).

One of the examiners' worst nightmares is the candidate who rushes through an examination and finishes in 3 or 4 minutes. This means the examination has not been thorough and leaves 12 minutes for discussion – this time can be very difficult to fill (not good!).

Presentation

Before presenting the findings, listen closely to the examiners' instructions. Candidates will often be asked: 'What did you find?' – at which point they are expected to describe the relevant signs first and then comment on possible causes. Sometimes candidates will be asked: 'What is your diagnosis?' – at which point they are expected to give a diagnosis or differential diagnosis first and then list the signs supporting the contention.

> ### HINT
> Formulate your diagnosis and differential diagnosis *based on the individual in front of you*.

Using a formulaic presentation of your findings might give you more time to think, but can be intensely irritating for the examiner if this is the fourth time they have heard 'Mr Smith is an elderly man lying comfortably in bed', and especially if the patient is no older than the examiners and is obviously breathless and not comfortable.

One useful method of presentation is to first repeat the examiners' introduction briefly, and then give the relevant findings, followed by the provisional diagnosis. For example: 'I was asked to examine Mr Jones, a 60-year-old man who has had problems with dyspnoea. On examination of his cardiovascular system, I found …' When describing the signs it is probably easiest to present them in the order they were looked for (e.g. for the cardiovascular system – pulse rate, then blood pressure, then jugular venous pressure). It is important to state all the positive signs and the important negative ones.

Be definite about each sign mentioned, or do not mention the sign at all. There is no place for expressions such as 'slightly asymmetrical' or 'minor'.

> **HINT**
>
> In neurological examinations, don't rush to undertake sensory testing, which is often frustrating and less reliable. Leave the sensory examination to the end if at all possible.

Confidence is critical to success in the short cases. Do not lose confidence if you make a minor error; just continue – the examiners may not even have noticed.

A short differential diagnosis is usually expected, even if the diagnosis is obvious. For example, a patient with fasciculation plus upper and lower motor neurone signs in the legs and no sensory loss almost certainly has motor neurone disease, but a non-metastatic manifestation of carcinoma must be considered. Always mention common diseases before rare ones and always consider the patient's age and sex. Never reel off any old list; the differential diagnosis must be tailored to the particular patient. Sometimes patients will have signs of two different problems. This should not be ignored. For example, a patient with proximal muscle weakness as a result of polymyositis may have unrelated Dupuytren's contractures.

After presentation of the signs, a few minutes or more are set aside for discussion. The examiners are not encouraged to take the candidate back for a second look at a sign, as this can be extremely unsettling for the candidate and perhaps not fair. However, this does happen occasionally and it is best to think of it as a genuine second chance.

> **HINT**
>
> A redirect represents a genuine second chance – grab hold of the opportunity. There are no tricks in the examination.

Understanding the role of the examiners

From the examiners' point of view, the candidate who is completely wrong presents a problem. This can occur because he or she has not read the stem properly – for example, when a request to examine the lower cranial nerves leads a candidate to begin to test visual acuity. Sometimes the examination depends on a spot diagnosis. For example, for an obvious acromegalic patient the stem might be: 'This man has noticed some changes in his hands. Have a look at his face, examine the hands and go on from there.' The risk here is that the acromegaly is not recognised and the candidate decides the diagnosis is, say, rheumatoid arthritis. The examination and discussion will then have nothing to do with what the examiners had expected and prepared for.

If the candidate's mistake is recognised early on, the examiners may attempt to redirect the examination. This can be surprisingly difficult. Some candidates persist in continuing the way they began, despite strong hints or even direction from the examiners. This is presumably because they think an attempt is being made to trick them. This never happens.

> **HINT**
>
> If your diagnosis is completely incorrect, a good discussion won't usually help you.

Sometimes the examination seems to be going well and then the candidate comes out with a completely wrong diagnosis. This makes the examiners' prepared discussion unusable. In this case the examiner will probably attempt to continue the discussion along the lines the candidate has begun. For example, the candidate appears to have examined a patient with small muscle wasting of the hands satisfactorily but then, against all the evidence, decides the problem is rheumatoid arthritis. The examiners may ask what was found that led to the diagnosis and were there any alternative possibilities, but if no alternatives can be extracted from the candidate then they will allow a discussion of rheumatoid arthritis.

This problem usually occurs when a candidate has decided on a diagnosis before looking at the patient. Deciding that because the stem was '"examine the hands", therefore this "can only rheumatoid" must be avoided.

One examiner will have introduced the patient and repeated the stem. This is likely to be the lead examiner. In many cases that examiner will conduct the discussion. There may or may not be an opportunity for the other examiner to ask some questions at the end. This may be a sign that the first one has run out of questions. This doesn't really tell you whether things are going very well or very badly.

Investigations

Relevant X-rays or an ECG may be shown to the candidate. Some diagnostic and therapeutic aspects are likely to be discussed in the short case. If a candidate has done well in a case and there are a few minutes left for extra questions, the score can only improve.

> **HINT**
>
> If you have done well, in the last few minutes of discussion your score can only go up, not down. So don't worry if the depth becomes overwhelming – press on talking about the problems in a mature, sensible fashion.

Short-case selection

Consider the short-case lottery as you prepare for the exam:
- cardiovascular 25%
- neurology 25%
- respiratory 15%
- rheumatology 10%
- gastroenterology 6%
- renal 5%
- haematology 5%
- endocrine 3%.
  The average frequencies of cardiovascular short cases is as follows:
- Most common: mitral regurgitation, aortic stenosis, aortic regurgitation, hypertrophic cardiomyopathy, aortic stenosis / aortic regurgitation (each about 10%)
- The rest:
  - pulmonary hypertension / tricuspid regurgitation
  - prosthetic valves, mitral valve prolapse, mitral stenosis / mitral regurgitation
  - pulmonary regurgitation.

The organising team are asked to find a variety of cases for each candidate, but when a patient drops out or is rejected by the examiners these arrangements can go astray. One candidate got three cases of interstitial lung disease in her exam! However, all types still crop up and a candidate must try to prepare for most possibilities. It is also true that the more straightforward the case, the higher is the standard of examination that will be expected, and vice versa. Trick cases are deliberately avoided.

Understanding the examiners' thinking

The value of some traditional clinical signs is now being questioned as *evidence-based* approaches to clinical examination help establish the validity and utility of signs. There is much work still to be done in this area, but an understanding of the value of signs is increasingly important. A tactful approach may be needed with the examiners to prevent any resentment at the candidate's failing to look for a traditional sign that is a particular favourite of theirs.

Six golden rules for the short cases

1. Do *everything* properly when you examine the patient – *never* take short cuts.
2. *Think* and *synthesise* as you examine the patient – be alert.
3. *Never* make up signs and *never* ignore signs because they don't fit neatly together.
4. Always *be sure of your facts* when presenting – it's better to say that you don't know than to guess.
5. Always show consideration for the patient and *never* cause the patient pain.
6. Wash your hands before and after the case.

Chapter 16

Common short cases

The trouble with doctors is not that they don't know
enough, but that they don't see enough.
Corrigan (1802–80)

In the short cases, candidates may be asked to examine a system or a particular part of
the patient. Fifteen minutes is available for each case. Unlike the approach of the MRCP
clinical exams, 'spot' diagnoses alone are not likely to be asked for by the examiners.
The following pages outline a system for examining major short-case possibilities. Use
this information to help develop your own system. Many useful lists are also included
in this section.

We have also provided examples of typical X-rays and scans related to particular
short-case examinations. At the end of each short-case discussion the examiners will often
ask: 'What investigations might be helpful in this case?', and in many cases X-rays, CT
scans or MRI scans will be indicated and available for you to look at and comment on.

Before you touch the patient, always wash your hands. After completing your examination, do the same. In all cases, before beginning a specific examination you should stand
back for a moment and carefully observe the patient. It is still important to look for an
associated 'spot' diagnosis, such as peripheral neuropathy in a myxoedematous patient
or aortic regurgitation in a patient with Marfan's syndrome.

The patient will normally be positioned and undressed ready for you to examine.
However, if either positioning or undressing is unsatisfactory, correct it. Ask the bulldog
or examiners for help. Remember that if you feel an irresistible urge to examine the
heart of a patient whose hands you have examined for rheumatoid arthritis and the
patient is in a chair and wearing several layers of clothing, it is unlikely the examiners
want you to do this. Rather than attempt an unsatisfactory examination, say that you
would normally examine the heart and ask whether you can get the patient into bed
and remove his or her top. The examiners will usually say that there is no need for this
and ask whether there is anything else you would like to do.

All hospitals have different bed mechanisms and trying to work out how to adjust
the bed when you are anxious is not worth it.

THE CARDIOVASCULAR SYSTEM

The cardiovascular examination

> **HINT**
>
> Many candidates worry about where they should start the examination – with the hands or at the praecordium. It rarely matters, but if the instruction is to examine the chest you should do that first. Otherwise, you can start with the hands, but this must be done quickly and efficiently. Some candidates take so long on the periphery that they scarcely have time to examine the praecordium.

Common stems

There are not many unless the examiners feel particularly imaginative.

1. 'This patient has been short of breath. Please examine him or her.' (Consider any left-sided valvular lesion, hypertrophic cardiomyopathy (HCM), ventricular septal defect (VSD) or cardiac failure.)
2. 'This patient has been found to have a murmur on a pre-anaesthetic assessment. Please examine him or her.' (This could be anything, but is not likely to be severe as the patient seems asymptomatic.)
3. 'This patient has hypertension. Please examine him or her.' (Consider secondary causes of HT.)
4. 'This patient has peripheral oedema. Please examine him or her.' (Consider right heart problems and congestive cardiac failure (CCF) – start at the legs.)
5. 'This patient has been unwell and had recurrent fever. Please examine him or her.' (Suspect endocarditis.)
6. 'This patient has had a cardiac problem from infancy. Please examine him or her.' (Try to remain calm in the face of congenital heart disease.)
7. 'This patient has been noticed to have some dysmorphic features. Please examine his or her cardiovascular system.' (Look for Marfan's, Down's, Noonan's, etc.)
8. 'Please examine this patient's cardiovascular system'. This is increasingly the stem for asymptomatic cardiac cases.

Method (Table 16.1)

1. Make sure the patient is positioned at 45° and that his or her chest and neck are fully exposed. For a woman, the requirements of modesty dictate that you cover her breasts with a towel or loose garment.
2. While standing back, inspect for the appearance of Marfan's, Turner's or Down syndrome. Also look for dyspnoea and cyanosis. It is also worth looking from a distance at the neck. Big *v* waves are sometimes more obvious from a distance.

> **HINT**
>
> Struggling unsuccessfully with an unfamiliar blood pressure cuff looks very bad – especially when the incorrectly placed cuff crackles and then bursts as you inflate it. Practise taking the blood pressure quickly with different sphygmomanometers.

Table 16.1 Cardiovascular system examination

Lying at 45°

1. GENERAL INSPECTION

Marfan's, Turner's, Down syndrome

Rheumatological disorders – ankylosing spondylitis (aortic regurgitation)

Acromegaly, etc.

Dyspnoea

2. HANDS

Radial pulses – right and left

Radiofemoral delay (if indicated)

Clubbing

Signs of infective endocarditis – splinter haemorrhages, Osler's nodes, etc.

Peripheral cyanosis

Xanthomata

3. BLOOD PRESSURE

4. FACE

Eyes:

Cornea: arcus cornea

Sclerae: pallor, jaundice

Pupils: Argyll Robertson (aortic regurgitation)

Xanthelasma

Malar flush (mitral stenosis, pulmonary stenosis)

Mouth:

Cyanosis

Palate (high arched – Marfan's)

Dentition

5. NECK

Jugular venous pressure:

Central venous pressure height

Wave form (especially large v waves)

Carotids:

Pulse character

6. PRAECORDIUM

Inspect:

Scars – whole chest, back

Deformity

Apex beat – position, character

Abnormal pulsations

Palpate:

Apex beat – position, character

Thrills

Abnormal impulses

Note: Beware of dextrocardia

Auscultate:

Heart sounds

Murmurs

Position patient left lateral position sitting forward (forced expiratory apnoea)

Note: Palpate for thrills again on positioning

Dynamic auscultation:

Respiratory phases

Valsalva manoeuvre

Exercise (isometric, e.g. handgrip)

Sitting forwards

7. BACK

Scars, deformity

Sacral oedema

Pleural effusion (percuss)

Left ventricular failure (auscultate)

Lying flat – 1 pillow only

8. ABDOMEN

Palpate liver (pulsatile, etc.), spleen, aorta

Percuss for ascites (right heart failure)

Femoral arteries – palpate, auscultate

9. LEGS

Clubbing toes

Cyanosis, cold limbs, trophic changes, ulceration (peripheral vascular disease)

All peripheral pulses

Oedema

Xanthomata

Calf tenderness

10. OTHER

Urine analysis (infective endocarditis)

Fundi (endocarditis)

Temperature chart (endocarditis)

3. Pick up the patient's hand. While feeling the radial pulse, ask whether you may take the blood pressure. The examiners will usually expect you to take the blood pressure.

Inspect the patient's hands for clubbing. Demonstrate Schamroth's sign (Fig. 16.1) to the delight of the examiners. If there is no clubbing, opposition of the index finger (nail to nail) demonstrates a diamond shape; in clubbing this space is lost. Also look for the peripheral stigmata of infective endocarditis. Splinter haemorrhages are common (and are usually caused by trauma), whereas Osler's nodes and Janeway lesions (Fig. 16.2) are rare (don't waste too much time searching for them). Look quickly, but

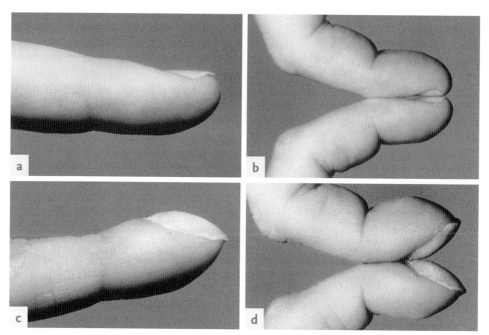

Figure 16.1 Lateral views of the index finger and Schamroth's sign in a healthy individual (a) and (b), and in an individual with severe clubbing (c) and (d).

L M Taussig, L I Landau. *Pediatric respiratory medicine*, 2nd edn. Fig 10-3. Mosby, Elsevier, 2008, with permission.

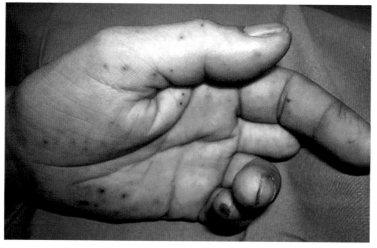

Figure 16.2 Janeway lesions.

Based on G L Mandell, J A Bennett, R Dolin. *Mandell, Douglas, and Bennett's principles and practice of infectious diseases*, 7th edn. Fig 195–15. Churchill Livingstone, Elsevier, 2009, with permission.

carefully, at each nail bed, otherwise it is easy to miss key signs. Note the presence of an intravenous cannula and, if an infusion is running, look at the bag to see what it is. There will usually be a peripheral or central line in situ if the patient is being treated for infective endocarditis. Note any tendon xanthomata (type II hyperlipidaemia).

4. The pulse at the wrist should be timed for rate and rhythm. Pulse character is poorly assessed here. This is also the time to feel for radiofemoral delay (which occurs in coarctation of the aorta) and radial–radial inequality.

> **HINT**
>
> Radiofemoral delay should be assessed very quickly or not at all, unless the stem suggests the patient has hypertension (or you find hypertension when taking the blood pressure).

5. Next inspect the face. Look at the eyes briefly for jaundice (valve haemolysis) and xanthelasma (type II or III hyperlipidaemia) (Fig. 16.3). You may also notice the classic 'mitral facies' (due to dilatation of malar capillaries associated with severe mitral stenosis and caused by pulmonary hypertension and a low cardiac output). Then inspect the mouth using a torch for a high-arched palate (Marfan's syndrome and the possibility of aortic regurgitation and mitral valve prolapse), petechiae and the state of dentition (endocarditis). Look at the tongue or lips for central cyanosis.

6. The neck is very important, so take time to examine here. The jugular venous pressure (JVP) must be assessed for height and character (Table 16.2 and Fig. 16.4). Use the right internal jugular vein to assess this. Look for a rise with inspiration (Kussmaul's sign).

7. Now feel each carotid pulse separately (never together). Assess the pulse character (Table 16.3).

8. Proceed to the chest. Look *everywhere* for scars. Previous mitral valvotomy may have been performed by a submammary or lateral thoracotomy approach. These patients slowly redevelop mitral stenosis over many years. Inspect for deformity, the site of the apex beat and visible pulsations. Do not forget about pacemaker and cardioverter-defibrillator boxes (Figs 16.5 and 16.6).

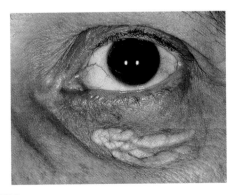

Figure 16.3 Xanthelasma.

M Yanoff, J S Duker. *Ophthalmology*, 3rd edn. Fig 12-9-18. Mosby, Elsevier, 2008, with permission.

Table 16.2 **Jugular venous pressure**

1. Wave form
   a. Causes of dominant *a* wave:
      i. tricuspid stenosis (also causes a slow y descent) (very rare)
      ii. pulmonary stenosis
      iii. pulmonary hypertension
   b. Causes of dominant *v* wave:
      i. tricuspid regurgitation (important and common)
   c. Causes of cannon *a* waves:
      i. complete heart block
      ii. paroxysmal nodal tachycardia with retrograde atrial conduction
      iii. ventricular tachycardia with retrograde atrial conduction or atrioventricular dissociation

2. Causes of an elevated central venous pressure:
   a. right ventricular failure
   b. tricuspid stenosis or regurgitation
   c. pericardial effusion or constrictive pericarditis
   d. superior vena caval obstruction
   e. fluid overload
   f. hyperdynamic circulation (e.g. fever, anaemia, thyrotoxicosis, arteriovenous fistula, pregnancy, exercise, beri beri, hypoxia, hypercapnia)

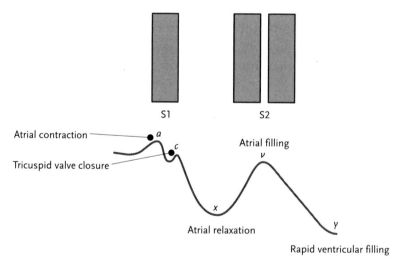

Figure 16.4 **The JVP and its relationship to the first (S1) and second (S2) heart sounds.**

Table 16.3 **Arterial pulse character**	
Anacrotic	Small volume, slow upstroke, plus *a* wave on the upstroke. Cause: aortic stenosis
Plateau	Slow upstroke. Cause: aortic stenosis
Bisferiens	Anacrotic plus collapsing. Cause: aortic stenosis plus aortic regurgitation
Collapsing	Cause: aortic regurgitation, hyperdynamic circulation, arteriosclerotic aorta (in elderly patients particularly), patent ductus arteriosus, peripheral arteriovenous aneurysm
Small volume	Cause: aortic stenosis, pericardial effusion
Alternans	Alternating strong and weak beats. Cause: left ventricular failure

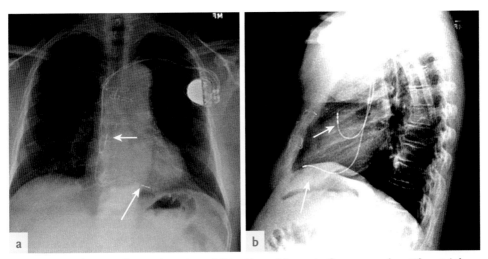

Figure 16.5 **Chest radiographs (a) and (b), PA and lateral of a pacemaker. The atrial pacing lead (top arrows) and the ventricular pacing lead (lower arrows) are smaller in diameter and less radiopaque than the leads associated with an ICD (see Fig 16.6).**

P E Parson, J P Wiener-Kronish. *Critical care secrets*, 5th edn. Figs 18.2a and b. Mosby, Elsevier, 2013, with permission.

HINT

Mitral valvotomy scars (under the left or right breast) can be quite lateral and easily missed (with ghastly repercussions in the test).

---

9. Palpate for the apex beat position. Be seen to count down the correct number of intercostal spaces. The normal position is the fifth intercostal space, 1 cm medial to the midclavicular line. The character of the apex beat is important. There are a number of types:
   a. A *pressure-loaded* (hyperdynamic, systolic-overloaded) apex beat is a forceful and sustained impulse (e.g. in aortic stenosis (AS), hypertension).
   b. A *volume-loaded* (hyperkinetic, diastolic-overloaded) apex beat is a forceful but unsustained impulse (e.g. in aortic regurgitation, mitral regurgitation).
   Don't miss the tapping apex beat of mitral stenosis (a palpable first heart sound) or the dyskinetic apex beat caused by a previous large myocardial infarction. The double or triple apical impulse in hypertrophic cardiomyopathy is very important too. Feel also for an apical thrill and time it.
10. Palpate with the heel of your hand for a left parasternal impulse, which indicates right ventricular hypertrophy or left atrial enlargement. Now feel at the base of the heart for a palpable pulmonary component of the second heart sound (P2) and aortic thrills. Percussion is usually unnecessary.
11. Auscultation begins with listening in the mitral area with both the bell and the diaphragm. Spend most time here. Listen for each component of the cardiac cycle separately. Identify the first and second heart sounds (Table 16.4) and decide whether they are of normal intensity and whether they are split. Now listen for extra heart

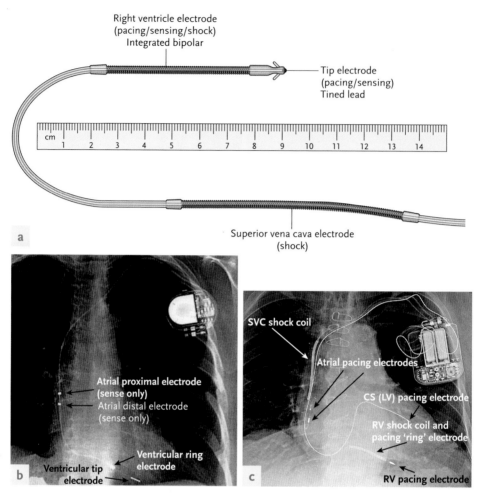

Figure 16.6 **Pacemaker. A conventional single lead pacemaker, an implantable cardioverter-defibrillator (ICD), and a right ventricular (RV) defibrillator lead. (a) Conventional pacemaker with one quadripolar lead that provides atrial and ventricular sensing and ventricular pacing. (b) Defibrillator system with biventricular pacing capability. Note the three leads: a conventional bipolar lead to the right atrium, a multipolar lead to the right ventricle, and a unipolar lead to the coronary sinus (CS). The bipolar lead in the right atrium will perform both sensing and pacing function. Likewise, the tip electrode in the right ventricle along with the shock coil performs RV pacing and sensing function. (c) Integrated bipolar RV defibrillator lead. The tip of this lead becomes enmeshed in the RV trabeculae (called a 'tined' lead) rather than engaging the myocardial wall with a screw ('active fixation').**

R D Miller. *Miller's anesthesia*, 7th edn. Fig 43-1. Churchill Livingstone, Elsevier, 2010, with permission.

Table 16.4 Heart sounds

FIRST HEART SOUND (S1)
Loud – mitral stenosis, tricuspid stenosis, tachycardia, hyperdynamic circulation
Soft – mitral regurgitation, calcified mitral valve, left bundle branch block, first-degree heart block

SECOND HEART SOUND (S2)
Aortic (A2)
Loud – congenital aortic stenosis, systemic hypertension
Soft – calcified aortic valve, aortic regurgitation (when the leaflets cannot coapt)
Pulmonary (P2)
Loud – pulmonary hypertension
Soft – pulmonary stenosis
Increased normal splitting (wider on inspiration)
Right bundle branch block, pulmonary stenosis, ventricular septal defect, mitral regurgitation (earlier A2)
Fixed splitting
Atrial septal defect
Reversed splitting (P2 first)
Left bundle branch block, aortic stenosis (severe), coarctation of aorta, patent ductus arteriosus (large)

THIRD HEART SOUND (S3)
Mechanism: possibly tautening of the mitral or tricuspid cusps at the end of rapid diastolic filling
Causes
Left ventricular third heart sound (S3) (louder at apex and on expiration)
Physiological (under 40 years of age or during pregnancy), left ventricular failure, aortic regurgitation, mitral regurgitation, ventricular septal defect, patent ductus arteriosus
Right ventricular third heart sound (S3) (louder at left sternal edge and on inspiration)
Right ventricular failure, constrictive pericarditis

FOURTH HEART SOUND (S4)
Mechanism: a high atrial pressure wave is probably reflected back from a poorly compliant ventricle; is always abnormal
Causes
Left ventricular fourth heart sound
Aortic stenosis, acute mitral regurgitation, systemic hypertension, ischaemic heart disease, hypertrophic cardiomyopathy
Right ventricular fourth heart sound
Pulmonary hypertension, pulmonary stenosis

or prosthetic heart sounds (see Table 16.4) and murmurs (Table 16.5). Mechanical valves include bileaflet, ball case and tilting disc. Ball case valves have a sharp opening sound and may rattle. Tilting disc valves have soft opening sounds and sharp closing sounds. All mechanical valves require anticoagulation. Biological valves may have a systolic murmur; anticoagulation is not required. Do not be satisfied at having identified one abnormality. However, remember that it is quite common to get simple rather than complex lesions in the examination.

12. Repeat the approach at the left sternal edge and then at the base of the heart (aortic and pulmonary areas). Time each part of the cycle with the carotid pulse. Listen below the left clavicle for a patent ductus arteriosus murmur, which may be audible here and nowhere else.

13. It is now time to reposition the patient, first in the left lateral position. Again feel the apex beat for character (particularly for tapping). Auscultate carefully for mitral stenosis with the bell. Next sit the patient forward and feel for thrills (with the patient in full expiration) at the left sternal edge and base. Then listen in those areas, particularly for aortic regurgitation.

Table 16.5 Differential diagnosis of murmurs	
Pansystolic	Mitral regurgitation, tricuspid regurgitation, ventricular septal defect, aortopulmonary shunts
Midsystolic	Aortic stenosis, pulmonary stenosis, hypertrophic cardiomyopathy, pulmonary flow murmur of an atrial septal defect
Early systolic	Ventricular septal defect (either very small, or large plus pulmonary hypertension), acute mitral regurgitation, tricuspid regurgitation
Late systolic	Mitral valve prolapse, papillary muscle dysfunction (e.g. hypertrophic cardiomyopathy)
Early diastolic	Aortic regurgitation, pulmonary regurgitation
Mid-diastolic	Mitral stenosis, tricuspid stenosis, atrial myxoma, Austin Flint murmur of aortic regurgitation, Carey Coombs murmur of acute rheumatic fever
Presystolic	Mitral stenosis, tricuspid stenosis, atrial myxoma
Continuous[a]	Patent ductus arteriosus Arteriovenous fistula (coronary artery, pulmonary, systemic), dialysis fistula Venous hum (situated over the right supraclavicular fossa and abolished by ipsilateral compression of the internal jugular vein) Rupture of a sinus of Valsalva into the right atrium or ventricle Aortopulmonary connection (e.g. Blalock shunt) 'Mammary soufflé' (in late pregnancy or early postpartum period)

[a]Aortic stenosis and aortic regurgitation or mitral stenosis and mitral regurgitation may be confused with a continuous murmur.

14. Dynamic auscultation should always be done if there is any doubt about the diagnosis. The Valsalva manoeuvre should be performed whenever there is a systolic murmur, otherwise hypertrophic cardiomyopathy is easily missed (p. 433).

HINT

A patient who seems familiar with the Valsalva manoeuvre may well have a murmur affected by it.

15. The patient is now sitting up. Percuss the back quickly to exclude a pleural effusion (e.g. due to left ventricular failure) and auscultate for inspiratory crackles (indicate left ventricular failure). If there is radiofemoral delay, also listen for a coarctation murmur here. Feel for sacral oedema and note any back deformity (e.g. ankylosing spondylitis (p. 513) with aortic regurgitation).

16. Next lay the patient flat and examine the abdomen properly (p. 460) for hepatomegaly (e.g. as a result of right ventricular failure) and a pulsatile liver (a reliable sign of tricuspid regurgitation). Perform the abdominojugular reflux test. Press over the upper abdomen for 10 seconds or so and watch for a rise in the JVP (abnormal if > 4 cm elevation for the duration of compression). This is a reliable sign of heart failure. Feel for splenomegaly (endocarditis) and an aortic aneurysm. Palpate both femoral arteries. Then examine all the peripheral pulses. Look particularly for peripheral oedema, clubbing of the toes, Achilles tendon xanthomata (Fig. 16.7), signs of peripheral vascular disease and the stigmata of infective endocarditis.

17. At the end, ask the examiners for the results of the urine analysis (haematuria in endocarditis) and a temperature chart (fever in endocarditis), and examine the fundi (for Roth's spots (Fig. 16.8) in endocarditis and for hypertensive changes).

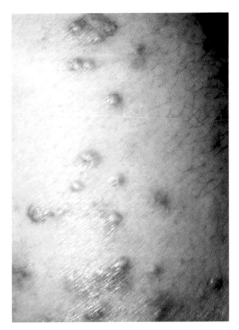

Figure 16.7 **Xanthomata.**

P Durrington. Dyslipidaemia, Reprinted with permission from Elsevier (*The Lancet*, 2003, vol no 362 (9385):717–31).

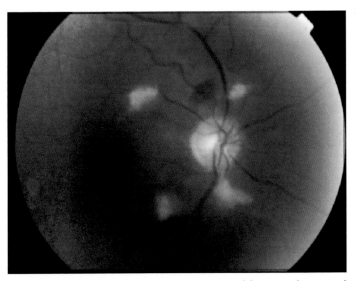

Figure 16.8 **A retina showing cotton-wool spots, retinal haemorrhage and Roth's spot in a septic bactereamic cancer patient.**

I Celik, M Cihangiroflu, T Yilmaz. The prevalence of bacteriaemia-related retinal lesions in seriously ill patients. *Journal of Infection* 2006; 52(2):97–104, Fig 1, with permission.

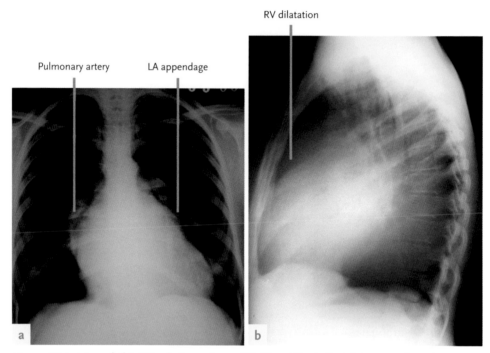

Figure 16.9 (a) and (b) Mitral stenosis on PA film. The left atrial appendage is dilated and there are prominent pulmonary arteries. The heart appears enlarged because of right ventricular enlargement, which is more obvious on the lateral film.

Figures reproduced courtesy of The Canberra Hospital.

Notes

1. It is fairly unlikely that you will have time to complete all aspects of your examination. If you are stopped, mention the list of things you would still like to do that are particularly relevant.
2. If you have auscultated and there is nothing obvious at first, consider the following and exclude them:
   a. mitral stenosis (Fig. 16.9) (position and exercise if necessary)
   b. atrial septal defect (ASD) (listen carefully for fixed splitting)
   c. mitral valve prolapse (perform a Valsalva manoeuvre)
   d. pulmonary hypertension (see below)
   e. constrictive pericarditis.

Notes on valve diseases

After you have made a diagnosis of a valve lesion, the following are the types of facts you should know. An assessment of the lesion's severity is usually required.

Candidates should be able to make some recommendation as to appropriate follow-up. Most patients with valve abnormalities should be reviewed regularly and have repeat echocardiograms. For patients with mild abnormalities about every 3–4 years is sufficient, but for more severe cases an annual review is usually recommended. Patients who are not symptomatic but have severe disease may need a 6-monthly review, usually with a repeat echocardiogram. Patients should be advised to return for earlier review if symptoms (e.g. dyspnoea, chest pain or exertional dizziness) occur.

Mitral stenosis

Valve area: normal, 4–6 cm^2; severe mitral stenosis, < 1 cm^2.

CAUSES

1. Rheumatic (in women more often than men).
2. Severe mitral annular calcification (sometimes associated with hypercalcaemia and hyperparathroidism (rare).
3. After mitral valve repair for mitral regurgitation (rare).

CLINICAL SIGNS OF SEVERITY

1. Small pulse pressure.
2. Early-opening snap (due to raised left atrial pressure).
3. Length of the mid-diastolic rumbling murmur (persists as long as there is a gradient).
4. Diastolic thrill at the apex (rare).
5. Presence of pulmonary hypertension, the signs of which are:
   a. prominent *a* wave in the JVP (only if the patient is in sinus rhythm)
   b. right ventricular impulse
   c. loud pulmonary component of the second heart sound (P2); a palpable P2 is more helpful
   d. pulmonary regurgitation
   e. tricuspid regurgitation.

RESULTS OF INVESTIGATIONS

1. ECG:
   a. *P* mitrale in sinus rhythm
   b. atrial fibrillation (a sign of chronicity)
   c. right ventricular systolic overload (severe disease)
   d. right axis deviation (severe disease).
2. Chest X-ray film (see Fig. 16.9):
   a. mitral valve calcification
   b. big left atrium:
      i. double left atrial shadow
      ii. displaced left main bronchus
      iii. big left atrial appendage
   c. signs of pulmonary hypertension:
      i. large central pulmonary arteries
      ii. pruned peripheral arterial tree
   d. signs of cardiac failure.

Note: If the investigations suggest that left ventricular dilatation is present in the presence of a mitral stenosis murmur, consider these other possibilities:
- associated mitral regurgitation
- associated aortic valve disease
- associated hypertension
- associated ischaemic heart disease.

Echocardiograph (M mode, two-dimensional (2D) Doppler and colour flow mapping)

The posterior mitral leaflet maintains its anterior position in diastole and this is pathognomonic. On 2D scanning the valve can be seen doming in diastole. The mitral valve area can be quite accurately determined by 2D echocardiography and Doppler measurements. The valve area is estimated using the pressure half-time measurement. This analysis of Doppler left ventricular inflow is performed routinely when mitral stenosis is suspected. Colour flow mapping makes finding the inflow jet easier and is very sensitive for the detection of any associated mitral regurgitation.

INDICATIONS FOR SURGERY

Exertional dyspnoea and falling valve area (when the valve area falls to about 1 cm^2) with signs of increasing right heart pressures are the usual indications for surgery. It should usually be performed before pulmonary oedema or major haemoptysis has occurred (when the valve area falls to about 1 cm^2).

Mitral regurgitation

CAUSES – CHRONIC

1. Degenerative disease.
2. Mitral valve prolapse.
3. Rheumatic (men more often than women) – rarely is mitral regurgitation the only murmur present.
4. Papillary muscle dysfunction:
   a. left ventricular failure
   b. ischaemia.
5. Connective tissue disease – rheumatoid arthritis, ankylosing spondylitis.
6. Congenital – endocardial cushion defect (including primum atrial septal defect and cleft mitral leaflet), parachute valve, corrected transposition.

CAUSES – ACUTE

1. Infective endocarditis (perforation of anterior leaflet), rupture of a myxomatous cord.
2. Myocardial infarction (chordae rupture or papillary muscle dysfunction).
3. Trauma

CLINICAL SIGNS OF SEVERITY

1. Enlarged left ventricle.
2. Pulmonary hypertension (a late sign).

3. Third heart sound (not always present).
4. Early diastolic rumble.
5. Soft first heart sound.
6. Aortic component of second heart sound (A2) is earlier.
7. Small-volume pulse (very severe).
8. Left ventricular failure.

RESULTS OF INVESTIGATIONS
1. ECG:
   a. *P* mitrale
   b. atrial fibrillation
   c. left ventricular diastolic overload
   d. right axis deviation.
2. Chest X-ray film:
   a. large (sometimes gigantic) left atrium
   b. increased left ventricular size
   c. mitral annular calcification (not always associated with significant MR)
   d. pulmonary hypertension (much less common).
3. Echocardiography (see Fig. 16.10) – this will give information about the possible aetiology, the severity and any associated valve or structural abnormalities:
   a. thickened leaflets – rheumatic aetiology
   b. prolapsing leaflet(s)
   c. left atrial size (a sign of chronicity and severity)
   d. left ventricular size and function (chronic MR cannot really be severe if the LV is not dilated)
   e. Doppler detection of the regurgitant jet in the left atrium; colour mapping of jet size and detection of reversal of flow in the pulmonary veins. Width of the vena contracta in the left atrium. Estimation of RV systolic pressure from TR jet velocity.
   f. other abnormalities (e.g. aortic valve disease as a result of rheumatic carditis or an ASD associated with mitral valve prolapse)
   g. calcification of the mitral annulus – common in elderly people. *Note:* the valve leaflets may not appear abnormal.
   h. Stress echocardiography may show a failure of the ejection fraction to increase during exercise (contractile reserve) in patients with severe MR.

INDICATIONS FOR SURGERY
In chronic mitral regurgitation, consider surgery if there are class III or IV symptoms, or if there is left ventricular dysfunction or the left ventricular dimensions have increased progressively. In acute mitral regurgitation, operate if there is haemodynamic collapse (there usually is). Repair of a prolapsing posterior and often anterior leaflet is now undertaken earlier than valve replacement. The short- and long-term results (1% recurrence per year) are so good that the operation should be recommended for even mild symptoms or once left ventricular dilatation occurs. Mitral valve replacement is usually with a mechanical valve. Tissue valves in the mitral position have a relatively short life (sometimes only 5–7 years).

Mitral valve prolapse (systolic click–murmur syndrome)
This is the most common heart lesion in the community (3% of adults) and is more common in women. When it occurs in men, it is more likely to progress to cause significant regurgitation.

Echocardiography Report

Reason for study: Middle and late systolic murmur ?MVP

Study quality: <u>Good</u>   Satisfactory   Poor

RV	18	(mm)	(N 10–26)
Sept.	8	(mm)	(N 7–11)
LVEDD	63	(mm)	(N 36–56)
LVESD	28	(mm)	(N 20–40)
LVPW	10	(mm)	(N 7–11)
Aorta	22	(mm)	(N 20–35)
LA	46	(mm)	(N 24–40)
FS	55	%	(N 27–40)
EF	85	%	(N 55–70)

Valves

Mitral   MR, prolapse posterior MV leaflet

Tricus.   Trivial TR

Aortic   Thickened, not stenosed

Pulm.   Appears normal

Doppler – 2D

The left ventricle is dilated. LV systolic function is preserved. LA is dilated. Severe prolapse of posterior MV leaflet. Possible flail segment.

Doppler – colour flow mapping

There is a large jet of mitral regurgitation extending into the left atrium.

Conclusions

Severe MR, possible flail mitral valve segment, severe MVP.

Comment

The echocardiography criteria for MVP have been tightened over the last several years. Redundancy of one or both of the MV leaflets is common and probably represents a variation of normal in many cases. Bowing of the leaflet into the left atrium of at least 1 cm must be present before the diagnosis of MVP can be made. In this case, the posterior leaflet appears very abnormal and seems to move into the left atrium in an unrestrained fashion. This suggests its chordal attachment may have been severed. The chords may be involved in the abnormality of the mitral leaflets in patients with prolapse and are at risk of rupture.

The left ventricle is dilated, suggesting that the mitral regurgitation is of haemodynamic significance. Left ventricular ejection remains high in cases of mitral regurgitation until late in the illness. This is because the left ventricular afterload is low. Part of the left ventricular ejection is into the left atrium, which is a low-resistance chamber.

The left atrial enlargement, present here, suggests that some mitral regurgitation has been present for some time. A large left atrium pleases the cardiac surgeons who have trouble getting their hands into the mitral valve through a normal-sized atrium.

Key

EF = ejection fraction; FS = fractional shortening; LA = left atrium; LV = left ventricle; LVEDD = left ventricular end-diastolic dimension; LVESD = left ventricular end-systolic dimension; LVPW = left ventricular posterior wall; MR = mitral regurgitation; MV = mitral valve; MVP = mitral valve prolapse; Pulm. = pulmonary; RV = right ventricle; Sept. = septal thickness; TR = tricuspid regurgitation; Tricus. = tricuspid.

Figure 16.10 Echocardiography report in a patient with mitral regurgitation and mitral valve prolapse.

DYNAMIC AUSCULTATION

The click murmur is affected by the:

1. Valsalva manoeuvre (decreases preload) – murmur longer, click earlier
2. handgrip (increases afterload) or squatting (increases preload) – murmur shorter.

ECHOCARDIOGRAPHY

There is now thought to be a considerable variation in the normal range of the appearance of the mitral leaflets on echocardiography. Some redundancy of one or both leaflets is commonly seen in normal people. Prolapse of a leaflet of 1 cm or more into the left atrium behind the attachment point of the valve is considered abnormal. Antibiotic prophylaxis, however, is not necessary for these patients unless mitral regurgitation is detected on Doppler interrogation.

ASSOCIATIONS

1. Marfan's syndrome.
2. ASD (secundum).

COMPLICATIONS (MORE COMMON FOR MEN WITH MITRAL VALVE PROLAPSE)

1. Mitral regurgitation.
2. Infective endocarditis.
    Arrhythmias, embolism and sudden death are probably not complications of mitral valve prolapse.

Aortic regurgitation

CAUSES OF CHRONIC AORTIC REGURGITATION

Valvular

1. Rheumatic (rarely the only murmur in this case).
2. Congenital (e.g. bicuspid valve; VSD – an associated prolapse of the aortic cusp is not uncommon).
3. Seronegative arthropathy, especially ankylosing spondylitis.

Aortic root (murmur may be maximal at the right sternal border)

1. Marfan's syndrome.
2. Aortitis (e.g. seronegative arthropathies, rheumatoid arthritis, tertiary syphilis).
3. Dissecting aneurysm.
4. Old age.

CAUSES OF ACUTE AORTIC REGURGITATION

Note: Murmur may be soft because of increased left ventricular end-diastolic pressure.

1. Valvular – infective endocarditis.
2. Aortic root – Marfan's syndrome, hypertension, dissecting aneurysm.

CLINICAL SIGNS OF SEVERITY IN CHRONIC AORTIC REGURGITATION

1. Collapsing pulse.
2. Wide pulse pressure.
3. Length of the *decrescendo* diastolic murmur.
4. Third heart sound (left ventricular).
5. Soft aortic component of the second heart sound (A2).
6. Austin Flint murmur (a diastolic rumble caused by limitation to mitral inflow by the regurgitation jet).
7. Left ventricular failure.

HINT

A loud systolic murmur, rarely with a thrill, may be present in patients with severe aortic regurgitation without any associated organic aortic stenosis. The peripheral signs of aortic regurgitation are the clue that this is the real lesion in this situation.

RESULTS OF INVESTIGATIONS

1. ECG – left ventricular hypertrophy (diastolic overload).
2. Chest X-ray film:
   a. left ventricular dilatation
   b. aortic root dilatation or aneurysm (Fig. 16.11)
   c. valve calcification.
3. Echocardiography:
   a. left ventricular dimensions and function
   b. Doppler estimation of size of regurgitant jet
   c. vegetations (endocarditis can be a cause of acute aortic regurgitation)
   d. aortic root dimensions
   e. valve cusp thickening or prolapse (associated AS).

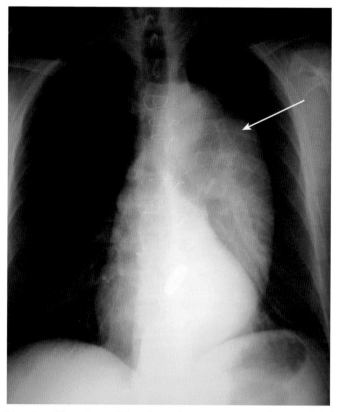

Figure 16.11 **Massive dilatation of the thoracic aorta (arrow) is seen in this patient with Marfan's syndrome and aortic regurgitation.**

Figure reproduced courtesy of The Canberra Hospital.

INDICATIONS FOR SURGERY

1. Symptoms – dyspnoea on exertion.
2. Worsening left ventricular function, such as low ejection fraction (in aortic regurgitation this is increased until late, severe disease intervenes).
3. Progressive left ventricular dilatation on serial echocardiograms – left ventricular end-systolic dimension of > 5.5 cm.

Aortic stenosis

Valve area: 1.5–2.0 cm^2. Significant stenosis at < 1 cm^2. In critical AS, less than 0.7 cm^2/m^2 or a valve gradient > 70 mmHg.

CAUSES

1. Degenerative senile calcific aortic stenosis (the most common cause in the elderly).
2. Rheumatic (rarely isolated).
3. Calcific bicuspid valve.

CLINICAL SIGNS OF SEVERITY

1. Plateau pulse.

HINT

The pulse character has been shown not to be useful in elderly patients; this fact may need to be put tactfully to the examiners.

2. Aortic thrill (very important sign of severe stenosis).
3. Length, harshness and lateness of the peak of the systolic murmur.
4. Fourth heart sound (S4).
5. Paradoxical splitting of the second heart sound (delayed left ventricular ejection and aortic valve closure).
6. Left ventricular failure (a late sign).

RESULTS OF INVESTIGATIONS

1. ECG – left ventricular hypertrophy (systolic overload).
2. Chest X-ray film (Fig. 16.12):
   a. left ventricular hypertrophy
   b. valve calcification.
3. Echocardiography (Fig. 16.13):
   a. Doppler estimation of gradient. (*Note:* Doppler estimation of peak gradient usually overestimates the value compared with cardiac catheterisation, Doppler mean gradient is more helpful.) Severe AS means a mean gradient of 40 mmHg or more
   b. calculation of valve area
   c. valve cusp mobility
   d. left ventricular hypertrophy
   e. left ventricular dysfunction.

INDICATIONS FOR SURGERY

1. Symptoms – exertional angina, exertional dyspnoea, exertional syncope (urgent).
2. Critical obstruction (based on catheterisation data) and severe left ventricular hypertrophy even if asymptomatic.

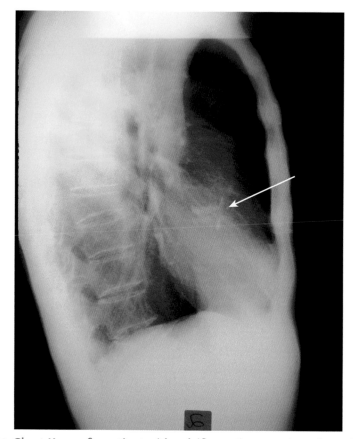

Figure 16.12 **Chest X-ray of a patient with calcific aortic stenosis; valve calcification is visible (arrow).**

Figure reproduced courtesy of The Canberra Hospital.

CHOICE OF VALVE

Tissue (bovine pericardial or porcine, or occasionally homograft) valves are usually offered to patients over the age of about 65 or to younger patients who wish to avoid warfarin. Their life expectancy before failing is up to 15 years or more. Transcatheter aortic valve replacement (TAVR) is increasingly used not only for patients too frail for surgery but for lower risk patients. This is a tissue valve.

Tricuspid regurgitation

Look for the following signs:
1. the JVP – large *v* waves: the JVP is elevated if right ventricular failure has occurred
2. palpation – right ventricular heave
3. auscultation – a pansystolic murmur, maximal at the lower end of the sternum and on inspiration, may be present, but the diagnosis can be made on the basis of the peripheral signs alone; multiple systolic clicks are characteristic of Ebstein's anomaly of the tricuspid valve
4. abdomen – a pulsatile, large and tender liver is usually present; ascites and oedema with pleural effusions may also occur.

Echocardiography Report

Reason for study: Systolic ejection murmur ?AS
Study quality: <u>Good</u>   Satisfactory   Poor

RV	13	(mm)	(N 10–26)
Sept.	13	(mm)	(N 7–11)
LVEDD	53	(mm)	(N 36–56)
LVESD	25	(mm)	(N 20–40)
LVPW	12	(mm)	(N 7–11)
Aorta	22	(mm)	(N 20–35)
LA	38	(mm)	(N 24–40)
FS	53	%	(N 27–40)
EF	83	%	(N 55–70)

Valves

Mitral	Trivial MR
Tricus.	Mild TR
Aortic	Thickened, calcified, reduced cusp movement
Pulm.	Appears normal

Doppler – 2D

There is mild symmetrical LV hypertrophy. The aortic valve is thickened and heavily calcified; it appears trileaflet. The mitral valve appears normal.

Doppler – colour flow mapping

The aortic outflow velocity is 4.6 m/s. The calculated peak aortic gradient is 85 mmHg. The mean gradient is 60 mmHg. Mild aortic regurgitation was detected. Mild MR is present. Mild TR. RV pressure = 24 mmHg.

Conclusions

Severe calcific aortic stenosis and mild LVH.

Comments

This echocardiography report gives considerable information about the patient's murmur. A candidate who had not diagnosed AS would be in some difficulty.

In AS the aortic valve is usually thickened and calcified unless the patient is young and has congenital AS. Stenosed aortic valves are often congenitally bicuspid and so the echocardiographer will often report the number of valve leaflets. Sometimes there is a comment about reduction in valve cusp movement. An almost immobile valve is more likely to be severely stenosed.

LVH is common when AS is significant. This LVH is mild; dimensions of 14 mm or more indicate severe LVH. Left ventricular dilatation and reduced fractional shortening are late signs.

Doppler measurement of the velocity of blood in the ascending aorta in systole allows calculation of the peak pressure difference across the valve (usually almost 0). This gradient tends to be higher than the gradient measured at cardiac catheterisation. The mean gradient is often closer to the catheter gradient.

Some AR is very often detected in the presence of significant AS. It is unlikely this mild AR would be audible and its presence on the report should not lead the candidate to panic.

Key

AR = aortic regurgitation; AS = aortic stenosis; EF = ejection fraction; FS = fractional shortening; LA = left atrium; LV = left ventricular; LVEDD = left ventricular end-diastolic dimension; LVESD = left ventricular end-systolic dimension; LVH = left ventricular hypertrophy; LVPW = left ventricular posterior wall; MR = mitral regurgitation; Pulm. = pulmonary; RV = right ventricle; Sept. = septal thickness; TR = tricuspid regurgitation; Tricus. = tricuspid.

Figure 16.13 **Echocardiography report for a patient with aortic stenosis.**

CAUSES

1. Functional (no disease of the valve leaflets) – right ventricular failure.
2. Rheumatic – only very rarely does tricuspid regurgitation occur alone; usually mitral valve disease is also present.
3. Infective endocarditis (right-sided endocarditis in intravenous drug abusers).
4. Congenital – Ebstein's anomaly.
5. Tricuspid valve prolapse (rare).
6. Right ventricular papillary muscle infarction.
7. Pacemaker or defibrillator lead.
8. Trauma (usually a steering-wheel injury to the sternum).

RESULTS OF INVESTIGATIONS

The chest X-ray film may show right ventricular enlargement or biventricular enlargement if the tricuspid regurgitation is secondary to heart failure. Patients with Ebstein's anomaly may have the characteristic box-shaped heart and narrow cardiac base (Fig. 16.14). Echocardiography enables detection of structural valve abnormality and estimation of

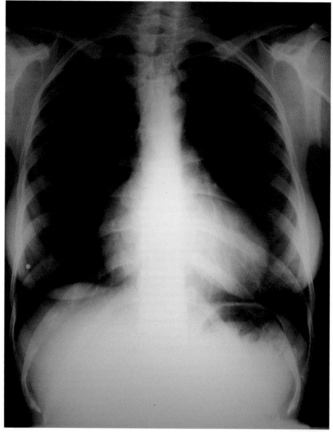

Figure 16.14 **Chest X-ray of a patient with Ebstein's anomaly, showing a narrow cardiac pedicle.**

Figure reproduced courtesy of The Canberra Hospital.

the size of the regurgitant jet in the right atrium. Measurement of the velocity of this jet allows estimation of the pressure gradient across the valve. As right atrial pressure is usually 5–10 mmHg, the right ventricular pressure can be estimated in any patient with tricuspid regurgitation by adding 5 to this pressure gradient. Trivial tricuspid regurgitation is a common and normal Doppler echocardiogram finding.

Pulmonary stenosis (in adults)

Look for the following signs:
1. General signs:
   a. peripheral cyanosis because of a low cardiac output
   b. the pulse – normal or reduced because of a low cardiac output
   c. the JVP – giant *a* waves because of right atrial hypertrophy; the JVP may be elevated
   d. palpation – right ventricular heave; thrill over the pulmonary area (common)
   e. auscultation – the murmur may be preceded by an ejection click; a harsh ejection systolic murmur maximal in the pulmonary area and on inspiration is present; S4 may be present (owing to right atrial hypertrophy)
   f. abdomen – presystolic pulsation of the liver may be present
2. Signs of severe pulmonary stenosis:
   a. an ejection systolic murmur peaking late in systole
   b. absence of an ejection click (also absent when the pulmonary stenosis is infundibular, i.e. below the valve level)
   c. presence of S4
   d. signs of right ventricular failure.

CAUSES
1. Congenital.
2. Carcinoid syndrome.

Chronic constrictive pericarditis

This is a difficult diagnosis; the clue is often that the patient appears cachectic and has ascites. Look for the following signs:
1. pulse and blood pressure – a low blood pressure and pulsus paradoxus are typical
2. JVP – this is raised; Kussmaul's sign is rare; the *x* and *y* descents are prominent
3. apex beat – impalpable
4. heart sounds – these are distant; there may be an early third heart sound and an early pericardial knock (as rapid ventricular filling is abruptly halted)
5. hepatosplenomegaly, ascites and oedema provide important clues
6. underlying aetiology (e.g. radiation, tumour, pericarditis after cardiac surgery (scar present), tuberculosis, connective tissue disease, chronic renal failure, trauma).

Hypertrophic cardiomyopathy

It is always important to consider this diagnosis – it is a popular 'trap'! The classical signs are as follows:
1. Pulse – this is typically sharp, rising and jerky, owing to rapid ejection by a hypertrophied ventricle early in systole, then followed by obstruction; it is not like the pulse of AS.
2. The JVP – there is a prominent *a* wave owing to forceful atrial contraction against a non-compliant ventricle.
3. Apex beat – there is typically a double or triple impulse owing to presystolic ventricular expansion following atrial contraction.

4. Auscultation:
   a. late systolic ejection murmur (left sternal edge)
   b. pansystolic murmur (apex) from mitral regurgitation
   c. fourth heart sound.
      Note: There are no diastolic murmurs.
5. Dynamic manoeuvres – the murmur is louder with the Valsalva manoeuvre, standing and isotonic exercise (e.g. jogging – not usually possible under examination conditions). The murmur is softer with squatting, raising the legs and isometric exercise (e.g. forceful handgrip).

RESULTS OF INVESTIGATIONS

1. ECG:
   a. left ventricular hypertrophy and lateral ST segment and T wave changes
   b. deep Q waves
   c. conduction defects.
2. Chest X-ray film:
   a. left ventricle enlarged with a hump along the border
   b. no valve calcification.
3. Echocardiography (Fig. 16.15):
   a. asymmetrical hypertrophy (ASH) of the ventricular septum
   b. systolic anterior motion (SAM) of the anterior mitral valve leaflet
   c. midsystolic closure of the aortic valve
   d. Doppler detection of mitral regurgitation
   e. Doppler estimation of the gradient in the left ventricular outflow tract (at rest and with the Valsalva manoeuvre).

Non-cyanotic congenital heart disease

These are difficult examination cases that not infrequently crop up in the test.

ATRIAL SEPTAL DEFECT

There are two types (sinus venosus defects are not often seen in adults): ostium secundum and ostium primum.

ASD: ostium secundum

This is the most common and presents in adult life with:
1. fixed splitting of the second heart sound (*Note:* Unfortunately, an ASD is still a possible diagnosis when some variation in splitting is detectable during the respiratory cycle.)
2. pulmonary systolic ejection murmur (increasing on inspiration)
3. pulmonary hypertension (late).

Results of investigations

1. ECG:
   a. right axis deviation
   b. right bundle branch block pattern
   c. right ventricular hypertrophy (systolic overload).
2. Chest X-ray film (Fig. 16.16):
   a. increased pulmonary vasculature
   b. enlarged right atrium and ventricle
   c. dilated main pulmonary artery
   d. small aortic knob.

Echocardiography Report

Reason for study: Systolic murmur, family history of hypertrophic cardiomyopathy

Study quality: <u>Good</u>   Satisfactory   Poor

RV	13	(mm)	(N 10–26)
Sept.	18	(mm)	(N 7–11)
LVEDD	54	(mm)	(N 36–56)
LVESD	30	(mm)	(N 20–40)
LVPW	10	(mm)	(N 7–11)
Aorta	22	(mm)	(N 20–35)
LA	40	(mm)	(N 24–40)
FS	44	%	(N 27–40)
EF	75	%	(N 55–70)

Valves

Mitral	Mild-to-moderate MR, SAM
Tricus.	Appears normal
Aortic	Appears normal
Pulm.	Appears normal

Doppler – 2D

There is asymmetrical septal hypertrophy. LV systolic function appears normal. LA upper limit of normal size.

Doppler – colour flow mapping

There is a gradient in the left ventricular outflow tract of 80 mmHg. Moderate MR jet – 1/2 LA.

Conclusions

Hypertrophic cardiomyopathy with LVOT gradient of 80 mmHg. Systolic anterior motion of anterior mitral valve leaflet. Moderate MR.

Comment

The typical echocardiograph findings in this condition are seen here. The septum is thicker than 11 mm and there is abnormal anterior movement of the anterior mitral valve leaflet in systole – SAM. This movement is, in part, responsible for any LVOT gradient. The LVOT gradient only correlates roughly with symptoms and prognosis in this condition. In some cases of hypertrophic cardiomyopathy there may be no LVOT gradient.

Key

EF = ejection fraction; FS = fractional shortening; LA = left atrium; LV = left ventricle; LVEDD = left ventricular end-diastolic dimension; LVESD = left ventricular end-systolic dimension; LVOT = left ventricular outflow tract; LVPW = left ventricular posterior wall; MR = mitral regurgitation; Pulm. = pulmonary; RV = right ventricle; SAM = systolic anterior motion; Sept. = septal thickness; Tricus. = tricuspid.

Figure 16.15 **Echocardiography report for a patient with hypertrophic cardiomyopathy.**

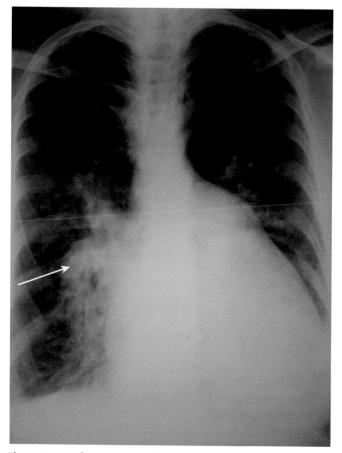

Figure 16.16 Chest X-ray of a patient with an ASD and right atrial and ventricular enlargement. The pulmonary arteries are very prominent (arrow).

Figure reproduced courtesy of The Canberra Hospital.

3. Echocardiography:
    a. paradoxical septal motion, right ventricular dilatation
    b. echo dropout in atrial septum
    c. Doppler detection of a shunt at the atrial level
    d. shunt (bubble) study using agitated saline
    e. transoesophageal echocardiogram.

Indication for surgery

Almost all ASDs need to be closed once RV dilatation has occurred. This can be done surgically or, if they are suitable, with a percutaneous closure device. A left-to-right shunt is measured to be at least 1.5 to 1 (unless there is reversal of the shunt) and is also an indication for closure. A nuclear cardiac shunt study may help estimation of the shunt size.

ASD: ostium primum

This is an endocardial cushion defect adjacent to the atrioventricular valves. The signs are the same as for ostium secundum, but associated mitral regurgitation, tricuspid regurgitation or VSD is common. The ECG is particularly helpful as there is left axis deviation and right bundle branch block (and sometimes a prolonged P–R interval). Look also for the presence of Down syndrome and skeletal upper limb defects (Holt–Oram syndrome).

VENTRICULAR SEPTAL DEFECT

The clues to the diagnosis of VSD are a thrill and a harsh pansystolic murmur confined to the left sternal edge. Sometimes mitral regurgitation is also present. Down syndrome is associated.

Results of investigations

The ECG and chest X-ray film may show left ventricular hypertrophy. The chest X-ray film may also show increased pulmonary vasculature and an enlarged right ventricle. The echocardiogram will show the defect and detect the shunt. Estimation of the pressure gradient between the ventricles will allow detection of right ventricular hypertension. As right ventricular pressure rises, the gradient across the defect falls (right ventricular pressure is closer to left ventricular) – a sign that the shunt is causing trouble.

Indication for percutaneous closure or surgery

Closure is indicated when the left-to-right shunt is moderate to large, with the pulmonary-to-systemic flow being > 1.5 to 1. Often the presence of right ventricular dilatation is taken as a sign that the shunt is large.

PATENT DUCTUS ARTERIOSUS

In patent ductus arteriosus (PDA) there is a vessel from the bifurcation of the pulmonary artery to the aorta. The shunt is usually from the aorta to the pulmonary artery. Reversal of the shunt leads to differential cyanosis and clubbing (of toes, *not* fingers). Often a continuous murmur is heard. Confusion with aortic stenosis and regurgitation commonly occurs when candidates examine these patients.

Results of investigations

1. The ECG may show left ventricular hypertrophy (diastolic overload).
2. The chest X-ray film may show:
   a. increased pulmonary vasculature
   b. calcification of the duct (trumpet-shaped calcification)
   c. an enlarged left ventricle.
3. Doppler echocardiography will demonstrate continuous flow in the main pulmonary artery. Left atrial size will be increased.

Indication for surgery

The indication for surgery or use of a closure device (surgery for this condition in adults is difficult and is now largely replaced by the use of percutaneous catheter closure devices) is the diagnosis of PDA with more than a trivial shunt (unless there is pulmonary hypertension).

HINT

The detection of a trivial shunt at echocardiography in a patient with a PDA but without a significant murmur or any symptoms is not an indication for closure.

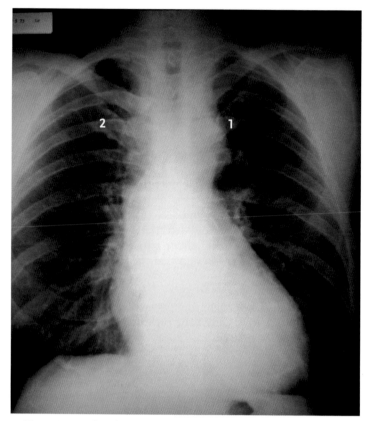

Figure 16.17 **Chest X-ray showing coarctation of the aorta. Note the small aortic knuckle (1) and rib notching (2).**

Figure reproduced courtesy of The Canberra Hospital.

COARCTATION OF THE AORTA

The most common site for this lesion is just distal to the origin of the left subclavian artery. Look for a better-developed upper body, radiofemoral delay, hypertension in the arms only, chest collateral vessels, a midsystolic murmur over the praecordium and back, and changes of hypertension in the fundi. Turner's syndrome may be associated in some cases.

Results of investigations
1. The ECG may show left ventricular hypertrophy (systolic overload).
2. The chest X-ray film (Fig. 16.17) may show:
   a. enlarged left ventricle
   b. enlarged left subclavian artery
   c. dilated ascending aorta
   d. aortic indentation
   e. aortic prestenotic and poststenotic dilatation
   f. rib notching – second to sixth ribs on the inferior border.
3. Echocardiography may show:
   a. left ventricular hypertrophy
   b. coarctation shelf in the descending aorta
   c. abnormal flow patterns in the same area.

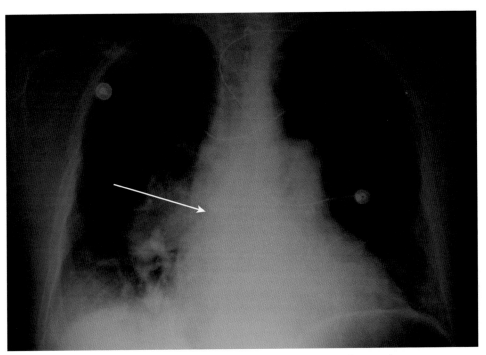

Figure 16.18 Chest X-ray of a patient with Eisenmenger's syndrome due to an untreated VSD: the pulmonary arteries are enormous centrally (arrow) but small in the periphery.

Figure reproduced courtesy of The Canberra Hospital.

Cyanotic congenital heart disease

This is a very difficult area. You probably will not be expected to identify the exact lesion. A cardiac cause should be suspected if the patient shows clubbing and cyanosis.

The common causes of the problem in adults are:

1. Eisenmenger's syndrome (see Fig. 16.18) – pulmonary hypertension plus a large communication between the left and right circulations (e.g. VSD, PDA, ASD)
2. tetralogy of Fallot
3. complex lesions – univentricular heart, Ebstein's anomaly (if there is an associated atrial septal defect with a right-to-left shunt).

You must decide while examining the patient whether pulmonary hypertension is present, as this distinguishes Eisenmenger's syndrome from the tetralogy of Fallot.

EISENMENGER'S SYNDROME

This syndrome may be found in older adults who had right-to-left shunting before the availability of open-heart surgery. The physical signs may include cyanosis, clubbing and polycythaemia. The JVP pattern may have a dominant *a* wave and sometimes a prominent *v* wave. A right ventricular heave and a palpable pulmonary component of the second heart sound (P2) may be found. On auscultation the S2 is normally single – there is persistent synchrony of A2 and P2. A fourth heart sound, a pulmonary ejection click, pulmonary regurgitation and, sometimes, tricuspid regurgitation may be present (but there may be no murmurs). The signs all add up to pulmonary hypertension in a cyanosed patient.

> **HINT**
>
> Despite traditional teaching, a loud P2 has little correlation with the presence of pulmonary hypertension, but a palpable P2 correlates well. It is said that a loud P2 is more a sign that a patient is thin than of anything else.

Results of investigations
1. The ECG may show:
   a. right ventricular hypertrophy
   b. *P* pulmonale.
2. The chest X-ray film (Fig. 16.18) may show:
   a. right ventricular and right atrial enlargement
   b. pulmonary artery prominence
   c. increased hilar vascular markings but attenuated peripheral vessels
   d. a heart that is *not* boot shaped.
3. Echocardiography will define the anatomy and enable measurement of pulmonary pressures.

TETRALOGY OF FALLOT

There are four features:
1. VSD
2. right ventricular outflow obstruction (which determines severity)
3. overriding aorta
4. right ventricular hypertrophy.

The physical signs may include cyanosis, clubbing, polycythaemia, a right ventricular heave and a thrill at the left sternal edge, but *not* cardiomegaly. On auscultation there may be a single second heart sound (A2) and a short pulmonary ejection murmur.

Results of investigations
1. The ECG may show:
   a. right ventricular hypertrophy
   b. right axis deviation.
2. The chest X-ray film (Fig. 16.19) may show:
   a. a normal-sized heart with a boot shape (i.e. a left concavity where the pulmonary artery is normally situated plus a prominent elevated apex)
   b. right ventricular enlargement
   c. decreased vascularity of lung vessels
   d. right-sided aortic knob, arch and descending aorta (25%).
3. Echocardiography will demonstrate the anatomical abnormalities.

The hypertensive examination

> **Common stem**
>
> 'This 30-year-old man has hypertension. Please examine him.'

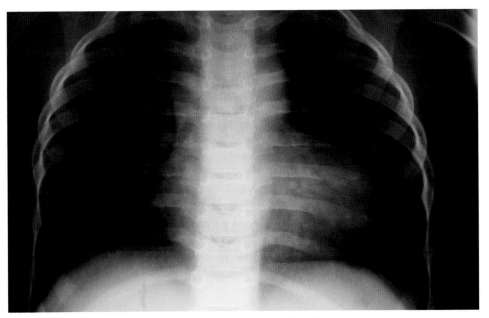

Figure 16.19 Chest X-ray of a child with tetralogy of Fallot.

Figure reproduced courtesy of The Canberra Hospital.

Method

1. Stand back and inspect the patient. Look for evidence of Cushing's syndrome, acromegaly, polycythaemia and uraemia (Table 16.6). If one of these is present, modify your examination appropriately.
2. Next, confirm that the blood pressure is elevated. Ask to measure it in both arms, and with the patient both lying and standing. Measurement in the legs in a young patient may be important.
3. Feel the radial pulse and very carefully feel for radiofemoral delay. Palpate for radial–radial asymmetry and inspect both hands for vasculitic changes.
4. Now look at the face. Inspect the conjunctivae for injection (polycythaemia), and then examine the fundi for hypertensive changes (Fig. 16.20). Describe what you see when presenting, rather than just giving a grade (Table 16.7).
5. Examine the rest of the cardiovascular system, looking especially for left ventricular failure and coarctation of the aorta. Usually a fourth heart sound is present in severe hypertension.
6. The abdomen should be examined for renal masses, adrenal masses and an abdominal aneurysm. Auscultate for renal bruits (as a result of fibromuscular dysplasia or atheroma). These may have a diastolic component. Listen first just to the right or left of the midline above the umbilicus. Then sit the patient up and listen in the flanks (a systolic–diastolic bruit in the costovertebral area suggests a renal arteriovenous fistula).
7. At the end, ask for the results of urine analysis (signs of renal disease). Also, remember that cerebrovascular accidents secondary to hypertension may cause other physical signs.

Table 16.6 Causes of hypertension		
ESSENTIAL (> 95%); SECONDARY (< 5%)		
Renal disease	Renovascular disease (renal artery atherosclerosis, fibromuscular disease, aneurysm, vasculitis)	
	Diffuse renal disease	
Endocrine	Conn's syndrome (primary aldosteronism), Cushing's syndrome (especially steroid treatment)	
	17- and 11-β-hydroxylase defects	
	Phaeochromocytoma	
	Acromegaly	
	Myxoedema	
	Contraceptive pill	
Coarctation of the aorta		
Other	Polycythaemia rubra vera	
	Toxaemia of pregnancy	
	Neurogenic (increased intracranial pressure, lead poisoning, acute intermittent porphyria)	
	Hypercalcaemia	
	Alcohol	
	Sleep apnoea	
Note: Alcohol consumption and obesity are associated with essential hypertension.		

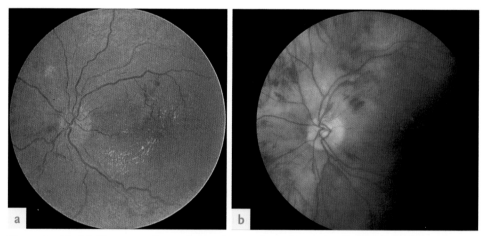

Figure 16.20 (a) Hypertensive retinopathy grade 3. Note the flame-shaped haemorrhages and cotton-wool spots. (b) Hypertensive retinopathy grade 4. Note AV nipping, silver wiring and papilloedema.

N Talley, S O'Connor, *Clinical examination*, 7th edn. Figs 7.4, 7.5. Elsevier Australia, 2013, with permission. Courtesy of Dr Chris Kennedy and Prof. Ian Constable. Copyright Lion's Eye Institute, Perth.

GRADE	CHANGES
Table 16.7 Fundoscopy changes in hypertension	
I	Silver wiring
II	Above change plus arteriovenous nipping
III	Above changes plus haemorrhages (characteristically flame-shaped) and exudates: soft exudates (also called cotton-wool spots) due to ischaemia, and hard exudates due to lipid residues from leaky vessels
IV	Above changes plus papilloedema

Marfan's syndrome

Common stem

'This 37-year-old man has a heart murmur. Please examine him.'

Method
Fortunately, you notice a Marfanoid habitus.
1. While performing your normal cardiovascular examination, look also for the following signs (and when reporting allude to the diagnostic criteria).
   a. *Hands and arms:* look for arachnodactyly (spider fingers) and joint hypermobility, as well as long, thin limbs.
   b. *Face:* you may notice a long and narrow face. Look for lens dislocation or lens replacement. The sclerae may be blue. Look in the mouth for a high-arched palate.
   c. *Chest:* note any pectus carinatum or excavatum.
   d. *Heart:* auscultate for aortic regurgitation and mitral valve prolapse. Also, look for the signs of dissecting aneurysm or coarctation of the aorta.
   e. *Back:* look for kyphoscoliosis and hypermobility.
2. At the end, always ask to measure the arm span, which will exceed the height. The upper segment to lower segment ratio will be less than 0.85 (the upper segment is from the crown to the symphysis pubis and the lower segment is from the symphysis pubis to the ground).

Investigations
1. Many of these patients will have had serial echocardiograms because the detection of progressive aortic root dilatation will warn of an increased risk of dissection before this occurs.
2. A slit-lamp examination may be required to diagnose lens dislocation.

Oedema

Common stem

'This man has oedema. Please assess him.'

Table 16.8 **Causes of oedema**
1. Drugs – calcium channel blockers
2. Cardiac – congestive cardiac failure, cor pulmonale, constrictive pericarditis
3. Renal – nephrotic syndrome (see Table 11.6, p. 315)
4. Hepatic – cirrhosis
5. Malabsorption or starvation
6. Protein-losing enteropathy
7. Myxoedema
8. Cyclical oedema

Method

1. First, stand back and look at the patient. Are there any clues if this is a cardiac, renal, liver or nutrition case?
2. Note whether the oedema is localised or generalised and whether it is gravitational or not.
3. Assess nutrition quickly (as hypoalbuminaemia and also beri beri due to vitamin B_1 deficiency[1] can cause oedema). Also, any obvious signs of myxoedema must never be missed.
4. If necessary, ask the patient to undress as appropriate and then further define the areas affected. Palpate for pitting. Proceed, depending on your findings (Table 16.8).

PITTING LOWER LIMB OEDEMA

1. Define the extent of the oedema.
2. Look for signs of DVT (2 cm difference in calf swelling, prominent superficial veins and increased warmth have minor diagnostic value; Homans' sign is unhelpful). Note the presence of varicose veins (a common cause of mild peripheral oedema) and of vein-harvesting scars (for coronary artery surgery).
3. Feel the inguinal nodes. Go to the abdomen and look for abdominal wall oedema, prominent abdominal wall veins (inferior vena caval obstruction), ascites, any abdominal masses and evidence of liver disease. A pulsatile liver (tricuspid regurgitation) or malignant involvement should be particularly sought.
4. Next, examine the JVP. Then examine for signs of right ventricular failure and constrictive pericarditis. Feel all the node groups.
5. Finally, examine for delayed ankle jerks (to exclude hypothyroidism) and look at the urine analysis. Remember that vasodilating drugs used for hypertension or angina are very common causes of oedema.

NON-PITTING LOWER LIMB OEDEMA

Consider the various causes, including lymphoedema (from malignant infiltration, congenital disease, filariasis, Milroy's disease) and myxoedema.

SUPERIOR VENA CAVAL OBSTRUCTION (TABLE 16.9, FIG. 16.21)

1. The patient may appear Cushingoid, from either a tumour or treatment with steroids. Note the plethoric cyanosed face with periorbital oedema. There may be exophthalmos and conjunctival injection.
2. Examine the pupils: a mass in the chest may have caused Horner's syndrome.

---

[1]Beri-Beri is rarely found in the exam.

Table 16.9 Causes of superior vena caval obstruction

1. Lung carcinoma (90%)
2. Retrosternal tumours – lymphoma, thymoma, dermoid
3. Retrosternal goitre
4. Massive mediastinal lymphadenopathy
5. Aortic aneurysm

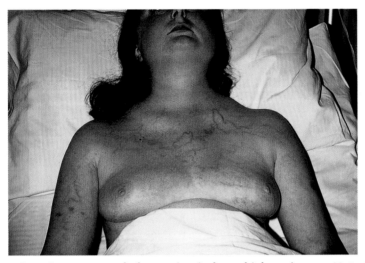

Figure 16.21 **Superior vena caval obstruction in bronchial carcinoma. Note the swelling of the face and neck and the development of collateral circulation in the veins of the chest wall.**

L Goldman, A I Schafer. *Goldman's Cecil medicine*, 24th edn. Fig 99.6. Elsevier, 2012, with permission.

3. Examine the fundi for venous dilatation. Examine the neck, which is enlarged. The JVP is raised, but the vein is not pulsatile.
4. Decide whether the thyroid gland is enlarged. Check Pemberton's sign (see Fig. 16.42).
5. Feel for supraclavicular lymphadenopathy and listen over the trachea for inspiratory stridor.
6. Examine the chest carefully for distended venous collaterals.
7. One or both arms may be oedematous.
8. Look for all the peripheral manifestations of lung carcinoma.

THE RESPIRATORY SYSTEM

The respiratory examination

Common stems

1. 'Please examine this patient's respiratory system. He or she has been breathless for …'
2. 'This patient has a cough. Please examine him or her.'
3. 'This man has had haemoptysis, Please examine him.'

Method (Table 16.10)

1. If necessary, ask the patient to undress to the waist and sit over the side of the bed or on a chair.
2. While standing back to make your usual inspection, ask whether sputum is available for you to look at. A large volume of purulent sputum is an important clue to bronchiectasis. Haemoptysis suggests lung carcinoma or pulmonary infection. Look for evidence of dyspnoea at rest and count the respiratory rate. Note the use of the accessory muscles of respiration and any intercostal indrawing of the lower ribs anteriorly (a sign of emphysema). General cachexia should also be noted.
3. Pick up the patient's hands. Note clubbing (Table 16.11), peripheral cyanosis, nicotine (actually tar) staining and anaemia, and look for wasting of the small muscles of the hands and weakness of finger abduction (which may be caused by a lower trunk brachial plexus lesion from apical lung carcinoma involvement). Palpate the wrists for tenderness, but only if there is clubbing (hypertrophic pulmonary osteoarthropathy

Table 16.10 Respiratory system examination

Sitting up	Expansion
1. GENERAL INSPECTION	Vocal fremitus
Sputum mug contents (blood, pus, etc.)	Percuss:
Type of cough	Supraclavicular region
Rate and depth of respiration	Back
Accessory muscles of respiration	Axillae
2. HANDS	Tidal percussion (diaphragm)
Clubbing	Auscultate:
Cyanosis (peripheral)	Breath sounds
Nicotine staining	Adventitial sounds
Wasting, weakness – finger abduction	Vocal resonance
Wrist tenderness (HPOA)	**7. CHEST ANTERIORLY**
Pulse (tachycardia; pulsus paradoxus)	Inspect
Flapping tremor (CO_2 narcosis)	Palpate:
3. FACE	Supraclavicular nodes
Eyes – Horner's syndrome (apical tumour), jaundice, anaemia	Vocal fremitus
	Axillary nodes
Mouth – central cyanosis	Percuss
Voice – hoarseness (recurrent laryngeal nerve palsy)	Auscultate
4. TRACHEA	**8. CARDIOVASCULAR SYSTEM (LYING AT 45°)**
5. FORCED EXPIRATORY TIME	JVP (SVC obstruction, etc.), Pemberton's sign (SVC obstruction)
6. CHEST POSTERIORLY	Apex beat
Inspect:	Pulmonary hypertension
Shape of chest and spine	Cor pulmonale
Scars	**9. OTHER**
Radiotherapy marks	Temperature chart (infection)
Prominent veins (determine direction of flow)	Fundi (CO_2 narcosis)
Palpate:	Evidence of malignancy or pleural effusion: examine breasts, abdomen, rectum, lymph nodes, etc.
Cervical lymph nodes	

HPOA = hypertrophic pulmonary osteoarthropathy; SVC = superior vena cava.

Table 16.11 **Causes of clubbing**

1. Respiratory:
   a. lung carcinoma (usually *not* small cell carcinoma)
   b. chronic pulmonary suppuration (e.g. bronchiectasis, lung abscess, empyema)
   c. idiopathic pulmonary fibrosis, asbestosis
   d. cystic fibrosis
   e. pleural fibroma or mesothelioma
   f. mediastinal disease (e.g. thymoma, lymphoma, carcinoma)

2. Cardiovascular:
   a. infective endocarditis
   b. cyanotic congenital heart disease

3. Other:
   a. inflammatory bowel disease
   b. cirrhosis
   c. coeliac disease
   d. thyrotoxicosis
   e. brachial arteriovenous aneurysm or arterial graft sepsis (unilateral)
   f. neurogenic diaphragmatic tumours
   g. familial (usually before puberty) or idiopathic
   h. hemiplegic stroke (unilateral)

Note: Clubbing does *not* occur with COPD, sarcoidosis, extrinsic allergic alveolitis, coal worker's pneumoconiosis or silicosis. With this important sign, decide whether it is definitely present or absent. Don't call it 'early' if in doubt.

(HPOA), see Fig. 16.27b and c). While holding the patient's hand, palpate the radial pulse for tachycardia or obvious pulsus paradoxus.

4. Go on to the face. Look closely at the eyes for ptosis and constriction of the pupils (Horner's syndrome, p. 526). Inspect the tongue for central cyanosis.
5. Palpate the position of the trachea.
6. Note the presence of a tracheal tug, which indicates gross over-expansion of the chest with airflow obstruction. Ask the patient to cough and note whether this is a loose cough, a dry cough or, because of recurrent laryngeal nerve palsy, a bovine cough.

HINT

Always ask the patient to cough.

HINT

Before feeling the trachea, apologise and warn the patient that the examination may be uncomfortable.

7. Next measure the forced expiratory time (FET). Tell the patient to take a maximal inspiration and blow out as rapidly and completely as possible. Note audible wheeze. Prolongation of expiration beyond 3 seconds is evidence of chronic airflow limitation. If you wish to impress the examiners use a peak flow meter – normal 600 L/min

for young men and 400 L/min for women. Doing these two tests can appear very impressive, but it must look smooth and practised.

8. The next step is to examine the chest. You may wish to examine this anteriorly first or go around to the back. The advantage of the latter is that there are usually more signs there, unless the trachea is obviously displaced.

> **HINT**
>
> Deviation of the trachea is a most important sign, so spend time on it. If the trachea is displaced, concentrate on the upper lobes for physical signs. Upper lobe fibrosis causes tracheal deviation to the same side.

9. Inspect the back. Look for kyphoscoliosis. Do not miss ankylosing spondylitis (p. 513), which causes decreased chest expansion and occasionally upper lobe fibrosis. Look for thoracotomy scars and prominent veins. Also note any skin changes from radiotherapy.

> **HINT**
>
> A large thoracotomy scar in a patient who looks Cushingoid suggests the possibility of a lung transplant. A unilateral transplant may leave signs on the other side, such as the crackles of interstitial lung disease (ILD, pulmonary fibrosis), whereas the side with the scar sounds normal.

10. Palpate the cervical nodes from behind. Then examine for expansion. First, upper lobe expansion is best seen by looking over the patient's shoulders at clavicular movement during moderate respiration. The affected side will show a delay or decreased movement. Then examine lower lobe expansion by palpation. Note any asymmetry and reduction of movement.

11. Ask the patient to bring his or her elbows together in front of the body so as to move the scapulae out of the way. Examine for vocal fremitus. Then percuss the back of the chest and include both axillae. Do not miss a pleural effusion (Table 16.12).

12. Auscultate the chest. Note breath sounds (whether bronchial or vesicular) and their intensity (normal or reduced) (Table 16.13). Listen for adventitial sounds (crackles and wheezes) (Table 16.14). Finally, examine for vocal resonance. If a localised abnormality is found, try to determine the abnormal lobe and segment.

13. Return to the front of the chest. Inspect again for chest deformity, symmetry of chest wall movement, distended veins, radiotherapy changes and scars. Palpate the supraclavicular nodes carefully. Palpate the apex beat and measure chest expansion. Then test for vocal fremitus and proceed with percussion and auscultation as before. Listen high up in the axillae too. Before leaving the chest, feel the axillary nodes and breasts.

> **HINT**
>
> If chronic obstructive pulmonary disease (COPD) seems likely, test for Hoover's sign: place your hands along the costal margins with your thumbs close to the xiphisternum. Normally inspiration causes your thumbs to separate, but the over-inflated chest of the COPD patient (Fig. 16.22) cannot expand any further and so the diaphragm pulls the ribs and your thumbs closer together.
>
> This sign is sensitive and specific.

Table 16.12 Pleural effusion

CAUSES

1. Transudate (pleural:serum protein < 0.5, and pleural LDH <⅔ upper limit of normal, and pleural:serum LDH < 0.6):
   a. cardiac failure
   b. nephrotic syndrome
   c. liver failure
   d. Meigs' syndrome (ovarian fibroma and pleural effusion)
   e. hypothyroidism (but classically an exudate)

2. Exudate (pleural:serum protein > 0.5, or pleural LDH >⅔ upper limit of normal, or pleural:serum LDH > 0.6):
   a. pneumonia
   b. neoplasm – lung carcinoma, metastatic carcinoma, mesothelioma
   c. tuberculosis, sarcoidosis
   d. pulmonary infarction
   e. subphrenic abscess
   f. pancreatitis
   g. connective tissue disease – rheumatoid arthritis, SLE
   h. drugs – nitrofurantoin (acute), methysergide (chronic), drugs causing lupus, chemotherapeutic agents, bromocriptine
   i. radiation

PLEURAL FLUID ANALYSIS: DIFFERENTIAL	DIAGNOSIS
pH < 7.2	Empyema, tuberculosis, neoplasm, rheumatoid arthritis, oesophageal rupture
Glucose < 3.33 mmol / L	Infection, carcinoma, mesothelioma, rheumatoid arthritis
Red blood cells > 5000 / mL	Pulmonary infarction, neoplasm, trauma, asbestosis, tuberculosis, pancreatitis
Amylase > 2000 U / L	Pancreatitis, abdominal viscera rupture, oesophageal rupture
Complement decreased	Rheumatoid arthritis, SLE
Chylous	Tumour (usually lymphoma), thoracic duct trauma, tuberculosis, tuberous sclerosis

LDH = lactate dehydrogenase; SLE = systemic lupus erythematosus.

Table 16.13 Breath sounds

1. **Vesicular:** normal, likened to wind rustling in the leaves
2. **Bronchial:** the expiratory phase is prolonged and has a blowing quality. The breath sounds heard over the trachea and right and left main bronchi are sometimes rather bronchial in quality
   Causes:
   a. lobar pneumonia (common) (see Fig. 16.24)
   b. localised fibrosis or collapse
   c. above a pleural effusion
   d. large lung cavity
3. **Reduced:** use this term rather than 'air entry'
   Causes:
   a. emphysema
   b. large lung mass
   c. collapse, fibrosis or pneumonia
   d. effusion
   e. pneumothorax

Table 16.14 Added sounds
WHEEZES (RHONCHI)
Inspiratory wheezes – characteristic of asthma or upper airway extrathoracic obstruction
Expiratory wheezes – occur in asthma and COPD
Fixed inspiratory wheeze (monophonic – does not change with respiration) – an important sign of fixed bronchial obstruction, usually due to a carcinoma
CRACKLES (CREPITATIONS)
Late or pan inspiratory crackles: <ul><li>fine – caused by fibrosis – dry crackles</li><li>medium – caused by left ventricular failure</li><li>coarse – caused by bronchiectasis or retained secretions</li></ul>Early inspiratory crackles: coarse – caused by COPD

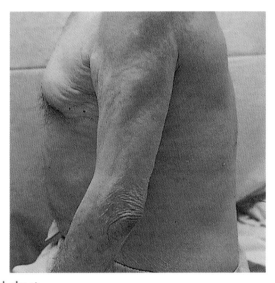

Figure 16.22 **Barrel chest.**

A Robins, R Rakhit, G A W Hornett et al. *Clinical Examination*, 4th edn. Fig. 5.36. Elsevier Ltd, 2008, with permission.

14. Ask the patient to lie down at 45° and then visually measure the JVP.
15. Examine the praecordium for signs of pulmonary hypertension and cor pulmonale. Finally, examine the liver and look for peripheral oedema. Check for Pemberton's sign (see Fig. 16.42).
16. Before leaving the patient, ask whether you may see the temperature chart.

HINT

Try to avoid finishing the examination by saying to the examiners, 'I now want to know the results of spirometry and pulse oximetry', as this may cause irritation.

HINT

Try to put the signs together. Common respiratory short cases include:
1. ILD (dry cough, crackles and clubbing)
2. bronchiectasis (loose cough, full sputum mug, coarse crackles and wheezes, clubbing)
3. COPD (over-inflated chest, possible cyanosis, pursed-lips breathing, reduced breath sounds and wheezes, Hoover's sign)
4. pleural effusion (stony dullness, bronchial breathing on top, needle marks from previous aspirations)
5. thoracoplasty (gross unilateral chest deformity, big scar)
6. cystic fibrosis (often young patient with signs of bronchiectasis and cachexia)
7. treated carcinoma (sometimes clubbing, scar, radiotherapy marks, signs of effusion or collapse, lymph nodes).

HINT

Although tracheal deviation to the side of upper lobectomy is usual, a total pneumonectomy may not cause deviation that can be detected clinically as it begins lower down – this will be apparent on the X-ray.

Chest X-ray films

Hints on how to read a chest X-ray film (Fig. 16.23)
This is a valuable investigation and some even consider a chest X-ray as an extension of the physical examination. It is essential to be familiar with the various radiographic appearances. As a physician, you should feel personally responsible for viewing all the patient's radiographs.
1. When first viewing the chest radiograph, check:
   a. film date, to ensure that it is current
   b. type of film – posteroanterior (PA) or anteroposterior (AP) film; the latter (which may be labelled 'portable') magnifies heart size, making assessment of cardiac diameter difficult
   c. correct orientation – the left side is most reliably determined by the position of stomach gas
   d. film 'centring' – the medial ends of each clavicle should be equidistant from the spines of the vertebrae; rotation affects the mediastinal and hilar shadows, causing undue prominence on the side opposite that to which the patient was turned.
2. Next, systematically examine the PA film, comparing right and left sides carefully for abnormalities of:
   a. soft tissues (e.g. mastectomy, subcutaneous emphysema) and bony skeleton (e.g. rib fractures, malignant deposits)
   b. tracheal displacement, paratracheal masses
   c. heart size, borders and retrocardiac density
   d. aorta and upper mediastinum (count the ribs, look for mediastinal shift, mediastinal masses – see Figs 16.23 and 16.24)

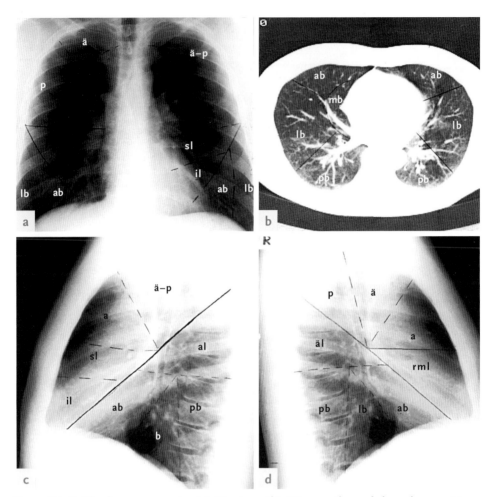

Figure 16.23 The lung segments. (a) PA view. (b) CT scan through lung bases. (c) Left lateral view. (d) Right lateral view. Right upper lobe: ä = apical segment; a = anterior segment; p = posterior segment. Left upper lobe: ä–p = apico-posterior segment; a = anterior segment; sl = superior lingular segment; il = inferior lingular segment. Right lower lobe: äl = apical segment; mb = medial basal segment; lb = lateral basal segment; ab = anterior basal segment; rml = right middle lobe; pb = posterior basal segment. Left lower lobe: äl = apical segment; lb = lateral basal segment; ab = anterior basal segment; pb = posterior basal segment.

The Canberra Hospital X-Ray Library, reproduced with permission.

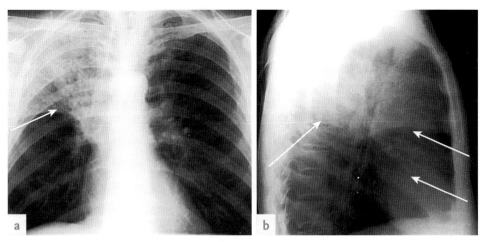

Figure 16.24 (a) and (b) Right upper lobe consolidation. The right upper lobe is opacified and is limited inferiorly by the horizontal fissure (arrows). There must be some collapse as well, as the fissure shows some elevation.

Figures reproduced courtesy of The Canberra Hospital.

e. diaphragm (right higher than left by 1–3 cm normally), cardiophrenic and costo-phrenic angles
f. lung hila (left normally above right by up to 3 cm, usually no larger than an average thumb)
g. lung fields – upper zone (to lower border of second rib), mid zone (from upper zone to lower border of fourth rib) and lower zone (from midzone to diaphragm)
h. pleura
i. gastric bubble (normally there should be no opacity > 0.5 cm above the air bubble)
j. the presence of monitoring leads, a permanent or temporary pacemaker, surgical clips central lines or other 'hardware'.
Learn to do all this rapidly and accurately.

3. Finally, always ask to look at a lateral film. Examine it just as carefully. The lateral film is used to help decide the exact anatomical site of an abnormality.

Candidates must learn the normal position of the fissures (the horizontal fissure, seen sometimes on the PA and lateral film, is a fine horizontal line at the level of the fourth costal cartilage, whereas the oblique fissure is seen only sometimes on the lateral, beginning at the level of the fifth thoracic vertebra and running downwards to the diaphragm at the junction of its anterior and middle thirds).

The lung segments must also be memorised (see Fig. 16.23). Remember: abnormalities in the lung fields are described by terms such as 'mottling', 'opacity' or 'shadow' – it is usually unwise to attempt to make a precise diagnosis of the underlying pathology in your initial assessment of the chest X-ray (Table 16.15).

Some common radiological abnormalities

The following X-rays and scans (Figs 16.24–16.33) show some important changes associated with pulmonary disease.

Text continued on p. 460

Table 16.15 Differential diagnosis of radiological appearances in chest X-ray film

HOMOGENEOUS OPACITY

Pneumonia – lobar or segmental

Collapse

Effusion (see Fig. 16.32)

LOCALISED NON-HOMOGENEOUS OPACITY

Pneumonia (see Fig. 16.24)

Pulmonary infarct

Carcinoma (see Fig. 16.27a and e)

Tuberculosis (see Fig. 6.13, p. 144)

DIFFUSE OPACITIES

Miliary (< 2 mm):

- miliary tuberculosis
- miliary metastases (especially breast, thyroid, melanoma, pancreas)
- sarcoidosis
- pneumoconiosis
- lymphoma, often with prominent hilar lymph nodes (see Fig. 16.33b)
- lymphangitis
- viral pneumonia
- vasculitis (e.g. polyarteritis, Wegener's granulomatosis – see Fig. 16.31)
- pulmonary haemorrhage (see Fig. 16.28)

Nodular (3–10 mm):

- pneumonia
- pneumoconiosis
- tuberculosis
- metastatic carcinoma (see Fig. 16.30)
- sarcoidosis (see Fig. 16.33a)

RETICULAR (LINEAR OPACITIES)

Fibrosis (see Fig. 16.26), bronchiectasis (thickened bronchial walls – see Fig. 16.25)

CAVITATED LESION

Lung abscess

Carcinoma (usually squamous cell) or Hodgkin lymphoma

Tuberculosis

Fungi (e.g. coccidioidomycosis)

CALCIFIED LESIONS IN THE LUNG FIELDS

Tuberculosis

Pneumoconiosis

Post-chickenpox pneumonia

Tularaemia

MILIARY CALCIFICATION

Post-chickenpox pneumonia

Histoplasmosis

Coccidioidomycosis

Ectopic calcification in chronic kidney disease, hyperparathyroidism

COIN LESION

Carcinoma (primary or metastatic – look closely for any rib lesion)

Tuberculoma

Hamartoma

Granuloma (e.g. fungus)

Arteriovenous fistula

Rheumatoid nodule

Lung abscess

Hydatid cyst

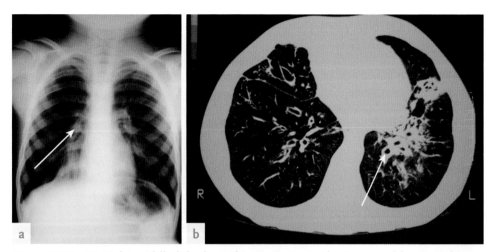

Figure 16.25 (a) Right middle lobe bronchiectasis. Note the increased lung markings and the thickened bronchial walls (arrow). (b) CT scan of the chest of a patient with bronchiectasis. Note the thickened bronchial walls (arrow).

Figures reproduced courtesy of The Canberra Hospital.

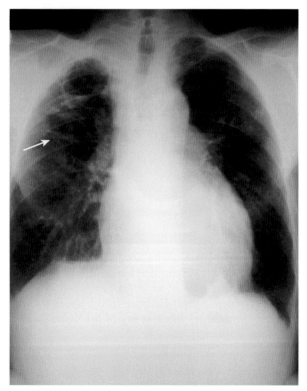

Figure 16.26 Right upper lobe fibrosis. Note the loss of volume and increased lung markings (arrow).

Figure reproduced courtesy of The Canberra Hospital.

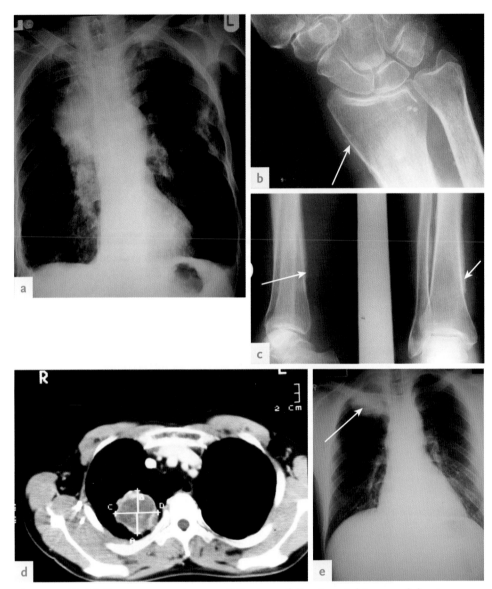

Figure 16.27 (a) Recurrent carcinoma of the lung following right upper lobectomy. Note mass and rib destruction. (b) Hypertrophic pulmonary osteoarthropathy (HPOA) of the ulna in the same patient as in (a) (arrow). (c) HPOA of the tibia in the same patient as in (a) (arrows). (d) CT scan of the chest showing a right upper lobe tumour – Pancoast tumour. (e) Chest X-ray of the same patient as in (d) showing right upper lobe tumour (arrow).

Figures reproduced courtesy of The Canberra Hospital.

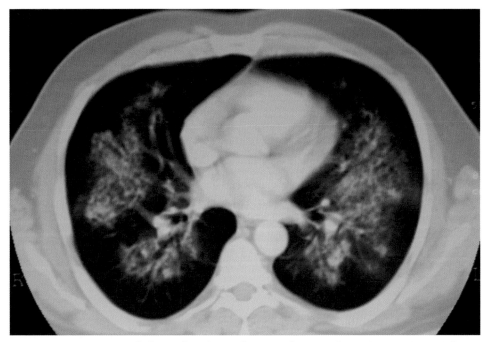

Figure 16.28 CT scan of chest showing pulmonary haemorrhage in a patient with Goodpasture's syndrome.

Figure reproduced courtesy of The Canberra Hospital.

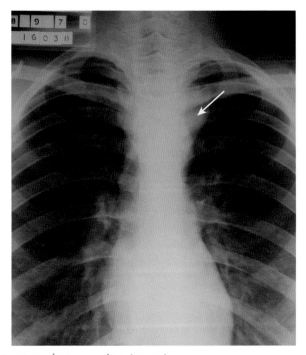

Figure 16.29 Retrosternal mass goitre (arrow).

Figure reproduced courtesy of The Canberra Hospital.

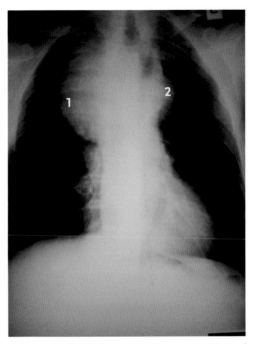

Figure 16.30 Retrosternal mass thoracic aortic aneurysm (1) and pulmonary metastases (2).

Figure reproduced courtesy of The Canberra Hospital.

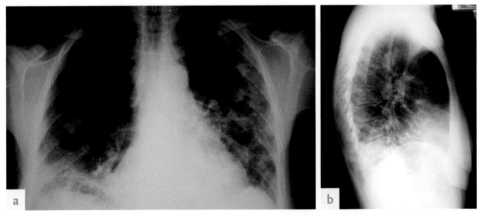

Figure 16.31 (a) Chest X-ray showing granulomatosis with polyangiitis (GPA, or Wegener's granulomatosis). Note infiltrates and destructive changes. (b) Lateral view. Note infiltrates and destructive changes.

Figures reproduced courtesy of The Canberra Hospital.

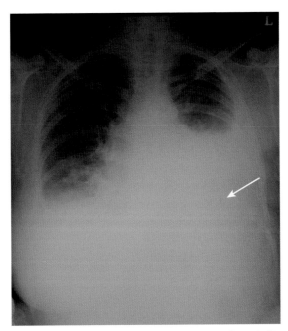

Figure 16.32 Large left pleural effusion (arrow). Note previous left mastectomy.

Figure reproduced courtesy of The Canberra Hospital.

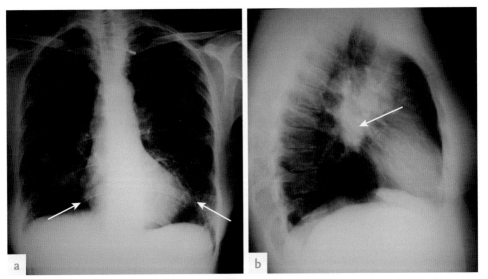

Figure 16.33 (a) Sarcoidosis basal infiltrate (arrows). (b) Hilar lymphadenopathy (arrow).

Figures reproduced courtesy of The Canberra Hospital.

THE GASTROINTESTINAL SYSTEM

The abdominal examination

> ### Common stems
>
> 1. 'This man has had episodes of abdominal discomfort. Please examine his abdomen.'
> 2. 'This woman has been found to have an abdominal mass. Please examine her.'
> 3. 'This woman has developed jaundice. Please examine her.'
> 4. 'This man has been losing weight recently. Please examine his abdomen.'
> 5. 'This man has had bloody diarrhoea. Please examine his abdomen.'
> 6. 'This woman has noticed abdominal distension. Please examine her.'

Method (Table 16.16)

1. Position the patient correctly, with one pillow for the head and complete exposure of the abdomen.
2. Briefly look at the patient's general appearance and inspect particularly for signs of chronic liver disease and renal disease.
3. Inspect the abdomen from the side, squatting to the patient's level. Large masses may be visible. Ask the patient to take slow, deep breaths – an enlarged liver or spleen may be seen to move downwards during inspiration. Stand up and look for scars, distension, prominent veins, striae, bruising and pigmentation.
4. Palpate lightly in each quadrant for masses (Tables 16.17–16.22). Ask first whether any particular area is tender (to avoid causing pain and also to obtain a clue to the site of possible pathology). Next palpate more deeply in each quadrant and then feel specifically for hepatomegaly and splenomegaly. A palpable liver may be a result of enlargement or ptosis. If there is hepatomegaly (see Table 16.17), confirm with percussion and estimate the span (normal span is approximately 12.5 cm). The same procedure is followed for splenomegaly (use a two-handed technique) (see Table 16.21). Percussion is useful to exclude splenomegaly (over the lowest intercostal space in the left anterior axillary line; if dull in full inspiration, suspect splenomegaly and palpate again[2]). Always roll the patient on to the right side and palpate again if no spleen is palpable. Be seen to watch the patient's face intermittently for signs that the examination is uncomfortable.
5. Carefully feel for the kidneys bimanually. Remember that any left-sided mass may arise from a number of sites.

HINT

Bimanual palpation of the kidneys (ballotting) will not work unless the hand under the patient is placed vertically (almost to the spine).

---

[2]Ludwig Traube described a space defined superiorly by the sixth rib, laterally by the mid-axillary line and inferiorly by the left costal margin, which is normally resonant to percussion. It becomes dull if the spleen is enlarged or there is a left-sided pleural effusion. If this area is resonant, it is very unlikely the spleen will be palpable by any other manoeuvre.

Table 16.16 Gastrointestinal system examination

Lying flat (1 pillow)

1. GENERAL INSPECTION

Jaundice (liver disease, etc.)

Pigmentation (e.g. haemochromatosis)

Xanthomata (e.g. primary biliary cholangitis, chronic biliary tract obstruction)

Mental state (encephalopathy)

2. HANDS

Nails – clubbing

    – leukonychia (white nails)

Palmar erythema

Dupuytren's contractures (alcohol)

Arthropathy

Hepatic flap

3. ARMS

Spider naevi

Bruising

Wasting

Scratch marks (chronic cholestasis)

4. FACE

Eyes – sclera: jaundice, anaemia, iritis

    – cornea: Kayser–Fleischer rings (Wilson's disease)

Parotids (alcohol)

Mouth – breath: fetor hepaticus

    – lips: stomatitis, leukoplakia, ulceration, localised pigmentation (Peutz–Jeghers syndrome), telangiectasia (hereditary haemorrhagic telangiectasia)

    – gums: gingivitis, bleeding, hypertrophy, pigmentation, *Candida*

    – tongue: atrophic glossitis, leukoplakia, ulceration

5. CERVICAL / AXILLARY LYMPH NODES

6. CHEST

Gynaecomastia

Spider naevi

7. ABDOMEN

Inspect:

    Scars

    Distension

    Prominent veins – determine direction of flow (caput medusae; inferior vena caval obstruction)

    Striae

    Bruising

    Localised masses

    Visible peristalsis

Palpate:

    Superficial palpation – tenderness, rigidity, outline of any mass

    Deep palpation – organomegaly (liver, gallbladder, spleen, kidney), abnormal masses

Roll on to right side (spleen)

Percuss:

    Viscera outline

    Ascites – shifting dullness

Auscultate:

    Bowel sounds

    Bruits, hums

    Rubs

8. GROIN

Genitalia

Lymph nodes

Hernial orifices (standing up and coughing)

9. LEGS

Bruising

Oedema

Neurological signs (alcohol)

10. OTHER

Rectal examination – inspect (fistulae, tags, blood on glove, etc.), palpate (masses)

Urine analysis (bile, etc.)

Blood pressure (renal disease)

Cardiovascular system (cardiomyopathy)

Neurological system (Wernicke's encephalopathy, etc.)

Temperature chart (infection)

HINT

If you have found hepatosplenomegaly, always consider the possibility of associated polycystic kidneys (a common trap for young players in the test).

Table 16.17 Differential diagnosis in liver palpation

HEPATOMEGALY

1. Massive
   a. metastases
   b. alcoholic liver disease with fatty infiltration
   c. myeloproliferative disease
   d. right heart failure
   e. hepatocellular carcinoma
2. Moderate
   a. the above causes
   b. fatty liver – obesity, diabetes mellitus, toxins
   c. haematological disease – chronic myeloid leukaemia, lymphoma
   d. haemochromatosis
3. Mild
   a. the above causes
   b. hepatitis (viral, drugs)
   c. cirrhosis
   d. biliary obstruction
   e. granulomatous disorders
   f. hydatid disease
   g. amyloidosis and other infiltrative diseases
   h. HIV infection
   i. ischaemia

FIRM AND IRREGULAR LIVER

Cirrhosis

Metastatic disease

Hydatid disease, granuloma, amyloid, cysts, lipoidoses

TENDER LIVER

Hepatitis

Rapid liver enlargement – right heart failure, Budd–Chiari syndrome

Hepatocellular carcinoma

PULSATILE LIVER

Tricuspid regurgitation

Hepatocellular carcinoma

Vascular abnormalities

Table 16.18 Causes of renal masses

BILATERAL

1. Polycystic kidneys (see Table 16.19)
2. Hydronephrosis or pyonephrosis (bilateral)
3. Hypernephroma (bilateral renal cell carcinoma)
4. Acute renal vein thrombosis (bilateral)
5. Amyloid, lymphoma and other infiltrative diseases
6. Acromegaly

UNILATERAL

1. Renal cell carcinoma
2. Hydronephrosis or pyonephrosis
3. Polycystic kidney (asymmetrical enlargement)
4. Acute renal vein thrombosis
5. Normal right kidney or a solitary kidney (uncommon)

Note: In very thin patients, bilateral renal enlargement due to early diabetic nephropathy or nephrotic syndrome is occasionally detectable.

Table 16.19 Adult polycystic kidneys

If you find polycystic kidneys, remember these very important points:

1. Take the blood pressure (75% have hypertension)
2. Examine the urine for haematuria (due to haemorrhage into a cyst) and proteinuria (usually less than 2 g/day when measured)
3. Look for evidence of anaemia (resulting from chronic kidney disease) or polycythaemia (due to high erythropoietin levels). *Note:* The haemoglobin level is higher than expected for the degree of chronic kidney disease
4. Note the presence of hepatic cysts (present in 30% of cases of polycystic renal disease) and splenic cysts (rare). These may cause confusion when examining the abdomen

Note: Subarachnoid haemorrhage occurs in 3% of patients as a result of intracranial aneurysm. As this is an autosomal dominant condition, all family members of patients with polycystic kidney disease should be assessed for kidney disease. Cerebral aneurysms can be screened for by MRI in patients with kidney disease, in the absence of a previous history of subarachnoid haemorrhage.

Table 16.20 Some other causes of abdominal masses

RIGHT ILIAC FOSSA	LEFT ILIAC FOSSA
Appendiceal abscess	Faeces (*note:* can be indented)
Carcinoma of the caecum	Carcinoma of sigmoid or descending colon
Crohn's disease	Diverticular disease
Pelvic kidney	Ovarian tumour or cyst
Ovarian tumour or cyst	Psoas abscess
Carcinoid tumour	**UPPER ABDOMEN**
Amoebiasis	Retroperitoneal lymphadenopathy (e.g. lymphoma, teratoma)
Psoas abscess	Abdominal aortic aneurysm (pulsatile)
Ileocaecal tuberculosis	Carcinoma of stomach
	Pancreatic pseudocyst or tumour
	Carcinoma of transverse colon

Table 16.21 Causes of splenomegaly

1. MASSIVE
a. chronic myeloid leukaemia
b. myelofibrosis
c. primary lymphoma of spleen, hairy cell leukaemia, malaria, kala-azar (all rare)

2. MODERATE
a. the above causes
b. portal hypertension
c. lymphoma
d. leukaemia (chronic or acute)
e. thalassaemia
f. storage diseases (e.g. Gaucher's disease)

3. SMALL
a. the above causes
b. other myeloproliferative disorders – polycythaemia rubra vera, essential thrombocythaemia
c. haemolytic anaemia
d. megaloblastic anaemia (rarely)
e. infection – viral (infectious mononucleosis (glandular fever), hepatitis), bacterial (infective endocarditis)
f. connective tissue disease or vasculitis – rheumatoid arthritis, systemic lupus erythematosus, polyarteritis nodosa
g. infiltration – amyloidosis, sarcoidosis

Note: Secondary carcinomatosis is a rare cause of splenomegaly.

Table 16.22 Causes of hepatosplenomegaly
1. Chronic liver disease with portal hypertension
2. Haematological disease – myeloproliferative disease, lymphoma, leukaemia, pernicious anaemia, sickle cell anaemia
3. Infection – acute viral hepatitis, glandular fever, cytomegalovirus
4. Infiltration – amyloidosis, sarcoidosis
5. Connective tissue disease – systemic lupus erythematosus
6. Acromegaly
7. Thyrotoxicosis

6. The usual distinguishing features of a spleen compared with a kidney are as follows.
   a. The spleen has no palpable upper border.
   b. The spleen has a notch.
   c. The spleen moves inferomedially on respiration.
   d. There is usually no resonance over a splenic mass.
   e. The spleen is not bimanually palpable (i.e. not ballottable).
   f. A friction rub may occasionally be heard over the spleen.
7. Percuss for ascites as a routine. If the abdomen is resonant out to the flanks on percussion, do not roll the patient over. Otherwise, look for shifting dullness. The technique is usually performed by percussing away from your side of the bed until you reach a dull note, then rolling the patient towards you and waiting at least a short time before percussing again for resonance.
8. Always auscultate briefly over the liver, spleen and renal areas. Listen for bruits, rubs and a venous hum. Note the presence of bowel sounds. An arterial systolic bruit over the liver is usually caused by either hepatocellular carcinoma or acute alcoholic hepatitis. A friction rub over the liver may be caused by tumour, recent liver biopsy, infarction or gonococcal perihepatitis (rather unusual); splenic rubs indicate infarction. A venous hum occurs uncommonly in portal hypertension.
9. Examine the groin next. Palpate for inguinal lymphadenopathy. Always ask if you may palpate the testes.

HINT

If you are asked to examine the gastrointestinal system rather than the abdomen, begin by examining the hands and go on to the arms, face, chest, abdomen and legs as described (see Table 16.16).

10. If you now suspect liver disease, you must go on and look for the peripheral stigmata of chronic liver disease. In this instance, it is probably better to proceed from the abdomen to the chest wall. Look for gynaecomastia, spider naevi (Fig. 16.34), hair loss (in men) and breast atrophy (in women). Examine the breasts if you suspect intra-abdominal malignant disease.
    a. Now sit the patient at 45° and measure the JVP so as not to miss constrictive pericarditis as a cause of cirrhosis. Palpate anteriorly for supraclavicular nodes, then sit the patient forwards and feel posteriorly for the other cervical nodes. Look at the back for sacral oedema and spider naevi. If ascites is present, examine the chest for pleural effusions.

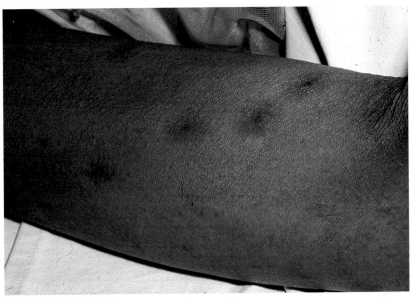

Figure 16.34 Chronic liver disease (spider naevi).

J J Kanski. *Clinical ophthalmology: a synopsis*, 2nd edn. Fig 24.23. Elsevier, 2009, with permission.

b. Look at the face next. Note any scleral abnormality (jaundice, anaemia or iritis) and look at the corneas for Kayser–Fleischer rings. Xanthelasma (see Fig. 16.3) are common in patients with advanced primary biliary cholangitis. Feel for parotid enlargement, which may be present soon after an acute alcoholic binge. Inspect the mouth with a torch and spatula for angular stomatitis, ulceration and atrophic glossitis. Smell the breath for fetor hepaticus.

c. Look at the arms for bruising and spider naevi. Next examine the hands. Ask the patient to extend his arms and hands and look for evidence of hepatic flap. Look also at the nails for clubbing and white nails (leukonychia) (Fig. 16.35), and note any palmar erythema and Dupuytren's contractures (the latter are associated with alcohol or trauma) (Fig. 16.36b). The arthropathy of haemochromatosis may also be present (a degenerative arthritis that particularly involves the second and third metacarpophalangeal joints).

d. Next, examine the legs for oedema, bruising and any rashes. If you have found Dupuytren's contractures in the hands, look for similar tendon thickening and shortening on the soles of the feet (see Fig. 16.36a); Dupuytren's contracture of the foot. Look for the nervous system signs of alcoholism – namely, peripheral neuropathy, proximal myopathy, cerebellar syndrome, Wernicke's encephalopathy (bilatera VI nerve palsies) and Korsakoff's psychosis.

HINT

Do not hurt patients while examining them.

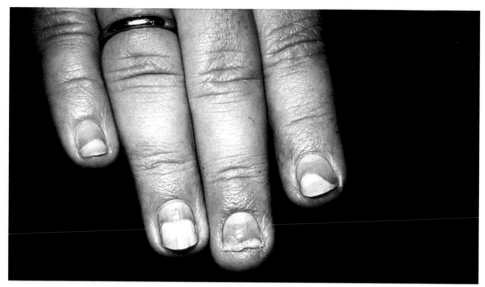

Figure 16.35 **Liver nails (leukonychia).**

Clinics in Dermatology, Fig 3. May / June 2008; 26(3):296–305, with permission.

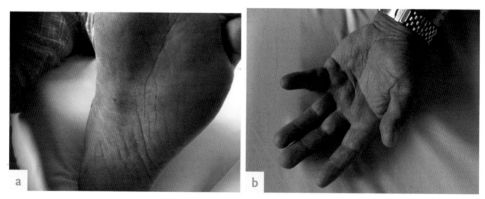

Figure 16.36 (a) **Dupuytren's contracture of the foot.** (b) **Dupuytren's contracture of the hand.**

   e. Candidates are almost always stopped well before this stage. Do not forget to ask to perform a rectal examination and urine analysis. Also ask to look at the temperature chart. Ask whether you may further examine for hernias by asking the patient to stand and cough.

11. If, on the other hand, you have found signs consistent with a haematological problem, proceed as described in that section.

12. If you find a pulsatile liver, examine the cardiovascular system and particularly note any other signs of tricuspid regurgitation.

13. If an enlarged kidney is present (see Table 16.19), ask to check the blood pressure and the urine.

14. If malignant disease is suspected, examine all the node groups, the lungs and the breasts after a thorough abdominal examination. Non-haematological malignant disease that causes hepatomegaly rarely leads to splenomegaly unless the portal vein is directly involved.

HINT

Haemochromatosis, an autosomal recessive disorder, is an important, but now uncommon, cause of liver disease. Consider this diagnosis if any of the following signs are present:

- pigmentation (bronze)
- arthropathy (typically degenerative arthritis of the MCP joints of the index and middle fingers, but any other joint may be involved; pseudogout may occur)
- testicular atrophy (due to iron deposition in the pituitary gland)
- dilated cardiomyopathy
- glycosuria (as a result of diabetes mellitus).

THE HAEMATOLOGICAL SYSTEM

The haemopoietic examination

Common stems

1. 'This 75-year-old man has had problems with tiredness. Please examine his haemopoietic system.'
2. 'This man has been anaemic. Please examine his haematological system.'
3. 'This woman has noticed abdominal fullness. Please examine her abdomen.'
4. 'This woman has noticed a rash on her arms and legs. Please examine her.'
5. 'This man has been found to have cervical lymphadenopathy. Please examine him.'

Method (Table 16.23)

1. If necessary, position the patient as for a gastrointestinal examination. Make sure he or she is fully undressed. Look for bruising, pigmentation, cyanosis, jaundice, scratch marks (due to myeloproliferative disease or lymphoma) and leg ulceration (see below). Also note the presence of frontal bossing and the racial origin of the patient (thalassaemia is more common in people of Asian or Greek background).
2. Pick up the patient's hands. Look at the nails for koilonychia (spoon-shaped nails, which are rarely seen today and which indicate iron deficiency) and the changes of vasculitis. Pale palmar creases suggest anaemia (usually the haemoglobin level is < 90 g/L). Evidence of arthropathy may be important – for example, rheumatoid arthritis and Felty's syndrome, recurrent haemarthroses in bleeding disorders or secondary gout in myeloproliferative disorders.
3. Examine the epitrochlear nodes. Do this by placing your palm under the patient's elbow – your thumb will be placed over the appropriate area (proximal and slightly anterior to the medial epicondyle). A palpable node is usually pathological and may

Table 16.23 Haematological system examination

Lying flat (1 pillow)	(marrow aplasia, etc.); atrophic glossitis, angular stomatitis (iron, vitamin deficiencies)
1. GENERAL INSPECTION	Tonsils – enlarged (lymphoma)
Bruising (thrombocytopenia, scurvy, etc.)	**Sitting up**
– petechiae (pinhead bleeding) (Fig. 16.37)	**5. CERVICAL NODES (PALPATE FROM BEHIND)**
– ecchymoses (large bruises)	**6. BONY TENDERNESS**
Pigmentation (lymphoma)	Sternum
Rashes and infiltrative lesions (lymphoma)	Clavicles
Ulceration (neutropenia)	Shoulders
Cyanosis (polycythaemia)	Spine
Plethora (polycythaemia) (Fig. 16.38)	**Lying flat**
Jaundice (haemolysis)	**7. ABDOMEN AND GENITALIA**
Scratch marks (myeloproliferative disease)	Detailed examination
Racial origin	**8. INGUINAL NODES**
2. HANDS	**9. LEGS**
Nails – koilonychia	Vasculitis (Henoch–Schönlein purpura – buttocks, thighs)
Palmar crease pallor (anaemia)	Bruising
Arthropathy (haemophilia, secondary gout, drug treatment, etc.)	Pigmentation
Pulse	Ulceration
3. ARMS	Neurological signs (subacute combined degeneration, peripheral neuropathy)
Epitrochlear nodes (non-Hodgkin lymphoma, chronic lymphocytic leukaemia, intravenous drug use, sarcoidosis)	**10. OTHER**
Axillary nodes	Fundi (hyperviscosity, haemorrhages, infection, etc.)
4. FACE	Temperature chart (infection)
Sclera – jaundice, pallor, conjunctival suffusion (polycythaemia)	Urine analysis (haematuria, bile, etc.)
Mouth – gum hypertrophy (acute leukaemia), ulceration, infection, haemorrhage	Rectal examination (blood loss)

indicate non-Hodgkin lymphoma. Note any arm bruising. Remember petechiae (see Fig. 16.37) are pinhead haemorrhages, whereas ecchymoses are larger bruises. Palpable purpura suggests vasculitis (idiopathic, hepatitis C, cancer), cryoglobulinaemia or bacteraemia (cutaneous emboli).

4. Go to the axillae and palpate the axillary nodes. Do this by raising the patient's arm and placing your fingers as high as possible in the axilla. Then position the patient's forearm comfortably over your own forearm. Use your left hand for the patient's right axilla, and vice versa. There are four main areas: central, lateral (above and lateral), pectoral (most medial) and subscapular (most inferior).

5. Look at the patient's face. Inspecting the eyes, note any jaundice, pallor or haemorrhage of the sclera, or the injected sclera of polycythaemia.

HINT

Anaemia is most accurately detected by pulling down one of the patient's lower eyelids and comparing the colour of the anterior part of the conjunctiva with the pearly white of the palpebral conjunctiva more posteriorly. The anterior conjunctiva should be distinctly redder in colour unless significant anaemia (<100 g/L) is present.

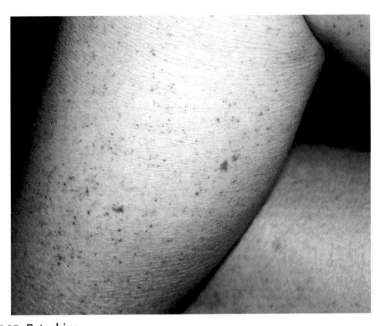

Figure 16.37 Petechiae.

J G Marks, J J Miller. *Lookingbill and Marks' principles of dermatology*, 4th edn. Fig 17.1. Saunders, Elsevier, 2006, with permission.

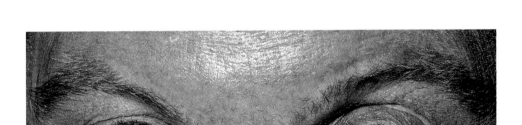

Figure 16.38 Plethora.

A V Hoffbrand, J E Pettite. *Color atlas of clinical hematology*, 3rd edn. p. 248. Mosby, Elsevier, 2000, with permission.

6. Examine the mouth. Note any gum hypertrophy (the differential diagnosis includes acute myeloid leukaemia – especially monocytic – and scurvy), ulceration, infection (e.g. *Candida*), haemorrhage, atrophic glossitis (secondary to iron, vitamin B_{12} or folate deficiency) and angular stomatitis. Look for tonsillar and adenoid enlargement (Waldeyer's ring).

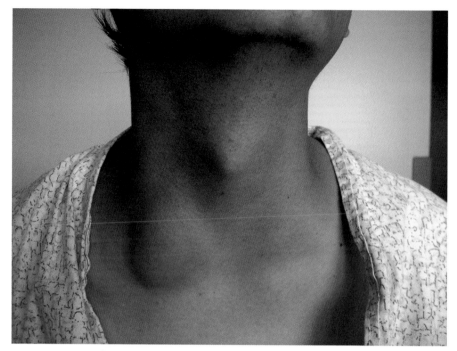

Figure 16.39 **Supraclavicular lymphadenopathy.**

7. Now sit the patient up. Examine the cervical nodes from behind (Fig. 16.39). There are seven groups: submental, submandibular, jugular chain, posterior triangle, postauricular, preauricular and occipital. Then feel the supraclavicular area from the front. Tap the spine with your fist for bony tenderness (which can be caused by an enlarging marrow – e.g. in myeloma, carcinoma). Also gently press the sternum, clavicles and shoulders for bony tenderness.

8. Lay the patient flat again. Examine the abdomen, particularly for splenomegaly (see Table 16.21) and hepatomegaly (see Tables 16.17 and 16.22).

9. Spring the hips for pelvic tenderness.

10. Palpate the inguinal nodes. There are two groups – along the inguinal ligament and along the femoral vessels. Remember to ask to feel the testes and ask to do a rectal examination (e.g. for melaena).[3]

11. Examine the legs. Note particularly leg ulcers, which may occur with hereditary spherocytosis, sickle cell syndromes, thalassaemia, macroglobulinaemia and Felty's syndrome. Ask to examine the legs from a neurological aspect for evidence of vitamin B_{12} deficiency. Remember, hypothyroidism and lead poisoning can cause anaemia and peripheral neuropathy. Do not miss Henoch–Schönlein purpura over the buttocks and legs (Fig. 16.40).

12. Finally, ask to examine the fundi (for engorged retinal vessels, papilloedema, haemorrhages, etc.) (Fig. 16.41a and b) and look at the temperature chart. Causes of generalised lymphadenopathy are presented in Table 16.24.

---

[3]The first is rarely allowed, the second never.

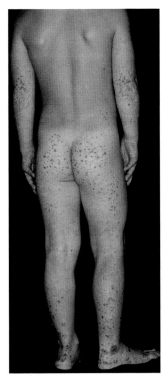

Figure 16.40 **Henoch–Schönlein purpura.**

J G H Dinulos. *Habif's Clinical Dermatology: A Color Guide to Diagnosis and Therapy*, 7th edn. Fig. 18.18. Elsevier Inc., 2021, with permission.

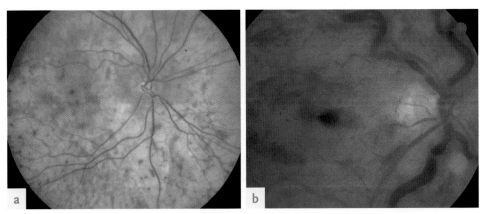

Figure 16.41 **Fundus changes in haematological disorders. (a) 'Leopard skin' appearance due to choroidal infiltration in chronic leukaemia. (b) Retinal and gross venous dilatation and segmentation in hyperviscocity.**

J J Kanski, Retinal vascular disease. *Clinical opthalmology: a systematic approach.* Elsevier, 2011, with permission.

Table 16.24 **Causes of generalised lymphadenopathy**
1. Lymphoma (rubbery and firm)
2. Leukaemia (chronic lymphocytic leukaemia, acute lymphoblastic leukaemia particularly)
3. Malignant disease (metastases or reactive changes usually causing asymmetrical, very firm nodes)
4. Infections – viral (e.g. cytomegalovirus, HIV, infectious mononucleosis (glandular fever)), bacterial (e.g. tuberculosis, brucellosis), protozoal (e.g. toxoplasmosis)
5. Connective tissue diseases – rheumatoid arthritis, systemic lupus erythematosus
6. Infiltrations – sarcoidosis
7. Drugs – phenytoin (pseudolymphoma)

THE ENDOCRINE SYSTEM

The thyroid gland

Common stems

1. 'This 40-year-old woman has noticed some discomfort in her neck. Please examine her.' (Look for a goitre but don't miss other neck pathology.)
2. 'This woman has noticed loss of weight and has a tremor. Please examine her.' (Think of thyrotoxicosis (obviously).)

HINT

The presence of a glass of water beside the patient suggests you are expected to examine the thyroid.

Method (Table 16.25)

The most likely problem is thyroid disease, but in the neck examination you should also consider the possibilities of superior vena caval obstruction, cervical lymphadenopathy, carotid aneurysm or bruit, JVP abnormalities and tracheal deviation.

1. Take time first to look at the face for signs of thyrotoxicosis or myxoedema (see point 7 below).
2. With the patient sitting up and the neck fully exposed, inspect for scars, swelling and prominent veins. Look at the front and the sides. Ask the patient to swallow a sip of water and look for thyroid enlargement. The thyroid moves up with swallowing.
3. Palpate gently from behind, with the neck flexed, feeling for any thyroid mass (Table 16.26). Use one hand to steady the gland and the other to feel. Note the shape, consistency and distribution of the thyroid enlargement. If a nodule is palpable, determine whether this is single or part of a multinodular goitre. Ask the patient whether the gland is tender (a clue to subacute thyroiditis) and note any hoarseness of

Table 16.25 Neck examination

Sitting up	Supraclavicular nodes
1. GENERAL INSPECTION	Trachea position
Face – thyrotoxicosis, myxoedema, other diagnostic facies (see Table 16.35)	Sternomastoid function
2. NECK	Percuss:
Inspect:	Upper manubrium
Scars	Auscultate:
Swelling	Thyroid bruit
Prominent veins	Carotid bruit
Swallowing (a glass of water)	Pemberton's sign (Fig. 16.42)
Palpate (from behind with neck flexed):	**3. OTHER**
Thyroid enlargement – note size, shape, consistency, borders, mobility	Signs of thyrotoxicosis / myxoedema elsewhere
Thyroid tenderness	Thyroidectomy scar – test for hypoparathyroidism (Chvostek's and Trousseau's signs)
Thyroid thrill	JVP – superior vena cava obstruction
Cervical nodes	Causes of localised cervical gland enlargement – chest, abdomen, head and neck examination
Palpate (from in front):	
Thyroid (as above)	
Carotid arteries	

Table 16.26 Causes of a diffuse goitre (Fig. 16.43)

1. Idiopathic (majority)
2. Puberty, pregnancy and postpartum
3. Graves' disease
4. Thyroiditis – Hashimoto's thyroiditis, subacute thyroiditis (tender), chronic fibrosing (Riedel's) thyroiditis (rare)
5. Simple goitre (iodine deficiency)
6. Goitrogens – iodine excess, drugs (e.g. lithium, phenylbutazone)
7. Inborn errors of thyroid hormone synthesis – Pendreds syndrome, an autosomal recessive condition associated with nerve deafness

the voice (which may be caused by recurrent laryngeal nerve palsy). Decide whether you can palpate the lower border of the gland (to exclude retrosternal extension) and whether there is a thrill. Feel for cervical lymphadenopathy from behind (see Fig. 16.39). Palpate each carotid artery (absence possibly indicating malignant infiltration). Test the sternocleidomastoid function, as malignant disease may infiltrate this muscle. Finally, palpate the gland from in front and note the tracheal position.

4. Percuss over the upper part of the manubrium from one side to the other, right across the bone, and note any change from resonant to dull (a sign of retrosternal extension).

5. Auscultate over the thyroid gland for bruits (a sign of active thyrotoxicosis) and also over the carotid arteries. A systolic flow murmur is common when patients are thyrotoxic.

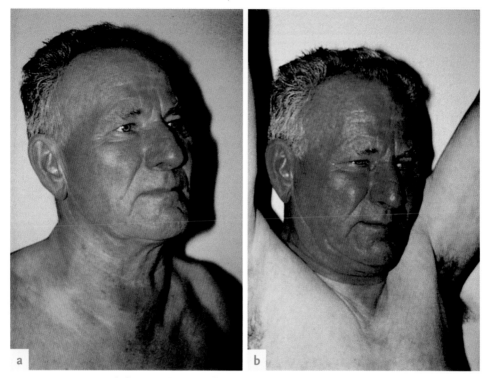

Figure 16.42 (a) and (b) Positive Pemberton's sign.

M H Swartz. *FACP – Textbook of physical diagnosis: history and examination*, 6th edn. Figs 9.14A and B, Elsevier, 2009, with permission.

6. Remember Pemberton's sign (see Fig. 16.42). Ask the patient to lift his or her arms over the head. Look for suffusion of the face, elevation of the JVP and inspiratory stridor. Any retrosternal mass may cause these changes.

7. If there is evidence of a goitre and obvious eye disease (indicating the presence of *thyrotoxicosis*; Table 16.27), proceed to the face. Examine the eyes for exophthalmos by noting the presence of sclera below the cornea when the patient is looking straight ahead. Note lid retraction by looking for the presence of sclera above the cornea. Then test for lid lag by asking the patient to follow your finger descending at a moderate rate. Now examine the conjunctiva for chemosis.

8. Test eye movements for ophthalmoplegia. In thyrotoxicosis the inferior oblique muscle power is lost first, then convergence is affected, followed by the other muscles. Examine the fundi because optic atrophy can occur late. Then look from behind, over the patient's forehead, when he or she is looking forward, for proptosis.

9. Examine the patient's outstretched hands for tremor. It is worthwhile placing a sheet of paper over the dorsal aspects of the fingers. Look at the nails for onycholysis (Plummer's nails) – distal separation of the nail from its bed – and thyroid acropachy (this looks like clubbing and is clubbing, but is not called clubbing). Note any palmar erythema. Feel for warmth and sweating. Feel the radial pulse for sinus tachycardia, atrial fibrillation or a collapsing pulse.

10. Test for proximal myopathy in the arms and tap the arm reflexes for briskness.

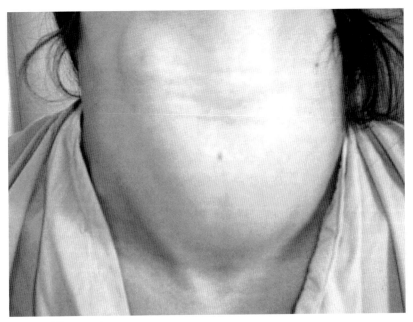

Figure 16.43 Diffuse goitre.

G Medeiros-Neto, R Y Camargo, E K Tomimori. Thyroid disorders and diseases: approach to and treatment of goiters. *Medical Clinics of North America* 2012; 96(2):351–68, Fig 3, with permission.

Table 16.27 Causes of thyrotoxicosis
PRIMARY
1. Graves' disease
2. Toxic adenoma or multinodular goitre
3. Hashimoto's thyroiditis (early in its course), subacute thyroiditis (transient) and painful (if granulomatous) or painless (if lymphatic)
4. Iodine-induced (after previous iodine deficiency) – termed the Jod-Basedow phenomenon
5. Excess thyroid hormone replacement
6. Postpartum thyroiditis (non-tender)
7. Drugs – amiodarone (via Jod-Basedow), lithium (rare)
SECONDARY
1. Pituitary or ectopic thyroid-stimulating hormone hypersecretion (very rare)
2. Hydatidiform mole or choriocarcinoma (human chorionic gonadotrophin secretion – rare)
3. Struma ovarii (rare)
4. Factitious
Note: The three components of Graves' disease – viz. eye signs, hyperthyroidism with goitre and pretibial myxoedema – run independent courses.

11. If there is time, proceed to the legs and look for skin manifestations: pretibial myxoedema – bilateral firm, elevated dermal nodules and plaques that can be pink, brown or skin-coloured and that are caused by mucopolysaccharide accumulation – and vitiligo. Test for proximal myopathy and hyperreflexia in the legs.
12. Ask to examine the chest for evidence of gynaecomastia (in men) and the heart for an ejection systolic murmur and signs of congestive cardiac failure.

Table 16.28 Causes of hypothyroidism
PRIMARY
Without a goitre (decreased or absent thyroid tissue)
Idiopathic atrophy
Treatment (e.g. iodine-131, surgery)
Agenesis or a lingual thyroid
Unresponsiveness to thyroid-stimulating hormone
With a goitre (decreased synthesis)
Chronic thyroiditis (e.g. late Hashimoto's disease, Riedel's thyroiditis)
Drugs (e.g. lithium, amiodarone)
Endemic iodine deficiency
Iodine-induced hypothyroidism
Inborn errors (enzyme deficiency)
SECONDARY
Pituitary lesions
TERTIARY
Hypothalamic lesions
TRANSIENT
Thyroid hormone treatment withdrawn
Subacute thyroiditis
Postpartum thyroiditis

13. Although it is rarely of importance, there may also be mild splenomegaly and hepatomegaly on abdominal examination (see Tables 16.17, 16.21 and 16.22), as well as generalised lymphadenopathy.

14. If a thyroidectomy scar is present, ask to look for the signs of hypocalcaemia (i.e. Chvostek's and Trousseau's signs). Chvostek's sign may be present in normal patients. It is tested by tapping over the facial nerve 3–5 cm below and in front of the ear. The facial muscle twitches briefly in the presence of hypocalcaemia. Trousseau's sign is tested by pumping up a sphygmomanometer cuff above systolic blood pressure and looking for *main d'accoucheur* (a strongly adducted thumb with fingers extended except at the MCP joints) that occurs within 2 minutes.

15. If you suspect *hypothyroidism* (when goitre is unusual) (Table 16.28), proceed as follows.

   a. Examine the hands. Note any peripheral cyanosis, swelling and dry, cold skin. Look at the palmar creases for anaemia (Table 16.29). Feel the pulse for bradycardia and a small volume. Test for carpal tunnel syndrome. Ask the patient to flex both wrists for 30 seconds – paraesthesiae will often be precipitated in the affected hand if this syndrome is present (Phalen's wrist flexion test).

   b. Test for delayed relaxation of the biceps jerk. Examine for proximal myopathy, which is rare.

   c. Proceed to the face. Note here any general swelling and periorbital oedema. Look for loss of the outer one-third of the eyebrows and periorbital xanthelasma. Note whether the skin is dry, fine and smooth. There may be signs of carotenaemia, alopecia or vitiligo (see Fig. 16.49). Look at the tongue, which may be swollen, then ask the patient to tell you his or her name and address, and note any hoarseness or slowness of speech. Test for nerve deafness, which may be bilateral.

Table 16.29 Causes of anaemia in patients with hypothyroidism

1. Chronic disease (direct or erythropoietin-mediated depressive effect on bone marrow)
2. Folate deficiency secondary to bacterial overgrowth
3. Pernicious anaemia associated with myxoedema
4. Iron deficiency in women owing to menorrhagia
5. Haemolysis secondary to hypercholesterolaemia-induced spur-cell anaemia

Table 16.30 Neurological associations of hypothyroidism

COMMON
1. Entrapment (e.g. carpal tunnel, tarsal tunnel)
2. Delayed relaxation phase of ankle jerks
3. Nerve deafness

UNCOMMON
1. Peripheral neuropathy
2. Proximal myopathy (with normal creatine kinase levels)
3. Hypokalaemic periodic paralysis
4. Eaton–Lambert syndrome or deterioration or unmasking of myasthenia gravis
5. Cerebellar syndrome
6. Psychosis
7. Coma
8. Cerebrovascular disease
9. High cerebrospinal fluid protein
10. Muscle cramps

d. Go to the legs next. Examine them neurologically, starting with the ankle jerks, noting particularly any evidence of slow relaxation, which is best seen with the patient kneeling on a chair. Then examine for peripheral neuropathy and look for other uncommon neurological abnormalities (Table 16.30).
e. Finally ask to examine the chest for pleural and pericardial effusions. There may be dry, rough 'sandpaper-like' skin over the chest.

Panhypopituitarism

Common stem

'This woman has lost her libido. Please assess her.'

Method
You cleverly note that this woman looks 'panhypopituitary' (Table 16.31, Fig. 16.44). Proceed as follows.

1. Ask her to stand and make sure she is fully undressed to her underwear. Note the pale skin and lack of hair.
2. The patient may be of short stature (failure of growth hormone secretion before growth is complete) with no secondary sexual characteristics (gonadotrophin failure before puberty).

Table 16.31 Causes of panhypopituitarism

1. Chromophobe adenoma (most common cause in males)
2. Other space-occupying lesion (craniopharyngioma, metastatic carcinoma, granuloma)
3. Iatrogenic (surgery, radiation)
4. Sheehan's syndrome (postpartum necrosis)
5. Head injury
6. Idiopathic

Note: Loss of function (in order):
60% pituitary loss: growth hormone, FSH and LH
80% pituitary loss: TSH
100% pituitary loss: ACTH

ACTH = adrenocorticotrophic hormone; FSH = follicle-stimulating hormone; LH = luteinising hormone; TSH = thyroid-stimulating hormone.

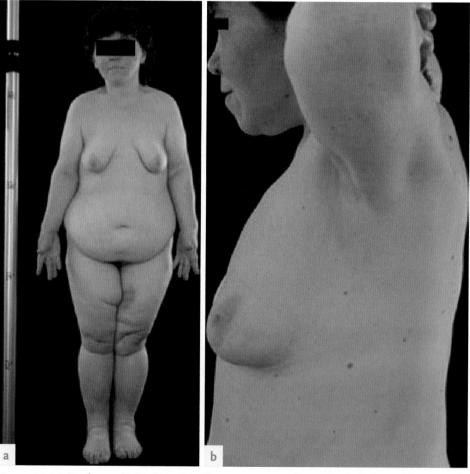

Figure 16.44 Panhypopituitarism. (a) Short stature, reduced body hair and increased abdominal fat are apparent. (b) Partial breast development results from oestrogen replacement. Failure of adrenal androgen production results in the absence of axillary hair.

F F Ferri. *Ferri's color atlas and text of clinical medicine*, 1st edn. Fig 263.2. Saunders, Elsevier, 2009, with permission.

3. Look at the face more closely. Multiple fine skin wrinkles around the eyes and mouth are characteristic of growth hormone deficiency. Look closely for a hypophysectomy scar on the forehead near the inner canthus of the eye. Examine the eyes for signs of a pituitary tumour (visual fields, especially for bitemporal hemianopia, fundi for optic atrophy) and assess cranial nerves III, IV and VI, as well as the first division of V (affected by tumour extension into the cavernous sinus). Feel the facial hair over the chin area.

4. Go to the chest and look for decreased body hair and pale skin (and gynaecomastia in men). Lay the patient down and look for loss of pubic hair and testicular atrophy (in males testes are small and soft – the normal size is 15–25 mL in volume).

5. Test the ankle jerks (for slow relaxation in hypothyroidism – there is no myxoedematous appearance) and ask to check the blood pressure with the patient lying and standing (hypotension with adrenocorticotrophic hormone (ACTH) deficiency).

Cushing's syndrome

Common stems

1. 'This woman has noted weight gain. Please examine her.'
2. 'This woman has difficulty standing up from a chair and changes in her appearance. Please examine her.'

Method (Table 16.32)

This type of introduction may mean Cushing's syndrome in the clinical examination (Fig. 16.45a–c). Make sure that the patient is undressed to her underwear and ask her to stand.

1. Look at the patient from the front, sides and behind. Note central obesity with peripheral sparing and look at the skin for bruising, atrophy and pigmentation of extensor areas. Hyperpigmentation suggests an ectopic ACTH-secreting tumour, or it may indicate an ACTH-secreting pituitary adenoma in a patient who has had a bilateral adrenalectomy (Nelson's syndrome).

2. Test for proximal myopathy of the arms and also of the legs (initially by getting the patient to squat). Examine the back for a buffalo hump and feel it. Look for kyphoscoliosis and tap the spine for bony tenderness as a result of osteoporotic vertebral crush fractures.

3. Ask the patient to sit on the side of the bed. Look at the face for plethora, hirsutism, acne, telangiectasia and a moon shape.

4. Test the eyes for visual field defects (which are uncommon) and look in the fundi for papilloedema (caused by benign intracranial hypertension or a pituitary tumour) and optic atrophy, as well as hypertensive or diabetic changes (see Tables 16.7 and 16.41). Then look at the neck for supraclavicular fat pads and acanthosis nigricans.

5. Ask the patient to lie down. Examine the abdomen for adrenalectomy scars, pigmentation, striae and adrenal masses. Ask the patient and the examiners if you may look at the genitalia. Virilisation in women or gynaecomastia in men suggests that adrenal carcinoma is more likely. Next, look at the legs for oedema, bruising and poor wound healing.

6. Do not forget to ask for the results of urine analysis (glucose) and take the blood pressure (hypertension). Diagnostic tests are summarised in Table 16.33.

Table 16.32 Cushing's syndrome examination

Standing

1. GENERAL INSPECTION

Central obesity and thin limbs

Skin bruising, atrophy

Pigmentation (ACTH tumour – rare – or bilateral adrenalectomy)

Poor wound healing

2. ARMS

Purple striae (proximally)

Proximal myopathy

Sitting

3. FACE

Plethora, hirsutism, acne, telangiectasia

Moon shape

Eyes – visual fields (pituitary tumour), fundi (atrophy, papilloedema, signs of hypertension or diabetes)

Mouth – thrush

Neck – supraclavicular fat pads, acanthosis nigricans

4. BACK

Buffalo hump (interscapular fat pad)

Kyphoscoliosis (osteoporosis)

Tenderness of vertebrae (osteoporotic fractures)

5. LEGS

Squat (proximal myopathy)

Striae (thighs)

Bruising, oedema

6. MENTAL STATE

Depression

Psychosis

Irritability

Lying flat

7. ABDOMEN

Purple striae

Adrenal masses, adrenalectomy scars

Liver (tumour deposits)

8. OTHER

Urine analysis (glycosuria, evidence of renal stone disease)

Blood pressure (hypertension)

Signs of ectopic tumour (e.g. lung small cell carcinoma or carcinoid) – rare

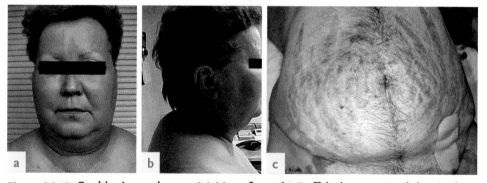

Figure 16.45 **Cushing's syndrome. (a) Moonface. (b) Buffalo hump. (c) Abdominal striae.**

C M Townsend. *Sabiston textbook of surgery: the biological basis of modern surgical practice*, 18th edn. Fig 39.11. Saunders, Elsevier 2007, with permission.

Table 16.33 Diagnosis of Cushing's syndrome[a]

SCREENING TESTS

1. Cortisol levels morning and evening (serum or salivary): loss of diurnal rhythm (evening cortisol level should be less than half the morning value) of little diagnostic value

2. 24-hour urine collection for urinary free cortisol determination (an indirect assessment of cortisol production). Should be threefold increased (above normal)

3. Overnight dexamethasone suppression test (1 mg dexamethasone at midnight causes suppression of cortisol in normal subjects at 9.00 am). No suppression is found in Cushing's syndrome, but this may also occur with alcoholism, induction of hepatic enzymes (e.g. phenytoin) or depression, in patients taking the contraceptive pill and in some obese patients

4. Blood count (secondary polycythaemia, neutrophil leukocytosis, eosinopenia)

5. Electrolyte levels (hypokalaemic alkalosis, particularly with ectopic ACTH-producing tumours)

6. Blood sugar level (hyperglycaemia)

DEFINITIVE TESTS

1. 2 mg dexamethasone suppression test (0.5 mg 6-hourly for 48 hours). No suppression of plasma cortisol or urinary free cortisol occurs in Cushing's syndrome, but usually suppression does occur in normal subjects, obese patients and depressed patients

2. 8 mg dexamethasone suppression test (2 mg 6-hourly for 48 hours). Suppression occurs in Cushing's disease, but no suppression is usually found in adrenal adenoma or carcinoma or in the presence of ectopic ACTH production. False-positive results can occur in patients taking anticonvulsants (which accelerate dexamethasone metabolism)

3. ACTH level – high in ectopic ACTH production; low with adrenal adenoma or carcinoma, high or normal in Cushing's disease. Ectopic secretion of CRH by tumours is a very rare cause of Cushing's syndrome

4. Petrosal sinus ACTH sampling – a central-to-peripheral venous cortisol ratio of > 2:1 is diagnostic of Cushing's disease; lateralisation of ACTH production helps the neurosurgeon plan trans-sphenoidal exploration of the sella

To diagnose Cushing's syndrome, at least two definitive tests should be abnormal

Note: If Cushing's disease is present, pituitary assessment is necessary. If adrenal disease is suspected, CT scanning is useful to assess the anatomy. Remember, ectopic ACTH production by a tumour (e.g. small cell carcinoma of lung, carcinoid of lung or thymus, pancreatic islet cell carcinoma, ovarian carcinoma) does not usually cause Cushingoid clinical features but may present with hyperpigmentation, hypokalaemic alkalosis and hypertension.

[a]Cushing's disease is specifically pituitary ACTH over-production.

Acromegaly

> ## Common stems
>
> 1. 'This man has noted some change in his facial appearance. Please examine him.' (Fig. 16.46a to c)
> 2. 'This man has acromegaly. Please examine him for activity and features of the disease.'

Method (Table 16.34)

The order and direction of the examination obviously depend on the stem. However, if a 'change of appearance' of any part of the body is mentioned in the stem it is likely you are expected to make a spot diagnosis. Look very carefully at the patient before deciding where to examine.

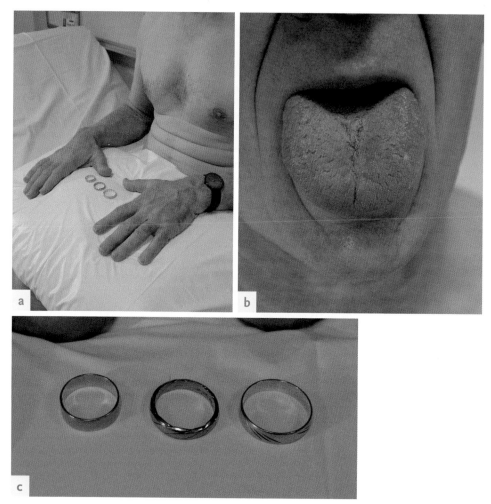

Figure 16.46 **(a) Acromegalic hands. (b) Macroglossia. (c) This patient has conveniently brought his rings with him.**

Courtesy of the Canberra course for basic trainees.

HINT

The change to a written stem has led to variations on this introduction. At one end of the spectrum the examiners may give the diagnosis: 'This 64-year-old man has acromegaly. Please examine him to assess the extent and activity of the condition.' At the other end of the spectrum the introduction may be more oblique: 'This 64-year-old man has had premature and severe arthritis. Please examine his knees.' The examiners have been advised at their calibration sessions to make the stem very clear.

---

1. Consider the possible diagnostic facies (Table 16.35). If the patient looks acromegalic, proceed as follows.
2. Have the patient stand or sit on the side of the bed. Look at the hands. Look for coarse features and spade-like shape, as well as increased sweating and warmth. Osteoarthritis-like changes are frequent in the hands, shoulders, hips and knees.

Table 16.34 **Acromegaly examination**	

1. GENERAL INSPECTION
   Diagnostic facies
2. HANDS
   Shape
   Sweat
   Phalen's test (carpal tunnel)
3. ULNAR NERVE
   Thickened
4. PROXIMAL MYOPATHY
5. AXILLAE
   Skin tags
   Acanthosis nigricans
   Greasy skin
6. FACE
   Frontal bossing
   Hirsutism
   Macroglossia
   Prognathism
   Hoarseness
7. EYES
	Visual fields
	      Cranial nerves III, IV, VI, V
	      Fundi
	8. NECK
	   Thyroid gland (diffuse or nodular goitre)
	9. HEART
	   Cardiac failure
	10. ABDOMEN
	   Organomegaly
	11. LOWER LIMBS
	   Hips } osteoarthritis, pseudogout
	   Knees
	   Entrapment neuropathy
	   Heel pad thickening
	12. OTHER
	   Urine analysis (glycosuria)
	   Rectal examination – colonic polyps (correlate with skin tags)
	   Blood pressure (hypertension)
	   Sleep apnoea

Table 16.35 **Common diagnostic facies**	
1. Acromegalic 2. Thyrotoxic 3. Myxoedematous 4. Cushingoid 5. Pagetic 6. Myopathic	7. Myotonic 8. Parkinsonian 9. Thalassaemic 10. Marfanoid 11. Mitral

Perform Phalen's wrist flexion test for the carpal tunnel syndrome (median nerve entrapment). Feel the ulnar nerve for thickening at the elbow.

3. Go to the arms and test for proximal myopathy. Also look in the axillae for skin tags (molluscum fibrosum), greasy skin and acanthosis nigricans (brown-to-black velvety elevation of the epidermis owing to multiple confluent papillomas).

4. Go on to the face. Look for frontal bossing as a result of a large supraorbital ridge (which may also occur in rickets, Paget's disease, hydrocephalus or achondroplasia). Note whether there is a large tongue (sometimes too big to fit into the mouth neatly). Enlargement of the lower jaw (called prognathism) and splaying of the teeth may be present. Notice any acne or hirsutism in women (see Table 16.44) and test the voice, which may be deep, husky and resonant.

5. The eyes must be carefully examined. Visual fields should be checked – look particularly for bitemporal hemianopia, but many field defects are possible (see Fig. 16.87). Examine the fundi for optic atrophy, papilloedema and angioid streaks (red, brown or grey streaks three to five times the diameter of the retinal veins appearing to emanate from the optic disc and resulting from degeneration of Bruch's membrane with resultant fibrosis). There may also be diabetic or hypertensive changes.

6. Examine the thyroid gland for diffuse enlargement or a multinodular goitre.

Table 16.36 Evidence of activity in acromegaly
1. Skin tag number
2. Excessive sweating
3. Presence of glycosuria
4. Increasing visual field loss or development of cranial nerve palsies of III, IV, VI and V
5. Enlarging goitre
6. Hypertension
7. Symptoms of headache, or increasing ring size, shoe size or dentures

Table 16.37 Diagnosis of acromegaly
BIOCHEMICAL
1. Insulin-like growth factor (IGF-I) (somatomedin C) level in plasma (elevated in active acromegaly)
2. Glucose tolerance test (no suppression or a paradoxical rise in growth hormone level)
ANATOMICAL (99% PITUITARY ADENOMA)
1. Skull X-ray film (enlarged sella, double floor) – not routine
2. MRI scan (if normal, exclude extrapituitary acromegaly)

Causes of angioid streaks (PASH)

Paget's disease, pseudoxanthoma elasticum (Fig. 16.47), poisoning (lead)
Acromegaly
Sickle cell anaemia
Hyperphosphataemia (familial)

7. Examine the cardiovascular system for signs of congestive cardiac failure, the abdomen for organomegaly – of liver, spleen and kidney – and for signs of hypogonadism (secondary to an enlarging pituitary adenoma).
8. Examine the lower limbs for osteoarthritis and pseudogout. Large osteophyte formation and ligamentous laxity are common features. Also look for foot drop (entrapment of the common peroneal nerve) and heel pad thickening.
9. If there is time, look for evidence of hypothyroidism and adrenocortical insufficiency (from an enlarging pituitary adenoma).
10. Do not forget to ask for the results of a urine analysis to exclude glycosuria secondary to glucose intolerance and to take the blood pressure (hypertension is an association). Decide whether the acromegaly is active (Table 16.36). Ask whether any photographs taken of the patient over the years are available for inspection (typically, manifestations begin in middle age). See Table 16.37 for the diagnostic evaluation.

Addison's disease

Common stems

1. 'This woman has weakness, anorexia and weight loss. Please assess her.'
2. 'This woman has had problems with low blood pressure. Please examine her.'

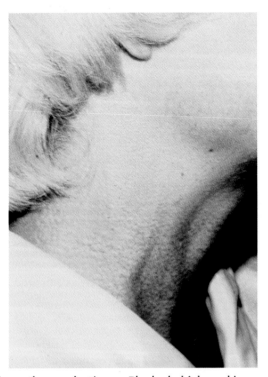

Figure 16.47 **Pseudoxanthoma elasticum. Plucked-chicken skin appearance on neck is characteristic of pseudoxanthoma elasticum.**

M Yanoff, J S Duker, J J Augsburger et al. *Ophthalmology*, 3rd edn. Fig 6-35-7. Elsevier, 2009, with permission.

Table 16.38 Autoimmune-associated diseases	
Addison's disease	Primary ovarian failure
Hypoparathyroidism	Pernicious anaemia
Mucocutaneous candidiasis	Vitiligo
Coeliac disease	Alopecia
Diabetes mellitus (type 1)	Hypophysitis
Hashimoto's thyroiditis	Myasthenia gravis
Graves' disease	

Method

Fortunately, you suspect Addison's disease.

1. Ensure the patient is appropriately undressed (to the underwear) and look for pigmentation (Fig. 16.48) (particularly in the palmar creases, elbows, gums and buccal mucosa, genital areas and scars) and vitiligo (Fig. 16.49), due to an autoimmune disease association. Ear lobe calcification occurs rarely.
2. Take the blood pressure and test for a postural drop. Ask for the results of a urine analysis, as diabetes is associated with Addison's disease. Remember that the rest of the autoimmune cluster may also be associated (Table 16.38) and consider the possible causes (Table 16.39). Diagnostic tests are summarised in Table 16.40.

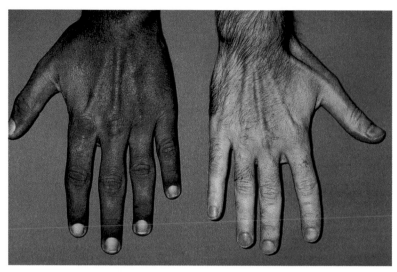

Figure 16.48 Hyperpigmentation in Addison's disease compared with a normal patient.

W D James. *Andrews' diseases of the skin: clinical dermatology*, 11th edn. Fig 24.3. Saunders, Elsevier, 2011, with permission.

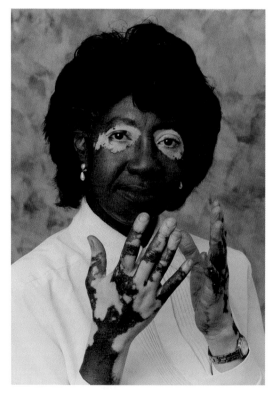

Figure 16.49 Vitiligo.

R A Spritz. The genetics of generalised vitiligo and associated autoimmune diseases. *Journal of Dermatological Science* 2006; 41(1):3–10, Fig 1, with permission

Table 16.39 **Causes of Addison's disease (chronic adrenal insufficiency)**[a]
1. IATROGENIC
2. PRIMARY
Autoimmune adrenal disease (> 80% of all cases)
Polyglandular syndromes:
Type I: Addison's disease, hypoparathyroidism, mucocutaneous candidiasis, primary hypogonadism
Type II: Addison's disease, type 1 diabetes mellitus, Hashimoto's thyroiditis or Graves' disease, primary hypogonadism
Tuberculosis, histoplasmosis
Infiltration (e.g. amyloidosis, sarcoidosis, metastatic malignant disease)
Demyelinating disease – adrenoleukodystrophy (asymmetrical cortical signs and Addison's disease), adrenomyeloneuropathy (spastic paraparesis and Addison's disease)
Drugs – heparin (bilateral adrenal haemorrhage), aminoglutethimide, ketoconazole, HIV infection
3. SECONDARY
Pituitary or hypothalamic disease (usually *no* mineralocorticoid deficiency)
[a]Acute adrenal insufficiency may follow any stress in a patient with chronic hypoadrenalism or abrupt cessation of prolonged high-dose steroid therapy.

Table 16.40 **Diagnosis of Addison's disease**
SCREENING TESTS
1. Electrolyte levels (hyponatraemia, hyperkalaemia, hyperchloraemic acidosis, hypercalcaemia)
2. Hypoglycaemia
3. Blood count (lymphocytosis, eosinophilia)
4. Chest X-ray film (tuberculosis, small heart)
5. Plain abdominal X-ray film (adrenal calcification)
DEFINITIVE TESTS
1. Short Synacthen test (0.25 mg synthetic ACTH given intramuscularly). Plasma cortisol measured at 0 and 30 minutes. Normal = plasma cortisol > 460 nmol/L at 0 or 30 minutes
2. Long Synacthen test (8-hour intravenous infusion or depot administration) if subnormal response
3. Plasma ACTH level

Diabetes mellitus

Common stems

1. 'This woman has diabetes. Please examine her.'
2. 'This man has diabetes. Please examine his eyes (or legs).'
3. 'This woman has gained weight and noticed changes in her appearance. She now has diabetes. Please examine her.'
4. 'This man who has developed diabetes has noticed changes in his skin colour.'

Method (Table 16.41)

1. General inspection may reveal a characteristic facial appearance (e.g. Cushing's syndrome or acromegaly) or pigmentation (e.g. rarely haemochromatosis), which will modify the examination approach. It is very likely the stem will make it clear

Table 16.41 Diabetes mellitus examination	

Lying
1. GENERAL INSPECTION
Weight – obesity
Hydration
Endocrine facies
Pigmentation – haemochromatosis, etc.
2. LEGS
Inspect:
    Skin – necrobiosis, hair loss, infection, pigmented scars, atrophy, ulceration, injection sites
    Muscle wasting
    Joint destruction – Charcot's joints
Palpate:
    Temperature of feet (cold, blue owing to small or large vessel disease)
Peripheral pulses:
    Femoral (auscultate)
    Popliteal
    Posterior tibial
    Dorsalis pedis
Oedema:
    Neurological assessment
    Femoral nerve mononeuritis
    Peripheral neuropathy
	3. ARMS
	Inspect:
	    Injection sites
	    Skin lesions
	Pulse
	4. EYES
	Fundi – cataracts, rubeosis, retinal disease, III nerve palsy, etc.
	5. MOUTH AND EARS
	Infection
	6. NECK
	Carotid arteries – palpate, auscultate
	7. CHEST
	Signs of infection
	8. ABDOMEN
	Liver – fat infiltration; rarely haemochromatosis
	Fat hypertrophy – insulin injection sites
	9. OTHER
	Urine analysis – glycosuria, ketones, proteinuria
	Blood pressure and pulse – lying and standing

    there is more going on than just diabetes. Otherwise, expose the patient's legs. This is the only case in which there is an advantage in starting at the legs.

2. Look for necrobiosis lipoidica over the shins (a central yellow scarred area with a surrounding red margin, if active, owing to atrophy of subcutaneous collagen – it is rare) (Fig. 16.50), pigmented scars, skin atrophy, small rounded plaques with raised borders lying in a linear fashion over the shins (diabetic dermopathy), ulceration and infection. Look at the thigh for injection sites, fat atrophy (owing to the use of impure insulin) or fat hypertrophy (repeated injections into the same site can lead to scarring and hypertrophy) and quadriceps wasting, from femoral nerve mononeuritis – called (inaccurately) diabetic amyotrophy.

3. Inspect the feet and toes very carefully. Look for loss of hair, skin atrophy and blue, cool feet (small vessel vascular disease), ulcers and foot deformity. Feel all the peripheral pulses and note capillary return. Feel for pitting oedema. Auscultate over the femoral artery for bruits.

4. Test proximal muscle power and test the reflexes. Assess for peripheral neuropathy, including dorsal column loss – called diabetic pseudotabes (see p. 566). Charcot's joints (Fig. 16.51) (due to proprioceptive loss) may be present. (*Note:* Neuropathic joint disease may occur when sensory loss (e.g. from diabetes, tabes dorsalis, amyloidosis, leprosy, meningomyelocele) allows repeated joint trauma, producing bony overgrowth, synovial effusion and joint distortion and instability.)

5. Go to the upper limbs. Look at the nails for *Candida* infection. Feel the upper arm injection sites. Ask for the blood pressure and take the pulse with the patient lying and standing to detect autonomic neuropathy (Table 16.42).

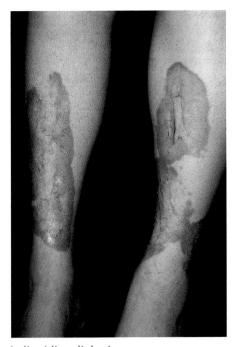

Figure 16.50 **Necrobiosis lipoidica diabeticorum.**

W D James et al. *Andrews' diseases of the skin*, 11th edn. Fig 26.29. Elsevier, 2011, with permission.

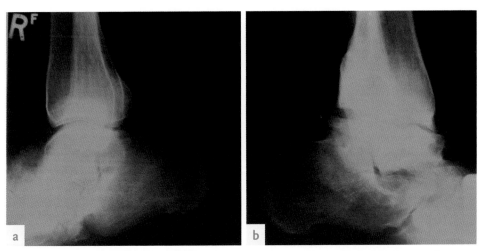

Figure 16.51 **(a) and (b) Gross destructive changes in the ankle joints in a patient with diabetic neuropathy – Charcot's joints.**

Figure reproduced courtesy of The Canberra Hospital.

Table 16.42 Autonomic neuropathy
CLINICAL FEATURES
Postural hypotension (a blood pressure fall of > 30/20 mmHg on standing upright from a supine position)
Loss of sinus arrhythmia
Valsalva manoeuvre causes no slowing of the pulse
Loss of sweating
Erectile dysfunction
Nocturnal diarrhoea
Urine retention, incontinence

Table 16.43 Features of diabetic retinopathy
NON-PROLIFERATIVE
Haemorrhages:
1. Dot-haemorrhage into the inner retinal areas
2. Blot-haemorrhage into more superficial nerve fibre layers
Hard exudates have straight edges – leakage of protein and lipids from damaged capillaries
Soft exudates (cotton-wool spots) have a fluffy appearance owing to microinfarcts
Microaneurysms
Dilated veins
PROLIFERATIVE
New vessels
Vitreous haemorrhage
Scar formation
Retinal detachment (opalescent sheet that balloons forward into the vitreous)
Laser scars (small brown or yellow spots)

6. Now examine the eyes for visual acuity. Remember, episodes of poor control cause lens abnormalities acutely. Look for Argyll Robertson pupils (which are rare). Remember, a diabetic third nerve palsy is usually pupil sparing – infarction affects the inner more than the outer fibres, whereas compressive lesions affect the outer fibres first and so involve the pupil early on.

7. Look in the fundi for diabetic retinopathy (Table 16.43, Fig. 16.52). While performing fundoscopy, also note the presence of cataracts and any new blood vessel formation over the iris (rubeosis).

8. Always test the III, IV and VI cranial nerves and remember that other cranial nerves may be affected. Periorbital and perinasal swelling with gangrene can occur with rhinocerebral mucormycosis, an opportunistic fungal infection.

9. Look in the mouth for *Candida* and other infections.

10. Look in the ears for infection (e.g. malignant otitis externa caused by *Pseudomonas aeruginosa*).

11. Feel and auscultate the carotid arteries.

12. Examine for hepatomegaly as a result of fatty infiltration and then ask for the results of urine analysis with respect to glucose and protein.

13. There may be signs of chronic kidney disease with advanced diabetes.

14. Ask whether you may weigh the patient.

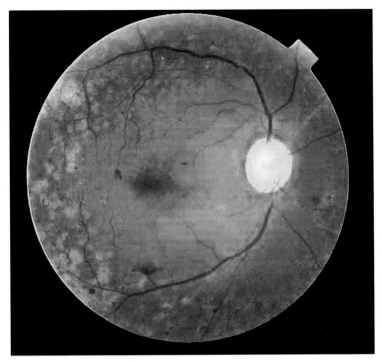

Figure 16.52 **Diabetic retinopathy.**

N Efron, *Contact lens practice*, 2nd edn. Fig 35.1. Elsevier, 2010, with permission.

Hirsutism

Common stem

'This woman has noticed an increase in facial and body hair. Please examine her.'

Method

A diagnostic approach is summarised in Table 16.44.

Table 16.44 **Hirsutism**
CLINICAL APPROACH General appearance – acromegaly, Cushingoid Skin changes of porphyria cutanea tarda (Fig. 16.53)
HAIR DISTRIBUTION Face Midline (front and back) Genital

Continued

Table 16.44 **Continued**
SIGNS OF VIRILISATION Receding hairline and increased oiliness of skin Breast atrophy Muscle bulk Clitoromegaly
ABDOMEN Adrenal masses (rarely palpable) Polycystic ovaries or ovarian tumour (rarely palpable)
BLOOD PRESSURE Raised in C-11-hydroxylase deficiency (potassium low)
CAUSES OF HIRSUTISM 1. Constitutional (normal endocrinology) 2. Polycystic ovarian syndrome 3. Adrenal – Cushing's syndrome, congenital adrenal hyperplasia (21- and 11-hydroxylase deficiency), virilising adrenal tumour 4. Ovarian (e.g. stromal ovarian cancer) 5. Drugs (e.g. phenytoin, diazoxide, streptomycin, minoxidil, androgen, glucocorticoids) 6. Other (e.g. acromegaly, porphyria cutanea tarda)

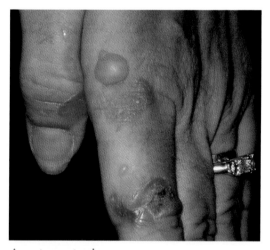

Figure 16.53 **Porphyria cutanea tarda.**

P Yachimski, N Shah, R T Chung. *Clinical gastroenterology and hepatology* 2007; 5(2):6, Fig 1, with permission.

THE RHEUMATOLOGICAL SYSTEM

In this section, only the common joints that are encountered in the examination are discussed.

The hands

Common stems

1. 'This 67-year-old woman has arthritis. Please examine her hands.' (Fig. 16.54)
2. 'This man has had pain in his hands, please examine him.' (The use of the word *pain* makes it likely the examination is a rheumatological rather than a neurological one.)
3. 'This patient has had difficulty using her hands. Please examine her.' (This stem is more ambiguous and the decision about which examination to perform will depend on what changes are seen during inspection of the hands.) Often the examiners, alarmed at the thought that candidates will begin to examine neurologically instead of rheumatologically, will say 'please perform a rheumatological examination'.

Method (see Table 16.45)

When you are asked to examine the hands consider the possibilities of arthropathy, acromegaly, a peripheral nerve lesion, a myopathy or a neuropathy. The stem will usually help.

Remember the principles of joint examination:
- Look (inspection)
- Feel (palpation) and move passively
- Test function
- Presence of extra-articular manifestations of arthritis.

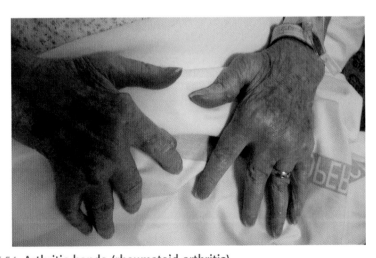

Figure 16.54 **Arthritic hands (rheumatoid arthritis).**

HINT – THE 'HAND DANCE'

A slick exam and presentation will always do wonders for your credibility to the examiners.

The 'hand dance' before you formally work through all the examination steps can be done in 20–30 seconds and gives you a lot of information early on.

With the patient sitting:

1. Ask the patient to lift his or her pronated open hands in front of the body. This will allow you to inspect the skin and joints of the dorsal aspects of the forearms, hands and nails, and assess for extensor weakness of the hands.
2. Ask them to turn their hands over. This tests supination of the wrist and you can inspect the palmar surfaces of the hands.
3. Ask 'Close the hand.' Any issue with weakness of finger flexors may become apparent and you will get a closer look at the interphalangeal joints (IPJs).
4. Ask 'Open the hand again.' Reduced range of motion in finger extension due to either weakness or contractures may be seen.
5. Ask 'Make the prayer sign.' Range of movement (ROM) of the wrist is assessed.
6. Ask 'Do the reverse prayer sign.' This also tests ROM of the wrists but if, in the short time the patient is performing this, pain or tingling develops in the median nerve distribution, this is suspicious for carpal tunnel syndrome.
7. Ask the patient to put his or her hands behind the head with elbows pointing towards the front of the body. This tests external rotation of the shoulder as well as function (relevant for being able to dress yourself or brush your hair). At this point, inspect the skin on the dorsal elbow joint.
8. Horizontally abduct both arms to 90°. This tests strength and ROM in the shoulders. If there is some arthritis in the larger joints, you will quickly find out without having to hurt the patient, something often missed in a focused hands exam.
9. Ask 'Put your hands down behind your back.' This tests internal rotation, which is another indication of function.

During the 'hand dance', look out for obvious rashes, muscle atrophy, scars and joint deformity. This is a *screening test* to help identify the major findings before going over them in more detail.

HINT

The diagnosis of arthritis is usually made during the inspection. Note the nature of the joint abnormalities and the pattern of joint involvement. Time spent on inspection is not wasted.

Start with the hand 'hand dance' (hint box). Then, if there is obvious joint disease, systematically examine as follows.

- **Look**
  1. Look at the patient for Cushingoid features (steroid treatment is more likely if the problem is rheumatoid arthritis or SLE).
  2. Look around the room for walking sticks, wheelie walkers or other aids to mobility.
  3. Make the patient comfortable; expose as much of the hands and forearms as possible.

Table 16.45 Hand examination

Sitting up (hands on a pillow)

1. GENERAL INSPECTION
  Cushingoid
  Weight
  Iritis, scleritis, etc.
  Obvious other joint disease

2. LOOK

Dorsal aspect
  Wrists:
    Skin – scars, redness, atrophy, rash, scleroderma (sclerodactyly)
    Swelling – distribution
    Deformity
    Muscle wasting
  Metacarpophalangeal joints:
    Skin
    Swelling – distribution
    Deformity – ulnar deviation, volar subluxation, etc.
  Proximal and distal interphalangeal joints:
    Skin
    Swelling – distribution
    Deformity – swan necking, boutonnière (see Fig. 16.58), Z, sausage-shaped, etc.
    Nails
    Psoriatic changes – pitting, ridging, onycholysis, hyperkeratosis, discoloration

Palmar aspect
  Skin – scars, palmar erythema (see Fig. 16.57), palm creases (anaemia), discolouration
  Muscle wasting

3. FEEL AND MOVE PASSIVELY
  Wrists:
    Synovitis
    Effusions
    Range of movement
    Crepitus
    Ulnar styloid tenderness
  Metacarpophalangeal joints:
    Synovitis
    Effusions
    Range of movement
    Crepitus
    Subluxation
  Proximal and distal interphalangeal joints:
    As above
    Palmar tendon crepitus
    Carpal tunnel syndrome tests

4. HAND FUNCTION
  Grip strength
  Key grip
  Opposition strength
  Practical ability

5. OTHER
  Elbows – subcutaneous nodules, psoriatic rash
  Other joints
  Signs of systemic disease

4. Ask the patient to show you his or her elbows. Look for ease of movement of the elbows and shoulders, and for rheumatoid nodules or a psoriatic rash on the elbows or extensor tendons.

5. Now place the patient's hands on a pillow, palms down.

6. Take some time to look at the hands, as the diagnosis is often made by inspection. Is there a symmetrical deforming polyarthropathy involving the wrists and hands? Are the DIP joints spared?

HINT

If the DIP joints are spared, the diagnosis is likely to be rheumatoid arthritis or SLE. If the DIP joints are involved, consider: nodal osteoarthritis, osteoarthritis, gouty arthritis or psoriatic arthritis.

7. Look at the skin for erythema, ecchymoses or skin atrophy (this may indicate steroid use), scars (tendon release or transfer) and rashes.

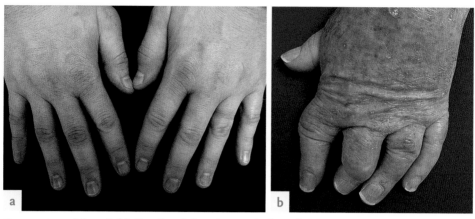

Figure 16.55 (a) and (b) Swollen joints in psoriatic arthritis over the second and third metacarpophalangeal joints of the hands.

A Garg, D Gladman. Recognizing psoriatic arthritis in the dermatology clinic. *Capsule Summary Journal of the American Academy of Dermatology* 2010; 63(5):733–48, Figs 3 and 5. American Academy of Dermatology Inc., with permission.

8. Then look for swelling and its distribution, wrist deformity and muscle wasting involving the forearms and interosseous muscles.

9. Go on to the metacarpophalangeal (MCP) joints. Note, if present, any skin abnormalities, swelling and deformity (Fig. 16.55), and particularly ulnar deviation and volar subluxation, 'swan necking' and boutonnière deformity of the fingers, and 'Z' deformity of the thumb. Sausage-shaped phalanges and telescoping of the fingers with predominant interphalangeal joint disease usually mean psoriatic arthropathy (Fig. 16.55) or Reiter's disease (reactive arthritis) (Fig. 16.56). Small joint ankylosis is common. Look for telangiectasiae.

10. Next look at the nails and describe any psoriatic nail changes (present in the great majority of patients with psoriatic arthritis) – namely pitting, onycholysis, hyperkeratosis, ridging and discoloration. Note the signs of vasculitis (splinter haemorrhages or black to brown 1–2 mm skin infarcts, usually in a periungual location) and mention this to the examiners.

11. Now ask the patient to open and close the hands. This will reveal tendon ruptures and fixed flexion deformities.

12. Turn the wrists over and look at the palms for scars (Fig. 16.57), palmar erythema and muscle wasting.

13. Next, describe the proximal and distal interphalangeal (PIP and DIP) joints. Symmetrical wrist, MCP and proximal joint swellings suggest rheumatoid arthritis. Swelling of the lateral aspects of the PIP and DIP joints is suggestive of osteoarthritis, and especially of nodal OA in women. These are Heberden's and Bouchard's nodes. These are hard and painless.

HINT

The DIP joints may look to be in the wrong position because of arthritis and deformity of the PIP and MCP joints, even when they are not involved.

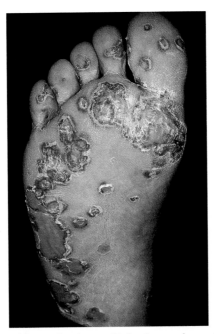

Figure 16.56 **Keratoderma blenorrhagicum (Reiter's syndrome). The palms and soles are commonly involved. There are keratotic papules, plaques, and pustules that coalesce to form circular borders like those seen on the penis.**

T P Habif. *Clinical dermatology*, 5th edn. Fig 8.13. Mosby, Elsevier, 2009, with permission.

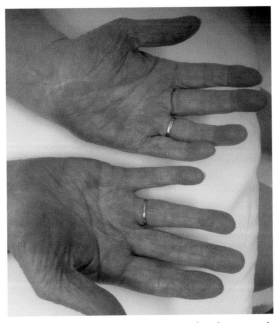

Figure 16.57 **Scars from previous tendon surgery and palmar erythema.**

HINT

Be gentle while examining – do not hurt the patient. Look up periodically during the examination at the patient's face for signs that the examination is uncomfortable.

- **Feel / move passively**
  1. Palpate each joint, starting with the wrists.
  2. Feel for synovitis (boggy swelling) and effusions. As you feel, remember that the joint line is the place where these changes occur.
  3. Note the range of passive movement of the joint.
  4. Feel for any joint crepitus.
  5. Palpate the ulnar styloid for tenderness.
  6. When examining the MCP joints, also feel for subluxation.
  7. Test for palmar tendon crepitus (tenosynovitis).
- **Test function**
  1. Test grip strength, key grip and opposition strength (thumb and little finger).
  2. Ask the patient to perform a practical procedure, such as undoing a button or writing something.
  3. A formal neurological examination of the hand is not required in assessing arthropathy. However, a ganglion or tenosynovitis may cause the carpal tunnel syndrome.
  4. Ask the patient to flex both wrists together for 30 seconds – paraesthesiae will often be precipitated in the affected hand if the carpal tunnel syndrome is present (Phalen's wrist flexion test). Tap over the carpal tunnel while the wrist is held in extension for Tinel's sign (paraesthesiae in the distribution of the median nerve). These tests have similar but limited specificity and sensitivity.
  5. If there is time, check sensation in the median and ulna nerve distributions.
- **Extra-articular manifestations and the extent of the disease**

At this point you need to decide whether to ask to examine other joints or look for other abnormalities.

1. If other joints seem obviously abnormal or are on display (e.g. shoes are off) ask to look at them.
2. Always look for psoriatic patches (hairline, behind the ears, extensor surfaces) as this may be an important clue to the diagnosis of psoriatic arthritis.
3. If the patient is seated in a chair with a number of layers of clothing covering the chest it is unlikely the examiners will want you to examine the heart or lungs. However, if you feel strongly that you want to do this, it is better to ask to put the patient onto the bed and remove the shirt rather than to try to examine the chest through layers of clothing.

You should now have an idea of the pattern and severity of the deformity, as well as the extent of the loss of function and the activity of the disease. Always consider the differential diagnosis of a deforming polyarthropathy:

- rheumatoid arthritis (see Figs 16.58, 16.59, 16.66 and 16.67)
- seronegative arthropathies – particularly psoriatic arthritis (see Figs 16.60, 16.61, 16.68 and 16.69)
- polyarticular gout (look for tophi) (see Figs 16.62a, b and 16.70) or pseudogout (Fig. 16.63)
- primary generalised osteoarthritis (where DIP and PIP joint involvement is common) (see Figs 16.64, 16.65 and 16.71).

Text continued on p. 504

HINTS

Severe osteoarthritis can cause hand deformity. Sometimes more than the DIP and PIP joints are involved, but these are usually the worst.

Destructive changes (especially shortening and telescoping of digits) and DIP disease suggest seronegative arthropathy – look carefully for psoriasis.

Practise highlighting the important features of arthritis early in your presentation (e.g. symmetrical / asymmetrical, mono / oligo or polyarthritis, associated nodules or rash, signs of activity, impact on function and extra-articular features) most consistent with your provisional diagnosis.

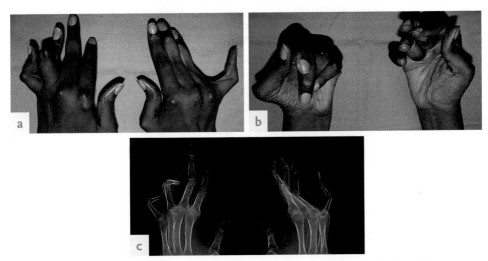

Figure 16.58 A 40-year-old patient with bilateral rheumatoid hand deformities. (a) Boutonnière deformities of the left small, left ring, and right small fingers with simultaneous swan neck deformities of the left long, right long, and right ring fingers. (b) Note the inability to make a fist on the right hand (predominantly swan neck deformity) compared with the left hand (predominantly boutonnière deformity). (c) Radiograph.

S J Sebastin, K C Chung. Reconstruction of digital deformities in rheumatoid arthritis. *Hand Clinics* 2011; 27(1):87–104, Fig 1, with permission.

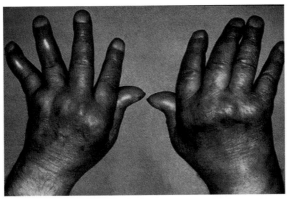

Figure 16.59 The hands of a patient with severe inflammatory arthritis, showing symmetrical deformity.

J E Dacre, J G. Worrall. Rheumatology part 1 of 2: the rheumatological history. *Medicine* 2010; 38(3):129–32, Fig 1, with permission.

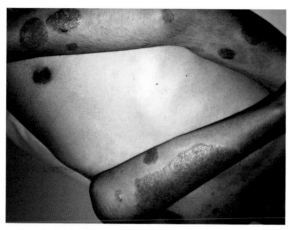

Figure 16.60 **Psoriasis.**

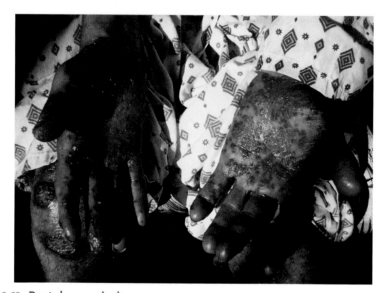

Figure 16.61 **Pustular psoriasis.**

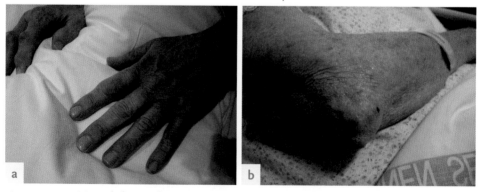

Figure 16.62 **(a) and (b) Tophaceous gout.**

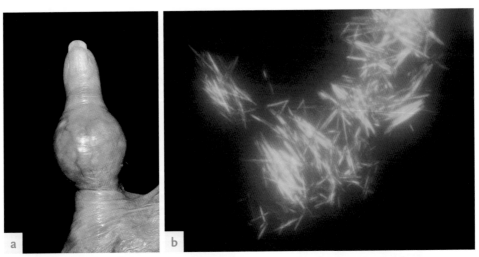

Figure 16.63 **(a) Pseudogout. The swollen interphalangeal joint. (b) Calcium pyrophosphate crystals.**

A Alexandroff, N Kirkham, N Nayak. Reprinted with permission from Elsevier (*The Lancet*, 2008, vol no 371(9618):1114).

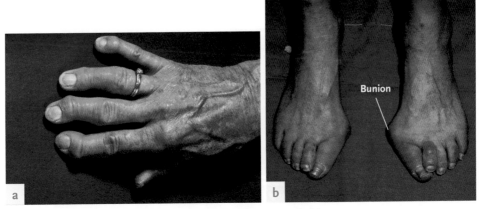

Figure 16.64 **(a) and (b) Primary generalised osteoarthritis.**

N Talley, S O'Connor, *Clinical examination*, 7th edn. Fig 24.5a and b. Elsevier Australia, 2013, with permission.

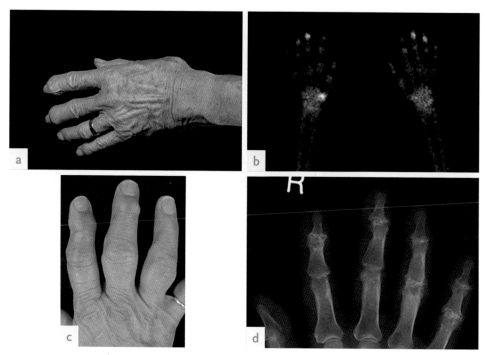

Figure 16.65 (a)–(d) Osteoarthritis of the hands.

T L Vincent, F E Watt. Rheumatology, part 1 of 2: osteoarthritis practice points, *Medicine* 2009; 38(3):151–6, Fig 2, with permission.

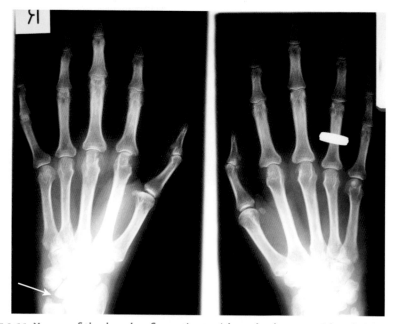

Figure 16.66 X-rays of the hands of a patient with early rheumatoid arthritis. Note the erosions of the metacarpal heads, reduced cartilage in the joint spaces and erosion of the ulnar styloid (arrow).

Figure reproduced courtesy of The Canberra Hospital.

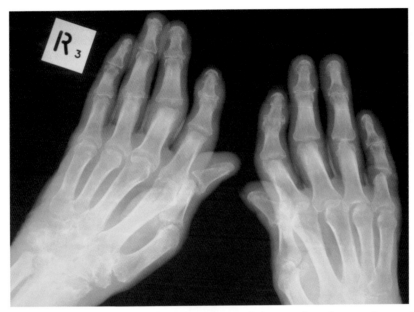

Figure 16.67 X-ray of the hands showing advanced destructive changes in a patient with rheumatoid arthritis. Note the ulnar deviation, Z deformity of the thumb, destruction of the PIP and MCP joints, and bone erosion.

Figure reproduced courtesy of The Canberra Hospital.

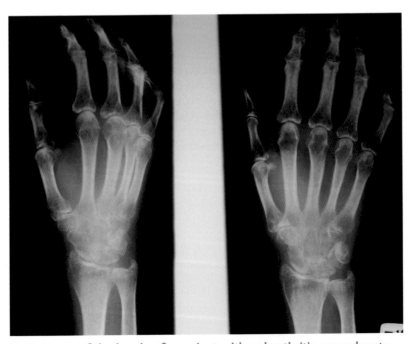

Figure 16.68 X-rays of the hands of a patient with polyarthritis secondary to connective tissue disease (CREST syndrome). There are destructive changes in all the joints (the DIP joints are not spared), and bony erosions are prominent.

Figure reproduced courtesy of The Canberra Hospital.

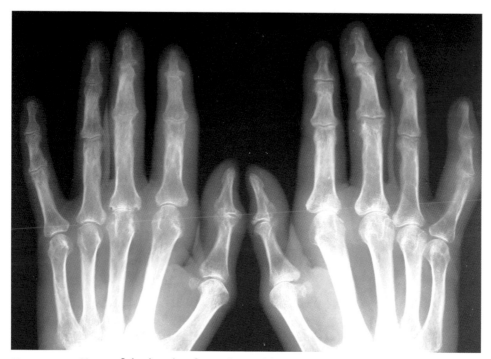

Figure 16.69 X-ray of the hands of a patient with psoriatic arthritis. Note bone erosion, loss of joint space and 'pencil in cup deformity' of the PIP joints.

Figure reproduced courtesy of The Canberra Hospital.

Look carefully while doing your hand examination for any of these possibilities.

At the end, ask whether you may examine all the other joints that are likely to be involved and the other systems likely to be affected.

Present your findings and give a differential diagnosis, in order of likelihood.

Say whether you think there are signs of active disease (e.g. synovitis).

Ask to look at X-rays of the hands (Figs 16.66–16.71) and point out the changes that are consistent with your clinical findings (assuming that there are some) including deformations, joints affected (mono or polyarthropathy) and any classic features (e.g. rheumatoid arthritis).

Ask for appropriate serological tests.

The knees

Common stems

1. 'This man has had painful knees. Please examine him.' (arthritis)

2. 'This woman has noticed swelling in her knees. Please examine her.' (arthritis or effusions)

3. 'This woman has had difficulty in walking. Please examine her knees.' (arthritis or muscle weakness)

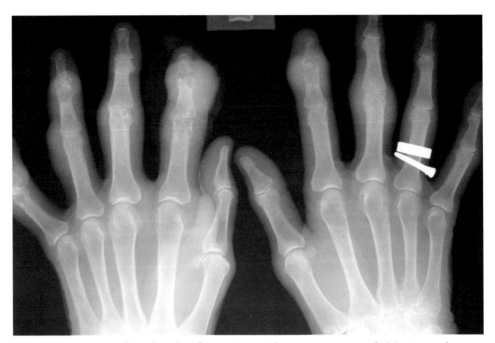

Figure 16.70 X-ray of the hands of a patient with severe gouty arthritis. Note the large soft-tissue masses and severe joint destruction.

Figure reproduced courtesy of The Canberra Hospital.

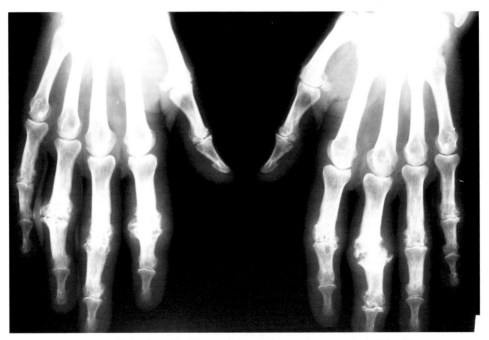

Figure 16.71 X-ray of the hands of a patient with severe osteoarthritis. Note Heberden's nodes and DIP joint involvement.

Figure reproduced courtesy of The Canberra Hospital.

Method

If walking has been mentioned in the stem, ask if you may begin by walking the patient and begin with a gait examination (p. 571). So that there will be time to examine the knees themselves, leave out Romberg's test.

Even if walking has not been mentioned, if the patient is sitting in a chair ask whether you may get him or her stand and walk. If the patient is already lying down, begin there but, if there is time, test knee function (walking) at the end.

Expose both knees and thighs fully and have the patient lie on his or her back.

- **Look**
  1. Look around the room for walking aids and at the patient's general appearance (e.g. for signs of Cushing's syndrome or acromegaly).
  2. Then look for quadriceps wasting.
  3. Then look over the knees for any skin abnormalities (scars or rashes), swelling and deformity; synovial swelling is seen medial to the patella and in the suprapatellar area.
  4. Fixed flexion deformity must be assessed; inspect the knee from the side (a space beneath the knee will be visible).
- **Feel / move passively**
  1. Feel the quadriceps for wasting.
  2. Ask the patient whether there is any pain or tenderness and palpate for warmth and synovitis over the knee joint.
  3. Examine for effusions – the patella tap (ballottement) is used to confirm a large effusion. The fluid from the suprapatellar bursa is pushed by the hand into the joint space by squeezing the lower part of the quadriceps and then pushing the patella downwards with the fingers. The patella will be ballottable if fluid is present under it. In patients with a smaller effusion, pressing over the lateral knee compartment may produce a noticeable medial bulge as a result of fluid displacement.
  4. Test flexion and extension passively and note the range of movement and the presence or absence of crepitus.
  5. Examine again for fixed flexion deformity by gently extending the knee.
  6. Test the ligaments next. The lateral and medial collateral ligaments are tested by having the knee slightly flexed, holding the leg with the right hand and arm, steadying the thigh with the left hand and moving the leg laterally and medially. Movements of more than 5°–10° are abnormal. The cruciate ligaments are tested by steadying the foot with your elbow and moving the leg anteriorly and posteriorly with the other hand. Again, laxity of more than 5°–10° is abnormal (Fig. 16.72 a and b).
  7. Use McMurray's test for meniscal integrity. Hold the lower leg and foot, flex and extend the knee while internally and externally rotating the tibia. Listen for a popping sensation and inability then to extend the knee in a meniscal tear.
  8. Ask the patient to stand up and examine for a Baker's cyst, which is felt in the popliteal fossa and is more obvious when the knee is extended.
- **Test function** i.e. ask the patient to walk.
- **Examine other joints** that may be involved.

  At the end, present your findings and differential diagnosis.

  Say whether the disease is active.

  Ask to look at X-rays (Figs 16.73 and 16.74).

  Ask for sensible blood tests to confirm the diagnosis and assess activity or severity (e.g. inflammatory markers, serology, ferritin (haemochromatosis)).

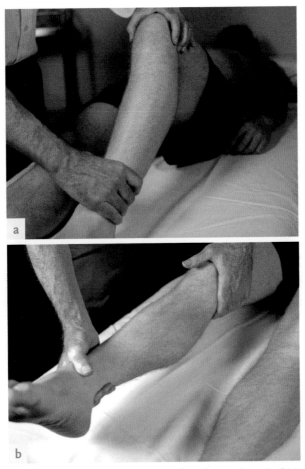

Figure 16.72 (a) Testing knee flexion – 'Let me bend your knee'. (b) Testing the collateral ligaments.

HINT

The knees and other hinge joints are commonly affected in patients with arthritis secondary to haemophilia. The pattern of joint involvement and juxta-articular bony sclerosis on X-ray film help to distinguish this from rheumatoid arthritis involving the knees (see Figs 16.73 and 16.74).

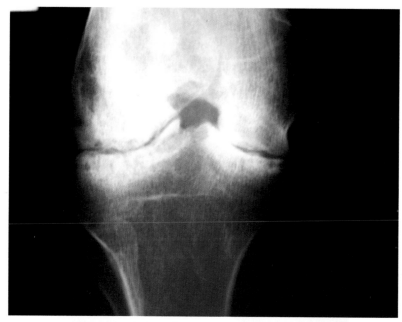

Figure 16.73 X-ray of the knee joint of a patient with arthritis secondary to haemophilia. Note the loss of joint space. The juxta-articular aspects of the tibia and femur appear sclerotic, but the bones are generally osteoporotic.

Figure reproduced courtesy of The Canberra Hospital.

The feet

Method

- **Look**
  1. As usual, glance around the room for walking aids and at the patient for signs of systemic disease, rashes, etc.

HINT

Although it is important to have a look around the room for clues, the examiners are a bit put out when some candidates prowl around the room and get down on their knees and look under the bed.

  2. Start by inspecting the ankles. Look at the skin of the feet and toes (for scars, ulcers and rashes), and look for swelling, deformity and muscle wasting.

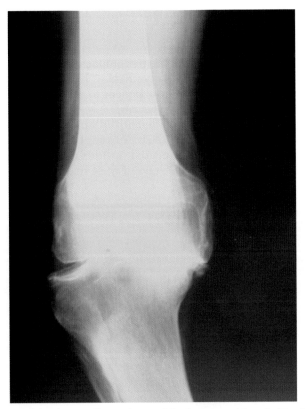

Figure 16.74 **X-ray of the knee of a patient with rheumatoid arthritis. Here there is more severe joint space loss.**

Figure reproduced courtesy of The Canberra Hospital.

3. Examine the midfoot and forefoot similarly. Deformities affecting the forefoot include hallux valgus and clawing and crowding of the toes (in rheumatoid arthritis). If pes cavus is present, consider an hereditary motor and sensory neuropathy. Pes cavus implies a long-term abnormality.
4. Note any psoriatic nail changes.
5. Look at the transverse and longitudinal arches.
6. Look for callus over the metatarsal heads, which occurs in subluxation.
7. Note any obvious gross deformities that suggest Charcot's joints.

- **Feel / move passively**
  1. Palpate, starting with the ankle, feeling for synovitis and effusion.
  2. Passive movement of the talar joints (dorsiflexion and plantarflexion) and subtalar joints (inversion and eversion) must be assessed.
  3. The best way to examine the subtalar and midtarsal joints is to fix the os calcaneus and ankle joint with the left hand while inverting and everting the midfoot with the right. Tenderness on movement is more important than range of movement. The midfoot (midtarsal joint) allows rotation of the forefoot on a fixed hindfoot.
  4. Squeeze the metatarsophalangeal joints for tenderness.
  5. Examining the individual toes is useful in seronegative spondyloarthropathies (a sausage-like swelling of the toe is characteristic of psoriatic arthritis).

6. Feel the Achilles tendon for nodules and palpate the inferior aspect of the heel for tenderness (plantar fasciitis).

• **Test function**
  1. Consider a neurological examination – test pinprick sensation and proprioception. Go on to examine other joints as appropriate.
  2. If this wasn't done at the start, ask the patient to walk. Try to associate the joint abnormalities with the character of the gait.

At the end, present the findings and differential diagnosis.

X-rays of the feet are the most likely investigations that will be available (Figs 16.75–16.79). Patients with rheumatoid arthritis can have involvement of the cervical spine, hips and shoulders, and X-rays of these may also be available.

Serological tests may be relevant.

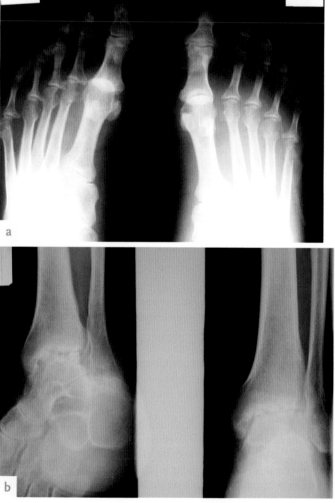

Figure 16.75 (a) X-ray of the feet of a patient with early rheumatoid arthritis. Note the joint erosions and deformity of some of the MTP and PIP joints. (b) X-ray of the ankles of a patient with rheumatoid arthritis. There is generalised loss of joint spaces, and early destructive changes are present.

Figures reproduced courtesy of The Canberra Hospital.

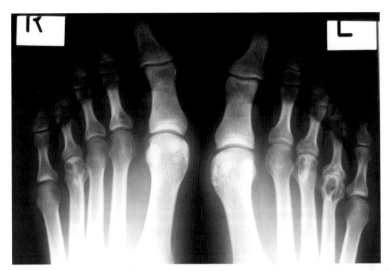

Figure 16.76 **X-ray of the feet of a patient with early psoriatic arthritis. Note the large erosions and absence of osteoporosis. There is already some joint deformity, and a spiculated bony growth is visible.**

Figure reproduced courtesy of The Canberra Hospital.

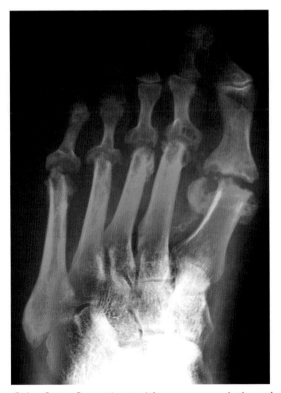

Figure 16.77 **X-ray of the feet of a patient with severe psoriatic arthritis: arthritis mutilans.**

Figure reproduced courtesy of The Canberra Hospital.

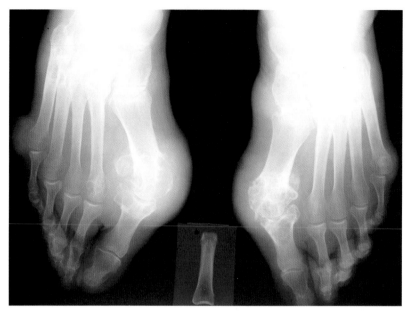

Figure 16.78 X-ray of the feet of a patient with severe gouty arthritis. Note the relative preservation of the joint spaces with erosions and overhanging edges. The area of the junction of the forefoot and midfoot has numerous erosions, which is a common finding.

Figure reproduced courtesy of The Canberra Hospital.

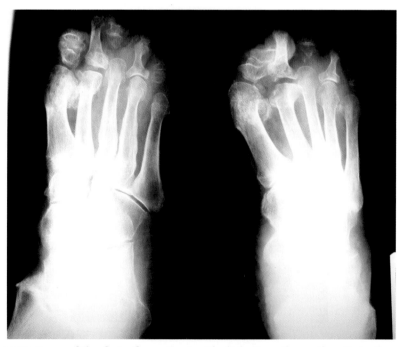

Figure 16.79 X-ray of the feet of a patient with diabetic arthropathy. Note the gross joint destruction – Charcot's joints.

Figure reproduced courtesy of The Canberra Hospital.

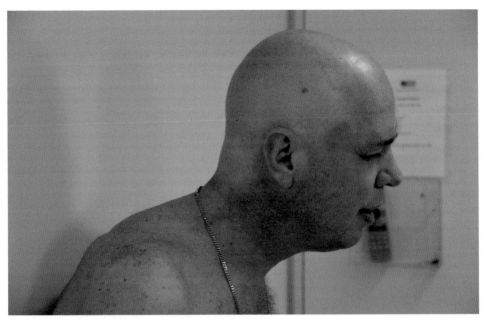

Figure 16.80 **Ankylosing spondylitis. Note the occiput-to-wall distance.**

Courtesy of the Canberra course for basic trainees.

The back

Common stems

1. 'This man has had back pain for many years. Please examine him.'
    The stem may not point you towards ankylosing spondylitis. Therefore, it is always important to stand back and observe the patient and surroundings before proceeding to the detailed examination, as you must be prepared to accommodate for unexpected findings – don't dismiss any clues.
2. 'This man has ankylosing spondylitis. Please examine him and assess the severity of his disease.' (Fig. 16.80)

Method
- **Look**
    1. The initial inspection confirms that this is a case of ankylosing spondylitis (Table 16.46). Ask the patient to undress to his underpants and stand up.
    2. Look for deformity, inspecting from both the back and the side, particularly looking for kyphosis and loss of lumbar lordosis.
- **Feel**
    1. Palpate each vertebral body for tenderness and palpate for muscle spasm.
- **Test function**
    1. Measure the finger–floor distance (inability to touch the toes suggests early lumbar disease).

Table 16.46 The seronegative spondyloarthropathies	
	HLA-B27 (%)
Ankylosing spondylitis	95
Psoriatic spondylitis	50
Reactive arthritis (Reiter's syndrome)	80
Enteropathic arthritis	75

2. Next, look at extension, lateral flexion and rotation of the back. Get the patient to run each hand down the corresponding thigh to test lateral flexion.
3. Ask whether you may perform a modified Schober's test. This involves identifying the level of the posterior iliac spine on the vertebral body (approximately at L5). Place a mark 5 cm below this point and another 10 cm above this point. Ask the patient to touch the toes. There should normally be an increase of 5 cm or more in the distance between the marks. In ankylosing spondylitis there will be little separation of the marks, since all the movement is taking place at the hips.

HINT

Small adhesive paper or plastic strips are popular as markers; do not mark the patient with a pen.

4. Next test the occiput-to-wall distance. Ask the patient to place his heels and back against the wall and ask him to touch the wall with the back of his head without raising his chin above the carrying level; inability to touch the wall suggests cervical involvement and the distance from occiput to wall is measured.

HINT

It is a good idea to know why testing of occiput-to-wall distance is performed: it is to assess progression of the disease at clinic visits.

5. Test for active sacroiliac disease by springing the anterior superior iliac spines. Pain felt in the region of the sacroiliac joints suggests activity. A simple (and unreliable) test for sacroiliac disease is to push with the heel of the hand on the sacrum and note the presence of tenderness in either sacroiliac joint. (*Note:* Usually there is bilateral disease in ankylosing spondylitis.)
6. Ask the patient to lie on his stomach. Examine the heels for Achilles tendinitis and plantar fasciitis, which are characteristic of the spondyloarthropathies. Evaluate the other large joints, particularly the knees, hips and shoulders.

• **Extra-articular manifestations**

If there is time, and especially if the patient seems to have been suitably undressed for these examinations:

1. Examine the chest for decreased lung expansion (chest expansion of less than 3 cm at the nipple line suggests early costovertebral involvement) and for signs of apical fibrosis (quite rare but you never know what exotic conditions might be found for

the clinical exams). Examine the heart for aortic regurgitation, mitral valve prolapse and evidence of conduction defects (palpate for the presence of implantable defibrillator), and the eyes for uveitis.

2. Examine the gastrointestinal system for evidence of inflammatory bowel disease and for signs of amyloid deposition (e.g. hepatosplenomegaly, abnormal urine analysis results).

3. Remember also to check for signs of psoriasis (scalp etc) and reactive arthritis, which may cause spondylitis and unilateral sacroiliitis.

4. Rarely, patients with ankylosing spondylitis have a cauda equina compression (see p. 517). X-ray changes are described in Table 16.47 and illustrated in Figs 16.81–16.83.
   Present your findings. If the stem has mentioned activity of the disease or limitation of function, make special mention of these.

Table 16.47 X-ray changes in ankylosing spondylitis		
SACROILIAC JOINTS		
1. Cortical outline lost (early)	3.	Erosions
2. Juxta-articular osteosclerosis	4.	Joint ankylosis
LUMBAR SPINE		
1. Loss of lumbar lordosis	4.	Bamboo spine (bony bridging of vertebrae) and osteoporosis
2. Squaring of vertebrae		
3. Syndesmophytes (thoracolumbar region)	5.	Apophyseal joint fusion

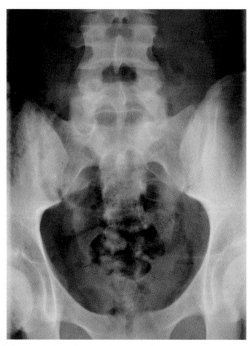

Figure 16.81 X-ray of the pelvis of a patient with Reiter's syndrome. Note the loss of joint space in the two sacroiliac joints and lumbar spine ankylosis.

Figure reproduced courtesy of The Canberra Hospital.

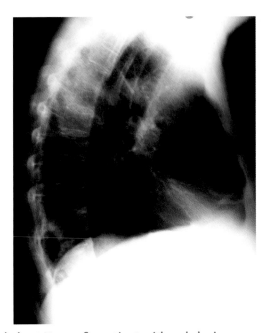

Figure 16.82 Lateral chest X-ray of a patient with ankylosing spondylitis. Note the loss of joint space and squaring of the vertebrae.

Figure reproduced courtesy of The Canberra Hospital.

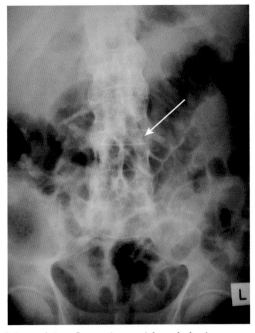

Figure 16.83 X-ray of the pelvis of a patient with ankylosing spondylitis. Note the lateral bridging syndesmophytes (arrow).

Figure reproduced courtesy of The Canberra Hospital.

Ask for X-rays (MRI scans may occasionally be available).
Ask for appropriate serology and inflammatory markers.
Features of the cauda equina syndrome are given below.

The cauda equina syndrome

Back, buttock and leg pain
Saddle sensory loss
Lower limb weakness
Loss of sphincter control

THE NERVOUS SYSTEM

Notes on the neurological short case

These examinations are often considered the most difficult short cases. However, when done well, they can also be the highest scoring. There are some principles to be kept in mind that can help, especially when presenting your findings. Create a framework and fill this in as you are examining, if possible. For example:

'I examined Mrs X, who presented with difficulty walking. In summary she has a:

- Symmetrical / asymmetrical
- Motor / sensory loss
- In a myotomal / dermatomal / stocking distribution
- Affecting __ root / up to the level of __
- With / without an associated __ motor / sensory loss
- Which would be most consistent with a diagnosis of **x**
- In further detail ...'

A cranial nerve deficit should point towards localising the lesion, and know your stroke syndromes before asking for imaging (see this website as a guide for revision: http://www.strokecenter.org/professionals/stroke-diagnosis/stroke-syndromes/).

1. Common neurological short cases include:
   - multiple cranial nerve palsies
   - pituitary lesions
   - cavernous sinus lesions
   - Parkinson's disease
   - motor neurone disease
   - facioscapulohumeral muscular dystrophy
   - multiple sclerosis, often with intranuclear ophthalmoplegia
   - gait disturbances
   - myasthenia gravis.
2. The initial inspection is extremely important.
3. Compare left and right sides ('symmetry is your friend').
4. Localisation of the lesion is what is required.
5. Think as you go along about what you are finding.
6. Speak to the patient clearly when you give instructions (but do not appear bossy or impatient).

7. The examiners are often taken in about your proficiency in general if your testing of reflexes looks good.

8. Leave the sensory examination until last. It is the most subjective part of the examination and its findings are more easily interpreted when you know what other abnormalities are present.

Cranial nerves

There will usually be some direction from the stem, sometimes to the upper or lower cranial nerves. The introduction may vary, from a problem with vision, speech or swallowing to a history of neck surgery or trauma.

> ### Common stems – II, III, IV, VI
>
> 1. 'This man has had problems with diplopia. Please examine his eyes.' (suggests III, IV, VI cranial nerve abnormality, myasthenia gravis or ocular myopathy)
> 2. 'This man has had some loss of vision. Please examine his relevant cranial nerves.' (suggests retinal or optic disc problem or field loss)
> 3. 'This woman has had blurred vision. Please examine her cranial nerves.' (consider retinopathy)

Method

1. Inspect the head and neck briefly first. Have the patient sit over the edge of the bed facing you and look for any craniotomy scars (often well disguised by hair), neurofibromata, Cushing's syndrome, acromegaly, Paget's disease, facial asymmetry and obvious ptosis, proptosis, skew deviation of the eyes or pupil inequality.

2. Look for the characteristic facies of myasthenia gravis or myotonic dystrophy.

FIRST NERVE

3. Ask the examiners whether they want you to test smell. They will rarely allow you to proceed as it is time-consuming and not usually fruitful in examinations. If you are required to test smell, a series of sample bottles will be provided by the examiners containing vanilla, coffee and other non-pungent substances. More recently, commercial 'scratch and sniff' cards are also available (see p. 527 for the causes of anosmia).

HINT

Testing upward gaze in the extreme lateral position will often reveal limitation in normal people.

SECOND NERVE

4. Test visual acuity (with the patient's spectacles on, as refractive errors are not cranial nerve abnormalities) using a visual acuity chart. Test each eye separately, covering

Table 16.48 Medical eye examination

Sitting up	Fields:
1. GENERAL INSPECTION	Red hatpin confrontation – each eye
Diagnostic facies (see Table 16.35)	Central vision
2. CORNEA	Fundi:
Corneal arcus	Cornea
Band keratopathy	Lens
Kayser–Fleischer rings	Humour
3. SCLERA	Colour of disc and state of cup
Jaundice	Retina – vessels, exudates, haemorrhages, pigmentation, etc.
Pallor	Pupils:
Injection	Shape, size, symmetry
4. PTOSIS	Light reflex – direct and consensual
5. EXOPHTHALMOS	Marcus Gunn phenomenon
6. EYELIDS	Accommodation
Xanthelasma	Eye movements:
7. LID LAG	III, IV, VI nerves – movement, diplopia, nystagmus
8. ORBITS	Gaze palsies (e.g. supranuclear lesions)
Palpate:	Fatiguability (myasthenia)
– tenderness	Corneal reflex (V)
– brow (for loss of sweating in Horner's syndrome)	**10. OTHER**
Listen for a bruit	Depends on findings – other cranial nerves, long-tract signs, urine analysis (diabetes)
9. NEUROLOGICAL EXAMINATION	
Acuity:	
Eye chart – each eye separately	

the other eye with a small card. If you ask the patient to cover the eye with his or her hand, make sure it is the palm and not the fingers that are used.[4]

5. Examine the visual fields by confrontation using a red-tipped hatpin, making sure your head is level with the patient's head. Explain before each step what it is you want the patient to do.[5] A red hatpin enables you to detect earlier peripheral field loss. Test each eye separately. If the patient has such poor acuity that a hatpin is difficult to use, map the fields with your fingers. When you are testing the patient's right eye, he or she should look straight into your left eye. The patient's head should be at arm's length and he or she should cover the eye not being tested with a hand. Bring the hatpin from the four main directions diagonally towards the centre of the field of vision. Ensure the pin stays midway between you and the patient. Apparently grossly increased peripheral fields suggest you have the pin incorrectly placed.

6. Next map out the blind spot by asking about disappearance of the hatpin lateral to the centre of the field of vision of each eye. Only a gross enlargement may be detectable by comparison with your own blind spot.

7. While using the red hatpin, ask about colour perception in each eye. Red desaturation suggests previous optic neuritis.

8. Look into the fundi (see Table 16.48). You will be provided with a conventional not a pan-optic ophthalmoscope.

---

[4]It is often possible to see between the fingers.

[5]The red hatpin is preferred as evidence suggests it is the most sensitive and specific method to assess fields. You can use your fingers as an alternative.

THIRD, FOURTH AND SIXTH NERVES

9. Look at the pupils. Note the shape, relative sizes and any associated ptosis. Use your pocket torch and shine the light from the side to gauge the reaction to light on both sides (normal : constriction). Do not bore the examiners by shining the light repeatedly into each eye – practise assessing the direct and consensual responses rapidly.

10. Look for a relative afferent pupillary defect (RAPD or Marcus Gunn phenomenon). Tell the patient 'I am going to test your pupils. Please look into the distance (at an object).' Move the torch from pupil to pupil. The movement should be quick, in an arc below the line of sight, though enough time should be allowed at each pupil for any constriction or dilatation to occur. The affected pupil will paradoxically dilate after a short time when the torch is moved from a normal eye to one with optic atrophy or decreased visual acuity from other causes. The test will be abnormal even when visual loss is only modest. An RAPD *should* be present if loss of acuity or colour saturation is present, unless the acuity is purely refractive.

11. Test accommodation by asking the patient to look into the distance and then at your red hatpin placed about 15 cm from his or her nose (normally: bilateral constriction).

12. Assess eye movements with both eyes first. Ask the patient to look voluntarily and quickly from left to right and then to follow the red hatpin in each direction – right and left lateral gaze, plus up and down in the central position. Look for failure of movement and nystagmus. While doing this, ask about diplopia as subtle ophthalmoplegia may be difficult to see. If diplopia is present then confirm that this improves if one eye is covered. Test the range of movement of each eye individually if necessary and undertake cover–uncover testing to confirm the paretic eye. If diplopia is variable then formally test for fatiguability by asking the patient to maintain gaze in one direction (myasthenia).

13. Subtle failure of normal eye movements can be detected by testing saccades (small, fast movements). The normal eye can move 600° a second, so only small degrees (about 7° is enough) of movement should be tested. Hold a finger up from one hand and a pen in the other – about 6 cm apart. Then get the patient to:
    a. look at your finger
    b. blink twice (to rest the eye)
    c. look at your finger
    d. look quickly at the pen.

    Watch eye movements for delay in one or both eyes. If the testing is difficult because of severe loss of movement (3rd or 6th nerve palsy), test one eye at a time. Do this in both horizontal and vertical directions. An undershoot or overshoot with a corrective saccade can be seen in cerebellar dysfunction ('past-pointing of the eyes').

HINT

Sometimes reduced eye movement will be detected only when the patient looks quickly from one side to the other.

14. Move the patient's head if he or she is unable to follow movements. Beware of strabismus.

HINT

Upward gaze is normally limited in elderly patients.

15. **Nystagmus**: the pattern of nystagmus, if present, provides substantial information regarding the underlying pathology. Nystagmus should have a fast phase (after which it is named), and a slow phase (the pathological part).

> **HINT**
>
> Subtle nystagmus is normal at the extremes of gaze.

- **Cerebellar nystagmus** can be unilateral or bilateral. It causes the eye to drift back (slow phase) to the centre, with the fast phase in the direction of gaze. It is therefore sometimes referred to as 'gaze-evoked nystagmus'. Other features include dysarthria, limb ataxia and hyper- or hypometric saccades.
- **Peripheral vestibular nystagmus** in acute peripheral vestibulopathies follows Alexander's law. It is unidirectional and frequently horizontal, though sometimes has a tortional element. It gets worse when the eyes move in the direction of the fast phase, and lessens as the eyes are allowed to move towards the direction of the slow phase. An abnormal head-impulse test should be present. This is performed by asking the patient to fixate on the bridge of your nose and relax his or her head. The head can then be moved gently from side to side before a few short, fast head movements are made towards to the midline. Watch the patient's eyes. In a normal patient, the patient should not lose fixation on the bridge of your nose owing to an intact vestibulo-ocular reflex (VOR). If the vestibular apparatus or nerve is disrupted then the eyes move with the head, and a corrective saccade can be seen after the head movement.
- Nystagmus can be **monocular** and occur in the setting of weakness of the opposite eye. Causes include neuropathies of cranial nerves III, IV and VI and internuclear ophthalmoplegia.
- **Vertical nystagmus** suggests a central disorder, and is virtually never peripheral.
- **Congenital nystagmus** is often dramatic, though the patient does not experience a sense of the world jumping.
- **Multidirectional nystagmus** in a gaze-evoked pattern suggests generalised cerebellar dysfunction or more commonly drug toxicity. Anticonvulsants in particular are a common cause.

Common stems – V, VII

1. 'This man has noticed numbness in the face. Please examine his cranial nerves, starting with the fifth.'
2. 'This woman has noticed some facial asymmetry, please examine her cranial nerves.'
3. 'This man has had difficulty with his speech. Please examine him.' (Consider dysarthria – cranial nerves, cerebellar speech, dysphasia.)

> **HINT**
>
> When asked to start with a particular cranial nerve, it is best to do just that. The instruction is given to help you. It is very common for candidates to ignore the request and start a routine cranial nerve examination.

16. Ask permission first to test the corneal reflexes. You can use cotton wool to touch the cornea (not the conjunctiva) gently. A better method is to use a syringe and do an air puff to avoid corneal injury. Warn the patient about what is to happen. Come in from the side and do this only once on each side. If the nerve pathways are intact, the patient will blink both eyes. Ask whether he or she can actually feel the air (V is the sensory component).

HINT

Corneal reflex: when there is an ipsilateral seventh nerve palsy, only the contralateral eye will blink – sensation is preserved – ask about this (nerve VII is the motor component). Also, with an ipsilateral seventh nerve palsy, the eye on the side of the lesion may roll superiorly with the corneal stimulus ('Bell's phenomenon').

17. Test facial sensation in the three divisions: ophthalmic, maxillary and mandibular. Use a neurotip first to assess pain. Map out any area of sensory loss from dull to sharp and check for any loss on the posterior part of the head (C2) and neck (C3). Light touch must be tested also, as there may be some sensory dissociation.

HINT

A medullary or upper cervical lesion of the fifth nerve causes loss of pain and temperature sensation with preservation of light touch. A pontine lesion may cause loss of light touch with preservation of pain and temperature sensation.

18. Examine the motor division by asking the patient to clench his or her teeth (feeling the masseter muscles) and open the mouth; the pterygoid muscles will not allow you to force it closed if the nerve is intact. A unilateral lesion causes the jaw to deviate towards the weak (affected) side.

HINT

Occasionally myasthenia affects the facial muscles. If you suspect myasthenia because of eye signs it might be worth testing for the *transverse smile* sign. Weakness of the levator muscles of the mouth makes an attempt at prolonged smiling look more like a grimace.

19. Always test the jaw jerk (with the mouth just open, the finger over the jaw is tapped with a tendon hammer). An increased jaw jerk occurs in pseudobulbar palsy. It may be absent in health.

SEVENTH NERVE

20. Look for facial asymmetry and then test the muscles of facial expression. Ask the patient to look up and wrinkle the forehead. Look for loss of wrinkling and feel the muscle strength by pushing down on each side. This is preserved in an upper motor neurone lesion because of bilateral cortical representation of these muscles.
21. Next, ask the patient to tightly shut the eyes – compare how deeply the eyelashes are buried on the two sides and then try to open each eye. Ask the patient to grin, and compare the nasolabial grooves.

22. If a lower motor neurone lesion is detected, quickly check for ear and palatal vesicles of herpes zoster of the geniculate ganglion – the Ramsay Hunt syndrome. Examining for taste on the anterior two-thirds of the tongue is not usually required.

Common stem – VIII

'This woman has noticed some hearing loss. Please examine her cranial nerves.'

EIGHTH NERVE

23. Whisper a number softly about 0.5 m away from each ear and ask the patient to repeat the number.

    An alternative method is to rustle your fingers together starting next to the ear and moving away. Ask the patient to tell you when they can no longer hear it. Compare the distance for each ear. This method allows you to compare relative hearing loss, not just a positive or negative result. It is no less arbitrary than whispering a number, and has the added advantage of being a good visual descriptor for those watching.

    Perform Rinne's and Weber's tests with a 256 Hz tuning fork.

    Always ask for an auriscope (wax is the most common cause of conductive deafness).

HINT

Look carefully for scars behind the ear. Surgery may have been performed for excision of a tumour (e.g. an acoustic neuroma).

24. The assessment of the vestibular portion of this nerve is typically done with eye assessment. However, if hearing loss is unilateral then assessment with a head-impulse test is critical. (This is covered above under 'Nystagmus'.)

Common stem – IX, X, XI, XII

'This man has noticed he has a hoarse voice. Please examine his lower cranial nerves.'

NINTH AND TENTH NERVES

25. Look at the palate and note any uvular displacement. Ask the patient to say 'aaah' and look for asymmetrical movement of the soft palate. When there is a unilateral tenth nerve lesion, the uvula is drawn towards the unaffected (normal) side.

26. Testing the gag reflex is traditional, but adds little to the examination. Ask if you may do this and warn the patient if you are given the go-ahead.

    If the palate moves normally and the patient can feel the spatula, the same information is obtained (the ninth nerve is the sensory component and the tenth nerve the motor component): touch the back of the pharynx on each side. Remember to ask the patient whether he or she feels the spatula each time. You may not attain top marks if the patient vomits all over the examiners. If the spatula is used correctly, the patient will gag only if the reflex is hyperactive.

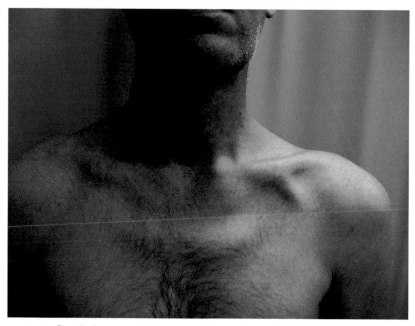

Figure 16.84 **Left-sided sternocleidomastoid wasting.**

27. Ask the patient to speak (to assess hoarseness) and to cough (listen for a bovine cough, which may occur with a recurrent laryngeal nerve lesion). *Note:* You will not usually be required to test taste on the posterior third of the tongue (i.e. ninth nerve).

ELEVENTH NERVE

28. Ask the patient to shrug his or her shoulders and then feel the trapezius bulk and push the shoulders down. Then instruct the patient to turn the head against resistance (your hand) and also feel the muscle bulk and note any sternocleidomastoid wasting (Fig. 16.84).

TWELFTH NERVE

29. While examining the mouth for cranial nerves IX and X, inspect the tongue for wasting and fasciculation (which may be unilateral or bilateral, and is best seen with the tongue not protruded).

HINT

Take time to inspect the tongue. Fasciculations and wasting are easily missed but are very important in the diagnosis of a lower motor neurone twelfth nerve palsy.

---

30. Then ask the patient to protrude the tongue. Look again for fasciculation and wasting. With a unilateral lesion it deviates towards the weaker (affected) side.
31. The way to finish your assessment depends entirely on your findings. For example, if you discover evidence of a particular syndrome (such as lateral medullary syndrome), you should proceed to confirm your impressions by examining more peripherally, if allowed (looking especially for sensory long tract and cerebellar signs; see below).

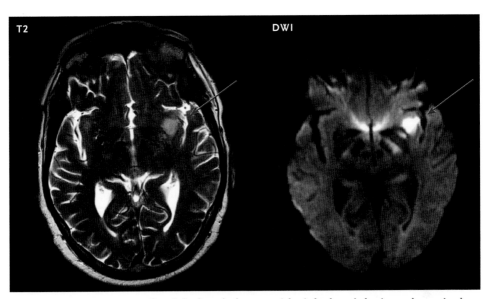

Figure 16.85 MRI scans of a right-handed man with right hemiplegia and nominal aphasia. There is a left middle cerebral artery stroke (red arrow) with increased signal in the insula cortex on the T2 image. The diffusion-weighted image (DWI) indicates this is an acute stroke.

Figure reproduced courtesy of The Canberra Hospital.

> **HINT**
>
> If you have discovered multiple lower cranial nerve palsies, you would want to assess, among other features, the nasopharynx for signs of tumour and the neck for scars and radiotherapy changes.

32. Auscultating for carotid or cranial bruits (over the mastoids, temples and orbits), as well as taking the blood pressure and testing the urine for sugar, are relevant.

    Relevant investigations are likely to be CT or MRI scans. These are not always easy for physicians to report. Candidates would hope to have a good idea where in the brain or the spinal cord the abnormality is likely to be present. Only scans with quite obvious abnormalities (Fig. 16.85) are likely to be used for the exam (because the examiners are otherwise more likely than not to have little idea of where the abnormality is).

Eyes

Common stems

1. 'This man has noticed loss of vision. Please examine his eyes.'
2. 'This woman is a diabetic. Please examine her eyes.'
3. 'Please examine this man's eyes.' (This is a deliberately vague stem, sometimes used when there is a specific ocular finding or something that should be obvious from inspection and would guide your exam.)

Method (Table 16.48)

1. Always inspect the eyes first, with the patient sitting over the end of the bed facing you at eye level if possible. Note any corneal abnormalities, such as band keratopathy (in hypercalcaemic states) or Kayser–Fleischer rings (Wilson's disease). Look at the sclerae for colour (e.g. jaundice, blue in osteogenesis imperfecta), pallor, injection and telangiectasia. Inspect carefully for subtle ptosis or strabismus. Look for exophthalmos from behind and above the patient, as well as in front.

2. Proceed then as for the cranial nerve eye examination, testing acuity, fields and pupils, and then performing fundoscopy.

3. You must do fundoscopy in this case. Begin by examining the cornea and lens, and then the retina. Note any corneal, lens or humour abnormalities. Look for retinal changes of diabetes mellitus (see Table 16.43) and hypertension (see Table 16.7). Also carefully inspect for optic atrophy, papilloedema, angioid streaks (see p. 484), retinal detachment, central vein or artery thrombosis and retinitis pigmentosa.

4. Test eye movements. Also, look for fatiguability of eye muscles by asking the patient to look up at your hatpin for half a minute (myasthenia gravis). Alternatively ask the patient to close the eyes tightly; if positive (the peek sign), within 30 seconds the lid margin will begin to separate, showing the sclera. Test for lid lag if you suspect hyperthyroidism.

5. Test the corneal reflex using a syringe with air (ask the examiners first and warn the patient).

6. Palpate the orbits for tenderness and auscultate the eyes with the bell of the stethoscope (the eye being tested is shut, the other is open and the patient is asked to stop breathing).

7. Do not forget that the patient may have a glass eye. Suspect this if visual acuity is zero in one eye and no pupillary reaction is apparent. Lengthy attempts to examine the fundus of a glass eye are embarrassing (and not uncommon).

One-and-a-half syndrome

This is rare but important to recognise. These patients have a horizontal gaze palsy when looking to one side (the 'one') plus impaired adduction on looking to the other side (the 'and-a-half'). Other features often include turning out (exotropia) of the eye opposite the side of the lesion (paralytic pontine exotropia).

When combined with a lesion of the fascicle of the ipsilateral facial nerve, causing a lower motor neurone facial weakness, it is termed the 'eight-and-a-half syndrome' (seven plus one-and-a-half).

The one-and-a-half syndrome can be caused by a stroke (infarct), plaque of multiple sclerosis or tumour in the dorsal pons. Once you have completed the task in the stem, focus your examination onto demonstrating other features of this differential diagnosis, including searching for other features of MS (e.g. spastic paraparesis).

Horner's syndrome

If you find a partial ptosis and a constricted pupil (which reacts normally to light), Horner's syndrome is likely (Fig. 16.86, Table 16.49).

Proceed as follows.

1. Test for a difference in sweating over each brow with the back of your finger (even though your brow is usually more sweaty than the patient's); this occurs only when the lesion is proximal to the carotid bifurcation. *Note:* Absence of sweating differences does not exclude the diagnosis of Horner's syndrome.

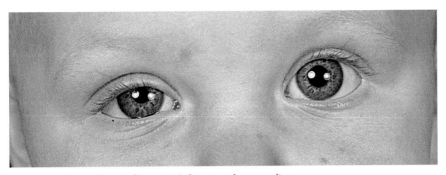

Figure 16.86 **Horner's syndrome (right eye abnormal).**

M Yanoff, J S Duker. *Ophthalmology*, 3rd edn. Fig 9.19.7. Mosby, Elsevier, 2008, with permission.

Table 16.49 Causes of Horner's syndrome
1. Carcinoma of the lung apex (usually squamous cell carcinoma)
2. Neck – thyroid malignancy, trauma
3. Carotid arterial lesion – carotid aneurysm or dissection, pericarotid tumour, cluster headache
4. Brain stem lesions – vascular disease (especially the lateral medullary syndrome), syringobulbia, tumour
5. Retro-orbital lesions
6. Syringomyelia (rare)

2. Next, examine the appropriate cranial nerves to exclude the lateral medullary syndrome:
   a. nystagmus (to the side of the lesion)
   b. ipsilateral fifth (pain and temperature), ninth and tenth cranial nerve lesions
   c. ipsilateral cerebellar signs
   d. contralateral pain and temperature loss over the trunk and limbs.
3. Ask the patient to speak and note any hoarseness (which may be caused by recurrent laryngeal nerve palsy from a chest lesion or a cranial nerve lesion).
4. Look at the hands for clubbing. Test finger abduction to screen for a lower trunk brachial plexus (C8, T1) lesion.
5. If there are signs of hoarseness or a lower trunk brachial plexus lesion, proceed to a respiratory examination, concentrating on the apices for signs of lung carcinoma.
6. Examine the neck for lymphadenopathy, thyroid carcinoma and a carotid aneurysm or bruit (e.g. fibromuscular dysplasia causing dissection).
7. As syringomyelia may rarely cause this syndrome, finish off the assessment by examining for dissociated sensory loss. Remember, this lesion may cause a *bilateral* Horner's syndrome (a trap for the unwary).

Notes on the cranial nerves

First (olfactory) nerve (p. 518)

CAUSES OF ANOSMIA

Bilateral

1. Upper respiratory tract infection (most common).
2. Meningioma of the olfactory groove (late).

3. Ethmoid tumours.
4. Head trauma (including cribriform plate fracture).
5. Meningitis.
6. Hydrocephalus.
7. Congenital – Kallmann's syndrome (hypogonadotrophic hypogonadism).
8. COVID-19.

Unilateral
1. Meningioma of the olfactory groove (early).
2. Head trauma.

Second (optic) nerve (p. 518)
LIGHT REFLEX
Constriction of the pupil in response to light is relayed via the optic nerve and tract, the superior quadrigeminal brachium, the Edinger–Westphal nucleus and its efferent parasympathetic fibres, which terminate in the ciliary ganglion. There is no cortical involvement.

ACCOMMODATION REFLEX
Constriction of the pupil with accommodation originates in the cortex (in association with convergence) and is relayed via parasympathetic fibres in the third nerve.

CAUSES OF ABSENT LIGHT REFLEX BUT INTACT ACCOMMODATION REFLEX
1. Midbrain lesion (e.g. Argyll Robertson pupil).
2. Ciliary ganglion lesion (e.g. Adie's pupil).
3. Parinaud's syndrome.
4. Bilateral anterior visual pathway lesions (i.e. bilateral afferent pupil deficits).

CAUSES OF ABSENT CONVERGENCE BUT INTACT LIGHT REFLEX
1. Cortical lesion (e.g. cortical blindness).
2. Midbrain lesions (rare).

PUPIL ABNORMALITIES
Causes of constriction
1. Horner's syndrome.
2. Argyll Robertson pupil.
3. Pontine lesion (often bilateral, but reactive to light).
4. Narcotics.
5. Pilocarpine drops.
6. Old age.

Causes of dilatation
1. Mydriatics, atropine poisoning or cocaine.
2. Third nerve lesion.
3. Adie's pupil.
4. Iridectomy, lens implant, iritis.
5. Post-trauma, deep coma, cerebral death.
6. Congenital.

VISUAL FIELD DEFECTS (FIG. 16.87)

1. Tunnel vision: concentric diminution (e.g. glaucoma, papilloedema)	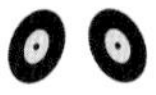
2. Enlarged blind spot: optic nerve head enlargement	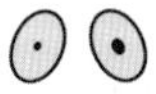
3. Central scotomata: optic nerve head to chiasmal lesion (e.g. demyelination, toxic, vascular, nutritional)	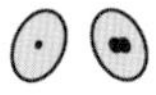
4. Unilateral field loss: optic nerve lesion (e.g. vascular, tumour)	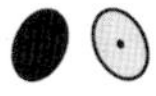
5. Bitemporal hemianopia: optic chiasma lesion (e.g. pituitary tumour, sella meningioma)	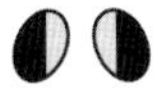
6. Homonymous hemianopia: optic tract to occipital cortex, lesion at any point (e.g. vascular, tumour). *Note:* Incomplete lesion results in macular (central) vision sparing	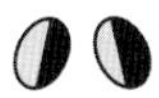
7. Upper quadrant homonymous hemianopia: temporal lobe lesion (e.g. vascular, tumour)	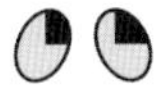
8. Lower quadrant homonymous hemianopia: parietal lobe lesion	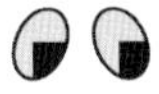

Figure 16.87 **Visual field defects associated with lesions of the visual system.**

ADIE'S SYNDROME

Cause

Lesion in the efferent parasympathetic pathway.

Signs
1. Dilated pupil.
2. Decreased or absent reaction to light (direct and consensual).
3. Slow or incomplete reaction to accommodation with slow dilation afterwards.
4. Decreased tendon reflexes.
5. Patients are commonly young women.

ARGYLL ROBERTSON PUPIL (FIG. 16.88)

Cause

Lesion of the iridodilator fibres in the midbrain, as in:
1. syphilis
2. diabetes mellitus
3. alcoholic midbrain degeneration (rarely)
4. other midbrain lesions.

Signs
1. Small, irregular, unequal pupil.
2. No reaction to light.
3. Prompt reaction to accommodation.
4. If tabes associated, decreased reflexes.

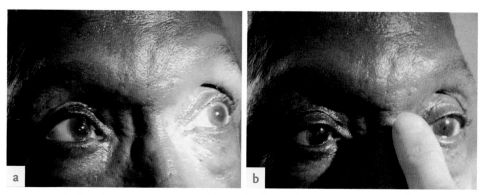

Figure 16.88 Argyll Robertson pupil. (a) Lack of pupillary constriction to light. (b) Pupillary constriction to accommodation.

T A Aziz, R P Holman. The Argyll Robertson pupil. *American Journal of Medicine* 2010; 123(2):120–1, Fig 1. Elsevier, with permission.

Table 16.50 Papilloedema versus papillitis	
PAPILLOEDEMA	**PAPILLITIS**
Optic disc swollen without venous pulsation	Optic disc swollen[a]
Acuity normal (early)	Acuity poor
Colour vision normal	Colour vision affected (particularly red desaturation)
Large blind spot	Large central scotoma
Peripheral constriction of visual fields	Pain on eye movement
Usually bilateral	Onset usually sudden and unilateral
[a]In retrobulbar neuritis and old papillitis the optic disc becomes pale.	

CAUSES OF PAPILLOEDEMA (TABLE 16.50)

1. Space-occupying lesion (causing raised intracranial pressure) or a retro-orbital mass.
2. Hydrocephalus (associated with large ventricles):
   a. obstructive (block in the third ventricle, aqueduct or outlet to fourth ventricle – e.g. tumour)
   b. communicating:
      i. increased formation – choroid plexus papilloma
      ii. decreased absorption – tumour causing venous compression, subarachnoid space obstruction from meningitis.
3. Idiopathic intracranial hypertension (pseudotumour cerebri):
   a. idiopathic
   b. contraceptive pill
   c. Addison's disease
   d. drugs – nitrofurantoin, tetracycline, vitamin A, steroids
   e. lateral sinus thrombosis
   f. head trauma.
4. Hypertension (grade IV).
5. Central retinal vein thrombosis.
6. Cerebral venous sinus thrombosis.
7. High cerebrospinal fluid protein level – Guillain–Barré syndrome.

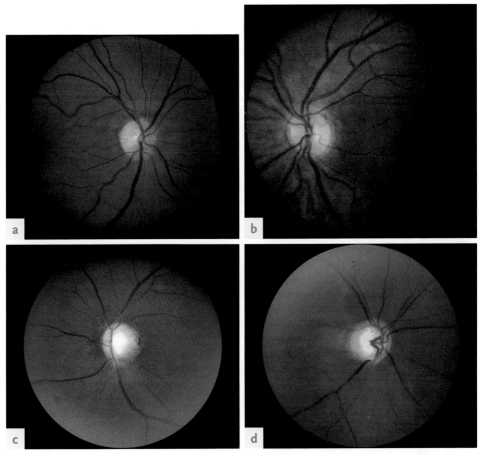

Figure 16.89 **Patterns of optic atrophy. (a) Superotemporal sector atrophy in a 59-year-old woman with a supraclinoid internal carotid artery aneurysm compressing the optic nerve. (b) Band ('bow-tie') atrophy in an 8-year-old boy with a craniopharyngioma compressing the optic chiasm. (c) Diffuse optic atrophy in a 41-year-old woman with neuromyelitis optica after a severe attack that left her with no light perception. (d) Glaucomatous cupping with atrophy of the superior and inferior neuroretinal rim appearing as 'notching' of the neuroretinal rim and vertical elongation of the cup.**

L A Levin, D M Albert (eds). *Ocular diseases: mechanisms and management.* Fig 44.1. Saunders, Elsevier, 2010, with permission.

CAUSES OF OPTIC ATROPHY (FIG. 16.89)

1. Chronic papilloedema or optic neuritis.
2. Optic nerve pressure or division.
3. Glaucoma.
4. Ischaemia.
5. Familial – retinitis pigmentosa, Leber's disease, Friedreich's ataxia.

CAUSES OF OPTIC NEUROPATHY

1. Multiple sclerosis (see Fig. 12.1, p. 336).
2. Toxic – ethambutol, chloroquine, nicotine, alcohol.

3. Metabolic – vitamin B_{12} deficiency.
4. Ischaemia – diabetes mellitus, temporal arteritis, atheroma.
5. Familial – Leber's disease.
6. Infective – infectious mononucleosis (glandular fever).

CAUSES OF CATARACT

1. Old age (senile cataract).
2. Endocrine – diabetes mellitus, steroids.
3. Hereditary or congenital – dystrophia myotonica, Refsum disease.
4. Ocular disease – glaucoma.
5. Irradiation.
6. Trauma.

CAUSES OF PTOSIS

1. With normal pupils:
   a. senile ptosis (common)
   b. myotonic dystrophy
   c. facioscapulohumeral dystrophy
   d. ocular myopathy, e.g. mitochondial myopathy
   e. thyrotoxic myopathy
   f. myasthenia gravis
   g. botulism, snake bite
   h. congenital
   i. fatigue.
2. With constricted pupils:
   a. Horner's syndrome
   b. tabes dorsalis.
3. With dilated pupils: third nerve lesion.

Third (oculomotor) nerve (p. 520)

> **HINT**
>
> When a patient has diplopia, ptosis and eye movement abnormalities not explained by cranial nerve problems, consider an ocular myopathy (e.g. mitochondrial myopathy). Unlike in myasthenia patients, these do not worsen with repetition or maintenance.

CLINICAL FEATURES OF A THIRD NERVE PALSY (FIG. 16.90)

1. Complete ptosis (partial ptosis may occur with an incomplete lesion).
2. Divergent strabismus (eye 'down and out').
3. Dilated pupil unreactive to direct or consensual light and unreactive to accommodation.

> **HINT**
>
> Always exclude a fourth (trochlear) nerve lesion when a third nerve lesion is present. Do this by tilting the patient's head to the same side as the lesion. The affected eye will intort if the fourth nerve is intact. Or ask the patient to look down and across to the opposite side from the lesion and look for intorsion. Remember **SIN**:
>
> **S**uperior (oblique muscle), supplied by the IV nerve, **IN**torts the eye

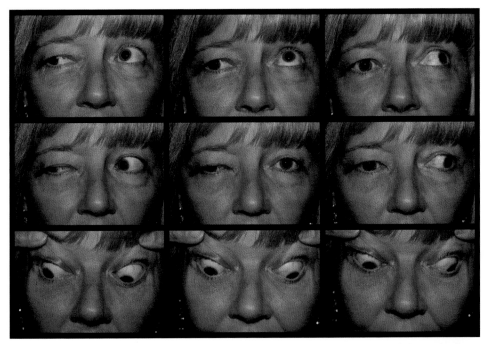

Figure 16.90 Third nerve palsy. A 52-year-old woman with right upper lid ptosis from a third nerve palsy. Note the marked limited adduction and elevation of the right eye. The patient has less limitation to depression of the right eye.

J A Nerad, K D Carter, M A Alford. Disorders of the eyelid: blepharoptosis and eyelid retraction. In *Rapid diagnosis in ophthalmology series: oculoplastic and reconstructive surgery*. Fig 5.6. Mosby, Elsevier, 2008, with permission.

AETIOLOGY
Central
1. Vascular (e.g. brain stem infarction).
2. Tumour.
3. Demyelination (rare).
4. Trauma.
5. Idiopathic.

Peripheral
1. Compressive lesions:
   a. aneurysm (usually on the posterior communicating artery)
   b. tumour causing raised intracranial pressure (dilated pupil occurs early)
   c. nasopharyngeal carcinoma
   d. orbital lesions – Tolosa–Hunt syndrome (superior orbital fissure syndrome – painful lesion of the third, fourth, sixth and the first division of the fifth cranial nerves)
   e. basal meningitis.
2. Infarction – diabetes mellitus, arteritis (pupil is usually spared).
3. Trauma.
4. Cavernous sinus lesions.

Sixth (abducens) nerve (p. 520)

CLINICAL FEATURES OF A SIXTH NERVE PALSY

1. Failure of lateral movement.
2. Affected eye is deviated inwards in severe lesions.
3. Diplopia – maximal on looking to the affected side; the images are horizontal and parallel to each other; the outermost image is from the affected eye and disappears on covering this eye (this image is also usually more blurred).

AETIOLOGY

Bilateral

1. Trauma (head injury).
2. Wernicke's encephalopathy.
3. Raised intracranial pressure.
4. Mononeuritis multiplex.

Unilateral

1. Central:
   a. vascular
   b. tumour
   c. Wernicke's encephalopathy
   d. multiple sclerosis (rare).
2. Peripheral:
   a. diabetes, other vascular lesions
   b. trauma
   c. idiopathic
   d. raised intracranial pressure.

HINTS

1. With the eye abducted: the elevator is the superior rectus (third nerve). The depressor is the inferior rectus (third nerve).
2. With the eye adducted: the elevator is the inferior oblique (third nerve). The depressor is the superior oblique (fourth nerve).

CAUSES OF NYSTAGMUS

Jerky

1. Horizontal:
   a. vestibular lesion (*Note:* Nystagmus is horizontal, with fast phase away from the side of the side of the lesion. Obeys Alexander's law.)
   b. cerebellar lesion (*Note:* Unilateral disease causes nystagmus to the side of the lesion. Drift is towards the midline with fast phase in direction of gaze.)
   c. internuclear ophthalmoplegia (Fig. 16.91). (*Note:* Nystagmus is in the abducting eye, with failure of adduction on the affected side. This is a result of a medial longitudinal fasciculus lesion. The most common cause in young adults with bilateral involvement is multiple sclerosis; in the elderly, consider brain stem infarction. When the medial longitudinal fasciculus and the abducens nucleus on the same side are affected, the only complete horizontal movement the patient can make is abduction of the contralateral eye – *one-and-a-half syndrome*.)

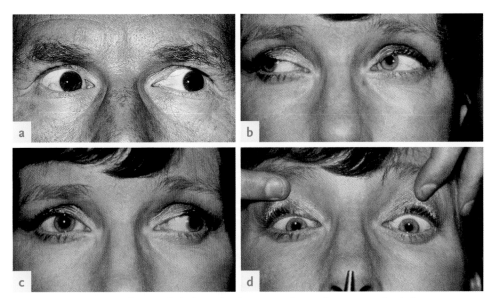

Figure 16.91 Internuclear ophthalmoplegia. (a) Unilateral, gaze to the left (abnormal). (b) Bilateral, gaze to the right (abnormal). (c) Bilateral, gaze to the left (abnormal). (d) Bilateral, convergence (normal).

A Compston, I McDonald, J Noseworthy et al. The symptoms and signs of multiple sclerosis. In *McAlpine's multiple sclerosis*, 4th edn. Fig 6.9, Churchill Livingstone, Elsevier, 2006, with permission.

2. Vertical:
   a. brain stem lesion
      i. upbeat nystagmus suggests a lesion in the floor of the fourth ventricle
      ii. downbeat nystagmus suggests a foramen magnum lesion
   b. toxic – phenytoin, alcohol (may be multidirectional).

Pendular
1. Retinal (decreased macular vision) – albinism.
2. Congenital.

SUPRANUCLEAR PALSY

Loss of vertical upward and / or downward gaze. (Isolated impairment of upward gaze is common with ageing owing to mechanical changes in the orbit.)

Clinical features (distinguishing it from third, fourth and sixth nerve palsy) are:
1. both eyes affected
2. pupils often unequal
3. no diplopia
4. reflex eye movements (e.g. on flexing and extending the neck) intact.

STEELE–RICHARDSON–OLSZEWSKI SYNDROME (PROGRESSIVE SUPRANUCLEAR PALSY)

1. Loss of vertical downward gaze first, later vertical upward gaze and finally horizontal gaze. Saccades are impaired before pursuit. Vergence is lost early.
2. Associated with pseudobulbar palsy, long-tract signs, extrapyramidal signs, dementia and neck rigidity.

PARINAUD'S SYNDROME

Loss of vertical upward gaze, which is often associated with convergence–retraction nystagmus on attempted convergence and pseudo Argyll Robertson pupils.

Causes of Parinaud's syndrome

1. Central:
   a. pinealoma
   b. multiple sclerosis
   c. vascular lesions.
2. Peripheral:
   a. trauma
   b. diabetes mellitus
   c. other vascular lesions
   d. idiopathic
   e. raised intracranial pressure.

Fifth (trigeminal) nerve palsy (p. 522) (Fig. 16.92)

AETIOLOGY

Central (pons, medulla and upper cervical cord)

1. Vascular.
2. Tumour.
3. Syringobulbia.
4. Multiple sclerosis.

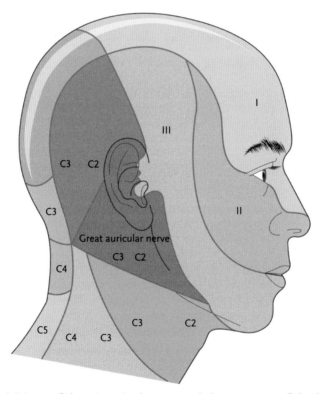

Figure 16.92 **Divisions of the trigeminal nerve and dermatomes of the head and neck.**

Peripheral (posterior fossa)
1. Aneurysm.
2. Tumour (skull base, e.g. acoustic neuroma).
3. Chronic meningitis.

Trigeminal ganglion (petrous temporal bone)
1. Meningioma.
2. Fracture of the middle fossa.

Cavernous sinus (associated third, fourth and sixth nerve palsies)
1. Aneurysm.
2. Thrombosis.
3. Tumour.

Other
1. Sjögren's syndrome.
2. SLE.
3. Toxins.
4. Idiopathic.

HINTS

1. If there is loss of all sensation in all three divisions of the fifth nerve – consider a lesion at the ganglion or sensory root.
2. If there is total sensory loss in one division – consider a postganglionic lesion.
3. If there is loss of pain but preservation of touch – consider a brain stem or upper cervical cord lesion.
4. If there is loss of touch but pain sensation is preserved – consider a pontine nucleus lesion.

Seventh (facial) nerve palsy (p. 522)
AETIOLOGY
Upper motor neurone lesion (supranuclear)
1. Vascular.
2. Tumour.

Lower motor neurone lesion
1. Pontine (often associated with nerves V, VI):
   a. vascular
   b. tumour
   c. syringobulbia
   d. multiple sclerosis.
2. Posterior fossa:
   a. acoustic neuroma
   b. meningioma.
3. Petrous temporal bone:
   a. Bell's palsy
   b. Ramsay Hunt syndrome

    c. otitis media

    d. fracture.

4. Parotid:

    a. tumour

    b. sarcoid.

CAUSES OF BILATERAL LOWER MOTOR NEURONE FACIAL WEAKNESS

1. Guillain–Barré syndrome.
2. Bilateral parotid disease (e.g. sarcoidosis).
3. Mononeuritis multiplex (rare).

HINT

Myopathy (usually genetic) and neuromuscular junction defects can cause bilateral facial weakness.

Eighth (vestibulo-cochlear) nerve (p. 523)

A careful assessment of eye movements followed by the head-impulse test and gait assessment allow clinical assessment of vestibular function. The Dix–Hallpike test is useful in the clinical setting of benign paroxysmal positioning vertigo (BPPV) but, although this element is clinically relevant, it is best grouped with ocular examination in the short case.

To differentiate nerve deafness from conductive deafness, use the following tests.

RINNE'S TEST

A 256 Hz vibrating tuning fork is placed first on the mastoid process, behind the ear, then, when the sound is no longer heard, in line with the external meatus.

Results

1. Normal – the note is audible at the external meatus.
2. Nerve deafness – the note is audible at the external meatus because air and bone conduction are reduced equally, so that air conduction is better (as is normal): positive result. Remember however that a severely deaf patient will not hear the tuning fork at all.
3. Conduction (middle ear) deafness – no note is audible at the external meatus: negative result.

WEBER'S TEST

A 256 Hz tuning fork is placed on the centre of the forehead.

HINT

The tines of the fork should be in line with the external auditory canal, so that the sound waves that leave the fork from two axes do not cancel each other out.

Results

1. Normal – the sound is heard in the centre of the forehead.
2. Nerve deafness – the sound is transmitted to the normal ear.
3. Conduction deafness – the sound is heard louder in the abnormal ear.

Note: Although these tests are of traditional importance, they are not very accurate and are now rarely used by neurologists. However, candidates must be able to perform them. Vestibular dysfunction *does* frequently present to the emergency department, though not to the examinations, and the ability to perform a head-impulse test is critical to assessment of vestibular function.

CAUSES OF DEAFNESS
1. Nerve (sensorineural) deafness:
   a. degeneration (e.g. presbycusis)
   b. trauma (e.g. high noise exposure, fracture of the petrous temporal bone)
   c. toxic (e.g. aspirin, alcohol, streptomycin)
   d. infection (e.g. congenital rubella syndrome, congenital syphilis)
   e. tumour (e.g. acoustic neuroma)
   f. brain stem lesions
   g. vascular disease of the internal auditory artery.
2. Conductive deafness:
   a. wax
   b. otitis media
   c. otosclerosis
   d. Paget's disease of bone.

Ninth (glossopharyngeal) and tenth (vagus) nerve palsy (p. 523)
AETIOLOGY
Central
1. Vascular (e.g. lateral medullary infarction due to vertebral or posterior inferior cerebellar artery disease).
2. Tumour.
3. Syringobulbia.
4. Motor neurone disease (vagus nerve only).

Peripheral – posterior fossa
1. Aneurysm.
2. Tumour.
3. Chronic meningitis.
4. Guillain–Barré syndrome (vagus nerve only).

Twelfth (hypoglossal) nerve palsy (see p. 524)
AETIOLOGY
Upper motor neurone lesion
1. Vascular.
2. Motor neurone disease.
3. Tumour.
4. Multiple sclerosis.

HINT
The syndrome of bilateral upper motor neurone lesions of the ninth, tenth and twelfth nerves is called *pseudobulbar palsy*.

Lower motor neurone lesion – unilateral
1. Central:
   a. vascular – thrombosis of the vertebral artery
   b. motor neurone disease
   c. syringobulbia.
2. Peripheral (posterior fossa):
   a. aneurysm
   b. tumour
   c. chronic meningitis
   d. trauma
   e. Arnold–Chiari malformation
   f. fracture or tumour of the base of the skull.

HINT

The Arnold–Chiari malformation is a protrusion of the cerebellar tonsils through the foramen magnum. The more severe types (II–IV) cause basilar compression with lower cranial nerve palsies, cerebellar limb signs (due to tonsillar compression) and upper motor neurone signs in the legs.

Lower motor neurone lesion – bilateral
1. Motor neurone disease.
2. Arnold–Chiari malformation.
3. Guillain–Barré syndrome.
4. Polio.

HINT

It is difficult to detect unilateral twelfth nerve lesions, as the tongue muscles (except the genioglossus) are bilaterally innervated.

Causes of multiple cranial nerve palsies

Think of *cancer* first.
1. Nasopharyngeal *carcinoma*.
2. Chronic meningitis (e.g. *carcinoma*, tuberculosis, sarcoidosis).
3. Guillain–Barré syndrome (spares nerves I, II and VIII), including the Miller Fisher variant.
4. Brain stem lesions – these are usually as a result of vascular disease causing crossed sensory or motor paralysis (i.e. cranial nerve signs on one side and contralateral long-tract signs); patients with brain stem *gliomas* may have similar signs and may live for many years.
5. Arnold–Chiari malformation.
6. Trauma.
7. Lesion of the base of the skull (e.g. Paget's disease, large *meningioma*, *metastasis*).
8. Rarely, mononeuritis multiplex (e.g. diabetes mellitus).
9. Myopathies and neuromuscular diseases – these cause weakness in muscles innervated by multiple cranial nerves.

Higher centres

Method (Table 16.51)

In this assessment especially, you must be guided by your findings. The introduction is important. For example, if you are told the patient also presents with right-sided weakness, you should concentrate on looking for dominant parietal lobe signs.

1. Shake the patient's hand, noting any obvious focal weakness and introduce yourself. Explain that you will be asking him or her some questions.
2. Examine speech systematically as outlined in Table 16.52.
3. Next, assess the parietal lobes. Begin with the dominant parietal lobe, as Gerstmann's syndrome is common in examinations.

HINT

Dominant parietal lobe evaluation: using the mnemonic AALF, examine for:

Acalculia (test mental arithmetic)

Agraphia (test for an inability to write)

Left–right disorientation (e.g. by asking the patient to put his or her right palm on the left ear, then vice versa)

Finger agnosia (inability to name individual fingers), which is caused by a left angular gyrus lesion in right-handed and about half of left-handed patients

---

4. Test general parietal functions (involving either lobe). Examine for sensory and visual inattention. Neglect and extinction tend to be more profound and persistent in non-dominant lesions. Also, test for agraphaesthesia (inability to appreciate numbers drawn on the palm) and astereognosis (inability to name objects placed in the hand). Assess constructional apraxia by asking the patient to draw a clock face and fill in the numbers.
5. The major specific non-dominant parietal dysfunction is dressing apraxia. This can be tested by turning the patient's pyjama top inside out and asking him or her to put it on correctly.
6. Assess memory, both short and long term. This is a medial temporal lobe function. Ask the patient to remember the name of three words of different groups (e.g. Brown, Tulip and Bicycle – choose some memorable to you) and repeat them immediately. Then assess long-term memory, such as by asking when World War II finished. Ask the names of the items again at the end of your higher centres' examination (remembering to do so can be difficult). If the patient cannot remember the

Table 16.51 Higher centres' examination	
Lying or sitting	Both
1. GENERAL INSPECTION	Sensory inattention
Diagnostic facies (see Table 16.35)	Visual inattention
Obvious cranial nerve or limb lesions	Cortical sensory loss (loss of graphaesthesia, two-point discrimination, joint position sense and stereognosis)
Ask patient about handedness, level of education	
Shake hands	Constructional apraxia
2. ORIENTATION	**5. MEMORY (TEMPORAL LOBE)**
Time	Short term (e.g. names of flowers)
Place	Long term (e.g. current US President)
Person	**6. FRONTAL LOBE**
3. SPEECH	Reflexes – grasp – pout – palmar – mental
Name objects (nominal dysphasia)	Proverb interpretation
4. PARIETAL LOBES	Smell
Dominant (AALF or Gerstmann's syndrome)	Fundi
Acalculia – (mental arithmetic)	Gait
Agraphia (write)	**7. OTHER**
Left–right disorientation	Visual fields
Finger agnosia (name fingers)	Bruits
Non-dominant	Blood pressure, etc.
Dressing apraxia	

Table 16.52 Examination of dysphasia
FLUENT SPEECH (USUALLY RECEPTIVE, CONDUCTIVE OR NOMINAL DYSPHASIA)
1. Naming of objects – patients with nominal, conductive or receptive aphasia name objects poorly
2. Repetition – conductive and receptive aphasics cannot repeat
3. Comprehension – only receptive aphasic patients cannot follow commands (verbal or written)
4. Reading – conductive and receptive aphasic patients have difficulty reading
5. Writing – conductive aphasic patients have impaired writing (dysgraphia), whereas receptive aphasic patients have abnormal content. Dysgraphia may also occur with dominant frontal lobe lesions
NON-FLUENT SPEECH (USUALLY EXPRESSIVE DYSPHASIA)[a]
1. Naming of objects – poor (but may be better than spontaneous speech)
2. Repetition – may be possible with great effort. Phrase repetition (e.g. 'no ifs, ands or buts') is poor
3. Comprehension – near normal (written and verbal commands are followed)
4. Writing – dysgraphia may be present
5. Look for hemiparesis – arm more affected than leg
[a]As the patient is aware of the deficit, he or she is often frustrated and depressed.

words then give categorical prompts (e.g. colour, flower and transport in the above example). If this does not help, you can give multiple options from which to choose. Distinguishing whether the words can be correctly selected may help to separate forms of dementia.

7. Test frontal lobe problems (Fig. 16.93), first by assessing the primitive reflexes normally not present in adults. The grasp reflex, pout reflex and palmar–mental reflex are usually all that need be tested. Then ask for interpretation of a common proverb, such as 'A rolling stone gathers no moss'. Ask if you may test for anosmia (cranial nerve I) and gait apraxia (a frontal gait abnormality is marked by gross

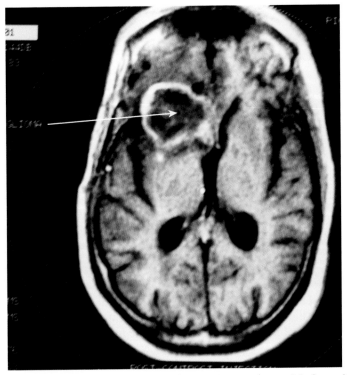

Figure 16.93 A frontal glioma found on MRI scan in a patient with frontal lobe signs (arrow).

Figure reproduced courtesy of The Canberra Hospital.

unsteadiness in walking – the feet typically behave as if glued to the floor, resulting in a hesitant shuffling gait with freezing).

8. If there is evidence of a frontal lobe lesion, look at the fundi to exclude the rare Foster Kennedy syndrome (optic atrophy on the side of the lesion and papilloedema in the opposite fundus).

9. Any abnormality of the parietal, temporal or occipital lobes may cause a characteristic visual field loss. This should be tested, if appropriate, at the conclusion of your examination. Other important signs to look for are carotid bruits, hypertension and relevant focal neurological signs.

10. MRI and CT scans may show cerebral atrophy consistent with dementia (Fig. 16.94), or sometimes a space-occupying lesion.

Speech

Common stems

1. 'Please assess this man's speech.'
2. 'This woman has had difficulty understanding speech. Please examine her.'

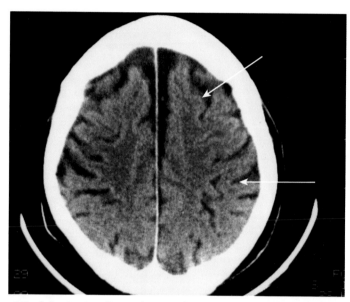

Figure 16.94 **CT of the brain of a patient with early dementia, showing generalised cerebral atrophy. There is obviously more CSF present than normal (arrows). Remember that frontal lobe atrophy is not specific for dementia.**

Figure reproduced courtesy of The Canberra Hospital.

Method

Take careful note of the stem as this may direct you. The first stem requires some initial assessment before choosing a path, whereas the second stem specifically indicates that language needs to be assessed.

Remember, if a patient does not hear you, cannot speak your language or does not understand you then the result will be the same: you will get nowhere. Therefore, when assessing language it is critical to follow a sequence that ensures you have established that the patient can understand and then process your instructions. If you do not follow an appropriate sequence it is very likely you will come to incorrect conclusions.

> **HINT**
>
> Remember to keep your instructions simple and concise. The longer and more complex your instruction, the easier it is for the patient to become confused.

1. First, assess the patient's comprehension (i.e. reception, Wernicke's area). Ensure you do not give leading cues with your body language. In other parts of the neurology examination this is very helpful, but in assessing language it is imperative you do not. *Start simple and increase complexity.* Begin by asking the patient to 'close your eyes'. Then ask the patient to 'poke out your tongue'. Watch for perseveration. Progress to some more complex commands, for example 'touch your left hand to your right ear'. This also gives helpful right–left information (which is lost in Gertmann syndrome). Ask the patient to 'touch your nose, then your chin, then your forehead'. Often patients with subtle deficits will touch their cheek in the place of their chin. Finally ask him or her to 'point to the ceiling *after* you point to the floor'. Stress 'after'. Remember that deficits may be incomplete or mild.

2. Next, assess repetition (i.e. conductive aphasia, arcuate fasciculus). This also allows an initial assessment for dysarthria. Again, start simple and move to the more complex. 'Say what I say' is a good first instruction as it is simple. Phrases may include 'blue sky', 'we went to the circus and had a good time' or 'the orchestra played and the audience applauded', 'hippopotamus' and finally 'no ifs, ands or buts'.

3. Then test naming function (nominal, parietal/temporal lobe). The same principle of simple to complex (low-frequency words) applies, for example naming parts of the 'hand' – e.g. 'thumb', then 'ring finger'; if they say just 'finger', ask which one. 'Knuckles' is a low-frequency, harder word. Or ask about the parts of a 'shirt' – 'collar', 'sleeve' and 'cuff' in order of increasing difficulty.

4. If the patient can complete these tests, then speech can be assessed more freely. Ask about the patient's handedness, and test orientation if you have not yet done so. Ask him or her to describe a picture. The examination room rarely has distinguishing features worth describing. Check that the patient is not neglecting part of the image, while listening to speech for fluency and errors.

5. The sequence from here on will depend upon your findings. If dysphasia is the finding, check for other parietal features as well as limb strength and visual fields. If the patient has dysarthria or dysphonia, proceed to examining the lower cranial nerves.

DYSPHASIA

1. If reception is severely impaired then further language assessment is very challenging. Consider giving written instructions to see whether the patient can comprehend them. Patients with impaired reception may generate fluent but content-poor speech, with many conjunctions but few verbs and nouns. They may be oblivious to the fact they are speaking nonsense.

2. If the speech is fluent but conveys information imperfectly, often with paraphasic errors (e.g. 'treen' for train – substitution of a word of similar sound – a phonemic error; 'bed' for chair – an error relating to identity of the word – a semantic error), the main possibilities are nominal and receptive dysphasia. Test for these by asking the patient to name objects, to repeat a statement after you and then follow commands. Then ask him or her to read and write if the above are abnormal (see Table 16.52).

3. If the speech is slow and non-fluent (hesitant), exactly the same procedure is followed, but an expressive dysphasia is likely. At the end, ask to assess for a hemiparesis (see Table 16.52).

4. Remember, large lesions may cause global aphasia, with inability to comprehend or speak, plus hemiparesis (Table 16.53).

Table 16.53 The sites of lesions in aphasia and dysphasia
RECEPTIVE
Wernicke's area – posterior part of first temporal gyrus in the dominant lobe
EXPRESSIVE
Broca's area – posterior part of the third frontal gyrus
CONDUCTIVE
Arcuate fasciculus (temporal lobe)
NOMINAL
Angular gyrus (temporal lobe) – small localised lesion
Other causes: encephalopathies (metabolic, toxic), pressure effects from a distant space-occupying lesion
Recovery phase from any dysphasia

5. Aim to perform a speech exam in 4 minutes. If you have time, try to elucidate the risk factors and aetiology for the lesions found. For instance, if your examination reveals a vascular territory cerebral lesion, check the patient's heart rate for atrial fibrillation, blood pressure, carotid bruits and previous carotid surgery, signs of diabetes mellitus or hypercholesterolaemia. Remember to ask for relevant investigations such as an ECG or HbA$_{1c}$.

DYSARTHRIA

1. This is a disorder of articulation with no disorder of the content of speech. Consider cerebellar disease and lower cranial nerve lesions particularly. Cerebellar speech is slurred or 'scanning' (i.e. irregular and staccato). Pseudobulbar palsy causes slow, hesitant, hollow-sounding speech with a harsh, strained voice, whereas bulbar palsy causes nasal speech with imprecise articulation. In motor neurone disease there may be mixed signs of bulbar and pseudobulbar palsy.
2. Ask the patient to say 'Hippopotamus', 'Constitution', 'Me Me Me' and 'Lah Lah Lah'.
3. If the speech is cerebellar, go on to this system (p. 572).
4. If palsy of a lower cranial nerve is likely, examine the lower cranial nerves carefully.
5. Do not forget to elicit the jaw jerk. Look in the mouth too for ulceration or other local lesions.
6. Less common causes of dysarthria include extrapyramidal disease and myopathies (p. 566).

DYSPHONIA

This is huskiness of the voice from a laryngeal disorder, recurrent laryngeal nerve palsy or focal dystonia. If this is found, assess the quality of the cough too.

Upper limbs

> **Common stems**
>
> 1. 'This man has noticed weakness in his arms. Please examine him.'
> 2. 'This woman has had difficulty combing her hair. Please examine her upper limbs.'

HINT

If told someone has trouble combing her hair, ask the patient to attempt to reach the back of her head with her hands. Possible causes include proximal muscle weakness (myopathic or upper motor neurone) and arthritis of the shoulder and occasionally elbow. Also consider the possibility of scapular winging, which you will miss if the arms are elevated to only 90°.

Method (Table 16.54)

1. Look at the whole patient briefly. Note particularly evidence of a muscle wasting, a myopathic face, Parkinsonian features or stroke.
2. Shake the patient's hand firmly and introduce yourself. If he or she cannot let go, you have made the diagnosis: myotonia (usually caused by dystrophia myotonica). Ask the patient to sit over the side of the bed facing you.

Table 16.54 **Upper limb neurological examination**	
1. GENERAL INSPECTION	Reflexes:
Diagnostic facies (see Table 16.35)	Biceps
Scars	Triceps
Skin (e.g. neurofibromata, café-au-lait)	Supinator
Abnormal movements	Coordination
2. SHAKE HANDS	Finger–nose test – intention tremor, past pointing:
3. MOTOR SYSTEM	
Inspect arms, shoulder girdle – extend both arms:	Dysdiadochokinesis
	Rebound
Wasting	**4. SENSORY SYSTEM**
Fasciculation	Temperature ± pain (pinprick)
Tremor	Vibration (128 Hz tuning fork)
Drift	Proprioception – DIP joint (each hand)
Palpate:	Light touch (cotton-wool)
Muscle bulk	**5. OTHER**
Muscle tenderness	Thickened nerves (wrist, elbow)
Tone:	Axillae
Wrist	Neck
Elbow	Lower limbs
Power:	Cranial nerves
Shoulder	Urine analysis, etc.
Elbow	
Wrist	
Fingers	
Ulnar, median nerve function	

MOTOR SYSTEM

Examine the motor system systematically every time.

1. Inspect first for wasting (both proximally and distally) and fasciculations. Do not forget to include the shoulder girdle in your inspection (p. 550).
2. Ask the patient to hold both hands out with the arms extended and to close the eyes. Look for drifting of one or both arms. There are only three causes for this drift:
   a. upper motor neurone weakness (usually downwards, owing to muscle weakness)
   b. cerebellar lesion (usually upwards, owing to hypotonia)
   c. posterior column loss (any direction, owing to loss of joint position sense).
3. Also note any tremor and pseudoathetosis resulting from proprioceptive loss.
4. Feel the muscle bulk next, both proximally and distally, and note any muscle tenderness. In the presence of wasting and weakness, fasciculation indicates lower motor neurone degeneration.
5. Test tone at the wrists and elbows by moving the joints at varying velocities.
6. Assess power next. Demonstrating the movement helps the patient to perform it correctly.
   a. Shoulder:
      i. abduction (C5, C6): tell the patient to abduct the arms with the elbows flexed and push up
      ii. adduction (C6–C8): tell the patient to adduct the arms with the elbows flexed and push in.

b. Elbow:
   i. flexion (C5, C6): tell the patient to bend the elbow and pull in
   ii. extension (C7, C8): tell the patient to bend the elbow and push away.
c. Wrist:
   i. flexion (C6, C7): tell the patient to bend the wrist and not to let you straighten it
   ii. extension (C7, C8): tell the patient to straighten the wrist and not to let you bend it.
d. Fingers:
   i. extension (C7, C8): tell the patient to straighten the fingers and keep them straight
   ii. flexion (C7, C8): tell the patient to squeeze two of your fingers
   iii. abduction (C8, T1): tell the patient to spread out the fingers and not to let you push them together
   iv. Grade the power (p. 554).
7. Test for an ulnar lesion (loss of finger abduction and adduction) and a median nerve lesion (loss of thumb abduction) (p. 559).
8. Examine the reflexes:
   a. biceps (C5, C6) – biceps muscle
   b. triceps (C7, C8) – triceps muscle
   c. supinator (C5, C6) – brachioradialis muscle (elbow flexion)
      Note: An inverted supinator jerk – when tapping the lower end of the radius, elbow extension and finger flexion are the only response; associated with an absent biceps and exaggerated triceps jerk this indicates an intraspinal lesion compressing the spinal cord and nerve roots at C5, C6
   d. Hoffman's reflex (C8) – flick the distal phalanx of the middle finger towards extension with the hand resting in a neutral position. A resulting flexion of the thumb indicates pathologically increased reflexes.
9. Assess coordination with finger–nose testing and look for dysdiadochokinesis and rebound (p. 573). Ensure, if testing rebound, that the patient is well supported and does not fall over.

Motor weakness can be caused by an upper motor neurone lesion, lower motor neurone lesion, neuromuscular junction disorder or myopathy. If there is evidence of a lower motor neurone lesion, consider anterior horn cell, nerve root and brachial plexus lesions, peripheral nerve lesions or a motor peripheral neuropathy.

SENSORY SYSTEM

Examine the sensory system after motor testing because this can be time-consuming (and confusing, even when assessed by experts). Less is more in sensation: over-zealous demarcation is seldom helpful and may be painful for the patient.

1. First, test the spinothalamic pathway (pain and temperature). Use the metal of a tuning fork to test cold, starting distally and moving proximally to detect a gradient or level. Temperature sensation is more specific than pain sensation, and less unpleasant to the patient.
2. To test pain, use a new blunt neurology pin. One candidate accidentally pricked his own finger during the examination with a sharp pin. By the time he stopped bleeding his short-case time was up. (In case you believe this might be a good ploy, the candidate failed.) Once again, move reasonably rapidly from distal to proximal. Avoid testing grossly oedematous legs with a pin. (Oedema fluid may leak everywhere). When using a tip with a sharp and a blunt end, there is seldom a good reason to use the blunt end; it will likely simply confuse you.

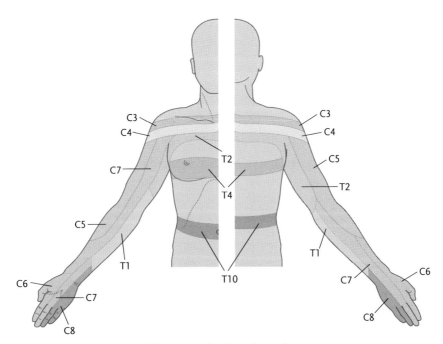

Figure 16.95 **Dermatomes of the upper limb and trunk.**

As you are assessing, try to fit any sensory loss into dermatomal (cord or nerve root lesion) (Fig. 16.95), peripheral nerve, peripheral neuropathy (glove) or hemisensory (cortical or cord) distribution. Also, remember that 'cape' sensory loss (neck, shoulders and arms) suggests syringomyelia, whereas 'shield' sensory loss (front of the chest) may occur with syphilis.

3. Next, test the posterior column pathway (vibration and proprioception). Use a 128 Hz tuning fork to assess vibration sense. Place this when vibrating on the nail bed of a finger when the patient has the eyes closed and ask whether he or she can feel it. If so, ask the patient to tell you when the vibration ceases and then stop the vibration. If the patient has deficient sensation, test at the ulnar head at the wrist, the elbow, and then the shoulder. Test both arms. Quantitative tuning forks are available, but unnecessary for short-case examinations.

4. Examine proprioception first with the DIP joint of the index finger. When the patient has the eyes open, grasp the distal phalanx from the sides and move it up and down to demonstrate, then ask him or her to close the eyes and repeat the manoeuvres. Start with large movements (to get the patient familiar with what you're asking) then test small movements. Normally, movement through even a few degrees is detectable (but this ability declines with age) and the patient can tell whether it is up or down. If there is any abnormality, proceed to test the wrist and elbows similarly.

HINT

Proprioceptive loss may be subtle. A normal person can detect movement and usually directional changes of 1°–2°. Ensure that you test small joint movements.

5. Light touch may be tested, but this is seldom useful if other modalities are examined properly. Test it with cotton-wool. Touch the skin lightly in each dermatome. Do *not* stroke.
6. Feel for thickened nerves – ulnar at the elbow, median at the wrist and radial at the wrist – and feel the axillae if there is evidence of a plexus lesion. Do not forget to mention any scars that may be present. Finally, examine the neck movements, if relevant, and look for surgical scars in the front and back of the neck and in the axillae.
7. To confirm a diagnosis, it may be necessary to examine further afield. Ask the examiners whether you can do this. For example, if there is evidence of motor neurone disease, assess the lower limbs as well as the tongue. If there is evidence of a C5, C6 root lesion, assess the lower limbs for an upper motor neurone lesion and the neck for cervical spondylosis.

Shoulder girdle examination

> **Common stem**
>
> 'This man has had difficulty lifting objects above his head and hanging out the washing. Please examine his shoulder girdle.'

> **HINT**
>
> This introduction is often used for facioscapulohumeral (FSH) muscular dystrophy. A careful inspection of the face from a distance will reveal wasting of the masseter and temporalis muscles, among others.

Method

This is likely to be a muscular dystrophy or a root lesion. Proceed by inspecting each muscle, palpating its bulk and testing function as follows.
1. From the back:
   a. trapezius (XI, C3, C4) – ask the patient to elevate the shoulders against resistance and look for winging of the upper scapula
   b. serratus anterior (C5–C7) – ask the patient to push the hands against the wall and look for winging of the lower scapula
   c. rhomboids (C4, C5) – ask the patient to pull both shoulder blades together, with hands on hips
   d. supraspinatus (C5, C6) – ask the patient to abduct the arms against resistance, beginning with the arms less than 15° from the sides
   e. infraspinatus (C5, C6) – ask the patient to rotate the upper arms externally against resistance with arms at the side
   f. teres major (C5–C7) – ask the patient to rotate the upper arms internally against resistance
   g. latissimus dorsi (C7, C8) – ask the patient to cough, and palpate on both sides.
2. From the front:
   a. pectoralis major, clavicular head (C5–C8) – ask the patient to lift the upper arms above the horizontal and push them forwards
   b. pectoralis major, sternocostal part (C6–T1) and pectoralis minor (C7) – ask the patient to adduct the upper arms against resistance
   c. deltoid (C5, C6) (and circumflex nerve) – ask the patient to abduct the arms against resistance, beginning with the arms more than 15° from the sides.
3. Go on to look for sensory changes, which will be absent if this is a muscular dystrophy.

HINT

If FSH is suspected (facial muscle wasting and winging of the scapulae), look for foot drop (see Fig. 16.100) and then test for facial weakness (inability to close the eyes tightly, whistle or puff out the cheeks).

Lower limbs

Common stems

1. 'This man has had difficulty in walking. Please examine his lower limbs.'
2. 'This woman has become unsteady when walking. Please examine her.'

HINT

If the stem mentions walking, *always* ask the patient to walk.

Method (Table 16.55)

1. Note the patient's general appearance. Especially look for upper limb girdle wasting and the presence of a urinary catheter. Look for pes cavus. Look around the room for a walking stick or frame and special shoes.
2. Begin by testing the gait. Ask the examiners whether this is possible – sometimes the patient may be unable to walk. If the patient can walk, ask him or her to walk

Table 16.55 **Lower limb neurological examination**	
Lying	Ankle
1. GENERAL INSPECTION	Plantar
Diagnostic facies (see Table 16.35)	Coordination:
Urinary catheter	Heel–shin test
Scars, skin	Toe–finger test
2. GAIT	Foot-tapping test
3. MOTOR SYSTEM	**4. SENSORY SYSTEM**
Inspect:	Pain
Wasting	Vibration
Fasciculation	Proprioception
Tremor	Light touch
Palpate:	**5. SADDLE REGION SENSATION**
Muscle bulk	**6. ANAL REFLEX**
Muscle tenderness	**7. BACK**
Tone:	Deformity
Knee – and test for clonus	Scars
Ankle – and test for clonus	Tenderness
Power:	Bruits
Hip	**8. OTHER**
Knee	Upper limbs
Ankle and foot	Cranial nerve
Reflexes:	Urine analysis, etc.
Knee	

across the room, turn around and walk back. If the patient appears to be in difficulty, ask the bulldog to help. Ask him or her (the patient, not the bulldog) to try heel-to-toe walking (for cerebellar disease) and then try standing and then walking on toes and heels (for an S1 or L4/L5 lesion, respectively), and to squat and stand (for proximal myopathy). Perform Romberg's test for ataxia before asking the patient to walk. The test is positive if the patient sways more when the eyes are closed – loss of visual clues makes the patient with proprioceptive loss more unsteady.

HINT

Specific testing of gait should help you decide whether there is an ataxic or high-stepping gait (cerebellar or proprioceptive problems) or muscle weakness (proximal or distal, or both).

Romberg's test helps you decide if the problem is due to proprioceptive loss or is cerebellar in origin.

---

3. Have the patient lie on the bed with the legs entirely exposed. Place a towel over the groin. Look at the patient's back for scars.
4. Look for muscle wasting and fasciculation. Note any tremor. Feel the muscle bulk of the quadriceps and run your hand up each shin, feeling for wasting of the anterior tibial muscles.
5. Test tone at the knees and ankles.
6. Test clonus at this time. Warn the patient first. Move the ankle gently to allow relaxation before sharply dorsiflexing the foot with the knee bent and the thigh externally rotated. Sustained rhythmical contractions indicate an upper motor neurone lesion. If there is ankle clonus, test at the knee by pushing the patella sharply downwards. Always test both sides!
7. Assess power next.
   a. Hip:
      i. flexion (L2, L3): ask the patient to lift up the straight leg and not let you push it down (having placed your hand above the knee)
      ii. extension (L5, S1, S2): ask the patient to keep the leg down and not let you pull it up
      iii. abduction (L4, L5, S1): ask the patient to abduct the legs and not let you push them together
      iv. adduction (L2, L3, L4): ask the patient to keep the legs adducted and not let you pull them apart.
   b. Knee:
      i. flexion (L5, S1): ask the patient to bend the knee and not let you straighten it
      ii. extension (L3, L4): with the patient's knee slightly bent, ask him or her to straighten the knee and not let you bend it.
   c. Ankle and foot:
      i. plantar flexion (S1): ask the patient to push the foot down and not let you pull it up
      ii. dorsiflexion (L4, L5): ask the patient to bring the foot up and not let you push it down
      iii. eversion (L5, S1): ask the patient to evert the foot against resistance; loss of this may also indicate a common peroneal (lateral popliteal) nerve palsy
      iv. inversion (L5): ask the patient to invert the plantarflexed foot against resistance.

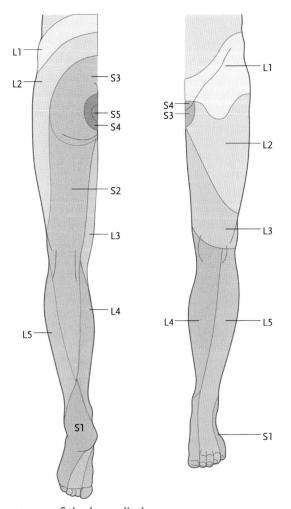

Figure 16.96 **Dermatomes of the lower limb.**

8. Elicit the reflexes:
   a. knee (L3, L4) – quadriceps muscle
   b. ankle (S1, S2) – calf muscle
   c. plantar response (S1).
9. Test coordination with the heel–shin test, toe–finger test[6] and tapping of the feet (p. 573).
10. Examine the sensory system (Fig. 16.96) as for the upper limbs: pin prick, then vibration and proprioception, and then light touch.

HINT

Sensory changes can be variable. If sensory loss is not quite consistent but seems generally to fit a pattern, it may be a good idea to describe it confidently as 'patchy'.

---

[6]Toe–nose testing is rarely practical.

11. If there is a peripheral sensory loss, attempt to establish a sensory level on the abdomen.
12. Examine the saddle region sensation (S3–5).
13. Ask to test the anal reflex (S2–4); if intact, there is brief contraction of the external sphincter of the anus to scratching of the perianal skin.[7]
14. If you have not done this already, go to the back. Look for deformity, scars and neurofibromata. Palpate for tenderness over the vertebral bodies and auscultate for bruits. Test straight leg raising.
15. It may be relevant to ask whether you can proceed to the upper limbs and cranial nerves.
16. Perform a urine analysis.

Notes on the neurological examination of the limbs

Grading muscle power (Medical Research Council)
0. Complete paralysis.
1. Flicker of contraction.
2. Movement with *no* gravity.
3. Movement against gravity only (any resistance stops movement).
4. Movement against gravity plus some resistance.
5. Normal power.
   This grading is weighted towards severe weakness (grades 0–3 are all severe). A more sensible scale would be the following:
1. Complete paralysis.
2. Severe weakness.
3. Moderate weakness.
4. Mild weakness.
5. Normal.

Signs of a lower motor neurone lesion
1. Weakness.
2. Wasting.
3. Decreased or absent reflexes.
4. Fasciculation (prominent in anterior horn cell diseases unless far advanced).

Signs of an upper motor neurone lesion
1. Weakness in an 'upper motor neurone pattern'; all muscle groups are weak, but may be more marked in upper limb abductor and extensor muscles – shoulder abduction, elbow and wrist extensors – and lower limb flexor muscles – hip flexion, knee flexion, ankle dorsiflexion.
2. Spasticity.
3. Clonus.
4. Increased reflexes and extensor plantar response.

An approach to peripheral neuropathy
This may be sensory (glove and stocking) or motor, or both. Autonomic nerves may be involved – check postural BP if possible.

---

[7]This will not be allowed, but you may be asked what you would expect to find.

Causes of peripheral neuropathy

But remember: diabetes 30%, hereditary 30%, idiopathic 30%, all others 10%.

1. Drugs and toxins – isoniazid, vincristine, phenytoin, nitrofurantoin, cisplatinum, amiodarone, large doses of vitamin B_6, heavy metals.
2. Alcohol (with or without vitamin B_1 deficiency); amyloidosis.
3. Metabolic – diabetes mellitus, chronic kidney disease, hypothyroidism, porphyria.
4. Immune-mediated – Guillain–Barré syndrome.
5. Tumour – lung carcinoma.
6. Vitamin B_{12} or B_1 deficiency or B_6 excess.
7. Idiopathic.
8. Connective tissue diseases or vasculitis – SLE, polyarteritis nodosa.
9. Hereditary (often over-represented in examinations).

CAUSES OF PREDOMINANTLY MOTOR NEUROPATHY

1. Guillain–Barré syndrome; chronic inflammatory demyelinating polyradiculoneuropathy (CIDP).
2. Hereditary motor and sensory neuropathy (Charcot–Marie–Tooth (CMT) disease) (see Figs 16.97 and 16.98).
3. Acute intermittent porphyria.
4. Diabetes mellitus.
5. Lead poisoning.
6. Multifocal motor neuropathy.

HINT

Motor neurone disease and neuromuscular junction disorders must always be considered in the differential diagnosis of distal motor weakness.

CAUSES OF PREDOMINANTLY SENSORY NEUROPATHY

This is unusual and results in sensory ataxia and pseudoathetosis. Causes include:

1. Diabetes mellitus
2. Carcinoma (e.g. lung, ovary, breast) (may be neuronopathy,[8] length independent)
3. Paraproteinaemia
4. Vitamin B_6 intoxication
5. Sjögren's syndrome (often a neuronopathy[8])
6. Syphilis
7. Vitamin B_{12} deficiency (occasionally)
8. Idiopathic.

CAUSES OF PAINFUL PERIPHERAL NEUROPATHY

1. Diabetes mellitus.
2. Alcohol.
3. Vitamin B_{12} or B_1 deficiency.
4. Carcinoma.
5. Porphyria.
6. Arsenic or thallium poisoning.
7. Heredity (most are not painful).

---

[8]Sensory neuronopathy – no motor involvement, profound sensory ataxia, often asymmetric, often idiopathic.

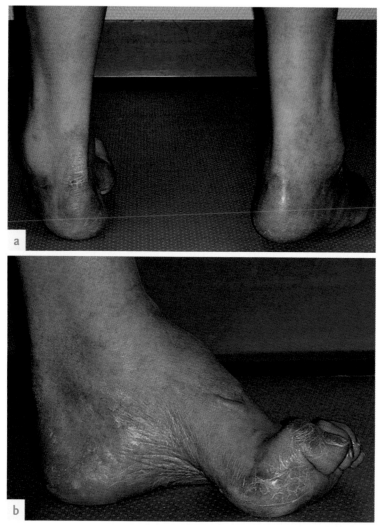

Figure 16.97 **Typical clinical manifestations of a cavovarus foot deformity in a 55-year-old man with hereditary motor and sensory neuropathy, which is characterised by different components: (a) hindfoot varus and equinus (hind- or forefoot) and forefoot pronation, and (b) cavus, flexion deformity of the first metatarsal, and claw toes.**

T Dreher, S Hagmann, W Wenz. Reconstruction of multiplanar deformity of the hindfoot and midfoot with internal fixation techniques. *Foot and Ankle Clinics* 2009; 14(3):489–531.

HINT

Remember the nerve conduction test findings for peripheral neuropathy:
- Demyelinating – e.g. diabetes, paraprotein, CMT, CIDP
  - Velocity < 75%
  - Distal latency > 130%
  - Amplitude normal
- Axonal – e.g. diabetes, toxins, metabolic, paraneoplastic
  - Amplitude < 50%
  - Velocity > 70%

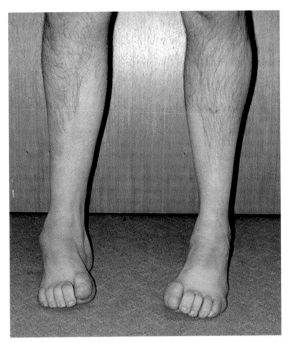

Figure 16.98 Classical appearance in the lower legs in a patient with Charcot–Marie–Tooth disease.

D W Howcroft, S Kumar, N Makwana. *Orthopaedics and Trauma* 23(4):274–7, Fig 1. Elsevier, 2009, with permission.

HINT

A burning sensation on the soles of the feet can be caused by a painful peripheral neuropathy. Small fibres may be involved in isolation, so ankle jerks may be preserved. Other causes include tarsal tunnel syndrome or an S1 lesion. An S1 lesion will cause a decreased or absent ankle jerk.

CAUSES OF MONONEURITIS MULTIPLEX

Mononeuritis multiplex refers to separate involvement of more than one peripheral or rarely cranial nerve (e.g. a common peroneal nerve palsy plus an axillary nerve palsy). Common causes include:

1. acute (usually vascular):
   a. diabetes mellitus
   b. polyarteritis nodosa or connective tissue diseases – SLE, rheumatoid arthritis.
2. chronic:
   a. multiple compressive neuropathies, especially with joint-deforming arthritis
   b. sarcoidosis
   c. acromegaly
   d. leprosy
   e. carcinoma (rare)
   f. idiopathic.

CAUSES OF THICKENED NERVES

1. Hereditary motor and sensory neuropathy.
2. Acromegaly.
3. Chronic inflammatory demyelinating polyradiculoneuropathy.
4. Amyloidosis.
5. Leprosy.
6. Others – sarcoidosis, neurofibromatosis.

CAUSES OF FASCICULATION

Fasciculation is *not* always motor neurone disease. Causes include:

1. benign idiopathic fasciculation (by far the most common, except possibly in the exam)
2. motor neurone disease
3. motor root compression
4. malignant neuropathy
5. spinal muscular atrophy / bulbospinal muscular atrophy (Kennedy syndrome)
6. any motor neuropathy (less commonly).

> **HINT**
>
> Myokymia resembles benign coarse fasciculation of the same muscle group (e.g. eyelids). Electromyographic myokymia can occur in multiple sclerosis, brain stem neoplasm, Bell's palsy, radiculopathy or radiation plexopathy, or chronic nerve compression.

Hereditary motor and sensory neuropathy (HMSN)

Charcot–Marie–Tooth disease (Figs 16.97 and 16.98) is usually autosomal dominant.

CLINICAL FEATURES

1. Pes cavus (short, high-arched feet with hammer toes) (see Fig. 16.97).
2. Distal muscle atrophy due to peripheral nerve degeneration, not usually extending above the elbows or above the middle one-third of the thighs (see Fig. 16.98).
3. Absent reflexes.
4. Slight to no sensory loss in the limbs (usually).
5. Thickened nerves.
6. Optic atrophy; Argyll Robertson pupils (rare).

An approach to brachial plexus lesions

COMPLETE LESION

1. Lower motor neurone signs affect the whole arm.
2. Sensory loss (whole limb).
3. Horner's syndrome (see Fig. 16.86) – an important clue, but only if the lesion is proximal in the lower plexus.

> **HINT**
>
> Remember always to feel for axillary lymphadenopathy at the end of your examination for a brachial plexus lesion.

UPPER TRUNK (ERB–DUCHENNE) (C5, C6) LESION

1. Loss of shoulder movement and elbow flexion – the hand is held in the 'waiter's tip' position.
2. Sensory loss is present over the lateral aspect of the arm and forearm, and over the thumb.

LOWER TRUNK (KLUMPKE) (C8, T1) LESION

1. True claw hand with paralysis of all the intrinsic muscles.
2. Sensory loss along the ulnar side of the hand and forearm.
3. Horner's syndrome.

CERVICAL RIB SYNDROME

1. Weakness and wasting of the small muscles of the hand (true claw hand).
2. Sensory loss over the medial aspect of the hand and forearm.
3. Unequal radial pulses and blood pressures.
4. Subclavian bruit and loss of the pulse on arm manoeuvring (this sign is often also present in the normal population).
5. Palpable cervical rib in the neck (uncommon).

Important peripheral nerves

RADIAL NERVE (C5–C8) LESION

Clinical features

1. Wrist and finger drop (wrist flexion normal).
2. Triceps loss (elbow extension loss) if lesion is above the spiral groove.
3. Sensory loss over the anatomical snuffbox.
4. Finger abduction *appears* to be weak because of the difficulty of spreading the fingers when they cannot be straightened.

MEDIAN NERVE (C6–T1) LESION

This nerve supplies all the muscles on the front of the forearm except for the flexor carpi ulnaris and half of the flexor digitorum profundus. It also supplies the following short muscles of the hand (LOAF):

Lateral two lumbricals
Opponens pollicis
Abductor pollicis brevis
Flexor pollicis brevis (this sometimes has ulnar innervation).

Clinical features

1. Loss of abductor pollicis brevis with a lesion at or above the wrist: pen-touching test – with the hand flat, ask the patient to abduct the thumb vertically to touch your pen.
2. Loss of flexor digitorum sublimis with a lesion in or above the cubital fossa: Ochsner's clasping test – ask the patient to clasp the hands firmly together; the index finger on the affected side fails to flex.
3. Sensory loss over the thumb, index, middle and lateral half of the ring finger (palmar aspect only).

> ## HINT
>
> Causes of carpal tunnel syndrome:
> 1. idiopathic
> 2. arthropathy – rheumatoid arthritis
> 3. endocrine disease – hypothyroidism, acromegaly
> 4. pregnancy
> 5. trauma and overuse.

ULNAR NERVE (C8–T1) LESION

Clinical features

1. Wasting of the intrinsic muscles of the hand (except LOAF muscles).
2. Weak finger abduction and adduction (loss of interosseous muscles).
3. Ulnar claw-like hand. (*Note:* A higher lesion causes less deformity, as an above-the-elbow lesion also causes loss of flexor digitorum profundus.)
4. Froment's sign: ask the patient to grasp a piece of paper between the thumb and lateral aspect of the forefinger with each hand – the affected thumb will flex (loss of thumb adductor).
5. Sensory loss over the little and medial half of the ring finger (both palmar and dorsal aspects).

WASTING OF THE SMALL MUSCLES OF THE HAND (FIG. 16.99)

Examine as for the upper limbs and make sure you feel the pulses and examine the neck, unless the cause is very obvious (e.g. rheumatoid arthritis).

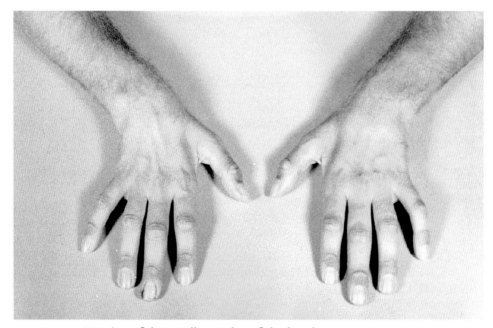

Figure 16.99 **Wasting of the small muscles of the hands.**

J Nicklin. Disorders of nerve II: polyneuropathies. In *Physical management in neurological rehabilitation*, 2nd edn. Fig 14.1. Mosby, Elsevier, 2004, with permission.

Causes
1. Nerve lesions:
   a. median and ulnar nerve lesions
   b. brachial plexus lesions
   c. peripheral motor neuropathy (in the examination, don't forget hereditary motor and sensory neuropathy).
2. Anterior horn cell disease:
   a. motor neurone disease
   b. polio
   c. spinal muscular atrophies (e.g. Kugelberg–Welander disease).
3. Myopathy:
   a. dystrophia myotonica – the forearms more affected than the hands
   b. distal myopathy.
4. Spinal cord lesions:
   a. syringomyelia
   b. cervical spondylosis with compression of the C8 segment
   c. other (e.g. tumour).
5. Trophic disorders:
   a. arthropathies (disuse)
   b. ischaemia, including vasculitis
   c. shoulder–hand syndrome.

HINT

When distinguishing an ulnar nerve lesion from a C8 root / lower trunk brachial plexus lesion, remember that the sensory loss of a C8 lesion extends proximal to the wrist and that the thenar muscles are involved with a C8 root or lower trunk brachial plexus lesion. Distinguishing a C8 root from a lower trunk brachial plexus lesion is difficult clinically, but the presence of Horner's syndrome or an axillary mass suggests that the brachial plexus is affected.

FEMORAL NERVE (L2, L3, L4) LESION

Clinical features
1. Weakness of knee extension (quadriceps paralysis).
2. Slight hip flexion weakness.
3. Preserved adductor strength.
4. Loss of knee jerk.
5. Sensory loss involving the inner aspect of the thigh and leg.

SCIATIC NERVE (L4, L5, S1, S2) LESION

Clinical features
1. Weakness of knee flexion (hamstrings involved).
2. Loss of power of all muscles below the knee causing a foot drop, so the patient may be able to walk, but cannot stand on the toes or heels.
3. Knee jerk intact.
4. Loss of ankle jerk and plantar response.
5. Sensory loss along the posterior thigh and total loss below the knee.

COMMON PERONEAL (LATERAL POPLITEAL) NERVE (L4, L5, S1) LESION
Clinical features
1. Foot drop and loss of foot eversion only.
2. Sensory loss (minimal) over the dorsum of the foot.
   Note: The reflexes are normal.

HINT

If there is a foot drop (see Fig. 16.100), test foot inversion and eversion. *Inversion* of the foot will be normal with a peroneal nerve compression but *absent* with a L5 radiculopathy. (Eversion is absent with both lesions.)

LATERAL CUTANEOUS NERVE OF THE THIGH LESION
Meralgia paraesthetica is caused by compression of this nerve, which may result in sensory loss or hyperaesthesia over the lateral aspect of the thigh, but no motor loss.

CAUSES OF FOOT DROP (FIG. 16.100)
1. Common peroneal nerve palsy.
2. Sciatic nerve palsy.
3. Lumbosacral plexus lesion.
4. L4, L5 root lesion.

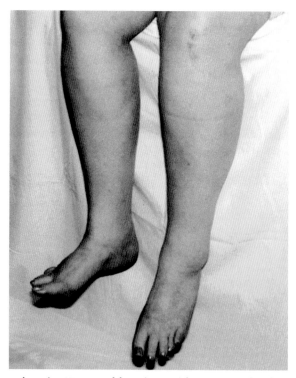

Figure 16.100 **Foot drop in 45-year-old patient with amyotrophic lateral sclerosis.**

R B Daroff. *Bradley's neurology in clinical practice*, 6th edn. Fig 74.5. Saunders, Elsevier, 2010, with permission.

5. Peripheral motor neuropathy.
6. Distal myopathy.
7. Motor neurone disease.
8. Precentral gyrus lesion.

> ### HINT
>
> Remember, if there is a foot drop, test the ankle jerk carefully. As a very rough rule of thumb, if it is absent then an S1 lesion should be suspected; if it is normal then a common peroneal palsy should be considered; if it is increased then an upper motor neurone lesion or motor neurone disease is likely.

Notes on spinal cord lesions

Assessment of the paraplegic patient

1. Is there also a sensory level? Do not forget to continue examining up the torso, especially if there is suggestion of a thoracic lesion. Patterns of sensory loss depend on the level and type of lesion. Consider:
   a. cord compression, which causes a loss of all modalities bilaterally below the level involved (*note:* extrinsic compression may spare the perineum); radicular pain and lower motor neurone weakness are present at the level of spinal compression
   b. transverse myelitis
   c. anterior spinal artery occlusion (posterior column function is spared)
   d. intrinsic cord lesion
   e. multiple sclerosis.
2. Back examination: for example, deformity, tenderness or bruits may provide clues about the underlying disease process.
3. Arm involvement? Consider:
   a. cervical spondylosis
   b. syringomyelia
   c. motor neurone disease
   d. multiple sclerosis.
4. Cranial nerve lesions? Consider:
   a. motor neurone disease
   b. multiple sclerosis.
5. Peripheral neuropathy? Consider:
   a. vitamin B_{12} deficiency
   b. Friedreich's ataxia
   c. carcinoma
   d. hereditary spastic paraplegia
   e. syphilis.

> ### HINT
>
> Intracranial lesions (e.g. parasagittal meningioma) cause paraplegia in extension only, whereas spinal cord lesions cause paraplegia in flexion or extension (i.e. flexor reflexes are released with spinal lesions).

Important motor and reflex changes of spinal cord and conus compression

Lower motor neurone signs occur at the level of the root lesion and upper motor neurone signs occur below the lesion.

UPPER CERVICAL

1. Upper motor neurone signs in the upper and lower limbs.
2. Paralysis of the diaphragm occurs with a lesion above C4.

C5

1. Lower motor neurone weakness and wasting of the rhomboids, deltoids, biceps and brachioradialis.
2. Upper motor neurone signs affect the rest of the upper and all the lower limbs.
3. The biceps jerk is lost.
4. The supinator jerk is 'inverted'.

C8

1. Lower motor neurone weakness and wasting of the intrinsic muscles of the hand.
2. Upper motor neurone signs in the lower limbs.

MIDTHORACIC

1. Intercostal paralysis (cannot be detected clinically).
2. Loss of upper abdominal reflexes at T7 and T8.
3. Upper motor neurone signs in the lower limbs.
4. Sensory level on the trunk (often missed).

T10–T11

1. Loss of the lower abdominal reflexes and upward displacement of the umbilicus on contraction (Beevor's sign).
2. Upper motor neurone signs in the lower limbs.

L1

1. Cremasteric reflexes lost (normal abdominal reflexes).
2. Upper motor neurone signs in the lower limbs.

L4

1. Lower motor neurone weakness and wasting of the quadriceps.
2. Knee jerk lost.

L5 AND S1

1. Lower motor neurone weakness of knee flexion and hip extension (S1) and abduction (L5), plus calf and foot muscles.
2. Knee jerk present.
3. No ankle jerk or plantar response.
4. Anal reflex present.

S3–S4

1. No anal reflex.
2. Saddle sensory loss.
3. Normal lower limbs.

Important syndromes

SUBACUTE COMBINED DEGENERATION OF THE CORD (VITAMIN B$_{12}$ DEFICIENCY)

Clinical features

1. Symmetrical posterior column loss (vibration and position sense), causing an ataxic gait.
2. Symmetrical upper motor neurone signs in the lower limbs with absent ankle reflexes; knee reflexes may be absent or, more often, exaggerated.
3. Peripheral sensory neuropathy (less common and mild).
4. Optic atrophy (occasionally).
5. Dementia (occasionally).
   The combination of upper motor neurone signs causing an extensor plantar response with peripheral neuropathy causing loss of knee and ankle jerks is a distinctive pattern.
   Causes of an extensor plantar response plus absent ankle jerk include:
1. subacute combined degeneration of the cord (vitamin B$_{12}$ deficiency)
2. conus medullaris lesion
3. combination of an upper motor neurone lesion with cauda equina compression or peripheral neuropathy
4. syphilis (taboparesis)
5. Friedreich's ataxia
6. diabetes mellitus (uncommon)
7. adrenoleukodystrophy or metachromatic leukodystrophy.

BROWN–SÉQUARD SYNDROME (HEMISECTION OF THE SPINAL CORD)

Clinical features

1. Motor changes:
   a. upper motor neurone signs below the hemisection on the *same* side as the lesion
   b. lower motor neurone signs at the level of the hemisection on the *same* side.
2. Sensory changes:
   a. pain and temperature loss on the *opposite* side of the lesion (*Note:* The upper level of sensory loss is usually a few segments below the level of the lesion.)
   b. vibration and proprioception loss on the *same* side
   c. light touch is often normal
   d. there may be a band of sensory loss on the same side at the level of the lesion (afferent nerve fibres).

Common causes

1. Multiple sclerosis.
2. Angioma.
3. Glioma.
4. Trauma.
5. Myelitis.
6. Postradiation myelopathy.

CAUSES OF DISSOCIATED SENSORY LOSS

(Usually indicates spinal cord disease, but may occur with peripheral neuropathy.)

Spinothalamic (pain and temperature) loss only

1. Syringomyelia ('cape' distribution).
2. Brown–Séquard syndrome (contralateral leg).
3. Anterior spinal artery thrombosis.
4. Lateral medullary syndrome (contralateral to the other signs).
5. Peripheral neuropathy (e.g. diabetes mellitus, amyloid, Fabry disease).

Dorsal column (vibration and proprioception) loss only

1. Subacute combined degeneration.
2. Brown–Séquard syndrome (ipsilateral leg).
3. Spinocerebellar degeneration (e.g. Friedreich's ataxia).
4. Multiple sclerosis.
5. Tabes dorsalis.
6. Sensory neuropathy or ganglionopathy (e.g. carcinoma).
7. Peripheral neuropathy from diabetes mellitus or hypothyroidism.

SYRINGOMYELIA (CENTRAL CAVITY IN THE SPINAL CORD)

Clinical triad

1. Loss of pain and temperature over the neck, shoulders and arms ('cape' distribution).
2. Amyotrophy (weakness, atrophy and areflexia) of the arms.
3. Upper motor neurone signs in the lower limbs.
   Note: There may also be thoracic scoliosis owing to asymmetrical weakness of the paravertebral muscles.

An approach to myopathy

CAUSES OF PROXIMAL MUSCLE WEAKNESS

1. Myopathic (see below).
2. Neuromuscular junction disorder: myasthenia gravis.
3. Neurogenic: Kugelberg–Welander disease (proximal muscle wasting and fasciculation as a result of anterior horn cell damage – autosomal recessive), motor neurone disease, polyradiculopathy.

CAUSES OF MYOPATHY

1. Hereditary muscular dystrophy.
2. Congenital myopathies (rare).
3. Acquired (mnemonic PACE PODS):
   Polymyositis or dermatomyositis (Figs 16.101 and 16.102)
   Alcohol
   Carcinoma
   Endocrine (e.g. hypothyroidism, hyperthyroidism, Cushing's syndrome, acromegaly, hypopituitarism)
   Periodic paralysis (hyperkalaemic, hypokalaemic or normokalaemic)
   Osteomalacia
   Drugs (e.g. clofibrate, chloroquine, steroids)
   Sarcoidosis

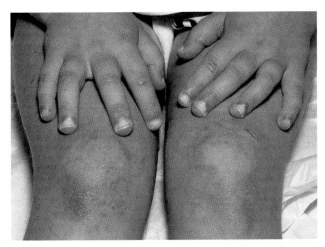

Figure 16.101 Dermatomyositis. Gottron's papules consisting of purplish-red, slightly scaling plaques on the extensor surfaces of the finger joints and knees.

H B Pride. *Pediatric dermatology*, 1st edn. Fig. 12-5. Saunders, Elsevier, 2008, with permission.

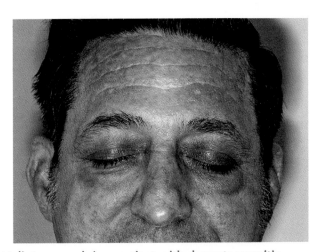

Figure 16.102 Heliotrope rash in a patient with dermatomyositis.

W D James et al. *Andrews' diseases of the skin: clinical dermatology*, 11th edn. Fig 8-15. Saunders, Elsevier, 2011, with permission.

Note: Causes of proximal myopathy and a peripheral neuropathy include:
1. paraneoplastic syndrome
2. alcohol
3. connective tissue disease.

MUSCULAR DYSTROPHIES
1. Duchenne's (pseudohypertrophic) (sex-linked recessive disorder) (Fig. 16.103):
    a. affects only males (or females with Turner's syndrome) (Fig. 16.104a and b)
    b. the calves and deltoids are hypertrophied early and weak later
    c. early proximal weakness

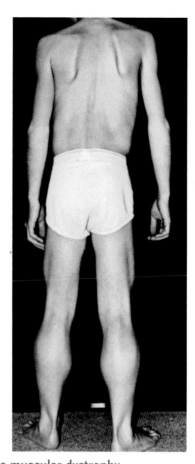

Figure 16.103 **Duchenne's muscular dystrophy.**

R B Daroff. *Bradley's neurology in clinical practice*, 6th edn. Fig 79.9. Saunders, Elsevier, 2010, with permission.

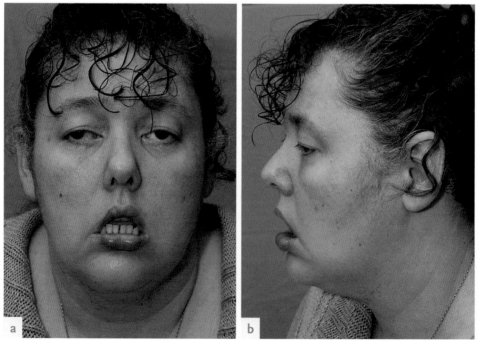

Figure 16.104 **(a) and (b) Muscular dystrophy facies.**

V Laina, A Orlando. Bilateral facial palsy and oral incompetence due to muscular dystrophy treated with a palmaris longus tendon graft. *Journal of Plastic, Reconstructive and Aesthetic Surgery* 2008; Figs 2a and b, with permission.

d. tendon reflexes are preserved in proportion to muscle strength
e. severe progressive kyphoscoliosis
f. heart disease (dilated cardiomyopathy)
g. creatine kinase level markedly elevated
h. patients die in the second decade, usually from heart disease.
2. Becker (sex-linked recessive disorder): same features as Duchenne's, but less severe, has a later onset and is less rapidly progressive.
3. Limb girdle (autosomal recessive):
a. shoulder or pelvic girdle affected (onset in the third decade)
b. face and heart are usually spared.
4. Facioscapulohumeral (autosomal dominant): facial and pectoral girdle weakness with hypertrophy of the deltoids (normal pelvic muscles early).
5. Distal dystrophies:
a. autosomal dominant disease, which is rare and causes distal muscle atrophy and weakness
b. dystrophia myotonica (autosomal dominant).

TESTS FOR MYOPATHY
1. Creatine kinase (highest in Duchenne's).
2. EMG.
3. ECG (particularly in Duchenne's and dystrophia myotonica).
4. Muscle biopsy.
5. Echocardiogram (cardiac involvement).

Dystrophia myotonica

Common stems

1. 'This man has noticed some arm weakness. Please examine him.'
2. 'This man has cramps. Please examine his upper limbs.'

Less common stem
'This man has difficulty shaking hands and is not an infectious diseases physician. Please examine him.'

Method
Standing back to observe the patient, you should notice the features of myotonic dystrophy (because now you have become, fortunately, an expert observer) (Fig. 16.105).
Proceed as follows:
1. Observe the face for frontal baldness (the patient may be wearing a wig), dull triangular facies ('hatchet' face), temporalis, masseter and sternomastoid atrophy, and partial ptosis. Note thick spectacles, as these patients develop cataracts (though a rare finding now that lens implantation is routine) and fine subcapsular deposits, which are virtually diagnostic.
2. Look at the neck for sternocleidomastoid atrophy, then test neck flexion (this is weak, whereas extension is normal).

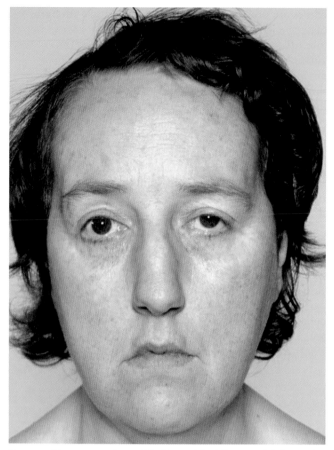

Figure 16.105 Dystrophia myotonica with frontal balding and bilateral ptosis.

G Douglas. The general examination. *Macleod's clinical examination*, 3rd edn. Fig. 3.11, 41–62. Churchill
Livingstone, Elsevier, 2013, with permission.

Table 16.56 **Causes of myotonia**
1. Dystrophia myotonica
2. Myotonia congenita (myotonia of the tongue and thenar eminence, the recessive form being more severe)
3. Paramyotonia congenita (episodic myotonia after cold exposure)
Note: Drugs (e.g. clofibrate) can also cause myotonic discharges on EMG, but do not cause clinical myotonia.

3. Go to the upper limbs. Shake the patient's hands (for grip myotonia) and test percussion
   myotonia. Tapping over the thenar eminence causes contraction then slow relaxation
   of the abductor pollicis brevis (Table 16.56).
4. Examine the arm now for signs of wasting and weakness, especially of the forearm muscles.
   Sensory changes from the associated peripheral neuropathy are usually very mild.
5. Go to the chest and inspect for gynaecomastia.
6. Ask to palpate the testes for atrophy.

7. Examine the lower limbs if there is time.
8. Always ask to test the urine for sugar (diabetes mellitus is more common in this disease) and to examine the cardiovascular system for cardiomyopathy. Finally, test mental status (mild mental retardation is usual).

HINT

Remember the classic EMG finding in dystrophia myotonica of a 'dive-bomber' effect with needle movement in the muscle at rest.

Gait

Common stems

1. 'Please examine this man's gait.'
2. 'This man has become unsteady when walking. Please examine his gait.'

Method (Table 16.57)

1. Scan the room for a walking stick or frame or special shoes.
2. Make sure the patient's legs are clearly visible. Ask him or her to 'hop out' of the bed or chair (look carefully for focal disease while this is being done); watch the patient walk normally for a few metres and then ask him or her to turn around quickly and walk back towards you.
3. Next ask the patient to walk heel-to-toe to exclude a midline cerebellar lesion.
4. Ask the patient to walk on the toes (an S1 lesion will make this difficult) and then on the heels (a lesion causing foot drop will make this difficult).
5. Test for proximal myopathy by asking the patient to squat and then stand up, or sit in a chair and then stand.
6. Look for Romberg's sign (posterior column loss causes inability to stand steadily when the feet are together with the eyes closed, whereas cerebellar disease also causes difficulty when the eyes are open).
7. Inspect the back for scars or deformity before lying or sitting the patient down.
8. Go on to formally examine the lower limbs depending on your findings.

Table 16.57 Gait examination	
Standing (legs fully exposed)	**2. ASK THE PATIENT TO:**
1. GENERAL INSPECTION	Walk normally and turn around quickly (abnormal gait)
Deformity	Walk heel-to-toe (cerebellar disease)
Diagnostic facies (see Table 16.35)	Walk on toes (S1)
Upper limb lesions	Walk on heels (L4 or L5)
Focal neurological disease (e.g. wasting)	Squat (proximal myopathy)
Fasciculation	Romberg's sign – feet together with:
Abnormal movements	eyes closed (posterior columns)
	eyes open (cerebellar disease)
	3. EXAMINE LOWER LIMBS

Table 16.58 **Typical gaits**
1. Hemiparetic (the foot is plantarflexed and the leg swung in a lateral arc)
2. Paraparetic (scissor gait)
3. Extrapyramidal (e.g. Parkinson's disease):
a. hesitation in starting
b. shuffling
c. freezing
d. festination (the patient hurries forward, trying to catch up with the centre of gravity)
e. propulsion (pull the patient towards you gently – he or she will be unable to stop), retropulsion
4. Cerebellar (a drunken gait that is wide based or reeling on a narrow base; the patient staggers towards the affected side)
5. Apraxic (prefrontal lobe) (feet appear glued to the floor when erect, but move more easily when the patient is supine; the arms may move well)
6. Posterior column lesion (clumsy slapping down of the feet on a broad base)
7. Distal weakness (high-stepping gait)
8. Proximal weakness (waddling gait)

9. You may find clues that direct you towards an extrapyramidal examination (Parkinson's disease).

The typical gaits to recognise are listed in Table 16.58.

Cerebellum

Common stems

1. 'This man has noticed a problem with his coordination. Please examine him.'
2. 'This woman finds walking difficult. Please examine her.' (This could be cerebellar, motor, extrapyramidal, sensory or rheumatological – but the type of examination required should be obvious from inspection. Otherwise the examiners will make the stem more specific.)

Method

If the patient seems likely to have a cerebellar problem (Table 16.59), proceed as follows for assessment of cerebellar disease.

1. Test the gait (the patient will stagger towards the affected side unless the problem is bilateral or involves the vermis).
2. Go on to perform a targeted examination of the legs. Pay attention to tone here.

HINT

If cerebellar testing seems normal but Romberg's test was positive, test position and vibration sense.

Table 16.59 Causes of cerebellar disease
UNILATERAL
1. Space-occupying lesion (tumour, abscess, granuloma)
2. Ischaemia (vertebrobasilar disease)
3. Paraneoplastic syndrome
4. Multiple sclerosis
5. Trauma
BILATERAL
1. Drugs (e.g. phenytoin)
2. Friedreich's ataxia
3. Hypothyroidism
4. Paraneoplastic syndrome
5. Multiple sclerosis
6. Trauma ('punch drunk')
7. Arnold–Chiari malformation
8. Alcohol
9. Large space-occupying lesion, cerebrovascular disease, rare metabolic diseases
MIDLINE
1. Paraneoplastic syndrome
2. Midline tumour
ROSTRAL VERMIS LESION (ONLY LOWER LIMBS AFFECTED)
1. Alcohol (most common cause of a cerebellar lesion)

3. Ask the patient to perform the heel–shin test, looking for accuracy of fine movement when the patient slides his or her heel down the shin quickly on each side for several cycles.

HINT

Subtle cerebellar changes may be obvious only if the test is made more difficult. Ask the patient to lift the leg in an arc before placing it back on the top of the shin.

4. Next, ask the patient to lift the big toe up to touch your finger, looking for intention tremor. Ask him or her to tap each foot rapidly on a firm surface.
5. Look now for nystagmus – usually jerky horizontal nystagmus with increased amplitude on looking towards the side of the lesion.
6. Assess speech – ask the patient to say 'Hippopotamus', 'Constitution' or 'West Register Street' (if working in London). Cerebellar speech is jerky, explosive and loud, with irregular separation of syllables.
7. Go to the upper limbs. Ask the patient to extend the arms and look for arm drift and static tremor as a result of hypotonia of the agonist muscles. Test tone. Hypotonia is caused by loss of a facilitatory influence on the spinal motor neurones in acute unilateral cerebellar disease.
8. Test rebound – ask the patient to lift his or her arms quickly from the sides and then stop. Hypotonia causes the patient to be unable to stop the arms. Always

demonstrate each movement for the patient's benefit, asking him or her to copy you. Ensure the patient does not fall over if the condition is severe.

9. Next, ask the patient to perform the finger–nose test – the patient touches his or her nose, then rotates the finger and touches your finger. Note any intention tremor (erratic movements increasing as the target is approached owing to loss of cerebellar connections with the brain stem) and past pointing (the patient overshooting the target).

10. Test rapid alternating movements – the patient taps alternately the palm and back of one hand on the other hand or thigh. Inability to perform this movement smoothly is called dysdiadochokinesis.

11. Look for truncal ataxia by asking the patient to fold the arms, sit up and then, while sitting, to put the legs over the side of the bed; then test for pendular knee jerks.

12. If there is time, look for possible causes of the problem. If there is an obvious unilateral lesion, auscultate over the cerebellum, then proceed to the cranial nerves and look for evidence of a cerebellopontine angle tumour (the fifth, seventh, eighth cranial nerves are affected) and the lateral medullary syndrome.

13. Always look in the fundi for papilloedema.

14. Next, examine for peripheral evidence of malignant disease.

15. If there is a midline lesion alone (i.e. truncal ataxia or abnormal heel–toe walking or abnormal speech), consider either a midline tumour or a paraneoplastic syndrome. If there is bilateral disease, look for signs of multiple sclerosis, Friedreich's ataxia (pes cavus being the most helpful initial clue) (Tables 16.60 and 16.61) and hypothyroidism (rare). Alcoholic cerebellar degeneration (which affects the anterior lobe of the cerebellar vermis) classically spares the arms.

16. If there are, in addition, upper motor neurone signs, consider the various causes in Table 16.62.

Table 16.60 Clinical features of Friedreich's ataxia (autosomal recessive)

Usually a young person with:
1. cerebellar signs (bilateral), including nystagmus
2. posterior column loss in the limbs
3. upper motor neurone signs in the limbs (although ankle reflexes are absent)
4. peripheral neuropathy
5. optic atrophy
6. pes cavus, cocking of the toes and kyphoscoliosis
7. cardiomyopathy (ECG abnormalities occur in more than 50% of cases)
8. diabetes mellitus

Table 16.61 Causes of pes cavus

1. Friedreich's ataxia or other spinocerebellar degenerations
2. Hereditary motor and sensory neuropathy
3. Neuropathies in childhood
4. Idiopathic

Table 16.62 Causes of spastic and ataxic paraparesis (upper motor neurone and cerebellar signs combined)
IN ADOLESCENCE
• Spinocerebellar degeneration (e.g. Friedreich's ataxia)
IN YOUNG ADULTS
• Multiple sclerosis
• Syphilitic meningomyelitis
• Spinocerebellar ataxia (SCA)
• Arnold–Chiari malformation or other lesions at the craniospinal junction
IN LATER LIFE
• Multiple sclerosis
• Syringomyelia
• Infarction (in upper pons or internal capsule bilaterally – 'ataxic hemiparesis')
• Lesion at the craniospinal junction (e.g. meningioma)
• SCA
Note: Don't forget, common unrelated diseases (e.g. cervical spondylosis and cerebellar degeneration from alcohol) may occur together by chance.

Parkinson's disease

Common stems

1. 'This woman has Parkinson's disease. Please assess the severity of the condition.'
2. 'This man has noticed a tremor. Please examine him.'
3. 'This man has difficulty in walking. Please examine him.'

Method

1. Look at the patient first. Note the obvious lack of facial expression ('mask-like') and paucity of movement.
2. Ask him or her to walk, turn quickly and stop, and restart. Note particularly any difficulty starting, shuffling, freezing and festination. It is probably a little dangerous to look for propulsion or retropropulsion (see Table 16.58).
3. Ask the patient to return to bed and look for a resting tremor with the arms relaxed (Table 16.63). The characteristic movement is described as 'pill rolling' and may be unilateral, or asymmetric when bilateral.
4. On finger–nose testing, a resting tremor diminishes, but an action tremor may appear. Test wrist tone, feeling for cogwheel or lead-pipe rigidity. Reinforce this by asking the patient to turn the head from side to side.
5. Test for abnormal rapid alternating movements. Look also for involuntary movements produced by medication use.
6. Go to the face. Note tremor, absence of blinking, dribbling of saliva and lack of expression. Test the glabellar tap: the sign is positive (Wilson's sign) when the patient continues to blink after the middle finger taps several times over the glabella from behind – it is important that your finger is out of the patient's line of vision.
7. Test speech, which is typically monotonous, soft, poorly articulated and faint.

Table 16.63 A classification of tremor
1. Parkinsonian – resting tremor
2. Action tremor – present throughout movement but resolves at rest: a. thyrotoxicosis b. anxiety c. drugs d. familial e. idiopathic (most common).
3. Intention tremor (cerebellar disease) – increases towards the target
4. Cerebellar outflow tract tremor ('red nucleus') – abduction–adduction movements of upper limbs with flexion–extension of wrists (usually associated with intention tremor, e.g. in multiple sclerosis or brain injury)
Note: Flapping (asterixis) is not strictly a tremor but rather a sudden brief loss of tone in hepatic failure, cardiac failure, respiratory failure or renal failure.

8. Look at the ocular movements for supranuclear gaze palsies. Feel for a greasy or sweaty brow (due to autonomic dysfunction).
9. Ask the patient to write (looking for micrographia) or draw a spiral (smaller than normal and lines closer together)
10. Test the frontal lobe reflexes and higher centres (looking for evidence of dementia).
11. Ask to test for postural hypotension.
12. Present your assessment of the degree of disability and whether the main problem is rigidity or tremor. Is there evidence of autonomic dysfunction or gaze palsy?

Causes of parkinsonism
1. Idiopathic (Parkinson's disease).
2. Drugs (e.g. phenothiazines, methyldopa).
3. Postencephalitis.
4. Other – toxins (carbon monoxide, manganese), Wilson's disease, Steele–Richardson syndrome, multisystem atrophy, syphilis, tumour. *Note:* Atherosclerosis is controversial as a cause of Parkinsonism.

Chorea

Common stem

'Please examine this man's arms.'

Less common stem:
'This man can't keep still. Please examine him.'

HINT

A stem that doesn't tell you what system to examine should mean there is an obvious diagnosis if you inspect carefully enough.

Table 16.64 **Causes of chorea**
1. Huntington's disease (autosomal dominant)
2. Sydenham's chorea (rheumatic fever)
3. Senility
4. Wilson's disease
5. Drugs (e.g. phenothiazines, the contraceptive pill, phenytoin, L-dopa)
6. Vasculitis or connective tissue disease (e.g. SLE)
7. Thyrotoxicosis (very rare)
8. Polycythaemia or other causes of hyperviscosity (very rare)
9. Viral encephalitis (very rare)

Method

Happily, you notice an extrapyramidal choreiform movement disorder. Choreiform movements are non-repetitive, abrupt, involuntary, more distal jerky movements, which the patient often attempts to disguise by completing the involuntary movement with a voluntary one. The condition is caused by a lesion of the corpus striatum.

- *Hemiballismus* is unilateral and usually involves rotary movements of proximal joints. It is caused by a subthalamic nucleus lesion on the opposite side.
- *Athetosis* means slow, sinuous distal writhing movements at rest. It is caused by a lesion of the outer segment of the putamen.

  If the patient has chorea, proceed as follows.

1. First, shake the patient's hand. Assess for a variability of sustained grip ('milkmaid grip').
2. Ask the patient to hold the hands out and look for a choreic posture (finger and thumb hyperextension and wrist flexion as a result of hypotonia). Note any signs of vasculitis.
3. Go to the face and look at the eyes for exophthalmos, Kayser–Fleischer rings and conjunctival injection (ataxia–telangiectasia). Ask the patient to poke the tongue out and note a serpentine tongue (moving in and out). Notice any rash (e.g. SLE).
4. Test the knee jerks (pendular) and the higher centres (for Huntington's disease). The causes of chorea are summarised in Table 16.64.
5. If the patient is young, examine the heart for signs of rheumatic fever.

Index

Page numbers followed by "f" indicate figures, "t" indicate tables, and "b" indicate boxes.